ENDOCRINOLOGY OF CRITICAL DISEASE

CONTEMPORARY ENDOCRINOLOGY

P. Michael Conn, SERIES EDITOR

6. *G Protein-Coupled Receptors and Disease,* edited by ALLEN M. SPIEGEL, 1997
5. *Natriuretic Peptides in Health and Disease,* edited by WILLIS K. SAMSON AND ELLIS R. LEVIN, 1997
4. *Endocrinology of Critical Disease,* edited by K. PATRICK OBER, 1997
3. *Diseases of the Pituitary: Diagnosis and Treatment,* edited by MARGARET E. WIERMAN, 1997
2. *Diseases of the Thyroid,* edited by LEWIS E. BRAVERMAN, 1997
1. *Endocrinology of the Vasculature,* edited by JAMES R. SOWERS, 1996

ENDOCRINOLOGY OF CRITICAL DISEASE

Edited by

K. PATRICK OBER, MD

Bowman Gray School of Medicine, Wake Forest University, Winston-Salem, NC

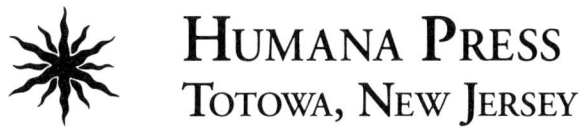

HUMANA PRESS
TOTOWA, NEW JERSEY

© 1997 Humana Press Inc.
999 Riverview Drive, Suite 208
Totowa, New Jersey 07512

For additional copies, pricing for bulk purchases, and/or information about other Humana titles, contact Humana at the above address or at any of the following numbers: Tel: 201-256-1699; Fax: 201-256-8341; E-mail: humana@mindspring.com or visit our website at http://www.humanapress.com

All rights reserved. No part of this book may be reproduced, stored in a retrieval system, or transmitted in any form or by any means, electronic, mechanical, photocopying, microfilming, recording, or otherwise without written permission from the Publisher.

All articles, comments, opinions, conclusions, or recommendations are those of the author(s), and do not necessarily reflect the views of the publisher.

This publication is printed on acid-free paper. ∞
ANSI Z39.48-1984 (American National Standards Institute)
Permanence of Paper for Printed Library Materials.

Cover design by Patricia F. Cleary.

Photocopy Authorization Policy:
Authorization to photocopy items for internal or personal use, or the internal or personal use of specific clients, is granted by Humana Press Inc., provided that the base fee of US $8.00 per copy, plus US $00.25 per page, is paid directly to the Copyright Clearance Center at 222 Rosewood Drive, Danvers, MA 01923. For those organizations that have been granted a photocopy license from the CCC, a separate system of payment has been arranged and is acceptable to Humana Press Inc. The fee code for users of the Transactional Reporting Service is: [0-89603-422-4/97 $8.00 + $00.25].

Printed in the United States of America. 10 9 8 7 6 5 4 3 2 1

PREFACE

All living organisms are relentlessly exposed to forces and events, both extrinsic and intrinsic, that have the potential to disrupt the essential functions supporting health and well-being; if unchecked and unbalanced, these perturbations can threaten the very survival of the individual. The endocrine system serves a role that is largely homeostatic, functioning to attenuate and compensate for the unending changes and disruptions threatening normal bodily function. The endocrine system is a complex hierarchical network designed to maintain and stabilize (and frequently to stimulate and encourage, but sometimes to suppress or inhibit) the innumerable metabolic activities involved in the life process; the endocrine system is repeatedly called upon to respond to a series of never-ending challenges that threaten the continuity of normal function. Among its countless functions, the endocrine system: promotes the growth and maturation of the immature individual; precisely controls the availability and flux of nutrients needed to provide the energy and raw materials that are essential for the functions of every tissue; maintains circulatory volume and blood pressure by means of complex interactions with the central nervous system, circulatory system, and kidneys; regulates the balance of water and electrolytes; tightly controls the critical mediators and signals of living processes (such as the circulating amounts of ionized calcium); determines the very structure of the living organism by controlling the multitude of factors involved in skeletal growth and remodeling; and controls those processes essential for reproduction. At a very basic level, every function of a living organism can be viewed as having a metabolic basis, with each function fastidiously regulated by endocrine processes—and, as a corollary, all disease ultimately can be defined as a disruption of the body's normal metabolic functions and regulatory processes.

In addition to the classic endocrine functions, it is becoming increasingly clear that the endocrine system is involved very intricately with nontraditional (i.e., non-"metabolic") activities, including interactions with the immune system and influences on neuropsychiatric function. All of these functions are poorly understood, even under circumstances in which the living organism is in a state of relative "calm" and equanimity (if such times truly exist); with severe and stressful illnesses, the extent of our comprehension of endocrine regulatory processes is even more primitive. Newer medical technology (dialysis, transplant, heart–lung bypass, and sophisticated ICU methodologies) and newer epidemics of disease have underscored our level of ignorance: current life-sustaining medical care often results in patients who survive catastrophic illnesses of a severity and duration that would not have been imaginable even a few years ago. The sophistication of the ICU and burn unit, the effectiveness of the dialysis unit, the potency of rejection-suppressing immunosuppressive drugs for the transplant patient, the increasing survival of patients with some malignancies, and the spread of the AIDS virus are all examples of situations that have led to the presence of a large number of patients with diseases at a truly phenomenal severity level. The study of each of these disorders (and other similarly severe and complex diseases) has given us great insight into the function of the endocrine system. Many mysteries remain: The interactions of the various segments of endocrine function are still unclear, and the immunological, psychological, and behavioral aspects of the endocrine responses to critical illness are even more occult. Traditionally, there has been intense focus on the understanding of *what* occurs in a particular endocrine response. Even more profound is the question of *why* the endocrine response has occurred: Is the endocrine response a compensatory activity, aimed at maintaining a steady state and providing the best strategy for survival (which has always been the classic teaching), or might the endocrine response at times be misguided and deleterious, wreaking havoc rather than alleviating, in the context of the complex disease states that are encountered in contemporary medicine?

The purpose of *Endocrinology of Critical Disease* is to review the complexity of the endocrine response to critical illness, explore the mechanisms and outcomes (both positive and negative) of the endocrine responses to severe illnesses, and even consider possible endocrine interactions that are not yet fully defined, while blending basic knowledge in these areas with discussion of the clinical relevance of this information.

K. Patrick Ober, MD

CONTENTS

Preface v

Contributors ix

1 General Adaptation Syndrome: *An Overview* 1
  David J. Torpy and George P. Chrousos

2 Developmental Considerations: *The Fetal and Neonatal
    Endocrine Response to Stress* 25
  C. Richard Parker, Jr.

3 Growth, Development, and Critical Disease 45
  Pamela A. Clark and Alan D. Rogol

4 Pituitary Response to Stress: *Growth Hormone and Prolactin* 67
  Mark E. Molitch

5 The Sympathoadrenomedullary Response to Critical Illness 87
  Otto Kuchel

6 The Adrenocortical Response to Critical Illness:
    The CRH–ACTH–Cortisol Axis 123
  Jay Watsky and Matthew C. Leinung

7 Adrenocortical Response to Critical Illness:
    The Renin–Aldosterone Axis 137
  Paul I. Jagger

8 Thyroid Response to Critical Illness 155
  Jonathan S. LoPresti and John T. Nicoloff

9 Pathophysiology of Water Metabolism During Critical Illness 175
  Mary H. Parks and Joseph G. Verbalis

10 Alterations in Fuel Metabolism in Critical Illness: *Hyperglycemia* ... 197
   Barry A. Mizock

11 Alterations in Fuel Metabolism in Critical Illness: *Hypoglycemia* 211
   K. Patrick Ober

12 Critical Illness and Calcium Metabolism 233
   Jack F. Tohme and John P. Bilezikian

13 Skeletal Metabolism in Critical Illness 249
   Steven R. Gambert and Stephen J. Peterson

14 Testicular Function in Critical Illness 271
   Stephen R. Plymate and Robert E. Jones

15 The Female Gonadal Response to Critical Disease 285
   Mark D. Nixon and Robert W. Rebar

16 Effects of Aging on the Hormonal Response to Stress **299**
Gary A. Wittert and John E. Morley

Index 311

CONTRIBUTORS

JOHN P. BILEZIKIAN, MD, *Department of Medicine, Columbia University, New York, NY*
GEORGE P. CHROUSOS, MD, *Developmental Endocrinology Branch, National Institute of Child Health and Human Development, Bethesda, MD*
PAMELA A. CLARK, MD, *Department of Pediatrics, University of Virginia, Charlottesville, VA*
STEVEN R. GAMBERT, MD, *Department of Medicine, University of Medicine and Dentistry of New Jersey, Newark, NJ*
PAUL I. JAGGER, MD, *Department of Medicine, University of California, San Diego School of Medicine, San Diego, CA (Retired)*
ROBERT E. JONES, MD, *Department of Medicine, University of Utah, Salt Lake City, UT*
OTTO KUCHEL, MD, *Clinical Research Institute of Montreal, Quebec, Canada*
MATTHEW C. LEINUNG, MD, *Division of Endocrinology and Metabolism, The Albany Medical College, Albany, NY*
JONATHAN S. LOPRESTI, MD, PHD, *Department of Medicine, University of Southern California, Los Angeles, CA*
BARRY A. MIZOCK, MD, FACP, *Medical Intensive Care Unit, Cook County Hospital, Chicago, IL*
MARK E. MOLITCH, MD, *Center for Endocrinology, Metabolism, and Molecular Medicine, Northwestern University Medical School, Chicago, IL*
JOHN E. MORLEY, MD, *Department of Internal Medicine, St. Louis University, St. Louis, MO*
JOHN T. NICOLOFF, MD, *Department of Medicine, University of Southern California, Los Angeles, CA*
MARK D. NIXON, MD, PHD, *Department of Obstetrics and Gynecology, University of Cincinnati Medical Center, Cincinnati, OH*
K. PATRICK OBER, MD, *Department of Endocrinology and Metabolism, Bowman Gray School of Medicine, Wake Forest University, Winston-Salem, NC*
C. RICHARD PARKER, JR., PHD, *Department of Obstetrics and Gynecology, University of Alabama at Birmingham, Birmingham, AL*
MARY H. PARKS, MD, *Division of Endocrinology and Metabolism, Georgetown University School of Medicine, Washington, DC*
STEPHEN J. PETERSON, MD, *Division of General Internal Medicine, Department of Medicine, New York Medical College, Westchester County Medical Center, Valhalla, NY*
STEPHEN R. PLYMATE, MD, *Department of Medicine, Universtiy of Washington, Seattle, WA*
ROBERT W. REBAR, MD, *Department of Obstetrics and Gynecology, University of Cincinnati Medical Center, Cincinnati, OH*
ALAN D. ROGOL, MD, PHD, *Department of Pediatrics and Pharmacology, University of Virginia, Charlottesville, VA*
JACK F. TOHME, MD, *Department of Medicine, Columbia University, New York, NY*
DAVID J. TORPY, MD, *Developmental Endocrinology Branch, National Institute of Child Health and Human Development, Bethesda, MD*

JOSEPH G. VERBALIS, MD, *Division of Endocrinology and Metabolism, Georgetown University School of Medicine, Washington, DC*

JAY WATSKY, MD, *Division of Endocrinology and Metabolism, Albany Medical College, Albany, NY*

GARY A. WITTERT, MD, *Department of Medicine, Royal Adelaide Hospital, Adelaide, Australia*

1 General Adaptation Syndrome
An Overview

David J. Torpy, MBBS, PhD
and George P. Chrousos, MD, DSs

CONTENTS

> INTRODUCTION
> GLUCOCORTICOIDS—MOLECULAR ACTIONS AND ROLE STRESS
> THE CIRCADIAN RHYTHM AND GLUCOCORTICOID FEEDBACK
> CRH—CENTRAL INTEGRATOR OF THE STRESS RESPONSE
> PRIMARY STRESS SYSTEM DISORDERS
> CRH AND VASOPRESSIN
> NEURAL CONTROL OF THE HPA AXIS
> HPA AXIS INTERACTIONS WITH THE IMMUNE SYSTEM
> AUTOIMMUNITY
> SEXUAL DIMORPHISM IN THE STRESS RESPONSE:
>   ROLE OF CENTRAL AND PERIPHERAL CRH SECRETION
> INTERACTIONS WITH OTHER NEUROENDOCRINE AXES
> STUDIES IN CRITICAL ILLNESS
> REFERENCES

INTRODUCTION

Stress may be defined as a threat to homeostasis or the stable internal environment. The physiologic response to stress involves activation of the central nervous system (CNS) with consequent stimulation of the hypothalamic–pituitary–adrenal (HPA) axis and the autonomic nervous system. Importantly, these systems respond to hormonal stimulation from the immune system; they also interact with other endocrine systems, such as those controlling gonadal, thyroid, and growth functions. The principal central control loci of the stress system are the corticotropin releasing hormone (CRH) and locus cerulus-norepinephrinergic neurons of the hypothalamus and brainstem; these neurons regulate the HPA axis and the sympathetic nervous system, respectively. The hormone products of these systems, cortisol and the catecholamines, act to maintain cardiovascular, metabolic, and immune homeostasis during stress.

Bernard *(1)* and Cannon *(2)*, coined the terms "internal milieu" and "homeostasis," respectively, to introduce the concept of a constant internal environment in living organisms. This internal environment is assiduously maintained despite a multitude of threats. These threats to homeostasis, or stressors, may originate internally or from the external environment. The modern study of stress owes much to the experiments of Hans Selye *(3)*. Selye noted as a medical student that patients with a diversity of diseases had signs and symptoms in common, such as anorexia, weight loss, reduced strength, and loss of interest in surroundings. Experiments in animals indicated that chronic stress produced similarly "stereotyped" morphological responses, independent of the nature of the stressor. These changes included adrenal hypertrophy, atrophy of the thymus and other lymphoid organs, and gastrointestinal ulcers; the latter had been observed many years earlier in patients who had extensive burn injuries *(4)*.

The "general adaptation syndrome" described by Selye was proposed to comprise three stages:

1. The alarm reaction characterized biochemically by acute catecholamine and glucocorticoid hypersecretion;
2. The stage of resistance, with reduced biochemical and behavioral stress responses; and
3. The stage of exhaustion, with the emergence of stress-induced disease.

It was the stereotypical nature of the clinical, physiologic, and pathologic outcomes of exposure to diverse stressors that led to the notion of a general adaptation syndrome. Stress-induced disease was thought to be a consequence of hormonal hyposecretion following depletion of stored hormones, but this has never been demonstrated. Recent studies in stress have characterized the hormone responses to a variety of acute and chronic stressors as well as the neurophysiologic mechanisms that control catecholamine and glucocorticoid release. These studies have refined the concepts of Cannon and Selye, have demonstrated a relative specificity in the stress system response to different stressors, and have pointed toward genetic and environmental influences on the ability of individuals to respond to stressful stimuli.

A number of common diseases are now thought to be secondary to disturbances in the regulation of the stress system, beginning with the observation of glucocorticoid hypersecretion *(5)* and the discovery that ACTH responses to CRH are blunted in melancholic depression *(6)*, suggesting central CRH hypersecretion. Further work has added to this hypothesis; a number of mood and inflammatory disorders may involve disturbed stress system function as a key part of their etiopathogenesis. Finally, the notion that the HPA axis and the immune system comprise a continuous feedback loop has arisen over the last 20 years; endocrine-immune relations are now a subject of intense investigation.

The hypothalamic hormones CRH and arginine vasopressin (AVP) are the major ACTH and, hence, cortisol secretagogs (Fig. 1). HPA axis basal hormone production is pulsatile and follows a circadian pattern, with peak activation at approx 8 AM. This axis is activated under the influence of stress, whereas glucocorticoids control their own secretion via several negative feedback loops.

GLUCOCORTICOIDS—MOLECULAR ACTIONS AND ROLE IN STRESS

Cortisol is produced by the zona fasciculata at the "resting," nonstressed rate of 12–15 mg/m^2 of body surface area per day; this production can increase up to fivefold during stress, such as critical illness. (For further discussion, refer to Chapter 6. Cortisol has a four-ring structure, similar to other steroid hormones, and contains 21-carbon atoms. The

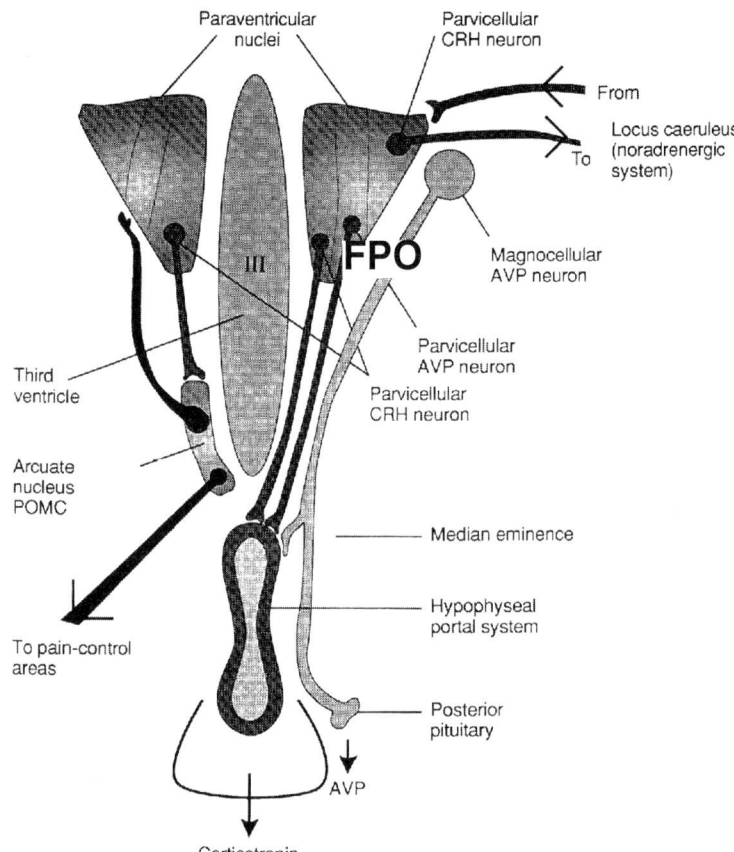

Fig. 1. The hypothalamic-hypophysial system. Parvicellular neurons of the paraventricular nuclei (PVN) secrete corticotropin releasing hormone (CRH) and arginine vasopressin (AVP) into the hypophysial-portal system. Magnocellular AVP-secreting neurons terminate in the posterior pituitary and secrete into the systemic circulation; they also have collateral terminals in the portal system. CRH and AVP act synergistically to stimulate ACTH release. The arcuate nucleus proopiomelanocortin (POMC) is shown along with mutual innervation between CRH and POMC peptide-secreting neurons. These neurons send projections to the brainstem and spinal cord to produce so-called stress-induced analgesia. (Adapted from ref. 7; with permission.)

3–10% of circulating cortisol that is not bound to cortisol binding globulin can readily diffuse through cell membranes and bind the cytoplasmic glucocorticoid receptor. This 777 amino acid cytoplasmic receptor consists of a ligand binding domain in the C-terminus, a DNA binding domain in the middle, and the N-terminal "immunogenic" region. After ligand binding, the receptor–ligand complex dissociates from a heteroligomer of heat-shock proteins, homodimerizes, and translocates into the nucleus. The DNA binding domain binds to sequences of DNA termed glucocorticoid-responsive elements (GREs); this leads to modulation of the transcription rates of glucocorticoid-responsive genes (8). Alternatively, the ligand-bound, activated glucocorticoid receptor can interact with other transcription factors, such as the c-*jun*/c-*fos* or NfkB heterodimers, to inhibit their effects on their responsive genes. Recently, a glucocorticoid nonligand binding receptor isoform, designated β, was described; this is a dominant negative inhibitor of the classic glucocorticoid receptor α *(9)*. This receptor isoform, along with other factors, may influence the sensitivity of target tissues to glucocorticoids *(10)*.

Under basal conditions, glucocorticoids maintain cardiac contractility and peripheral vascular tone by permissively allowing catecholamines and other vasopressor hormones to exert their effects *(11)*. Therefore, glucocorticoid deficient patients may exhibit postural hypotension, persistent systemic hypotension, or even collapse. Attempts to develop an integrated overview of the physiological functions of elevated cortisol secretion during stress, however, have aroused controversy over several decades. Selye emphasized the role of glucocorticoids in intermediary metabolism-mobilizing glucose, free fatty acids, and amino acids, as well as their permissive effects on vascular tone *(3)*. However, recent attention has focused on the physiological importance of glucocorticoids as agents of restraint, protecting tissues from the effects of an unrestrained stress response *(12)*. Glucocorticoids do this by suppressing the effects of many noninflammatory and inflammatory mediators, such as their own regulatory hormones, CRH and ACTH, the other stress hormones adrenaline and noradrenaline, as well as the inflammatory cytokines and the lipid mediators of inflammation. (Fig. 2).

THE CIRCADIAN RHYTHM AND GLUCOCORTICOID FEEDBACK

Cortisol levels peak at about the time of waking and have their nadir around midnight. The daily circadian variation in cortisol secretion may serve a primary role, or simply reflect an intrinsic rhythm of the nervous system, vital for other processes, or for normal brain function. A "free-running" circadian rhythm occurs in totally blind persons, with peak cortisol levels occurring in different individuals at various times of the day *(13)*. This suggests that light, rather than other time cues such as activity or meals, is the major zeitgeber (entrainer) of the rhythm. Jet-lag produces a disturbance of this rhythm relative to the day–night cycle, which then takes several days to be re-entrained *(14)*.

ACTH, a 39 amino acid peptide, binds adrenocortical cell-surface receptors to effect cortisol release. This process is dependent on extracellular calcium, and leads to activation of a cAMP/protein kinase A second messenger system *(15)*. Cortisol feedback acts on the pituitary to inhibit ACTH release, on the hypothalamus to inhibit release of hypothalamic ACTH secretagogs, and on suprahypothalamic centers to influence their input to the hypothalamus. All these sites contain glucocorticoid receptors. There is evidence from in vivo studies in rats to indicate that the brain, rather than the pituitary, is the site at which physiological levels of glucocorticoids suppress ACTH secretion and, hence, "fine-tune" their own secretion *(16)*. Remarkable plasticity of feedback inhibition of the HPA axis is evident from studies that reveal that the quality and quantity of stressor can alter sensitivity to feedback in both animals *(17)* and humans *(18,19)*. This plasticity is probably expressed at various levels in the brain.

In humans, the phenomenon of prolonged HPA axis suppression, which lasts up to 24 mo after as little as 2–4 wk of exogenous glucocorticoid treatment, probably relates to suppression of CRH neuronal activity or higher pathways that regulate such activity. This conclusion is based on a study of successfully treated Cushing's disease patients with suppressed HPA axes; it was possible to normalize ACTH secretion with a 24-h ovine CRH infusion in these patients *(20)*.

Glucocorticoid feedback is mediated by the classic glucocorticoid receptor type 2, and by the type 1 or mineralocorticoid receptor. Glucocorticoids are present in much higher concentration in the circulation than mineralocorticoids. Type 1 receptors in the brain are not protected from glucocorticoids by the enzyme 11β-hydroxysteroid dehydrogenase, as in the renal tubule; therefore, brain type-1 receptors are not mineralocorticoid-specific *(21)*. Whereas type 2 receptors are widespread in the brain and anterior pituitary, type 1 receptors are mainly found in the limbic system, particularly the hippocampus *(22)*. Type 1 receptors have a glucocorticoid affinity that is 10-fold higher than that of type 2 receptors *(23)*. In humans, studies with mifepristone (RU 486), a type 2 glucocorticoid receptor antagonist, suggest that type 2 receptors are only activated by the high cortisol concentrations that occur in the morning *(24)* or during stress.

Local brain disruptions in glucocorticoid receptor sensitivity may be associated with psychiatric symptoms and reduced sensitivity to glucocorticoid feedback, with consequent glucocorticoid hypersecretion. Indeed, tricyclic antidepressants upregulate corticosteroid receptor activity; the time-course of this phenomenon matches the delayed (several weeks) clinical efficacy observed with these agents *(25,26)*.

CRH—CENTRAL INTEGRATOR OF THE STRESS RESPONSE

Ovine CRH, a 41 amino acid peptide, was sequenced in 1981 *(27)*. Human CRH differs from ovine CRH by seven amino acids and is metabolized much more rapidly. Both have been synthesized and used in clinical research. The discovery of ovine and human CRH led to the characterization of CRH as a hypothalamic hormone in humans *(28–30)*, followed by clinical trials of its use as a diagnostic agent in pituitary-adrenal and related disorders *(31)*. CRH has proven useful in the differential diagnosis of Cushing's syndrome, as a provocation test and a stimulator of ACTH release during inferior petrosal sinus sampling; these tests are aimed at separating Cushing's disease from ectopic ACTH production *(32)*. The same peptide has proven useful in the differential diagnosis of adrenal insufficiency *(33)*.

Paraventricular nucleus (PVN)-CRH neurons innervate cell bodies of the central control nuclei of the sympathetic nervous system in the brainstem *(34)*. CRH stimulates noradrenergic neurons of the locus cerulus *(35)*, one of the central control nuclei that regulate arousal. Therefore, CRH is the central controller of both the HPA axis and the sympathetic nervous system, the two hormonal elements of the stress response. CRH may also mediate behavioral phenomena under stress conditions. Delivery of intracerebroventricular CRH to rats, mice, and primate species leads to a constellation of behavioral and endocrine abnormalities reminiscent of acute stress, intense anxiety, and melancholic depression. These include tachycardia, increased arterial pressure, reduced appetite and sexual activity, social withdrawal, and psychomotor retardation or agitation, depending on the context *(36–39)*. CRH receptors, which mediate these effects, are widespread in the central nervous system; they are found at the PVN-CRH/locus cerulus cell bodies and limbic structures *(40)*. Specific sites of CRH neurons may have discrete roles; for example there is evidence that the anxiogenic effects of alcohol withdrawal may be mediated by CRH acting at the central nucleus of the amygdala *(41)*. CRH availability at the receptor is regulated by specific binding of the peptide to CRH binding protein *(42)*.

PRIMARY STRESS SYSTEM DISORDERS

An inappropriately hyperactivated or underactivated stress system may be responsible for thus far unexplained human disorders. Major melancholic depression is associated with slight cortisol hypersecretion, and in about 50% of cases with resistance to dexamethasone suppression *(5)*. The anterior pituitaries *(43)* and adrenals *(44)* of depressed patients are enlarged. The ACTH response to CRH is blunted *(6)*, suggesting endogenous CRH hypersecretion and consequent CRH receptor downregulation. Increased CRH levels in lumbar CSF have been reported *(45)*. Autopsy studies of human depressed subjects have revealed decreased CRH binding sites in limbic areas *(46)* and increased numbers of CRH neurons in the hypothalamic PVN *(47)*. Circadian cortisol release in depressed patients tends to be "phase advanced" with peak/trough levels occurring earlier in the day than in healthy subjects *(47a)*. There is also evidence of chronic CRH hypersecretion in the posttraumatic stress disorder of the young, who are particularly prone to anxiety and depression *(48)*. Therefore, central CRH hypersecretion may be a primary biological event leading to melancholic depression and anxiety disorders.

Central CRH hyposecretion, on the other hand, has been inferred in atypical/seasonal depression *(49)*, the chronic fatigue/fibromyalgia syndromes *(50–52)*, the mood and immune phenomena occurring in the postpartum period *(53,54)*, and in subjects who have increased vulnerability to alcoholism *(55)*. Patients with the fibromyalgia and chronic fatigue syndromes have decreased urinary free cortisol secretion, perhaps owing to low central CRH secretion *(50–52)*. Paraventricular CRH neurons also innervate pain control areas of the arcuate nucleus of the hypothalamus, brainstem, and spinal cord; lack of CRH input to these neurons may participate in the decreased pain threshold and/or pain syndrome associated with the chronic fatigue and fibromyalgia syndromes. In the postpartum period, the "blues" consisting of a mild transient depression whose onset is within 3 wk of parturition and a more severe depressive syndrome are well described. During late pregnancy, glucocorticoid hypersecretion occurs, probably owing to high circulating CRH of placental origin acting in the anterior pituitary. The abrupt withdrawal of placental CRH at childbirth would be expected to result in a low hypothalamic CRH secretory state, until recovery from hypercortisolism occurs. This low CRH period may be expected to result in mood disturbances, including atypical depression, and a surge in autoimmune phenomena, secondary to transient hypocortisolism. Both mood and autoimmune disturbances in the postpartum fit the model of CRH secretory disturbances developed from a number of other conditions (Table 1).

Acute and chronic alcohol ingestion causes activation of the HPA axis *(56–58)*. Lewis rats, which have a hypoactive CRH neuron, are prone to alcohol addiction *(59)*. Offspring of alcoholic subjects have increased vulnerability to alcoholism and a hypoactive HPA axis *(55)*. Therefore, central CRH hyposecretion may predispose alcoholism in humans, and chronic active alcoholism may represent a maladaptive self-treatment, leading to excessive CRH secretion and hypercortisolism with all its long-term sequelae.

CRH AND VASOPRESSIN

CRH neurons are widespread within the brain, and although they may all subserve a general stress function, they are likely to be differentially regulated in accordance with a diversity of roles. Although PVN-CRH neuron firing is inhibited by glucocorticoids, other CRH neurons are not inhibited by glucocorticoids *(59a)*, and may even be activated by them *(60)*. Similarly, activation of CRH neurons by stress may not lead to ACTH and cortisol release. Psychological stress in rats can increase arousal through a CRH-mediated mechanism, with CRH originating from the central nucleus of the amygdala; exposure to foot-shocked rats reduces phenobarbital-induced sleep duration. This effect of psy-

Table 1
States Associated with Dysregulation or Altered Regulation of the HPA Axis

Increased HPA activity	Decreased HPA activity	Disrupted HPA activity
Severe chronic disease	Atypical depression	Cushing's syndrome
Melancholic depression	Seasonal depression	Glucocorticoid deficiency
Anorexia nervosa	Chronic fatigue syndrome	Glucocorticoid resistance
Obsessive-compulsive disorder		
Panic disorder	Hypothyroidism	
Chronic excessive exerise	Adrenal suppression	
Malnutrition	Obesity (hyposerotonergic forms)	
Diabetes mellitus	Nicotine withdrawal	
Hyperthyroidism	Vulnerability to inflammatory disease (Lewis rat)	
Premenstrual tension syndrome	Rheumatoid arthritis	
Central obesity	Postpartum mood and inflammatory disorders	
Childhood sexual abuse	Vulnerability to alcoholism	
Pregnancy		

chic stress on sleep can be blocked by the CRH antagonist α-helical CRH, although this stress did not induce ACTH and cortisol release into the systemic circulation *(61)*.

CRH and CRH receptor genes are also expressed outside the central nervous system as well. Peripheral CRH secreted in inflammatory sites acts as a paracrine/autocrine proinflammatory modulator, hence its designation "immune CRH" *(62)*. Reproductive organs, such as the ovaries, endometrium, and placenta, can exhibit "aseptic" inflammatory processes. They also contain immunoreactive CRH designated "reproductive" CRH *(63)*.

CRH levels in human peripheral plasma are very low and probably are derived from both hypothalamic and extrahypothalamic sources. These levels do not exhibit circadian variation or increase after metyrapone *(59a)*. Thus, they cannot be used to assess hypothalamic CRH release relevant to the HPA axis. Cerebrospinal fluid (CSF) levels of CRH have been used to assess PVN CRH activity, although a proportion of this CRH is extrahypothalamic in origin *(64)*. As the hypothalamic-hypophysial portal circulation is inaccessible in humans, it is not currently possible to assess hypothalamic secretion directly.

Two corticotropin releasing factor receptor (CRF) genes have been characterized in the rat, with the α and β-subtypes of the CRF R_2 receptor representing different splicing products. Specific receptor localization has been determined in the rat; CRF R_1 is found in the pituitary and brain *(65–68)*, CRF $R_{2\alpha}$ has a specific limited brain distribution *(69)*, whereas CRF $R_{2\beta}$ is found in peripheral tissues and brain vasculature *(70,71)*. A rat neuropeptide that shows 45% sequence identity with CRH and is 10 times more potent than CRH in binding and activating type CRF $R_{2\beta}$ receptors has been named urocortin, reflecting its 63% sequence identity with fish urotensin *(72)*. The relative importance of CRH and urocortin for their various effects at the three known CRF receptors has not yet been established. Preliminary data suggest that CRH is much more anxiogenic and less anorexigenic than urocortin. It may also be that residual ACTH secretion in the CRH gene "knockout" mouse *(73)* is owing to urocortin action at the pituitary. CRH has cognition-enhancing properties in rodents; low cortical CRH levels in postmortem brains of Alzheimer's disease patients coexist with normal levels of CRH-BP, further lowering active, unbound CRH levels. Like the rat, humans also have two CRH receptor genes (hCRH R_1 and hCRH R_2) *(74)*. Human urocortin has also been cloned and shown to be a more potent stimulator of CRF $R_{2\alpha}$ (40X) and CRF $R_{2\beta}$ (20X) receptor-mediated cyclic AMP production than CRH in cells stably transfected with these CRF receptors *(75)*. Therapeutically, CRH-BP agonists may displace mature CRH and enhance the agonistic effects of CRH at its target tissues *(76)*.

The hypothalamus secretes the nonapeptide arginine vasopressin and CRH from axons terminating at the zona externa of the median eminence (Fig. 1). The median eminence is outside the blood–brain barrier *(77)*. Secretion occurs after secretory granules undergo membrane fusion at terminal axons, thereby discharging hormones into the hypothalamic-hypophysial portal circulation, which transports these hormones to the adenohypophysis. Some 2000 CRH-containing neurons can be found in the parvicellular region of the PVN of the hypothalamus, close to the third ventricle *(78)*. Many of these neurons also contain AVP *(79)*. The perikarya of neurons that send AVP-secreting axons to the neurohypophysis, and are involved in water balance regulation are found in the magnocellular region of this nucleus. In addition, some magnocellular AVP-secreting neurons may contribute to ACTH regulation by providing projections to the median eminence *(80)*.

AVP may be important in maintaining pituitary-adrenal responsiveness to acute stressors in chronic physical stress conditions, where there is a significant decrease in the CRH:AVP ratio *(81,82)*. Animal models of chronic stress have implicated a stimulus-specific attenuation of ACTH/cortisol responses to repeated acute stress; novel stressors, however, elicit a normal or exaggerated glucocorticoid response *(83,84)*. Studies using plasma sampling from the hypophysial portal circulation of rats *(85)* and sheep *(86–88)* suggest a stimulus-specific variation in the CRH:AVP ratio, as well as a variation in this ratio according to the magnitude and/or duration of the stressor. The finding of populations of corticotropes with different sensitivities to CRH and AVP suggests that the range of hypothalamic CRH or AVP secretory responses, produced by qualitatively and quantitatively different stressors, can be interpreted at the pituitary level *(89)*. Stimulatory doses of CRH and AVP produce a synergistic ACTH response in humans *(28)*. CRH and AVP both act to increase ACTH release from corticotropes; The AVP response to stress is discussed further in Chapter 9. CRH also stimulates transcription of the proopiomelanocortin (POMC) gene in the anterior pituitary *(90)*.

NEURAL CONTROL OF THE HPA AXIS

Studies of the neural control of the HPA axis are important for at least two reasons. First, measurement of hormones, such as ACTH and cortisol, allows access to brain function and extends our knowledge of the crucial central control of this stress system. Second, such studies may help shed light on the pathogenesis of common mental and autoimmune disorders, where there is a substantial body of evidence for concomitant brain–HPA axis dysfunction.

Much of the current understanding of the neural control of hypophysiotropic factor release arises from:

1. In vitro studies of explanted hypothalamic fragments;
2. Measurement of CRH/AVP in hypophysial portal blood of rats, sheep, and horses; and
3. In vivo pharmacologic studies in animals and humans.

Each of these techniques has limitations. For example, in vitro studies involve deafferentation that may enhance end-organ sensitivity, and portal sampling involves anesthesia and major surgery in the rat and invokes species differences in the sheep. Studies of intact organisms during pharmacologic manipulation are limited by the specificity of the drugs used, both with regard to site and mechanism of action.

The available human studies with pharmacologic agents indicate a stimulatory role for brain noradrenergic pathways on ACTH release *(91)*, an inhibitory role for γ-aminobutyric acid (GABA$_{A1}$) pathways linked to the GABA$_A$/benzodiazepine receptor *(92)*, and an inhibitory role for central opioidergic *(93)* and substance P-ergic *(94)* pathways. Serotonin, acetylcholine, histamine, and neuropeptide Y(NPY), which is colocalized in adrenergic projections or is present in NPY-containing neurons of the arcuate nucleus of the hypothalamus, have all been stimulatory in animal studies, but the human data are contradictory or limited in interpretation by the specificity of the pharmacologic probe used *(95)*.

Noradrenergic pathways to the CRH neuron are thought to link the sympathetic nervous system and HPA axis. The neuroanatomical substrate for this is well defined, with direct synaptic connections between noradrenergic and CRH neurons *(96)*. Noradrenergic and adrenergic terminals arise from A_1, A_2, and A_6 areas or C_1, C_2 and C_3 areas, respectively, in the brainstem. The locus cerulus and/or its vicinity has *rich* CRH fiber innervation *(97)* and locus cerulus firing is activated by application of CRH *(35)*. A reciprocal stimulatory relationship between PVN CRH neurons and locus cerulus noradrenergic neurons coordinates the sympathetic nervous system (adrenomedullary and sympathoneural) and HPA responses to stress.

A number of neurotransmitters known to affect the HPA axis have been postulated to play a role in the development of psychiatric and other idiopathic syndromes. These include serotonin deficiency in depression, obsessive-compulsive disorder, and some forms of obesity; these hypotheses were based on the success of serotoninergic drugs in these entities. Attempts to find a suitable pharmacologic probe of a serotonin-neuroendocrine system to study these disorders have proven difficult because of a lack of drug specificity *(95)* and, perhaps, redundant neural pathways. A noradrenergic mechanism has been proposed for panic disorder, based on measures of autonomic function and interactions with agents, such as yohimbine and clonidine *(98)*. Hypersecretion of neuropeptide Y, detected on CSF measurements *(99)*, may be pathogenic in anorexia nervosa *(100)* and has been hypothesized to be pathogenic in obesity. It definitely appears pathogenic in Zucker rats, which have an apparently deficient leptin receptor, leading to hypersecretion of NPY *(101)*. Further examination of these hypotheses in humans may need more specific pharmacologic probes and/or more sensitive functional brain imaging.

HPA AXIS INTERACTIONS WITH THE IMMUNE SYSTEM

Glucocorticoids have potent anti-inflammatory and immunosuppressive effects' and this has led to their use in many inflammatory diseases. Glucocorticoids influence the traffic of circulating leukocytes, and inhibit many functions of leukocytes and immune accessory cells *(8)*. They suppress the immune activation of these cells, inhibit the production of cytokines and other mediators of inflammation, and cause resistance to cytokines. Glucocorticoids preferentially suppress certain subgroups of T-lymphocytes; they suppress the function of type 1 helper T-lymphocytes, and stimulate apoptosis of eosinophils and certain groups of T-cells. These effects depend on alterations of the transcription rates of glucocorticoid-responsive genes and/or changes in the stability of messenger RNA of several inflammatory proteins. These effects of glucocorticoids may be direct through binding to glucocorticoid-response elements of DNA, or indirect through blockade of transcription factors, such as AP-1 or NFκB.

T-helper cell subtypes have recently been described. T-helper 1 (Th1) cells produce interleukin (IL)-12, IL-2, and interferon γ and favor a cellular response such as that seen in tissue rejection or certain autoimmune diseases. T-helper 2 (Th2) cells produce IL-10, IL-4, and tumor necrosis factor-α (TNF-α)–and favor a humoral (antibody) response *(102,103)*. The balance of Th1/Th2 cell responses may influence susceptibility to infection or autoimmunity *(103)*. Recent evidence suggests that stress may, through hypersecretion of glucocorticoids and catecholamines, alter cytokine secretion *(104)*, and result in a shift from a Th1- to a Th2-type predominant response (Fig. 3). Such an effect of stress could help explain enhanced susceptibility to infections, such as tuberculosis *(105)* and the common cold *(106)*. Conversely, an underactive stress system (and shift to Th1 predominance) is associated with autoimmunity in rats *(107)*, and in human states, such as the postpartum and after cure of Cushing's syndrome *(7,54)*.

Conversely, activation of the immune system beyond a certain threshold leads to activation of the HPA axis. The link between the immune system and the HPA axis is the inflammatory cytokines, especially TNF-α, IL-1 and IL-6. At inflammatory sites, TNF-α is secreted first, then IL-1, followed by IL-6 (Fig. 2). TNF-α and IL-1 stimulate each other's secretion, whereas IL-6 inhibits secretion of both TNF-α and IL-1. CRH-neutralizing antisera and/or antagonists block the effects of each of the three inflammatory cytokines on the HPA axis. An immune-HPA negative feedback loop is closed by glucocorticoids, which inhibit synthesis and secretion of these cytokines. Systemic IL-6 concentrations also increase during stress unrelated to inflammation, presumably stimulated by catecholamines acting through $β_2$-adrenergic receptors *(108,109)*. IL-6 acts synergistically with glucocorticoids in stimulating the production of acute-phase reactants *(8,110)*.

Administration of IL-6 to humans can acutely and chronically activate the HPA axis; in fact, the ACTH response to a single Sc dose of IL-6 is the highest ever seen in response to any stimulus. This may become a useful test of HPA axis function, since (unlike IL-1 and TNF-α, which are believed to produce many of the cardiovascular effects seen in septic shock) IL-6 can be administered safely, with only minor side effects in studies to date *(111,112)*. It may also be a useful probe of immune–neuroendocrine relations in disorders where dysregulation of this link is postulated.

The primary site of cytokine action on the HPA axis is suprahypophysial, although prolonged cytokine exposure can activate corticotropin *(113,114)* and glucocorticoid *(111,115)* release directly. It is not known how inflammatory cytokines reach the hypothalamic CRH and AVP neurons, given that the neuronal bodies are protected by the blood–brain barrier. Inflammatory cytokines may permeate the barrier, there may be a special transport system for cytokines, or cytokines may act on CRH and AVP axon ter-

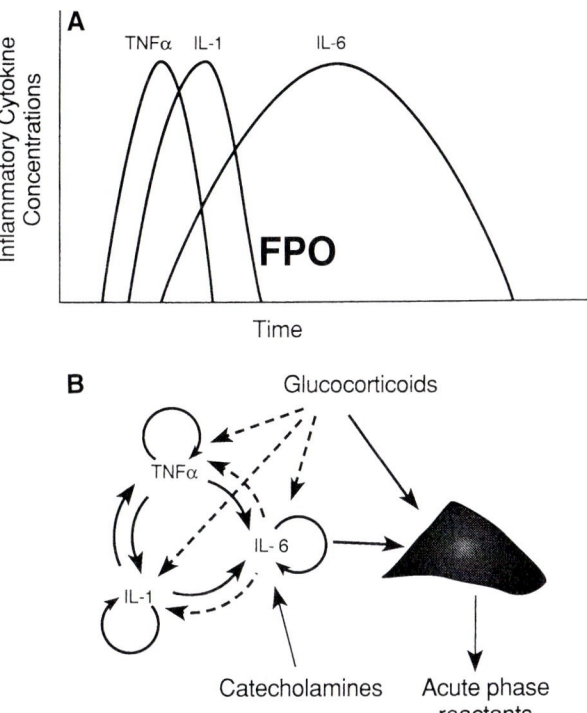

Fig. 2. Interactions among the inflammatory cytokines and the effects of glucocorticoids and catecholamines. The upper panel shows the sequence of events at an inflammatory site. TNF-α, IL-1, and IL-6 are secreted sequentially. Both TNF-α and IL-1 stimulate IL-6 secretion. IL-6 inhibits the secretion of both TNF-α and IL-1. Glucocorticoids, the end products of the HPA axis, inhibit the production of all three cytokines and inhibit their effects on target tissues, except for the effect of IL-6 on the production of acute-phase reactants, which is potentiated by glucocorticoids. Catecholamines, the other end products of the stress system, have a major role in the control of inflammation through the stimulation of IL-6, which inhibits the other cytokines, stimulates glucocorticoids, and induces the acute-phase response. The solid lines indicate stimulation, and the broken lines inhibition. (Adapted from ref. 7 with permission.)

minals at the median eminence, which is outside the blood–brain barrier. Alternatively, and quite likely, endothelial, glial, and neuronal cells may produce cytokines and other mediators of inflammation within the brain, in a cascade-like fashion, starting with circulating cytokines affecting the nonfenestrated endothelium of the blood–brain barrier, and proceeding to activate glial and neural cells.

Early work established the presence of CRH, ACTH, and glucocorticoid-releasing bioactivities in serum or supernatants of stimulated immunocytes. These findings relate to the presence of cytokines or other mediators of inflammation; three cytokines—TNF-α, IL-1, and IL-6, account for most of the HPA axis-stimulating activity in plasma (7). Recently, peptide inhibitors of glucocorticoid release were also isolated from the leukocytes of several species, including humans. Known as corticostatins, their physiological role in the stress response is not known (116).

Chronic activation of the HPA axis or chronic inflammation results in reciprocally protective adaptations. For instance, patients with endogenous Cushing's syndrome

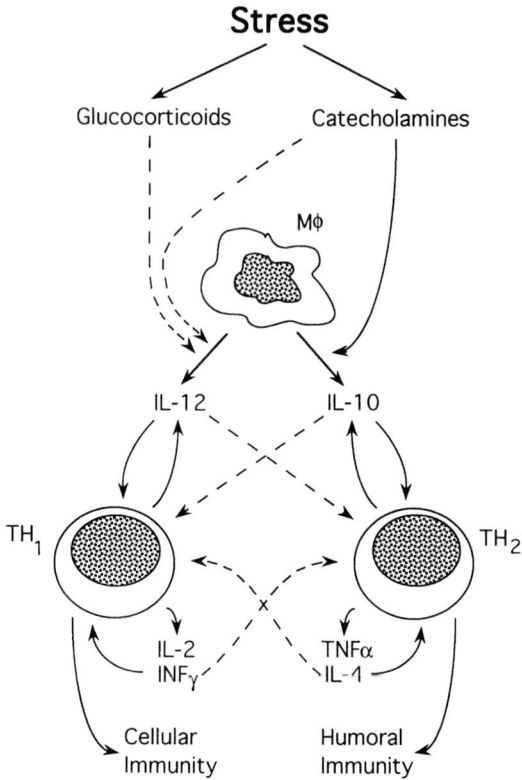

Fig. 3. The effects of stress on the Th1/TH2 balance. The final effectors of stress system activation, the glucocorticoids and catecholamines, inhibit IL-12 production, reducing Th1 cell function. Catecholamines also increase IL-10 production, inhibiting Th2 cell function. The net effect is a shift from Th1 to Th2 cell activity, favoring humoral over cellular immunity. Such a shift in immune function may be detrimental when the stress system is inappropriately activated or inhibited. (Continuous lines denote stimulation, broken lines inhibition; Th1, T helper 1; Mφ, macrophage; IL interleukin, INF, interferon; TNF, tumor necrosis factor.)

have mild rather than severe immune suppression; animals with chronic inflammation have only mild hypercortisolism (7). There may be adaptive inhibitory neural mechanisms at the hypothalamus to reduce CRH production, such as elevation of substance P, an inhibitor of CRH secretion (94,117,118).

AUTOIMMUNITY

It has been suggested that immune activity unrestrained by glucocorticoids may induce excessive inflammatory responses or autoimmunity (119,120). Several animal models of autoimmune disorders exist that exhibit such HPA axis dysregulation. Lewis rats develop Th1 cell-mediated inflammatory disorders, such as erosive polyarthritis following a bacterial cell-wall antigen, experimental allergic encephalomyelitis induced by basic myelin protein, and uveitis in response to a retinol binding epitope. These inbred rats have defective pituitary-adrenal responses, secondary to deficient PVN-CRH synthesis and secretion (121). They have compensatory magnocellular AVP hypersecretion (122). Other animal models in which hypoactivity of the HPA axis appears to contribute to autoimmune/inflammatory disease include the obese strain chicken (autoimmune thyroiditis), and several animal models of systemic lupus and insulin-dependent diabetes mellitus *(123)*. Parallel abnormalities occur in human rheumatoid arthritis patients, including low or normal circadian corticotropin and cortisol, despite elevated IL-1 and IL-6 *(124,125)*; a poor HPA axis response to surgery *(125)*; increased synovial fluid CRH *(126)*; and elevated plasma AVP.

Excessive immune-mediated inflammation may also arise from glucocorticoid resistance in target tissues. This has been suggested in rheumatoid arthritis, steroid-resistant asthma, and osteoarthritis *(7,10)*.

Interestingly, Lewis rats exhibit a behavioral syndrome consistent with atypical depression, a condition that has been linked to CRH hyposecretion *(127)*, and patients with rheumatoid arthritis have premorbid personalities compatible with subclinical atypical depression.

SEXUAL DIMORPHISM IN THE STRESS RESPONSE: ROLE OF CENTRAL AND PERIPHERAL CRH SECRETION

Generally, female animals and humans exhibit greater basal and stimulated HPA axis activity and more pronounced immune/inflammatory reactions than males. In addition, there is a relatively high incidence of autoimmune disorders in women compared to men. Gonadal steroid regulation of both the HPA axis and inflammatory mediators may account for this. The CRH gene contains functional estrogen-responsive elements *(128)*, and estrogen increases PVN CRH levels and CRH mRNA *(129,130)*. Human female hypothalami contain higher CRH levels than male ones *(131)*. Women have greater plasma ACTH responses to ovine CRH and more prolonged cortisol elevations, findings that may relate to increased central tone of the stress system in women, possibly secondary to CRH activation *(132)*. As discussed earlier, central CRH hypersecretion is strongly implicated in human depression; the increased risk of depression and other emotional disorders seen in women may, thus, also relate to CRH neuron activation by estradiol.

Estradiol downregulates glucocorticoid receptor binding in the anterior pituitary, hypothalamus and hippocampus, which would tend to increase HPA axis activity, by interfering with glucocorticoid feedback *(133–135)*. It is not known if the changes in CRH neuronal activity and central glucocorticoid receptor activity induced by estrogen are mechanistically related; however, they alter the system in the same direction.

Peripheral or "immune" CRH appears to act as a paracrine proinflammatory mediator; this role is implied by the finding of elevated levels of CRH in inflammatory sites in Lewis rats *(136–138)*, Sprague-Dawley rats *(62,137)*, mice *(138)*, and humans *(136,139)*. Despite high levels of CRH at the inflammatory site, concomitant plasma levels of CRH are very low *(62)*; therefore, direct stimulation of corticotropes from locally produced CRH does not occur. CRH immunoneutralization inhibits inflammation at these sites *(62,138)*. Immune CRH levels and the attendant inflammation are greater in female animals *(137–140)*. The presence of immune CRH in human inflammatory sites has been demonstrated by Crofford et al. *(126)* in rheumatoid arthritis and osteoarthritis, and by Scopa et al. *(139)* in Hashimoto's thyroiditis. These high levels of immune CRH may partly represent CRF-like peptides, such as the newly discovered urocortin *(72)*, since only low levels of CRH mRNA have been detected in inflamed synovial tissue *(136,141)*. Alternatively, the major source of CRH at inflammatory sites may be the postganglionic sympathetic neurons or sensory afferent fibers.

Androgen withdrawal in males increases HPA axis responsiveness, an effect reversed by subsequent androgen replacement *(142)*. Castration increases hypothalamic CRH levels and the number of immunohistochemically positive CRH neurons, an effect probably mediated at distant CNS sites, since very little androgen receptor is found in the PVN *(143)*.

INTERACTIONS WITH OTHER NEUROENDOCRINE AXES

The hypothalamic–pituitary–gonadal, thyroid, and growth axes interact with the HPA axis and the immune system. Gonadotropin-releasing hormone (GnRH) neurons of the hypothalamic arcuate nucleus are regulated by estradiol/testosterone feedback; GnRH is stimulatory to the pituitary gonadotropins, follicle stimulating hormone (FSH) and luteinizing hormone (LH). FSH stimulates ovarian follicle development and consequent estradiol secretion in females and spermatogenesis in males. LH produces cellular changes in the follicle and luteinization, leading to progesterone production, a midcycle LH surge induces ovulation, and LH stimulates Leydig cell testosterone production in males. Thyroid hormones, thyroid (T_4) and triiodothyronine (T_3), act on the pituitary to inhibit thyroid-stimulating hormone (TSH) secretion and conversion of T_4 to the more active T_3 in the pituitary increases this feedback effect. Hypothalamic thyrotropin-releasing hormone (TRH) stimulates TSH release from the pituitary; somatostatin inhibits TSH release. Secretion of growth hormone from the pituitary is regulated by the hypothalamic factors growth hormone-releasing hormone (GHRH), which stimulates, and somatostatin, which inhibits growth hormone release. Negative feedback signaling to these hypothalamic factors occurs from growth hormone itself and somatomedin C, an endocrine (and paracrine) product of growth hormone secretion that is responsible for much of the growth-promoting effects of growth hormone.

During stress, available resources are directed toward survival through maintenance of homeostasis and alteration of behavior. The gonadal, thyroid, and growth axes are inhibited at many sites by the HPA axis as shown in Fig. 4. In addition, the immune system interacts reciprocally with these axes, both directly and indirectly via the HPA axis.

With regard to the hypothalamic–pituitary–gonadal axis, CRH inhibits the GnRH neuron of the hypothalamic arcuate nucleus directly and via β-endorphin *(53,144)*. As the GnRH neuron has no estradiol receptor *(145)*, estradiol may act through hypothalamic CRH to inhibit GnRH secretion and, hence, may exert its negative feedback effects through this mechanism. Glucocorticoids inhibit GnRH secretion as well as gonadotropin and gonadal steroid hormone production and action. Conversely, estradiol appears to exert positive effects on CRH production, both in the hypothalamus and peripheral tissues (Fig. 4; *128*).

Direct hypothalamic–pituitary–gonadal axis immune effects were recently reviewed *(107)*. Sex steroids directly influence thymocyte development in a sexually dimorphic fashion. GnRH itself is produced in immune tissues where it directly influences immune function *(145a)*. Estradiol stimulates the expression of adhesion molecules by immune cells *(146)*, whereas it inhibits the production of IL-6 *(147)*, an inflammatory cytokine that plays a major role in the control and termination of inflammation directly via inhibition of TNF-α and IL-1 production, and indirectly, via stimulation of glucocorticoid secretion and activation of the acute-phase reaction *(7)*.

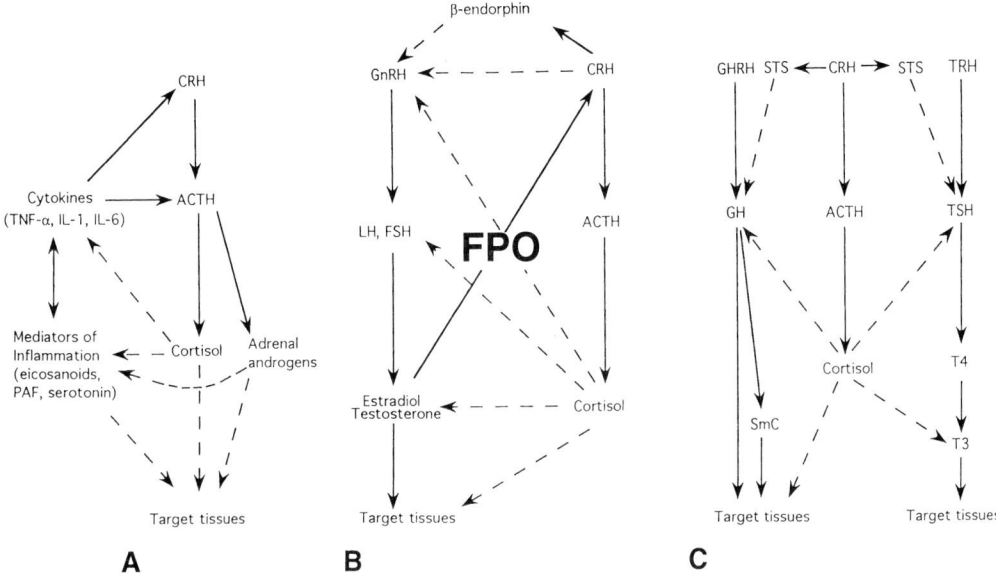

Fig. 4. A heuristic representation of the interactions between the HPA axis and other neuroendocrine systems, including the immune system (**A**), the reproductive axis (**B**), and the growth and thyroid axes (**C**). CRH, corticotropin-releasing hormone; ACTH, corticotropin; TNF-α, tumor necrosis factor-α; IL-1, interleukin-1; IL-6, interleukin-6; PAF, platelet-activating factor; GnRH, gonadotropin-releasing hormone; LH, leutinizing hormone; FSH, follicle-stimulating hormone; GHRH, growth hormone-releasing hormone; STS, somatostatin; TRH, thyrotropin-releasing hormone; GH, growth hormone; TSH, thyroid-stimulating hormone; T_4, thyroxine; T_3, triiodothyronine; SmC, somatomedin C. (Adapted from ref. *53* with permission.)

Cytokines of the immune system directly stimulate the HPA axis as described earlier, and directly inhibit TSH production *(148)*. The mechanism of stress inhibition of hypothalamic TSH secretion may involve a portion of pre-pro TRH (178–199), which is also a putative corticotropin-release inhibiting factor (CRIF); central activation of the HPA axis may reduce CRIF production and TRH production concomitantly *(149)*. In addition, glucocorticoids inhibit hypothalamic TRH gene expression *(150)*, perhaps via a GRE on the TRH gene *(151)*; glucocorticoids also inhibit deiodination of T_4 to T_3 in peripheral tissues.

Acute stress initially provokes growth hormone and prolactin secretion (as discussed in detail in Chapter 4), both of which bind specific receptors on immunocompetent cells, such as monocytes, lymphocytes, and macrophages. These hormones are immunostimulatory: they increase thymic growth and activity, and lymphocyte proliferation *(152)*. However, chronic stress, which increases somatostatin and glucocorticoid secretion, is associated with decreases of both growth hormone and prolactin. Also, very importantly, glucocorticoids prevent the actions of somatomedin C locally at the level of the target tissues. One mechanism is by interference with the actions of the AP-1 transcription factor.

STUDIES IN CRITICAL ILLNESS

In severe illness, many of the general principles described above are observed; emotional and physical stimuli lead to hypersecretion of ACTH *(18)* and cortisol *(153)*. An attenuation of the diurnal rhythm is noted *(154)*. More detailed biochemical testing of the HPA axis in these highly stressed individuals has revealed a unique state, quite different from that which develops from simple autonomous ACTH hypersecretion. Specifically, the changes noted in critical illness involve a shift away from adrenal androgen and aldosterone production toward cortisol release, suggesting alteration in relative activities of adrenal enzymes. Chronically ill individuals exhibit an exaggerated response to ACTH 1–24, suggesting adrenal hypertrophy. An increased cortisol response to exogenous human CRH and diminished suppression of cortisol after dexamethasone administration represents a unique set of parameters described only in critical illness and Cushing's disease *(154)*.

The details of HPA axis regulation under critical conditions are beginning to be understood or inferred from animal studies. Correlation of cortisol and IL-6 levels in critical illness *(155)* confirms the importance of the immune system in HPA axis activation. A change in relative importance of hypothalamic secretagog, from CRH to AVP, as observed in animal chronic physical stress models or humans with inflammatory stress, (such as patients with multiple sclerosis) may underlie the reduced responsiveness of cortisol secretion to dexamethasone suppression *(82,156,157)*.

During sepsis, glucocorticoids ensure metabolic substrate availability, elevate blood pressure, and restrain the immune system from producing host tissue damage. Sepsis can lead to septic shock, a state of overwhelming systemic infection where tissue hypoperfusion and dysfunction occur and are associated with a mortality in excess of 50%. Although controlled clinical trials of the once popular use of a short-term (<48 h) course of glucocorticoids were negative *(158)*, recent case series have identified critically ill patients with clinical features consistent with hypoadrenalism, such as hypotension, who exhibit relatively low plasma cortisol levels (<15 mcg/dL) and respond clinically to glucocorticoid therapy *(159,160)*. This syndrome may be much more frequent than is currently recognized, since the cortisol response to the standard 250 µg cosyntropin test may be normal whereas the response to the 1 µg test may be subnormal *(160)*.

Resistance of tissues to circulating glucocorticoids may contribute to the septic shock syndrome. Cytokines, including IL-1, IL-6, interferon-γ *(161)* and the combination of IL-2 and IL-4 *(162)*, can cause glucocorticoid resistance by reducing glucocorticoid receptor binding affinity. This may occur through interaction of cytokine-stimulated transcription factors AP-1 and NF-κB with the glucocorticoid receptor. Acquired tissue resistance to glucocorticoids also contributes to the late stages of acquired immune deficiency syndrome *(163)*. This area was recently extensively reviewed by Bamberger et al. *(10)*.

In summary, the coordinated hypercortisolemic and sympathetic nervous response to stress, with attendant changes in the gonadal, thyroid, and growth axes and the inflammatory reaction, comprise a crucial adaptive response to life-threatening illness, redirecting metabolic energies, and preventing excessive tissue damage from the immune system. Whereas all these changes are adaptive for limited periods of time, they may become detrimental when they persist beyond a certain period of time. Observations of a suboptimal stress system response in some critically ill patients and the possibility of tissue resistance to glucocorticoids may open fruitful new avenues for therapeutic intervention.

The recent notion of a disturbed stress system actually producing specific disease, including mood, inflammatory, and some other poorly understood disorders, may represent the "tip of the iceberg." Many of these "stress system disorders" and other disorders may be initiated or exacerbated by the stress of critical illness. In addition, chronic repeated or unrelenting environmental activation of the stress system at a population and societal level may produce detrimental changes in the individual organism, such as increased visceral fat, hyperinsulinism, hyperlipidemia, and osteoporosis, the extent of which probably varies depending on individual genetic constitution relevant to the stress system and susceptible end organs. This may contribute significantly to the prevalence of disease by predisposing to common disorders.

REFERENCES

1. Bernard C. An introduction to the Study of Experimental Medicine. Henry Schuman, New York, 1949.
2. Cannon W. The wisdom of the body. Norton, New York, 1932.
3. Selye H. General adaptation syndrome and the diseases of adaptation. J Clin Endocrinol 1946;6:117–230.
4. Curling TB. On acute ulceration of the duodenum in cases of burns. Trans Med-Chir Soc London 1842;25:260.
5. Carroll BJ, Feinberg M, Greden JF, Tarika J, Albala AA, Haskett RF, James NM, Kronfol Z, Lohr N, Steiner M, de Vigne JP, Young E. A specific laboratory test for the diagnosis of melanholia. Standardization, validation and clinical utility. Arch Gen Psychiatry 1981;38:15–22.
6. Gold P, Chrousos G, Kellner C, Post R, Roy A, Avgerinos P, Schulte H, Oldfield E, Loriaux DL. Psychiatric implications of basic and clinical studies with CRF. Am J Psychiatry 1984;141:619–627.
7. Chrousos GP. The hypothalamic–pituitary–adrenal axis and immune mediated inflammation. N Engl J Med 1995;332:1351–1362.
8. Boumpas DT, Chrousos GP, Wilder RL, Cupps TR, Balow JE. Glucocorticoid therapy for immune-mediated diseases: basic and clinical correlates. Ann Intern Med 1993;119:1198–1208.
9. Bamberger CM, Bamberger A-M, de Castro M, Chrousos GP. Glucocorticoid receptor β, a potential endogenous inhibitor of glucocorticoid action in humans. J Clin Invest 1995;95:2435–2441.
10. Bamberger CM, Schulte HM, Chrousos GP. Molecular determinants of glucocorticoid receptor function and tissue sensitivity to glucocorticoids. Endocrine Rev 1996;17:245–261.
11. Udelsman R, Ramp J, Gallucci WT, Gordon A, Lipford E, Norton JA, Loriaux DL, Chrousos GP. Adaptation during surgical stress. A reevaluation of the role of glucocorticoids. J Clin Invest 1986;77:1377–1381.
12. Munck A, Guyre PM, Holbrook NJ. Physiological functions of glucocorticoids in stress and their relation to pharmacological actions. Endocrine Rev 1984;5:25–44.
13. Sack RL, Lewy AJ, Blood ML, Keith LD, Nakagawa H. Circadian rhythm abnormalities in totally blind people: incidence and clinical significance. J Clin Endocrinol Metab 1992;75:127–134.
14. Desir D, Van Cauter E, Fang VS, Martino E, Jadot C, Spire JP, Noel P, Refetoff S, Copinschi G, Golstein J. Effects of "jet-lag" on hormonal patterns. I. Procedures, variations in total plasma proteins, and disruption of adrenocorticotropin-cortisol periodicity. J Clin Endocrinol Metab 1981;52:628–641.
15. Orth DN, Kovacs WJ, Debold CR. The adrenal cortex. In: Wilson JD, Foster DW, eds. Williams Textbook of Endocrinology, 8th ed. Saunders, Philadelphia, 1992, pp. 489–619.
16. Levin N, Shinsako J, Dallman M. Corticosterone acts on the brain inhibit adrenalectomy-induced adrenocorticotropin secretion. Endocrinology 1988;122:694–701.
17. Keller-Wood ME, Dallman MF. Corticosteroid inhibition of ACTH secretion. Endocr Rev 1984;5:1–24.
18. Reincke M, Allolio B, Wurth G, Winkelmann W. The hypothalamic-pituitary-adrenal axis in critical illness: response to dexamethasone and corticotropin-releasing homone. J Clin Endocrinol Metab 1993;77:151–156.
19. Petrides JS, Mueller GP, Kalogeras KT, Chrousos GP, Gold PW, Deuster PA. Exercise-induced activation of the hypothalamic-pituitary-adrenal axis: marked differences in the sensitivity to glucocorticoid suppression. J Clin Endocrinol Metab 1994;79:377–383.
20. Gomez T, Magiakou MA, Mastorakos G, Chrousos GP. The pituitary corticotrope is not the rate limiting step in the postoperative recovery of the hypothalamic–pituitary–adrenal axis in patients with Cushing's syndrome. J Clin Endocrinol Metab 1993;77:173–177.
21. Edwards CRW, Stewart PM, Burt D, Brett L, McIntyre MA, Sutanto WS, de Kloet ER, Monder C. Localization of 11-beta-hydroxysteroid dehydrogenase tissue-specific protector of the mineralocorticoid receptor. Lancet 1988;ii:986–989.

22. McEwen BS, de Kloet ER, Rostene W. Adrenal steroid receptors and actions in the nervous system. Physiol Rev 1986;66:1121–1188.
23. Reul JHM, de Kloet ER. Two receptor systems for corticosterone in rat brain: microdistribution and differential occupation. Endocrinology 1985;117:2505–2511.
24. Gaillard R, Riondel A, Muller AF, Herrmann W, Baulieu EE. RU 486: a steroid with anti-glucocorticosteroid activity that only disinhibits the human pituitary–adrenal system at a specific time of day. Proc Natl Acad Sci USA 1984;81:3879–3882.
25. Brady LS, Whitfield HJ Jr, Fox RJ, Gold PW, Herkenham M. Long-term antidepressant administration alters corticotropin-releasing hormone, tyrosine hydroxylase, and mineralocorticoid receptor gene expression in rat brain. Therapeutic implications. J Clin Invest 1991;87, 831–837.
26. Peiffer A, Veilleux S, Barden N. Antidepressant and other centrally acting drugs regulate glucocorticoid receptor messenger RNA levels in rat brain. Psychoneuroendocrinology 1991;16:505–515.
27. Vale W, Spiess J, Rivier C, Rivier J. Characterization of a 41-residue ovine hypothalamic peptide that stimulates secretion of corticotropin and beta-endorphin. Science 1981;213:1394–1397.
28. De Bold CR, Sheldon WR, DeCherney GS, Jackson RV, Alexander AN, Vale W, Rivier J, Orth DN. Arginine vasopressin potentiates adrenocorticotropin release induced by ovine corticotropin-releasing factor. J Clin Invest 1984;73:533–538.
29. Schurmeyer TH, Averginos PC, Gold PW, Gallucci WT, Tomai TP, Cutler GB Jr, Loriaux DL, Chrousos GP. Human corticotropin-releasing factor in man: pharmacokinetic properties and dose response of plasma adrenocorticotropin and cortisol secretion. J Clin Endocrinol Metab 1984;59:1103–1108.
30. Schulte HM, Chrousos GP, Oldfield EH, Gold PW, Cutler GB, Loriaux DL. Ovine corticotropin-releasing factor administration in normal men. Pituitary and adrenal responses in the morning and evening. Horm Res 1985;21:69–74.
31. Orth DN. Corticotropin-releasing hormone in humans. Endocr Rev 1992;13:164–191.
32. Oldfield EH, Doppman JI., Nieman LK, Chrousos GP, Miller DL, Katz DA, Cutler GB Jr, Loriaux DL. Petrosal sinus sampling with and without corticotropin releasing hormone for the differential diagnosis of Cushing's syndrome. N Engl J Med 1991;325:897–905.
33. Schulte HM, Chrousos GP, Avgerinos P, Oldfield EH, Gold PW, Cutler GB Jr, Loriaux DL. The corticotropin releasing hormone stimulation test: a possible aid in the evaluation of patients with adrenal insufficiency. J Clin Endocrinol Metab 1984;58:1064–1067.
34. Saper CB, Lowey AD, Swanson LW, Cowan WM. Direct hypothalamic-autonomic connections. Brain Res 1976;117:305–312.
35. Valentino RJ, Foote SL. Corticotropin releasing hormone increases tonic but not sensory-evoked activity of noradrenergic locus ceruleus neurons in unanesthetized rats. J Neurosci 1988;8:1016–1025.
36. Kalin NH. Behavioural effects of ovine corticotropin-releasing factor administered to rhesus monkeys. Fed Proc 1985;44:249–253.
37. Koob GF, Bloom FE. Corticotropin-releasing factor and behavior. Fed Proc 1991;44:259–263.
38. Rivier C, Rivier J, Vale W. Stress-induced inhibition of reproductive function: role of endogenous corticotropin releasing factor. Science 1986;231:607–609.
39. Sutton RE, Koob GF, Le Moal M, Rivier J, Vale W. Corticotropin releasing factor produces behavioural activation in rats. Nature 1982;297:331–333.
40. Aguilera G, Millan MA, Hauger RL, Catt KJ. Corticotropin-releasing factor receptors: distribution and regulation in brain and peripheral tissues. Ann NY Acad Sci 1987;512:48–66.
41. Menzaghi F, Rassnick S, Heinrichs S, Baldwin H, Pich EM, Weiss F, Koob GF. The role of corticotropin-releasing factor in the anxiogenic effects of ethanol withdrawal. Ann NY Acad Sci 1996;176–184.
42. Behan DP, Linton EA, Lowry PJ. Isolation of the human plasma corticotropin-releasing factor-binding protein. J Endocrinol 1989;122:23–31.
43. Krishnan KRR, Doraiswamy PM, Lurie SN, Figiel GS, Husain MM, Boyko OB, Ellinwood EH Jr., Nemeroff CB. Pituitary size in depression. J Clin Endocrinol Metab 1991;72:256–259.
44. Amsterdam J, Marinelli D, Arger P, Winokur A. Assessment of adrenal gland volume by computed tomography in depressed patients and healthy volunteers: a pilot study. Psychiatry Res 1987;21:189–197.
45. Gold PW, Goodwin FK, Chrousos GP. Clinical and biochemical manifestations of depression. Relation to neurobiology of stress. N Engl J Med 1988;319:348–353, 413–420.
46. Nemeroff CB, Owens MJ, Bissette G, Audoin AC, Stanley M. Reduced corticotropin releasing factor binding sites in the frontal cortex of suicide victims. Arch Gen Psychiatry 1988;45:577–579.

47. Raadsheer FC, Hoogendijk WJG, Stam FC, Tilders FJH, Swaab DF. Increased numbers of corticotropin-releasing hormone expressing neurons in the hypothalamic paraventricular nucleus of depressed patients. Neuroendocrinology 1994;60:436–444.
47a. Wehr TA, Wirz-Justice A. Circadian rhythm mechanisms in affective illness and in anti-depressant drug action. Pharmacopsychiatry 1982;15:31–39.
48. De Bellis MD, Chrousos GP, Dorn LD, Burke L, Helmers K, Kling MA, Tricket PK, Rutnam FW. Hypothalamic–pituitary–adrenal axis dysregulation in sexually abused girls. J Clin Endocrinol Metab 1994;78:249–255.
49. Joseph-Vanderpool JR, Rosenthal NE, Chrousos GP, Wehr TA, Skwerer R, Kasper S, Gold PW. Evidence for hypothalamic CRH deficiency in patients with seasonal affective disorder. J Clin Endocrinol Metab 1991;72:1382–1386.
50. Demitrack MA, Dale JK, Straus SE, Laue L, Listwak SJ, Kruesi MJ, Chrousos GP, Gold PW. Evidence of impaired activation of the hypothalamic–pituitary–adrenal axis in patients with chronic fatigue syndrome. J Clin Endocrinol Metab 1991;73:1224–1234.
51. Griep EN, Boerdma JW, de Kloet ER. Altered reactivity of the hypothalamic–pituitary–adrenal axis in the primary fibromyalgia syndrome. J Rheumatol 1993;20:469–474.
52. Crofford LJ, Pillemer SR, Kalogeras KT, Cash JM, Michelson D, Kling MA, Sternberg EM, Gold PW, Chrousos GP, Wilder RL. Hypothalamic–pituitary–adrenal axis perturbation in patients with fibromyalgia. Arthritis Rheum 1994;37:1583–92.
53. Chrousos GP, Gold PW. The concepts of stress snd stress system disorders. Overview of physical and behavioral homeostasis. J Am Med Assoc 1992;267:1244–1252.
54. Magiakou MA, Mastorakos G, Rabin D, Dubbert B, Gold PW, Chrousos GP. Hypothalamic corticotropin releasing hormone suppression during the postpartum period: Implications for the increase of psychiatric manifestations in this period. J Clin Endocrinol Metab 1996;81:1912–1917.
55. Waltman C, McCaul ME, Wand GS. Adrenocorticotropin responses following administration of ethanol and ovine corticotropin-releasing hormone in the sons of alcoholics and control subjects. Alcohol Clin Exp Res 1994;18:826–830.
56. Rivier C, Imaki T, Vale W. Prolonged response to alcohol: effect on CRF mRNA levels, and CRF- and stress-induced ACTH secretion in the rat. Brain Res 1990;520:1–5.
57. Wand GS, Dobs AS. Alterations in the hypothalamic-pituitary-adrenal axis in actively drinking alcoholics. J Clin Endocrinol Metab 1991;72:1290–1295.
58. Waltman C, Blevins LS, Boyd G, Wand GS. The effects of mild ethanol intoxication on the hypothalamic–pituitary–adrenal axis in nonalcoholic men. J Clin Endocrinol Metab 1993;77:518–522.
59. Sternberg EM, Chrousos GP, Wilder RL, Gold PW. The stress response and the regulation of inflammatory disease: NIH combined clinical staff conference. Ann Intern Med 1992;117:854–866.
59a. Ur E, Grossman A. Corticotropin-releasing hormone in health and disease: an update. Acta Endocrinol 1992;127:193–199.
60. Makino S, Gold PW, Schulkin J. Effects of corticosterone on CRH mRNA and content in the bed nucleus of the stria terminalis; comparison with the effects in the central nucleus of the amygdala and the paraventricular nucleus of the hypothalamus. Brain Res 1994;657:141–149.
61. Shibasaki T, Imaki T, Hotta M, Ling N, Demura H. Psychological stress increases arousal without significant increase in adrenocorticotropin and catecholamine secretion. Brain Res 1993;618:71–75.
62. Karalis K, Sano H, Redwine J. Autocrine or paracrine inflammatory actions of corticotropin-releasing hormone in vivo. Science 1991;254:421–423.
63. Makrigiannakis A, Margioris AN, Le Goascogne C, Zoumakis E, Nikas G, Stournaras C, Psychoyos A, Gravanis A. Corticotropin-releasing hormone (CRH) is expressed at the implantation sites of early pregnant rat uterus. Life Sci 1995;57:1869–1875.
64. Geracioti TD Jr., Orth DN, Ekhator NN, Blumenkopf B, Loosen PT. Serial cerebrospinal fluid corticotropin-releasing hormone concentrations in healthy and depressed humans. J Clin Endocrinol Metab 1992;74:1325–1330.
65. Chang CP, Pearse R 2d, O'Connell S, Rosenfeld MG. Identification of a seven transmembrane helix receptor for corticotropin-releasing factor and sauvagine in mammalian brain. Neuron 1993;11:1187–1195.
66. Chen R, Lewis KA, Perrin MH, Vale WW. Expression cloning of a human corticotropin-releasing-factor receptor. Proc Natl Acad Sci USA 1993;90:8967–8971.

67. Perrin MH, Donaldson CJ, Chen R, Lewis KA, Vale WW. Cloning and functional expression of a rat brain corticotropin releasing factor (CRF) receptor. Endocrinology 1993;133:3058–3061.
68. Vita N, Laurent P, Lefort S, Chalou P, Lelias JM, Kaghad M, LeFur G, Caput D, Ferrara P. Primary structure and functional expression of mouse pituitary and human brain corticotrophin releasing factor receptors. FEBS Lett 1993;335:1–5.
69. Potter E, Sutton S, Donaldson C, Chen R, Perrin M, Lewis K, Sawchenko PE, Vale W. Distribution of corticotropin-releasing factor receptor mRNA expression in the rat brain and pituitary. Proc Natl Acad Sci USA 1994;91:8777–8781.
70. Lovenberg TW, Chalmers DT, Liu C, De Souza EB. CRF (2 alpha) and CRF (2 beta) receptor mRNAs are differentially distributed between the rat CNS and peripheral tissues. Endocrinology 1995;136:3351–3355.
71. Perrin M, Donaldson C, Chen R, Blount A, Berggren T, Bilezikjian L, Sawchenko P, Vale W. Identification of a second corticotropin-releasing factor receptor gene and characterization of a cDNA expressed in heart. Proc Natl Acad Sci USA 1995;92:2969–2973.
72. Vaughan J, Donaldson C, Bittencourt J, Perrin MH, Lewis K, Sutton S, Chan R, Turnbull AV, Lovejoy D, Rivier C. Urocortin, a mammalian neuropeptide related to fish urotensin I and to corticotropin-releasing factor. Nature 1995;378:287–292.
73. Muglia L, Jacobson L, Dikkes P, Majzoub J. Corticotropin-releasing hormone deficiency reveals major fetal but not adult glucocorticoid need. Nature 1995;373:427–432.
74. Liaw CW, Lovenberg TW, Barry G, Oltersdorf T, Grigoriadis DE, De Souza EB. Cloning and characterization of the human corticotropin releasing factor (CRF)$_2$ receptor complementary deoxyribonucleic acid. Endocrinology 1996;137:72–77.
75. Donaldson CJ, Sutton SW, Perrin MH, Corrigan AZ, Lewis KA, Rivier JE, Vaughan JM, Vale WW. Cloning and characterization of human urocortin. Endocrinology 1996;137:2167–2170.
76. Behan DP, Heinrichs SC, Troncosa JC, Liu KJ, Kawas CH, Ling N, DeSouza EB. Displacement of corticotropin-releasing factor from its binding protein as a possible treatment for Alzheimers disease. Nature 1995;378:284–287.
77. Pardridge WM. Receptor-mediated peptide transport through the blood–brain barrier. Endocr Rev 1986;7:314–330.
78. Sawchenko PE, Swanson LW. The organization of noradrenergic pathways from the brainstem to the paraventricular and supraoptic nuclei in the rat. Brain Res Rev 1982;4:275–325.
79. Whitnall MH. Stress selectively activates the vasopressin-containing subset of corticotropin-releasing hormone neurons. Neuroendocrinology 1989;50:702–707.
80. Holmes MC, Antoni FA, Aguilera G, Catt KJ. Magnocellular axons in passage through the the median eminence release vasopressin. Nature 1986;319:326–329.
81. Hashimoto K, Suemaru S, Takao T, Sugawara M, Makino S, Ota Z. Corticotropin-releasing hormone and pituitary-adrenocortical responses in chronically stressed rats. Regul Pept 1988;23:117–126.
82. Harbuz MS, Lightman SL. Stress and the hypothalamo–pituitary–adrenal axis: acute, chronic and immunological activation. J Endocrinol 1992;134:327–339.
83. Spencer RL, McEwen BS. Adaptation of the hypothalamo-pituitary-adrenal axis to chronic ethanol stress. Neuroendocrinology 1990;52:481–489.
84. Scribner KA, Walker C, Cascio CS, Dallman MF. Chronic streptozotocin diabetes in rats facilitates the acute stress response without altering pituitary or adrenal responsiveness to secretagogues. Endocrinology 1991;129:99–108.
85. Plotsky PM. Pathways to the secretion of adrenocorticotropin: a view from the portal. J Neuroendocrinol 1991;3:1–9.
86. Canny BJ, Funder JW, Clarke IJ. Glucocorticoids regulate ovine hypophysial portal levels of corticotropin-releasing factor and arginine vasopressin in a stress specific manner. Endocrinology 1989;125:2532–2539.
87. Engler D, Pham T, Fullerton MJ, Ooi G, Funder JW, Clarke IJ. Studies of the secretion of corticotropin-releasing factor and arginine vasopressin into the hypophysial-portal circulation of the conscious sheep. I. Effect of an audiovisual stimulus and insulin-induced hypoglycemia. Neuroendocrinology 1989;49:367–381.
88. Caraty A, Grino M, Locatelli A, Guillaume V, Boudouresque F, Coute-Devolx B, Oliver C. Insulin-induced hypoglycemia stimulates corticotropin-releasing factor and arginine vasopressin secretion into hypophysial portal blood of conscious rams. J Clin Invest 1990;85:1716–1721.

89. Jia LG, Canny BJ, Orth DN, Leong DA. Distinct classes of corticotropes mediate corticotropin-releasing hormone- and arginine vasopressin-stimulated adrenocorticotropin release. Endocrinology 1991;128:197–203.
90. Aguilera G, Harwood JP, Wilson JX, Morell J, Brown JH, Catt KJ. Mechanisms of action of corticotropin-releasing factor and other regulators of corticotropin release in rat pituitary cells. J Biol Chem 1983;258:8039–8045.
91. Al-Damluji S, Perry L, Tomlin S, Bouloux P, Grossman A, Rees LH, Besser GM. Alpha adrenergic stimulation of corticotropin secretion by a specific central mechanism in man. Neuroendocrinology 1987;45:68–76.
92. Torpy DJ, Grice JE, Hockings GI, Walters MM, Crosbie GV, Jackson RV. Alprazolam blocks the naloxone-stimulated hypothalamo-pituitary-adrenal axis in man. J Clin Endocrinol Metab 1993;76:388–391.
93. Delitala G, Grossman A, Besser GM. Differential effects of opiate peptides and alkaloids on anterior pituitary hormone secretion. Neuroendocrinology 1983;37:275–279.
94. Larsen PJ, Jessop D, Patel H, Lightman SL, Chowdrey HS. Substance P inhibits the release of anterior pituitary adrenocorticotrophin via a central mechanism involving corticotrophin-releasing factor-containing neurons in the hypothalamic paraventricular nucleus. J Neuroendocrinol 1993;5:99–105.
95. Al-Damluji S, Rees LH. The neuroendocrine control of corticotropin secretion in normal humans and in Cushing's disease. In: Collu R, Brown GM, Van Loon GR, eds. Clinical Neuroendocrinology. Blackwell Oxford, 1988, pp.251–286.
96. Liposits Z, Phelix C, Paull WK. Electron microscopic analysis of tyrosine hydroxylase, dopamine-β-hydroxylase and phenylethanolamine-N-methyltransferase immunoreactive innervation of the hypothalamic paraventricular nucleus in the rat. Histochemistry 1986;84:105–120.
97. Cummings S, Elde R, Ells J, Lindall A. Corticotropin-releasing factor immunoreactivity is widely distributed within the central nervous system of the rat: an immunohistochemical study. J Neurosci 1983;3:1355–1368.
98. Charney DS, Heninger GR. Noradrenergic function and the mechanism of antianxiety treatment: I. The effect of long term alprazolam treatment. Arch Gen Psychiatry 1985;42:458–467.
99. Kaye H, Berrittini W, Gwirtsman H, George DT. Altered cerebrospinal fluid neuropeptide Y and peptide YY immunoreactivity in anorexia and bulimia nervosa. Arch Gen Psych 1990;47:548–556.
100. Engler D, Liu J, Clarke IJ, Funder JW. Corticotropin-release inhibitory factor. Evidence for dual stimulatory and inhibitory hypothalamic regulation over adrenocorticotropin secretion and biosynthesis. Trends Endocrinol Metab 1994;5:272–283.
101. Pacak K, McCarty R, Palkovits M, Cizza G, Kopin IJ, Goldstein DS, Chrousos GP. Decreased central and peripheral catecholaminergic activation in obese zucker rats. Endocrinology 1995;136:4360–4367.
102. Paul WE, Seder RA. Lymphocyte responses and cytokines. Cell 1994;76:241–251.
103. Mosmann TR, Sad S. The expanding universe of T-cell subsets:Th1, Th2 and more. Immunol Today 1996;17:138–146.
104. Elenkov IJ, Papanicolaou DA, Wilder RL, Chrousos GP. Effects of glucocorticoids and catecholamines on human interleukin-12 and interleukin-10 production: Implications for the effect of stress on immunity and the Th1/Th2 balance. Proc Am Assoc Physicians, 1996;108:374–381.
105. Lerner BH. Can stress cause disease? Revisiting the tuberculosis research of Thomas Holmes 1949–1961. Ann Intern Med 1996;124:673–680.
106. Cohen S, Tyrrell DA, Smith AP. Psychological stress and the common cold. N Engl J Med 1991;325:606–612.
107. Wilder RL. Neuroendocrine-immune system interactions and autoimmunity. Ann Rev Immunol 1995;13:307–338.
108. Kowaki G, Gottschall PE, Somogyvari-Vigh A, Tatsuno I, Yatohgo T, Arimura A. Rapid increase in plasma IL-6 after hemorrhage, and posthemorrhage reduction of the IL-6 response to LPS in conscious rats: interrelations with plasma corticosterone levels. Neuroimmunomodulation 1994; 1:127–134.
109. van Gool J, van Vugt H, Helle M, Aarden LA. The relation among stress, adrenaline, interleukin 6 and acute phase proteins in the rat. Clin Immunol Immunopathol 1990;57:200–210.
110. Hirano T, Akira S, Taga T, Kishimoto T. Biological and clinical aspects of interleukin 6. Immunol Today 1990;11:443–449.

111. Mastorakos G, Chrousos GP, Weber J. Recombinant interleukin-6 activates the hypothalamic–pituitary–adrenal axis in humans. J Clin Endocrinol Metab 1993;77:1690–1694.
112. Mastorakos G, Weber JS, Magiakou MA, Gunn H, Chrousos GP. Hypothalamic–pituitary–adrenal axis activation and stimulation of vasopressin secretion by recombinant interleukin-6 in humans: potential implications for the syndrome of inappropriate vasopressin secretion. J Clin Endocrinol Metab 1994;79:934–939.
113. Bernton EW, Beach LE, Holaday JW, Smallridge RC, Fein HG. Release of multiple hormones by a direct effect of interleukin-1 on pituitary cells. Science 1987;238:519–521.
114. Fukata J, Usui T, Naitoh Y, Nakai Y, Imura H. Effects of recombinant interleukin-1α, 1β, -2 and -6 on ACTH synthesis and release in the mouse pituitary tumour cell line AtT-20. J Endocrinol 1988;122:33–39.
115. Salas MA, Evans SW, Levell MJ, Whicker JT. Interleukin-6 and ACTH act synergistically to stimulate the release of corticosterone from adrenal gland cells. Clin Exp Immunol 1990;79:470–473.
116. Solomon S. Corticostatins. Trends Endocrinol Metab 1993;4:260–264.
117. Culman J, Tschope C, Jost N, Itoi K, Unger T. Substance P and neurokinin A induced desensitization to cardiovascular and behavioral effects: evidence for the involvement of different tachykinin receptors. Brain Res 1993;625:75–83.
118. Jessop DS, Chowdrey HS, Larsen PJ, Lightman S. Substance P: mulitifunctional peptide in the hypothalamo–pituitary system? J Endocrinol 1992;132:331–337.
119. Besedovsky H, Sorkin E. Network of immune-neuroendocrine interactions. Clin Exp Immunol 1977;27:1–12.
120. Craddock CG. Corticosteroid-induced lymphopenia, immunosuppression and body defense. Ann Intern Med 1978;88:564–566.
121. Calogero AE, Sternberg EM, Bagdy G, Smith C, Bernardini R, Acsentijeych S, Wilder RL, Gold PW, Chrousos GP. Neurotransmitter-induced hypothalamic–pituitary adrenal axis responsiveness is defective in inflammatory disease-susceptible Lewis rats: in vivo and in vitro studies suggesting globally defective hypothalamic secretion of corticotropin-releasing hormone. Neuroendocrinology 1992;55:600–608.
122. Patchev VK, Kalogeras KT, Zelazowski P, Wilder RL, Chrousos GP. Increased plasma concentrations, hypothalamic output, and in vivo release of arginine vasopressin in inflammatory disease-prone, hypothalamic corticotropin-releasing hormone-deficient Lewis rats. Endocrinology 1992;131:1453–1457.
123. Wick G, Hu Y, Schwarz S, Kroemer G. Immunoendocrine communication via the hypothalamo-pituitary-adrenal axis in autoimmune diseases. Endocr Rev 1993;14:539–563.
124. Neeck G, Federlin K, Graef V, Rusch D, Schmidt KL. Adrenal secretion of cortisol in patients with rheumatoid arthritis. J Rheumatol 1990;17:24–29.
125. Chikanza IC, Petrou P, Kingsley G, Chrousos G, Panayi GS. Defective hypothalamic response to immune and inflammatory stimuli in patients with rheumatoid arthritis. Arthritis Rheum 1992;35:1281–1288.
126. Crofford LJ, Sano H, Karalis K, Friedman TC, Epps HR, Remmers EF, Mathern P, Chrousos GP. Corticotropin-releasing hormone in synovial fluids and tissues of patients with rheumatoid arthritis and osteoarthritis. J Immunol 1993;151:1587–1596.
127. Sternberg EM, Glowa JR, Smith MA, Calogero AE, Listwak SJ, Aksentijevich S, Wilder RL, Chrousos GP. Corticotropin releasing hormone related behavioral and neuroendocrine responses to stress in Lewis and Fisher rats. Brain Res 1992;570:54–60.
128. Vamvakopoulos NC, Chrousos GP. Hormonal regulation of human corticotropin-releasing hormone gene expression: implications for the stress response and immune/inflammatory reaction. Endocr Rev 1994;15:409–420.
129. Haas DA, George SR. Gonadal regulation of corticotropin releasing factor in hypothalamus. Brain Res Bull 1988;20:361–367.
130. Bohler HC Jr, Zoeller RT, King JC, Rubin BS, Weber R, Merriam GR. Corticotropin releasing hormone mRNA is elevated in the afternoon of proestrus in the parvocellular paraventricular nuclei of the female rat. Mol Brain Res 1990;8:259–262.
131. Fredericksen SO, Ekman R, Gottfries CG, Widerlov E, Jonsson S. Reduced concentrations of galanin, arginine vasopressin, neuropeptide Y and peptide YY in the temporal cortex but not the hypothalamus of brains from schizophrenics. Acta Psychiatr Scand 1991;83:273–277.

132. Gallucci WT, Baum A, Laue L, Rabin DS, Chrousos GP, Gold PW, Kling MA. Sex differences in sensitivity of the hypothalamic–pituitary–adrenal axis. Health Psychol 1993;12:420–425.
133. Peiffer A, Barden N. Estrogen-induced decrease of glucocorticoid receptor messenger ribonucleic acid concentration in rat anterior pituitary gland. Mol Endocrinol 1987;1:435–440.
134. Turner BB. Sex difference in glucocorticoid binding in rat pituitary is estrogen dependent. Life Sci 1990;46:1399–1406.
135. Turner BB. Sex differences in the binding of type I and type II corticosteroid receptors in rat hippocampus. Brain Res 1992;581:229–136.
136. Crofford LJ, Sano H, Karalis K, Webster EL, Goldmuntz EA, Chrousos GP, Wilder RL. Local secretion of corticotropin-releasing hormone in the joints of Lewis rats with inflammatory arthritis. J Clin Invest 1992;90:2555–2564.
137. Karalis K, Crofford L, Wilder RL, Chrousos GP. Glucocorticoid and/or glucocorticoid antagonist effects in inflammatory disease-susceptible Lewis rats and inflammatory disease-resistant Fischer rats. Endocrinology 1995;136:3107–3112.
138. Mastorakos G, Bouzas EA, Silver PB, Sartani G, Friedman TC, Chan CC, Caspi CC, Chrousos GP. Immune corticotropin-releasing hormone is present in the eyes of and promotes experimental autoimmune uveoretinitis in rodents. Endocrinology 1995;136:4650–4658.
139. Scopa CD, Mastorakos G, Friedman TC, Melachrinou M, Merino MJ, Chrousos GP. Presence of immunoreactive corticotropin releasing hormone in thyroid lesions. Am J Pathol 1994;145:1159–1167.
140. Allen JB, Blatter D, Calandra GB, Wilder RL. Sex hormone effects on the severity of streptococcal wall-induced polyarthritis in the rat. Arthritis Rheum 1983;26:560–563.
141. Lightman SL. From stress to cognition. Nature 1995;378:233–234.
142. Gaskin JH, Kitay JI. Adrenocortical function in the hamster: sex differences and effects of gonadal hormones. Endocrinology 1970;87:779–786.
143. Handa RJ, Burgess LH, Kerr JE, O'Keefe JA. Gonadal steroid hormone receptors and sex differences in the hypothalamo–pituitary–adrenal axis. Horm Behav 1994;28:464–476.
144. Ferin M, Van Vugt DA, Wardlaw SL. The hypothalamic control of the menstrual cycle and the role of endogenous opioid peptides. Rec Prog Horm Res 1984;40:441–485.
145. Shivers BD, Harlan RE, Morrell JI, Pfaff DW. Absence of estradiol concentration in cell nuclei of LHRH-immunoreactive neurons. Nature 1983;304:345–347.
145a. Jacobson JD, Nisula BC, Steinberg AD. Modulation of the expression of murine lupus by gonadotropin-releasing hormone analogs. Endocrinology 1994;134:2516–2523.
146. Cid MC, Kleinman HK, Grant DS, Schnaper HW, Fauci AS, Hoffman GS. Estradiol enhances leukocyte binding to tumor necrosis factor (TNF)-stimulated endothelial cells via an increase in TNF-induced adhesion molecules E-selectin, intercellular adhesion molecule type 1, and vascular cell adhesion molecule type 1. J Clin Invest 1994;93:17–25.
147. Stein B, Yang MX. Repression of the interleukin-6 promoter by estrogen receptor is mediated by NF-kappa B and C/EBP beta. Mol Cell Biol 1995;15:4971–4979.
148. Reichlin S. Neuroendocrinology. In: Wilson JD, Foster DW, eds. Williams Textbook of Endocrinology. 8th ed. Saunders, Philadelphia, 1992, pp. 135–219.
149. Redei E, Hilderbrand H, Aird F. Corticotropin release-inhibiting factor is preprothyrotropin-releasing hormone-(178–199). Endocrinology 1995;136:3557–3563.
150. Kakucska I, Yanping Q, Lechan RM. Changes in adrenal status affect hypothalamic thyrotropin-releasing hormone gene expression in parallel with corticotropin-releasing hormone. Endocrinology 1995;136:2795–2802.
151. Lee SL, Stewart K, Goodman RH. Structure of the gene encoding thyrotropin releasing hormone. J Biol Chem 1988;263:16,604–16,609.
152. Blalock JE. A molecular basis for bidirectional communication between the immune and neuroendocrine systems. Physiol Rev 1989;69:1–32.
153. Wade CE, Lindberg JS, Cockrell Jl, Lamiell M, Hunt MM, Ducey J, Jurney TH. Upon-admission adrenal steroidogenesis is adapted to the degree of illness in intensive care unit patients. J Clin Endocrinol Metab 1988;67:223–227.
154. Reincke M, Lehmann R, Karl M, Magiakou A, Chrousos GP, Allolio B. Severe illness. Neuroendocrinology. Ann NY Acad Sci 1996;771:556–569.
155. Reincke MM, Magiakou MA, Wurth G, Winkelmann W, Chrousos GP, Allolio B. Activation of the

hypothalamic-pituitary-adrenal axis in patients with critical illness: role of TNF-alpha, IL-1β and IL-6. Exp Clin Endocrinol 1993;101(Suppl.1):89.
156. Bilezikjian VM, Blount AL, Vale WW. The cellular actions of vasopressin in corticotrophs of the anterior pituitary: Resistance to glucocorticoid actions. Mol Endocrinol 1987;1:451–458.
157. Michelson D, Stone L, Galliven E, Magiakou MA, Chrousos GP, Sternberg EM, Gold PW. Multiple sclerosis is associated with alterations in hypothalamic–pituitary–adrenal function. J Clin Endocrinol Metab 1994;79:848–853.
158. Cronin L, Cook DJ, Carlet J, Heyland DK, King D, Math B, Lansang MAD, Fisher CJ Jr. Corticosteroid treatment for sepsis: A critical appraisal and meta-analysis of the literature. Crit Care Med 1995;23:1430–1439.
159. Kidess A, Caplan R, Reynertson R, Wickus G, Goodnough D. Transient corticotropin deficiency in critical illness. Mayo Clin Proc 1993;68:435–441.
160. Merry W, Caplan R, Wickus G, Reynertson R, Kisken W, Cogbill T, Landercasper J. Postoperative acute adrenal failure caused by transient corticotropin deficiency. Surgery 1994;116:1095–1100.
161. Almawi WY, Lipman ML, Stevens AC, Zanker B, Hadro ET, Strom BT. Abrogation of glucocorticosteroid-mediated inhibition of T cell proliferation by the synergistic action of Il-1, Il-6, and IFN-γ. J Immunol 1991;146:3523–3527.
162. Kam JC, Szefler SJ, Surs W, Sher ER, Leung DYM. Combination IL-2 and IL-4 reduces glucocorticoid receptor binding affinity and T cell response to glucocorticoids. J Immunol 1993;151:3460–3466.
163. Norbiato G, Bevilacqua M, Vago T, Baldi G, Chebat E, Bertora P, Moroni M, Galli M, Oldenburg M. Cortisol resistance in acquired immunodeficiency syndrome. J Clin Endocrinol Metab 1992;74:608–613.

2 Developmental Considerations
The Fetal and Neonatal Endocrine Response to Stress

C. Richard Parker, Jr., PhD

CONTENTS

   INTRODUCTION
   HYPOTHALAMIC–PITUITARY AXIS DEVELOPMENT
   ADRENAL CORTEX
   ADRENAL MEDULLA
   THYROID
   REFERENCES

INTRODUCTION

The morphologic and physiologic bases for an endocrine response to critical illnesses, which is an important adaptive mechanism for homeostatic balance and recovery during postnatal life, are established during fetal development and in many instances become competent prior to birth. This chapter will explore the structural and functional development of several key elements of the endocrine system during intrauterine life and in infancy. Although clearly of importance in homeostasis and response to illness, the endocrine pancreas, parathyroid, and gastrointestinal hormone systems will not be addressed herein. Additionally, development and regulation of the gonads, which are adversely impacted by many illnesses, will not be discussed since their responses do not appear to be of critical importance to survival in serious illnesses. Rather, emphasis will be placed on the development of hypothalamic endocrine control, the anterior and posterior pituitary, adrenal cortex, adrenal medulla, and thyroid.

HYPOTHALAMIC–PITUITARY AXIS DEVELOPMENT

Morphologic Maturation of the Hypothalamus, Anterior Pituitary, and Posterior Pituitary

The hypothalamus serves as the principal site of integration of peripheral and central signals that control function of the endocrine system. Hypothalamic control of endocrine tissues is exerted via control of the anterior pituitary gland (the pars distalis), and is achieved by means of neuropeptides and catecholamines (chiefly dopamine) that

From *Contemporary Endocrinology: Endocrinology of Critical Disease*
Edited by K. P. Ober   Humana Press Inc., Totowa, NJ

stimulate or inhibit synthesis and secretion of pituitary hormones. The hypothalamus also is the site of neural elements having cell bodies in the supraoptic and paraventricular nuclei, and axons that terminate in the anterior pituitary (pars nervosa). The embryonic development of the hypothalamus, anterior pituitary, and posterior pituitary, as detailed by others (1–3), is briefly described below. In the human, the diencephalon and the telencephalon arise from the prosencephalon during the fifth developmental week. The hypothalamus arises by proliferation of neuroblasts in the ventral diencephalon and forms on either side of the third ventricle. By the seventh week of development, the infundibulum (the precursor of the hypothalamic–pituitary stalk) can be readily recognized and the posterior pituitary, also derived from neural ectoderm, is formed soon thereafter. The anterior pituitary is classically considered to arise from the oral ectoderm by means of a dorsally formed diverticulum (Rathke's pouch) during the fourth week. By the fifth week, Rathke's pouch begins to become separated from the roof of the oral cavity and is in contact with the infundibulum. By the seventh week of development, the floor of the sella turcica is formed and completely separates the pituitary from the oral cavity. The hypothalamic–pituitary vascular system is in place near the end of the first trimester of gestation. Hypothalamic nuclei and fiber tracts are discernible soon thereafter. The vascular connections among the hypothalamus, anterior pituitary, and posterior pituitary provide for interesting functional interrelationships (4). A portal system connecting a capillary bed in the median eminence region of the hypothalamus via long vessels to a capillary bed in the anterior pituitary provides one route of hypothalamic communication with the anterior pituitary. Another portal system, composed of short vessels, connects capillary beds in the posterior pituitary, and thus hypothalamic nerve terminals ending there, with those in the anterior pituitary.

Biochemical Development of Hypothalamic and Posterior Pituitary Neuropeptides

The development of the chemical signals in the hypothalamus that regulate anterior pituitary function occurs by the end of the first trimester. Substantial quantities of the thyrotropin-releasing hormone (TRH): pyroglutamyl-histidyl-proline amide (5) have been found in the human fetal hypothalamus beginning as early as 10–11 wk and even earlier in extrahypothalamic brain tissue (3,6). TRH is synthesized in the hypothalamus by means of posttranslational processing of a large precursor polypeptide that contains several copies of the tripeptide sequence (7). In the human fetus, as in the adult, TRH is present in highest concentrations in the hypothalamus, but also is found in other regions of the brain (6,8). Within the hypothalamus, the median eminence has the highest concentrations of TRH, whereas lesser amounts are found in the arcuate, ventromedial, periventricular, and dorsomedial nuclei. Over the interval of 10–19 wk of gestation, we found that TRH in homogenates of fetal hypothalamus was present mainly in particulate fractions, with the synaptosomal fraction (isolated nerve terminals) having the highest concentration (9), suggesting that the hypothalamic neuronal elements are competent to release TRH upon stimulation during this developmental period.

Corticotropin-releasing hormone (CRH), the neuropeptide that has been determined to regulate pituitary synthesis and secretion of proopiomelanocortin (10), has been detected in fibers of the rostral median eminence at the 16th gestational week, but not in hypothalami from fetuses at 11–15 wk (11). Immunopositive perikarya were first noted at 19 wk of gestation, with fibers terminating near the blood vessels of the pituitary portal system. A few CRH-positive neurons were found also to immunostain with anti-vasopressin antisera; no costaining in CRH neural elements was observed with anti-methionine enkephalin antisera. In newborn infants, there was no obvious correlation between their ages and the amount of CRH in the median eminence, whereas there was much more striking immunostaining intensity in the hypothalami of older infants and adults. The production of CRH in the hypothalamus appears to be negatively regulated by glucocorticoid feedback mechanisms.

Of potential relevance to both the maternal and fetal compartments is an extrahypothalamic source of CRH, namely the placenta *(12)*. The production of placental CRH is likely to be determined largely by placental mass, although placental CRH secretion also appears to be modulated by other factors as well. Interestingly, placental CRH production appears to be stimulated rather than inhibited by glucocorticoids *(13)*. Several investigators have reported the presence of substantial concentrations of CRH in maternal plasma, which rise over the course of pregnancy *(14,15)*. Fetal blood also contains much lower, but clearly measurable, quantities of CRH *(14)*. Increased concentrations in maternal and fetal plasma have been noted in circumstances considered to be associated with stress to the developing fetus *(16–18)*. The significance of increased levels of CRH in maternal or fetal blood is unclear. Interestingly, however, we have found that CRH stimulates cortisol production by cultured human fetal adrenal cells *(19)*, and many stressed infants have been found to have increased umbilical cord plasma levels of cortisol at delivery *(20)*.

Also of relevance to a consideration of hypothalamic control of the pituitary and posterior pituitary function in stress is the development of the vasopressin secretory apparatus in the developing human. Arginine vasopressin (AVP) is one of several nonapeptides found in the posterior pituitary of various species that derive from nuclei originating in the hypothalamus. AVP, like oxytocin, is synthesized from a large precursor, and during transport down axons from the hypothalamus to the posterior pituitary, the precursor is processed in secretory granules to yield AVP and its associated carrier protein—human neurophysin-I. AVP is produced in both parvocellular and magnocellular neurons. AVP-containing parvocellular neurons project to the median eminence where they release their neuropeptides into the pituitary portal blood. The major site of AVP production is in magnocellular neurons in the supraoptic and paraventricular nuclei; those from the supraoptic nucleus project to the posterior pituitary, and are responsive to osmotic and pressure fluctuations *(21)*. AVP is detectable in the fetal hypothalamus and pituitary by 11–12 wk of gestation, and its concentration increases strikingly thereafter through 28 wk in both tissues *(22)*. Both AVP and its neurophysin are detectable 3–4 wk prior to oxytocin in both tissues. Based on studies in experimental animals, it seems likely that AVP derived from parvocellular neurons participates in the regulation of pituitary ACTH secretion by means of modulating CRH effects on POMC-producing cells in the anterior pituitary *(23)*. Interestingly, a significant proportion of CRH-containing neurons in the parvocellular region coexpress AVP *(24)*. It has been noted that AVP potentiates ACTH secretion by cultured human fetal pituitary cells in response to CRH *(25)*.

Development of Anterior Pituitary Hormones

Adrenocorticotropin (ACTH), which is the key regulator of adrenal steroidogenesis, is synthesized as part of a larger polypeptide hormone, proopiomelanocortin (POMC)

(26,27). By means of immunohistochemistry *(28,29)*, it has been determined that ACTH is detectable in the anterior lamina of Rathke's pouch at 8 wk of development and in the anterior pituitary thereafter. Immunopositive cells also were Periodic acid Schiff (PAS) positive; other non-ACTH-containing pituicytes also were PAS-positive, obviating this characteristic as useful for identification of ACTH-containing cells. Whereas ACTH interfered with immunostaining, pretreatment of the antiserum with other POMC-derived peptides did not. In a more recent, comprehensive study of the ontogeny of pituitary hormones, it was determined that as early as the eighth gestational week, ACTH-containing cells also were immunopositive for β-endorphin *(30)*. ACTH has been reported to be secreted by cultures of pituitary tissues as early as 5 wk of gestation *(31)*. The fetal pituitary has been demonstrated to be competent to secrete ACTH in response to CRH near the end of the first trimester of gestation by some investigators *(25,32)*, whereas others failed to observe responsiveness until after 20 wk of gestation *(33)*. AVP also was found to stimulate ACTH secretion from cultured and superfused fetal pituitary tissue *(25)*. In these studies, it was noted that glucocorticoid treatment of pituitary cells blunted the secretory response of corticotrophs to CRH, AVP, and cAMP. In anencephaly, it has been found that the pituitary does contain ACTH *(28,34)*. ACTH secretion from the anencephalic pituitary is extremely limited, though responsive to exogenous secretogogs, such as AVP *(34)*. The presence of ACTH in pituitaries of anencephalic fetuses and term infants is suggestive that the hypothalamus is not necessary for synthesis of POMC and its posttranslational processing. The low levels of ACTH found in the circulation of the anencephalic *(34)*, however, suggests that the hypothalamus is important for regulation of ACTH secretion during intrauterine development.

Thyrotropin-stimulating hormone (TSH), like the other glycoproteins—luteinizing hormone and follicle-stimulating hormone, is composed of an α- and a β-subunit. The α-subunit is common to all three of these hormones, whereas each has a unique β-subunit. Although immunostaining with antisera directed against the α-subunit has been found in the fetal pituitary as early as 9 wk, staining for the β-subunit of TSH has not been detected until about 12 wk of development *(29,30,35)*. Pituitary content of TSH rises steadily from 12 wk through the latter part of gestation; pituitary TSH concentration (relative to body weight) is highest between 12 and 17 wk *(36)*.

Secretion of ACTH, AVP, and TSH in the Fetus and Newborn

The gestational regulation of fetal pituitary ACTH secretion is not well characterized. The most comprehensive study *(37)* reported that immunoreactive ACTH levels in umbilical cord blood plasma were about twofold higher in 15 fetuses and newborns delivered at 12–34 wk of gestation than in infants delivered at 35–42 wk of gestation. The antiserum used in this study was specific for the midportion of the ACTH sequence. Among the infants delivered at term ($n = 376$), there were only slight differences in ACTH concentrations as a function of labor and delivery method. The umbilical cord plasma ACTH levels were about 70% of those in maternal plasma during labor, but were three- to fourfold higher than in normal adults. Interestingly, it was noted that ACTH levels in a group of infants sampled between 1 and 7 d after birth were only slightly lower that at delivery. On the other hand, as discussed later, the adrenal gland displays a significant degree of involution during this time. In a subsequent study employing another antiserum that was also most reactive against a midportion of the ACTH molecule, reasonably similar concentrations of umbilical cord plasma ACTH were found in a group of normal, vaginally delivered term infants *(38)*. In this study, however, it was found that infants delivered by cesarean section prior to the onset of labor had lower ACTH levels than the above infants. Also, infants who were found to be acidemic had higher ACTH levels than normal infants, regardless of delivery method. Other investigators who evaluated other POMC products, β-endorphin and β-lipotropin, also found evidence for increased fetal production in association with indices of hypoxia *(39)*. As had been noted for ACTH, umbilical cord concentrations of these peptides also were higher than in normal adults. Other investigators have found that ACTH levels in umbilical cord blood are higher in term infants delivered vaginally after an average of 13 h of labor than in infants delivered vaginally after only 6 h of labor *(40)*. The above examples all suggest that intrauterine stress in the peripartum period causes increased secretion of fetal pituitary POMC peptides. Further study is, however, necessary for a more complete understanding of the developmental pattern of fetal pituitary ACTH production. Based on prior studies, it is conceivable that only with extreme care in blood handling (use of peptidase inhibitors and rapid chilling and centrifugation) and possibly the use of an assay that utilizes antisera directed against both the N- and C-terminal peptide sequences of ACTH will it be possible to rationalize the paradoxical findings of decreasing immunoreactive ACTH levels in the fetus over the time period of substantial adrenal growth and steroid production (described later).

In healthy infants, plasma levels of ACTH and β-endorphin decline over the first few days of life *(41)*. On the other hand, there is evidence for enhanced pituitary secretion of POMC peptides in association with several neonatal stress situations *(42,43)*.

Maximal levels of TSH in fetal serum occur between 18 and 22 wk. The subsequent decline in circulating levels late in gestation probably is reflective of the maturation of the negative feedback regulation of TSH secretion *(44)*. TSH is usually low to undetectable in blood of anencephalics, but does respond to TRH administration *(34,45,46)*. Shortly after delivery, there is a dramatic, transient TSH surge in the neonate that is mediated by TRH and is considered to be in response to cooling of the neonate once exposed to the extrauterine environment *(47)*.

At the time of delivery, AVP levels are usually quite high in umbilical cord blood. It is assumed that the high levels are representative of a fetal stress response in association with labor *(48,49)*. As was seen with POMC products, there is an inverse correlation between umbilical cord plasma levels of AVP and pH *(50)*. Acidotic infants have clearly elevated AVP levels compared to similarly delivered, normal infants *(38,50)*. Also, nonacidemic infants delivered vaginally of women whose pregnancies were complicated by pre-eclampsia are increased over those of normal infants of normal women, but not as much as were those of acidemic infants *(51)*. In normal infants, plasma AVP levels decline rapidly after birth, and are similar to those of adults by 1–3 d of life *(49)*. Inappropriate secretion of AVP, i.e., that seen in the absence of the normal osmolar stimuli, is inferred in infants in whom there is hyponatremia and serum hypoosmolality in the absence of other endocrine/regulatory anomalies; such excessive secretion of AVP has been found in many circumstances of impaired respiration, including pneumothorax *(52,53)*, respiratory infections *(54)*, and neonatal asphyxia *(55)*, among others. It is not clear in such situations whether the stimulus for AVP is via intrathoracic baroreceptors or other mechanisms, such as pain. AVP secretion, as would be expected, also is increased in response to surgery in infancy *(56)*. In both term as well as preterm infants, the capacity for AVP secretion in response to the usual stimuli, though not necessarily fully matured, is normally adequate for homeostatic regulation.

ADRENAL CORTEX

Embryonic Development

The adrenal cortex in the adult is composed of three morphologic zones, which also display differing functional phenotypes: the outer cortical zone, the zona glomerulosa, is characterized by the production of aldosterone; the large middle cortical zone, the zona fasciculata, primarily produces 17 hydroxylated corticosteroids, such as cortisol; the inner zona reticularis produces large quantities of conjugated C_{19}-steroids, such as dehydroepiandrosterone sulfate (DS). The adrenal cortex during fetal life is different, being composed of two morphologic and functional zones, the thin outer neocortical zone (also termed the definitive or permanent zone) and the large inner fetal zone.

The early development of the human adrenal gland has been elegantly described based on studies of Carnegie staged embryos (57). The primitive adrenal cortex begins to form from cells derived from the coelomic epithelium during the fifth developmental week. At the Carnegie stages 15–16 (7–11 mm embryonic size; postconceptional days 33–37), one can see substantial migration of cells into the adrenal primordium. According to Crowder, a single progenitor cell gives rise to both the outer and inner cortical cells, whereas others give rise to the stroma and adrenal capsule. By the eighth developmental week, the two distinct cellular zones of the fetal cortex are present. The inner cortical cells are large eosinophilic cells that have pale nuclei, whereas the outer neocortex cells are smaller, and have darkly staining nuclei and scant cytoplasm (Fig. 1A).

Once formed, the principal site of cortical cell mitotic activity in the fetal adrenal appears to be in the subcapsular region, in which we also find the cell nuclei to immunostain prominently with antiproliferating cell nuclear antigen (PCNA) antisera (not shown). The fetal adrenal undergoes extensive growth and achieves a maximal size relative to total body size during the third to sixth gestational month. By term, 40 wk of gestation, the fetal adrenal is as large as that of adults and the cortex is composed roughly of 80% fetal zone cells. The stimulus to early fetal adrenal growth is unknown. It has been observed in a few instances that the adrenals of anencephalic fetuses, in whom the hypothalamus is usually absent, are within normal size limits at about 20 wk of gestation, but are clearly subnormal at term (58). Other investigators suggest, however, that the fetal zone tissue also is reduced in anencephalic's adrenals from 15–21 wk of gestation (59). The adrenal of the term anencephalic infant usually has a very thin fetal zone, but has a neocortical zone that is as broad as in normal infants. Owing, however, to its substantially reduced overall size, there are also fewer neocortical cells than in the normal adrenal. The impact of such reductions in cortical cells of the anencephalic adrenal has a predictable impact on adrenal steroid production in vivo. Based on these observations, it seems plausible that early development of the neocortex, but not the fetal zone, may be independent of the hypothalamic–pituitary axis, whereas steroid production, detailed below, requires an intact hypothalamus and anterior pituitary. One possible source of trophic stimuli for the fetal adrenal prior to midgestation may be the placenta, in which both CRH and POMC (the precursor of ACTH, β-endorphin, MSH, and β-lipotropin) production has been described (60,61). It also is possible that chorionic gonadotropin or luteinizing hormone (LH) plays a role in early fetal adrenal growth (62,63).

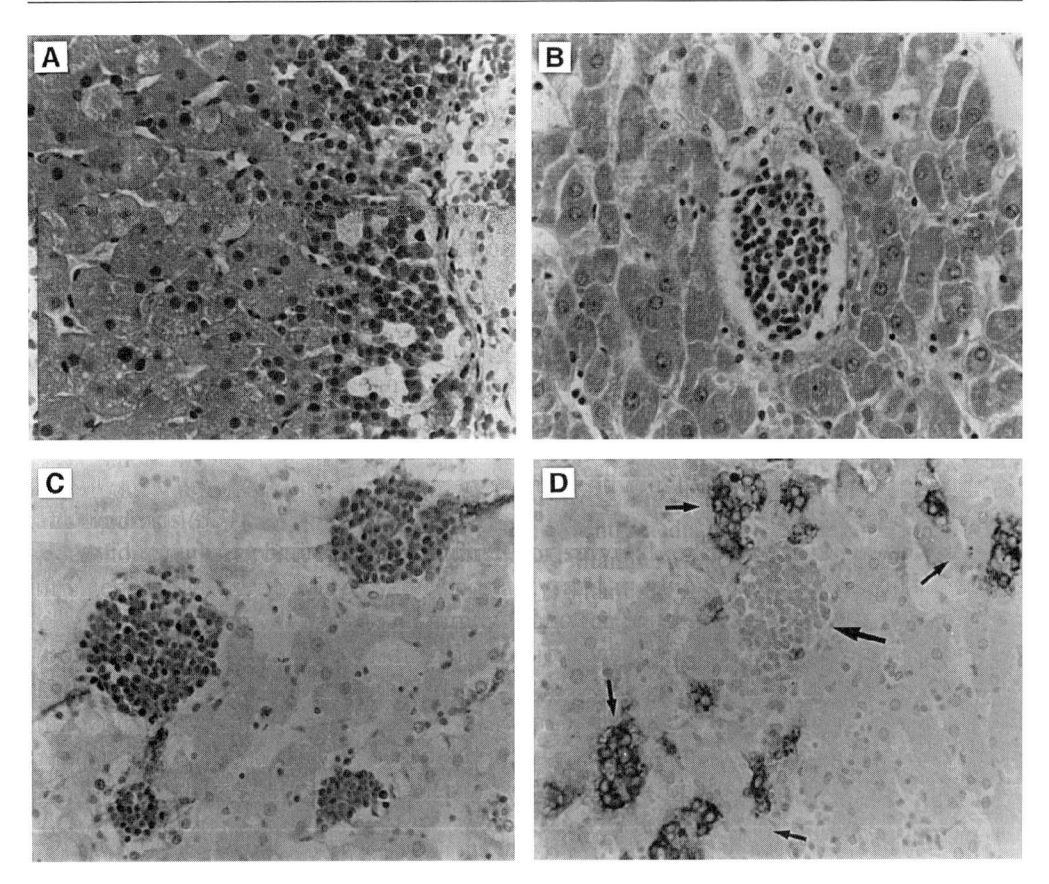

Fig. 1. Histologic and immunohistochemical characterization of the human fetal adrenal. (A) Photomicrograph of a hematoxylin and eosin stained section from the adrenal at 16 wk of gestation (weeks since last menstrual cycle). In the left portion of the figure are the large pale staining cells of the fetal zone; in the right half are neocortical zone cells, which have scant cytoplasm, and the adrenal capsule. (B) Photomicrograph of a hematoxylin and eosin stained section from the adrenal at 19 1/2 wk of gestation in which a large cluster of neuroblasts is prominently shown in the middle of the fetal zone. (C) Photomicrograph of a section of the adrenal at 12 wk that was immunostained for the presence of neuron-specific enolase. Two large and two small clusters of neuroblasts that were immunostained are shown. Immunostained nerve fibers in association with some of the clusters also are apparent. (D) Photomicrograph of a section of the adrenal at 23 wk of gestation that was immunostained for chromogranin A. Whereas the cluster of neuroblasts (large arrow) did not appear to contain chromogranin A, several groups of pheochromocytes (small arrows) were prominently immunostained for this antigen that is associated with the neurosecretory granules of mature medullary chromaffin cells. All photographs were taken using a 40× objective. The immunostaining procedure employed the horseradish peroxidase method and diaminobenzidene as chromogen (unpublished observations of O. Faye-Petersen and C. R. Parker, Jr.).

Fetal Adrenal Steroid Production

The adrenal has an evolving steroidogenic potential during fetal development. Fetal adrenal DS production during gestation parallels the growth of the adrenal *(64)*. The fetal adrenal has enormous capacity for synthesis of DS from early gestation through term, but has limited potential for production of cortisol until late in development. At midgestation, we *(65)* and others *(66,67)* find that the fetal adrenal has little if any 3β-hydroxysteroid dehydrogenase (3β-HSD), which is essential for the *de novo* synthesis of Δ 4 steroids, such as cortisol. On the other hand, both the inner and outer fetal zones appear to posses dehydroepiandrosterone sulfotransferase (DST), which not only sulfurylates steroids, such as pregnenolone and dehydroepiandrosterone, but also effectively interferes with their conversion into Δ 4,3 ketosteroids *(68)*. Later in gestation, there is a gradual appearance of 3β-HSD in the neocortical zone, but not in the fetal zone cells *(65,66)*. Thus, only a small portion of the adrenal has the capacity to produce cortisol or mineralocorticoids, such as aldosterone at delivery. Soon thereafter, there is remodeling of the adrenal with a substantial reduction in mass owing to the involution of the fetal zone and the ultimate evolution of the remaining neocortex into the cortical zones seen in adults *(69,70)*. The cause for the regression of the fetal cortex is unknown, but is likely owing to the removal of some trophic support rather than the action of a inhibitory substance. During the involution phase, fetal plasma levels of DS are reduced in parallel to the reduction in adrenal mass; there is no known alteration in plasma cortisol levels over this period. Production of DS as a major adrenal secretory product does not reoccur until near the time of puberty; this reacquisition of substantial rates of DS production is correlated with the growth of the zona reticularis and is independent of gonadal maturation.

The factors that regulate the development of the steroidogenic apparatus necessary for cortisol and aldosterone production are not clear, since the adrenal of the term anencephalic has virtually normal levels of several key steroidogenic enzymes and their mRNAs *(71)*. On the other hand, in contrast to the adrenals of normal infants, the adrenals of anencephalic fetuses have significantly reduced capacity for cholesterol synthesis and lipoprotein-cholesterol transport into the cell *(71)*, thus severely limiting its steroidogenic capacity *(72,73)*, regardless of the presence of steroidogenic enzymes. In vitro, the most effective peptide stimulator of steroidogenesis by cultured fetal adrenal cells is ACTH, which enhances both DS and cortisol production. One mechanism of action of ACTH is likely via activation of the protein kinase, A pathway in fetal adrenal cells, which augments production of DST, 3β-HSD, and 17 hydroxylase enzymes *(74–76)*. Cholesterol synthesis and lipoprotein cholesterol uptake by fetal adrenal cells also are stimulated by ACTH *(77)*. It is not well established to what extent the fetal adrenal is exposed to circulating ACTH during most of gestation. Based on the above findings, however, one would anticipate that if bioactive ACTH is present, its action is modulated such that cortisol production is limited, whereas DS production is massive. Several investigators believe that the estrogenic milieu of the fetus, possibly coupled with paracrine actions of the high adrenal levels of insulin-like growth factor-II *(78)*, interfere with ACTH's effect on formation of Δ 4 steroids, such as cortisol, thus shunting steroid substrate into the DS synthetic pathway *(79,80)*. It also is possible that during the latter stages of gestation, there is maturation of the posttranslational processing of POMC, such that there is proportionately less of the high-mol-wt forms produced, but more ACTH1-39 is available for secretion *(81)*, as seems likely from the studies of others in experimental animals *(82,83)*. In the third trimester of gestation, fetal adrenal steroidogenesis is clearly dependent on pituitary ACTH production, and there is an active negative feedback mechanism involving glucocorticoids in place *(84)*.

As mentioned earlier, the fetal adrenal produces prodigious quantities of DS, which serves as the principal precursor for placental estrogen formation *(85)*. In adulthood, the

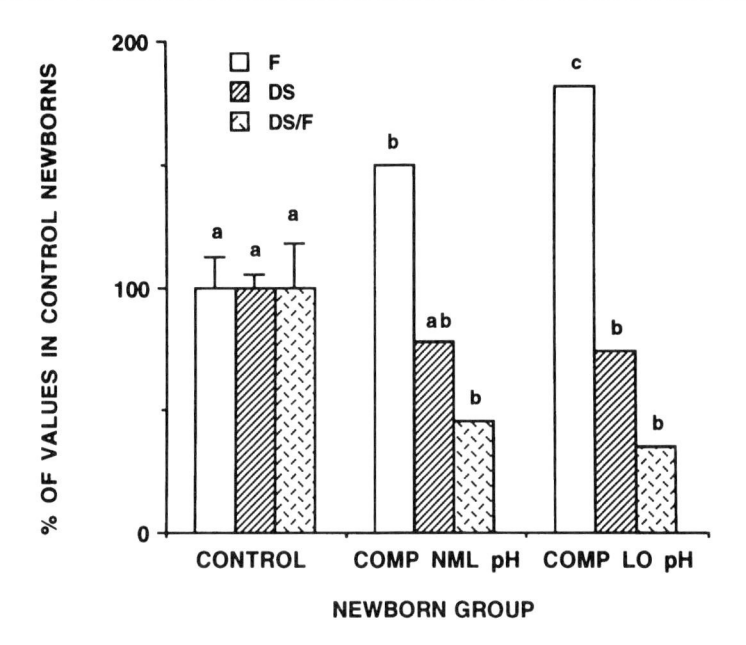

Fig. 2. Effects of pregnancy complications or pregnancy complications plus acidemia on the fetal adrenal steroid production at term: Divergence in DS vs cortisol synthetic pathways. These data are derived from one of the author's studies (ref. *91*). The data are plotted as a percentage of values in a group of 36 normal term newborns who were pair-matched to two other groups of term infants: those having respiratory acidemia, many of whom were delivered of women having pregnancy complications, and infants of women with the same pregnancy characteristics as the acidemic newborns, but who had normal umbilical cord pHs. The SE of the control values are shown as an index of group variability. Values for each parameter having different letters differed significantly from each other. DS, dehydroepiandrosterone sulfate; F, cortisol.

adrenal responds to many stressors by activation of cortisol production, whereas there often is reduction in adrenal DS secretion. It appears that the fetus responds in a similar fashion to intrauterine stress, particularly with regard to reduced DS formation, which leads to reductions in placental estrogen synthesis. For example, reduced levels of maternal estrogen levels and low estrogen concentrations in amniotic fluid have been reported in association with many pregnancy complications *(86)*. Subnormal levels of DS have been noted at delivery in newborns of women having complications such as pregnancy-induced hypertension *(87,88)*, fetal growth retardation *(89,90)*, and hypoxemia *(91)*. On the other hand, in many of the above circumstances, there is evidence for increased cortisol levels in umbilical cord blood. In a study of respiratory acidemia, we found that acidemic infants had higher cortisol levels, lower DS levels and, thus, lower DS/cortisol molar ratios than did normal infants of normal women (Fig. 2). Many of these infants were delivered of women having various pregnancy complications. To control for the possible independent effect of these complications, we also analyzed adrenal status in a group of pair-matched newborns of complicated pregnancies in which the umbilical cord pH was, nevertheless, completely normal. In these infants, intermediate values for cortisol, DS, and the DS/cortisol ratio were found (Fig. 2). The mechanisms for the divergence in the corticoid vs DS pathway in the fetus are not established, but are possibly similar to that in adults, which is also ill-defined. It appears that the fetal hypothalamic–

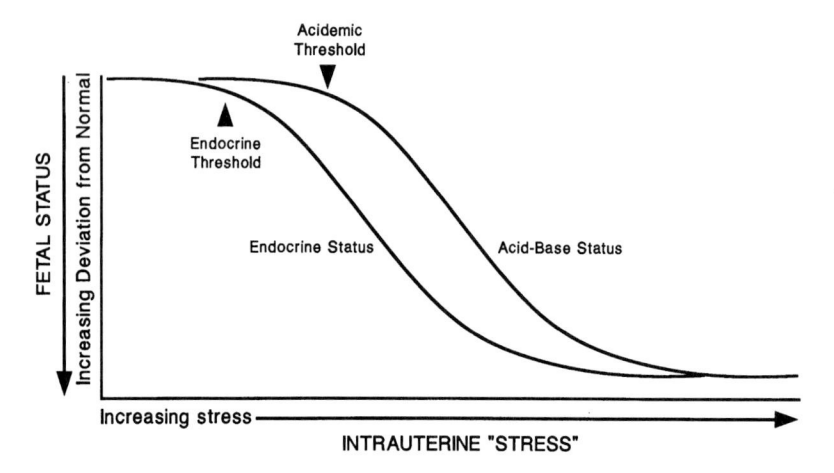

Fig. 3. Fetal endocrine and acid–base response to intrauterine stressors. The hypothalamic–pituitary–adrenocortical axis of the fetus appears to respond to pregnancy complications that compromise fetal well-being at a lower degree of stress than is reflective of altered pH, PO_2, and PCO_2. This conceptualization is derived from data generated in studies of the author and several other investigators as well.

pituitary–adrenocortical axis is very sensitive to alterations in nutrient and oxygen transport that characterize placental insufficiency associated with various stressors, responding at stress levels that are not sufficient to cause noticeable changes in other metabolic parameters, such as acid-base balance (Fig. 3).

Adrenal Steroid Secretion in Newborns

In infancy, the adrenal responds to stress by increased secretion of cortisol. Interestingly, however, subnormal levels of cortisol have been noted at delivery in newborns who subsequently develop serious complications, such as respiratory distress syndrome (RDS) *(92)*. Based on the above observation and other data, in pregnant women in whom preterm delivery is expected, it is common practice to administer glucocorticoids that will cross the placenta into the fetus and hopefully accelerate lung maturation. There was concern that in such infants, whose own adrenal steroid production is downregulated during and for a few days after completion of such treatment *in utero (84)*, there might be a lingering suppression of the pituitary–adrenal axis during the newborn period; such a response could put these infants at risk for adrenal insufficiency during a crisis situation. It appears, however, that the hypothalamic–pituitary–adrenal axis recovers quickly from the effects of antenatal glucocorticoid treatment in the neonatal period *(93)*. It also has been reported that despite potentially lower than normal cortisol levels during fetal life, infants who develop RDS have higher than normal plasma levels of adrenal corticoids *(94)*. Very premature infants having bronchopulmonary dysplasia are being treated with glucocorticosteroids in an attempt to improve their clinical status. As was observed in fetuses treated *in utero*, such neonates also experience adrenal suppression. In many preterm infants treated with glucocorticosteroids postnatally, there is evidence for secondary adrenal insufficiency in that the adrenal responds poorly to exogenous ACTH *(95)*, and resistance of the pituitary to stimulation with CRH also can develop *(96)*. It is possible, however, that such infants already have a predisposition for insufficient adrenocortical function *(97)*.

In normal infants, plasma levels of adrenal steroids and progestins decrease to variable extents over the course of the first week of life *(98,99)*. Whereas neonatal concentrations of DS continue to decline during the first month, cortisol levels are fairly constant after reaching a nadir during the first 24 h of life. In carefully studied infants who had an indwelling umbilical arterial line for monitoring of respiratory status, and who were otherwise clinically stable, it was recently found that several characteristics of cortisol production were similar in preterm and term infants: 6-h mean plasma concentration, plasma corticosteroid binding globulin level, and plasma half-life. In both groups, pulsatile secretion of cortisol was documented, as occurs in later life. The premature infants, however, were found to have longer secretory episodes and a lower maximal secretory rate for cortisol *(100)*. Both premature and term infants have been found to be capable of mounting a response to operative stress *(101)*. Newborns also mount a pituitary–adrenal response to other procedures, such as exchange transfusion *(102)*. Because of the potential for pain or disturbance-related activation of the adrenal in newborns, it is difficult to state with confidence how certain disease states affect adrenal steroidogenesis. It should be possible, however, for a relatively noninvasive procedure, such as collection of saliva *(103)* or urine, or use of indwelling catheters to evaluate longitudinal cortisol responses to disease states in infancy. The renin–angiotensin–aldosterone axis is also competent in the newborn infant, responding to intrauterine conditions and adapting to extrauterine circumstances *(104,105)*. The importance of aldosterone in the human fetus is not clear, considering the high concentrations of progesterone and deoxycorticosterone, which can be produced in considerable amounts by extraglandular 21–hydroxylation of progesterone under the influence of estrogen *(106)*.

ADRENAL MEDULLA

Embryonic Development

The autonomic nervous system is composed of the sympathetic and parasympathetic systems; the adrenal medulla, along with sympathetic nerves comprise the sympathetic (or sympathoadrenal) system. In contradistinction to the parasympathetic nervous system, which has cholinergic transmission in both the pre- and postganglionic components, the sympathetic system uses cholinergic transmission in the preganglionic component and adrenergic transmitters in the postganglionic nerves and the medulla.

The anlage of the adrenal medulla and the extra-adrenal sympathetic elements are derived from common precursors in the neural crest. As detailed by Crowder *(57)* and confirmed later by O'Rahilly *(107)*, neuroblastic cells migrate from the neural crest along the aorta and form collections that later develop into the paravertebral sympathetic ganglia (para-aortic bodies). Two of the three cell types noted by Crowder in the paraglanglia are destined to give rise to the adrenal medulla. Once the condensation of primordial cells that will become the adrenal cortex is initiated, neurogenic cells and fibers from the thoracico-lumbar region invade the primitive cortex beginning at around Carnegie developmental stages 16–17 (36–42 developmental days; 8–14 mm embryonic size). The primitive sympathetic cells, neuroblasts, appear to migrate into the cortical primordium along nerves and begin to proliferate, forming clusters of neuroblasts. These neuroblast clusters can be seen scattered throughout the fetal adrenal, of which about 80% is composed of the large inner fetal zone cells (Fig. 1B,C). Histologically, the neuroblasts have dense, basophilic nuclei and scant cytoplasm. Over the period of 8–17 wk of gestation, Turkel et al. *(108)* found that both the number and size of neuroblast clusters increase in the adrenal; thereafter, a reduction in the size and number of such aggregates occurs. Also during the interval of 8–20 wk, the proportion of superficial neuroblast clusters declines from about 20–3%, whereas those located within the inner cortical region rise from about 80 to over 95%. By term, 40 wk of gestation, there are usually no noticeable neuroblast clusters in the periphery of the cortex, and the cortical elements of the medulla are coalesced in the medial portion of the gland around the central vein.

The morphologic conversion of neuroblasts into mature pheochromocytes occurs gradually during the interval of about 8–25 wk gestation. The pheochromocytes in the fetal adrenal are histologically distinct from the neuroblasts. These mature cells have somewhat larger and less dense appearing nuclei in which chromatin granules and threads are apparent along with a small nucleolus. There also is more cytoplasm in such cells. These cells often are seen at the periphery of the neuroblast clusters, and also are found as isolated single cells or small groups not adjoining neuroblasts. In the latter instance, one gets the sense that such isolated, mature-looking cells budded off from neuroblast clusters and then migrated further themselves, or else remained in place while the clusters of immature cells continued moving toward the central parts of the gland. It has been noted that although the pheochromocytes look differentiated, some display the characteristic brown appearance on reaction with potassium dichromate and look like the chromaffin cells of the mature gland, whereas other cells that appear indistinguishable do not yet display this feature *(109)*. When immunostained with antisera against chromogranin A, we find that the pheochromocytes are immunopositive, whereas the clusters of neuroblasts are negative during the interval of 11 wk (the earliest time-point examined) to 23 wk of gestation (Fig. 1D). Interestingly, others *(110)* have noted that tyrosine hydroxylase is detectable as early as embryonic stage 18 (44 developmental days) in the adrenal, whereas chromogranin A was not evident. Subsequently, certain cells described by these authors as neuroblasts were immunopositive for both markers, but other similar appearing cells were negative for both. These latter cells were most abundant at midgestation, but soon thereafter were not identifiable throughout the remainder of development.

The factors that influence the initial expression of enzymes necessary for catecholamine synthesis (Fig. 4) and proteins involved in catecholamine storage in the medulla are not clear. The developmental appearance of tyrosine hydroxylase and dopamine β-hydroxylase in pheochromocytes precedes that of phenylethanolamine N-methyl transferase (PNMT) *(111)*. Based on studies in experimental animals, it seems likely that glucocorticoids influence the production in the developing adrenal of PNMT, which is required for the conversion of norepinephrine to epinephrine *(112)*. It is not clear whether glucocorticoids of fetal adrenal origin or those derived from transplacental passage of maternal corticosteroids are responsible for differentiation of subpopulations of pheochromocytes into epinephrine-producing cells. Interestingly, it has been proposed that medullary development in anencephalic fetuses is accelerated compared to that in normal fetuses *(113)*. Recall that at least in the latter half of gestation, adrenal cortical growth and steroidogenesis clearly are severely impaired in such

```
            TH         DDC          DBH              PNMT
Tyrosine----->Dopa------->Dopamine-------->Norepinephrine---------->Epinephrine
```

Fig. 4. Biosynthetic pathway involved in the formation of catecholamines. Abbreviations: TH, tyrosine hydroxylase; DDC, Dopa decarboxylase; DBH, Dopamine β hydoxylase; PNMT, phenylethynolamine N-methyl transferase.

fetuses owing to the maldevelopment of the hypothalamus and, therefore, lack of hypothalamic regulation of pituitary ACTH secretion. Thus, a paracrine role of fetal adrenal corticosteroids may not be required for some aspects of early medullary development. Thereafter, however, it seems that the local environment of the medulla is important for the fine-tuning of the production and release of catecholamines *(114)*, and probably influences synthesis of the numerous bioactive peptides present in the medulla *(115–118)*.

Direct neural control of the medulla is achieved via the splanchnic nerve, which employs acetylcholine as the preganglionic transmitter. The hypothalamus serves as the organizing center of the sympathetic nervous system and thus plays an important role in regulating adrenal medullary activity. Various stressors cause activation of the sympathoadrenal system in postnatal life. In the developing fetus, this system also is capable of adaptive responses, as detailed below.

Sympathoadrenal Activity in the Fetus and Newborn

Since the sympathetic nervous system is not completely developed at birth, catecholamines in blood, urine, and amniotic fluid are relatively good indices of the activity of the adrenal medulla and the paraglanglia compared to the situation in the adult. There is, however, continued maturation of the adrenal medulla after birth, since epinephrine does not predominate over norepinephrine during early infancy as it does in adults *(119)*. Since maternal plasma catecholamines are extensively metabolized in the placenta, catecholamines in the fetus are largely if not exclusively of fetal origin. In normal pregnancies, amniotic fluid catecholamine levels and those in the first voided urine of infants delivered at or near term correlate well *(120)*. The concentrations of dopamine in amniotic fluid and urine were about 10 times those of norepinephrine and about 50–100 times those of epinephrine. Amniotic fluid levels of norepinephrine and epinephrine in infants considered to have experienced intrauterine stress (as indicated by abnormal heart rate patterns, meconium stained amniotic fluid, and/or low 1-min Apgar scores) were increased over those in normal infants. Moreover, infants considered to have experienced severe stress had higher amniotic fluid levels of these catecholamines than infants experiencing moderate stress *(120)*.

Catecholamine levels in the fetal circulation increase substantially during the stress of labor *(121)* and are particularly high in umbilical cord blood of hypoxic newborns *(122)*, even in the absence of labor *(123)*. After birth, catecholamine levels in normal newborns decrease rapidly and soon are as low as are those in adults. On the other hand, infants who are ill may have increased catecholamine levels. In addition, it seems likely that the stress of many procedures may cause increased release of catecholamines, since sedation tends to reduce catecholamine levels in the infant *(124)*. Epinephrine and norepinephrine levels typically rise substantially during the stress of surgery in the newborn *(125)* and also increase to variable extents in response to hypoglycemic episodes *(126).*

THYROID

Embryonic Development

The development of the thyroid gland *(107,127)* begins early in human embryogenesis from two anlagens, a midline thickening of the pharyngeal floor and paired extensions of the fourth pharyngobranchial pouch; the thyroid primordium is identifiable by Carnegie stage 10–11 (22–24 d of development), and by 28 developmental days, the thyroid is bilobed and connected to the pharynx by a hollow pedicle. The parathyroid glands develop from the third and fourth pouch, and the thymus gland develops from the third pharyngeal pouch. The parafollicular C cells of the thyroid, which produce calcitonin and the calcitonin gene-related peptide, develop from elements of the fourth pharyngeal pouch. By stage 15–16 (the fifth developmental week), the thyroid becomes detached from the pharynx and begin to curve around the carotid arteries. During the seventh week, the thyroid assumes its definitive shape. The histologic differentiation of the fetal thyroid has been divided into three phases: the precolloid (7–13 wk of gestation), the early colloid (13–14 wk), and the follicular phase (beyond the 14th wk). The thyroid is innervated by both sympathetic and parasympathetic nerves. Development of the thyroid in the fetus appears to be independent of the fetal hypothalamic–pituitary axis, since that of anencepahalic infants is essentially normal *(2).*

The functional unit of the thyroid is composed of follicular cells surrounding the follicular lumina. Thyroid hormones are produced as mono- and diiodotyrosyl residues within thyroglobulin, which is synthesized in the follicle cells and stored in the lumen. The process of thyroid hormone synthesis is comprised of the thyroidal trapping of iodine, synthesis of thyroglobulin, and thence, iodination of the tyrosine moieties and oxidative conversion of the iodotyrosines into iodothyronines. Secretion of thyroid hormones involves hydrolytic cleavage of thyroglobulin in the thyroid cell to liberate thyroid hormones. Synthesis of thyroid hormones in the fetus begins at about the 12th gestational week; prior to that time, any thyroid hormones in the fetal compartment would be derived from the limited transplacental passage and metabolism of maternal hormones. After the fetal thyroid develops synthetic capacity, the fetal milieu is reflective almost exclusively of fetally produced thyroid hormones.

Thyroid Hormone Production in the Fetus and Newborn

The principal thyroid hormone in the maternal and fetal blood is thyroxine (3,5,3′,5′ tetraiodothyronine, T_4). Triiodothyronines exist as T_3 and reverse T_3 (rT_3). The principal bioactive thyroid hormone is T_3. At midgestation, fetal plasma levels of T_4, rT_3, and T_3 are about 3000, 250, and 10 ng/DL, respectively. By term, T_4 and T_3 levels increase about fourfold, whereas those of rT_3 are virtually unchanged *(127,128).* Umbilical cord serum levels of T_4 over the interval of 20–30 wk of gestation continue to be reduced in relation to those at term *(129).* Thyroid hormones circulate in plasma largely bound to a thyroxinebinding globulin (TBG), thyroxinebinding prealbumin (TBPA), and albumin; the proportionate distribution of T_4 and T_3 bound to these proteins is about 70–75% TBG, 20–25% TBPA, and 5–10% albumin. Only a fraction of a percent of T_4 and T_3 circulate as unbound hormones *(130).* The reason for the inordinately low level of T_3 in the fetus, but increased levels of rT_3 compared to the adult is that monodeiodination in the 5′-position is limited in the fetus *(131)*.

In the early neonatal period, there is a massive, though transient activation of thyroid hormone production; levels of T_4 rise about 70% and those of T_3 increase about 10-fold over the first 48 h of life in term newborns. This activation is dependent on hypothalamic–pituitary integrity and likely is responsive to postpartum cooling of the newborn. A similar postnatal activation of thyroid hormone production also occurs, though of lesser magnitude, in preterm infants. The excessive increase in blood levels of T_3 relative to that of T_4 is probably reflective of augmented hepatic conversion of T_4 to T_3. The period of relative hyperthyroidism extends for the first few weeks of life *(132)*. Thyroid hormone levels in umbilical cord blood of premature infants who develop respiratory distress syndrome have been reported to be lower than in those who did not have respiratory problems in several studies. Subnormal levels of thyroid hormones also appear to persist in premature infants having respiratory distress or other illnesses, and also in ill term newborns *(133)*. Such deficiencies seem similar to that noted to occur frequently in adults with nonthyroidal illnesses. Moreover, it seems likely that reduced production of thyroid hormones during illness in infants does not have any significant untoward effects and is transient in nature. Thus, thyroid hormone supplementation is probably not warranted in such circumstances.

REFERENCES

1. Moore KL, Persuad TVN. The Developing Human. WB Saunders, Co, Philadelphia, 1993.
2. Kaplan SL, Grumbach MM, Aubert ML. The ontogenesis of pituitary hormones and hypothalamic factors in the human fetus: Maturation of central nervous system regulation of anterior pituitary function. Rec Prog Horm Res 1976;32:161–234.
3. Mulchahey JJ, DiBlasio AM, Martin MC, Blumenfeld Z , Jaffe RB. Hormone production and peptide regulation of the human fetal pituitary gland. Endocr Rev 1987;8:406–425.
4. Page RB, Bergland RM. Pituitary vasculature. In: Allen MB, Mahesh VB, eds. The Pituitary. Academic, New York, 1977, pp. 9–17.
5. Folkers K, Ensmann, Boler FJ, Bowers CY, Schally AV. Discovery of the synthetic tripeptide-sequence of the thyrotropin releasing hormone having activity. Biochem Biophys Res Commun 1969;37:123–26.
6. Winters AJ, Eskay RL, Porter JC. Concentration and distribution of TRH and LHRH in the human fetal brain. J Clin Endocrinol Metab 1974;39:960–63.
7. Lechan RM, Wu P, Jackson IMD, et al. Thyrotropin-releasing hormone precursor: characterization in rat brain. Science 1986;231:159–61.
8. Parker CR Jr, Griffin WST, Porter JC. Age-dependent extinction of thyrotropin-releasing hormone in the human cerebellum. J Clin Endocrinol Metab 1981;53:1233–37.
9. Parker CR Jr, Porter JC, MacDonald PC. Subcellular localization of LHRH and TRH in the human fetal brain. Proceedings of the 25th annual meeting of the Society for Gynecologic Investigation (Abstract 102), 1978.
10. Vale W, Spiess, Rivier JC, Rivier J. Characterization of a 41-residue ovine hypothalamic peptide that stimulates secretion of cortocotrophin and β-endorphin. Science 1981;213:1394–97.
11. Breeson J-L, Clavequin M-C , Bugnon C. Anatomical and ontogenetic studies of the human paraventriculo-infundibular corticoliberin system. Neuroscience 1985;14:1077–90.
12. Frim DM, Emanuel RL, Robinson BG, Smas CM, Adler GK, Majzoud JA. Characterizaion and gestational regulation of corticotropin-releasing hormone messenger RNA in human placenta. J Clin Invest 1988;82:287–292.
13. Robinson BG, Emanuel RL, Frim DM, et al. Glucocorticoid stimulates expression of corticotropin-releasing hormone in human placenta. Proc Natl Acad Sci USA 1988;85:5244–5248.
14. Goland RS, Wardlaw SL, Stark RI, Brown LS Jr, Frantz AG. High levels of corticotropin-releasing

hormone immunoreactivity in maternal and fetal plasma during pregnancy. J Clin Endocrinol Metab 1986;63:1199–1203.
15. Campbell EA, Linton EA, Wolfe CDA, Scraggs PR, Jones MT, Lowry PJ. Plasma corticotropin-releasing-hormone concentration during pregnancy and partuition. J Clin Endocrinol Metab 1987;64:1054–1059.
16. Goland RS, Jozak S, Warren WB, Conwell IM, Stark RI, Tropper PJ. Elevated levels of umbilical cord plasma corticotropin-releasing hormone in growth-retarded fetuses. J Clin Endocrinol Metab 1993;77:1174–1179.
17. Goland RS, Tropper PJ, Warren WB, Stark RI, Jozak SM, Conwell IM. Umbilical cord corticotropin releasing hormone concentrations in pregnancies complicated by pre-eclampsia. J Dev Physiol 1994;20:127–130.
18. Laatikainen T, Virtanen T, Kaaja R, Salminen-Lappalainen K. Corticotropin releasing hormone in maternal and cord plasma in preeclampsia. Eur J Obstet Gynecol Repre Biol 1991;39:19–24.
19. Stankovic AK, Parker CR Jr. Corticotropin releasing hormone enhances steroidogenesis by cultured human adrenal cells. Proceedings of the 77th annual meeting of the Endocrine Society (Abstract 468), 1995.
20. Parker CR Jr. Endocrinology of pregnancy. In: Carr BR, Blackwell RE, eds. Textbook of Reproductive Medicine. Appleton and Lange, East Norwalk CT, 1992, pp. 17–44.
21. Brownstein MJ, Russell JT, Gainer H. Synthesis, transport, and release of posterior pituitary peptides. Science 1980;207:373–378.
22. Burford GD, Robinson ICAF. Oxytocin, vasopressin and neurophysins in the hypothalamo-neurohypophysial system in the fetus. J Endocrinol 1982;95:403–408.
23. Aguilera G. Regulation of pituitary ACTH secretion during chronic stress. Front Neuroendocrinol 1994;15:321–350.
24. Whitnall M, Mezey E, Gainer H. Colocalization of corticotropin releasing factor, vasopressin in median eminence secretory vesicles. Nature 1985;317:248–250.
25. Blumenfeld Z, Jaffe RB. Hypophysiotropic and neuromodulatory regulation of adrenocorticotropin in the human fetal pituitary gland. 1986;78:288–294.
26. Mains RE, Eipper BA, Ling N. Common precursor to corticotropins and endorphins. Proc Natl Acad Sci USA 1977;74:3014–3018.
27. Roberts JL, Herbert E. Characterization of a common precursor to corticotropin and β-lipotropin: Cell free synthesis of the precursor and identification of corticotropin peptides in the molecule. Proc Natl Acad Sci USA 1977;74:4826–4830.
28. Begeot M, Dubois MP, Dubois PM. Growth hormone and ACTH in the pituitary of normal and anencephalic human fetuses: Immunocytochemical evidence for hypothalamic influences during development. Neuroendocrinology 1977;24:208–220.
29. Baker BL, Jaffe RB. The genesis of cell types in the adenohypophysis of the human fetus as observed with immunocytochemistry. Am J Anat 1975;143:137–161.
30. Asa SL, Kovacs K, Laszlo FA, Domokos I, Ezrin C. Human fetal adenohypophysis. Histologic and immunocytochemical analysis. Neuroendocrinology 1986;43:308–316.
31. Siler-Khodr TM, Morgenstern LL, Greenwood FC. Hormone synthesis and release from human fetal adenohypophyses in vitro. J Clin Endocrinol Metab 1974;39:891–905.
32. Gyevai AT, Kuznetsova LV, Stark E, Bukulya B, Acs Z. Invitro study of functional maturation of CRF-ACTH axis in man, in the intrauterine period. Translated from Byull Eksp Biol Med 1982;94:88.
33. Gibbs DM, Stewart RD, Vale W, Rivier J, Yen SSC. Synthetic corticotropin-releasing factor stimulates secretion of immunoreactive β-endorphin/β-lipotropin and ACTH by human fetal pituitaries in vitro. Life Sci 1983;32:547–550.
34. Allen JP, Greer MA, McGilvra R, Castro A, Fisher DA. Endocrine function in an anencephalic infant. J Clin Endocrinol Metab 1974;38:94–98.
35. Dubois PM, Begeot M, Dubois MP, Herbert DC. Immunocytochemical localization of LH, FSH, TSH and their subunits in the pituitary of normal and anencephalic human fetuses. Cell Tiss Res 1978;191:249–265.
36. Fukuchi M, Inoue T, Abe H, Kumahara Y. Thyrotropin in human fetal pituitaries. J Clin Endocrinol Metab 1970;31:565–569.
37. Winters AJ, Oliver C, Colston C, MacDonald PC, Porter JC. Plasma ACTH levels in the human fetus and neonate as related to age and partuition. J Clin Endocrinol Metab 1974;39:269–273.

38. Ramin SM, Porter JC, Gilstrap LC III, Rosenfeld CR. Stress hormones and acid-base status of human fetuses at delivery. J Clin Endocrinol Metab 1991;73:182–186.
39. Wardlaw SL, Stark RI, Baxi L, Frantz AG. Plasma β-endorphin and β-lipotropin in the human fetus at delivery: Correlation with arterial pH and pO2. J Clin Endocrinol Metab 1979;49:888–891.
40. Bacigalupo G, Langner K, Schmidt S, Saling E. Plasma immunoreactive beta-endorphin, ACTH and cortisol concentrations in mothers and their neonates immediately after delivery- their relationship to the duration of labor. J Perinat Med 1987;15:45–52.
41. Gemelli M, Mami C, Manganaro, De Luca F, Saja A, Costa G. Correlation between plasma levels of ACTH and β-endorphin in the first seven days of postnatal life. J Endocrinol Invest 1988;11:395–398.
42. Hindmarsh KW, Sankaran K, Watson VG. Plasma beta-endorphin concentrations in neonates associated with acute stress. Dev Pharmacol Ther 1984;7:198–204.
43. Milner RDG, Cser A, Goode M, Ratcliffe JG. Adrenocorticotrophin and glucocorticoid response to exchange transfusion. Acta Paediatr Scand 1976;65:439–444.
44. Fisher DA, Dussault JH, Sack J, Chpora IJ. Ontogenesis of hypothalamic-pituitary-thyroid flunction and metabolism in man, sheep and rat. Rec Prog Horm Res 1977;33:59–116.
45. Hayak A, Driscoll SG, Warshaw JB. Endocrine studies in anencephaly. J Clin Invest 1973;52:1636–1641.
46. Cavallo L, Altomare M, Palmieri P, Licci D, Carnimeo F, Mastro F. Endocrine function in four anencephalic infants. Hormone Res 1981;15:159–166.
47. Fisher DA. Maternal-fetal thyroid function in pregnancy. Clin Perinatol 1983;10:615–626.
48. DeVane GW, Porter JC. An apparent stress-induced release of arginine vasopressin by human neonates. J Clin Endocrinol Metab 1980;51:1412–1416.
49. Leung AKC, McArthur RG, McMillan DD, et al. Circulating antidiuretic hormone during labor and in the newborn. Acta Paediatr Scand 1980;69:505–510.
50. Parboosingh J, Lederis K, Singh N. Vasopressin concentration in cord blood: Correlation with method of delivery and cord pH. Obstet Gynecol 1982;60:179–183.
51. Ruth V, Fyhrquist F, Clemons G, Raivio KO. Cord plasma vasopressin, erythropoietin, and hypoxanthine as indices of asphysia at birth. Pediatr Res 1988;24:490–494.
52. Stern P, LaRochelle FT, Little GA. Vasopressin and pneumothorax in the neonate. Pediatrics 1981;68:499–503.
53. Paxson CL Jr, Stoerner JW, Denson SE, Adcock EW III, Morriss FJ Jr. Syndrome of inappropriate antidiuretic hormone secretion in neonates with pneumothorax or atelectasis. J Pediatr 1977;91:459–463.
54. van Steensel-Moll HA, Hazelzet JA, van der Voort E, Neijens HJ, Hackeng WHL. Excessive secretion of antidiuretic hormone in infections with respiratory syncytial virus. Arch Dis Child 1990;65:1237–1239.
55. Khare SK. Neurohypophyseal dysfunction following perinatal asphyxia. J Pediatr 1977;90:628–629.
56. Hoppenstein JM, Miltenberger FW, Moran WH Jr. The increase in blood levels of vasopressin in infants during birth and surgical procedures. Surg Gynecol Obstet 1968;127:966–974.
57. Crowder RE. The development of the adrenal gland in man, with special reference to origin and ultimate location of cell types and evidence in favor of the "cell migration" theory. Contributions to Embryology 1957;36:193–210.
58. Benirschke K. Adrenals in anencephaly and hydrocephaly. Obstet Gynecol 1956;8:412–425.
59. Gray ES, Abramovich DR. Morphologic features of the anencephalic adrenal gland in early pregnancy. Am J Obstet Gynecol 1980;137:491–95.
60. Kreiger DT. Placenta as a source of "brain" and "pituitary" hormones. Biol Reprod 1982;26:55–71.
61. Grino M, Chrousos GP, Margioris AN. The corticotropin-releasing hormone gene is expressed in human placenta. Biochem Biophys Res Commun 1987;148:1208–1214.
62. Seron-Ferre M, Lawrence CC, Jaffe RB. Role of hCG in regulation of the human fetal adrenal gland. J Clin Endocrinol Metab 1978;46:834–837.
63. Burke BA, Wick MR, King R, et al. Congenital adrenal hypoplasia and selective absence of pituitary luteinizing hormone; a new autosomal recessive syndrome. Am J Med Genet 1988;31:75–97.
64. Parker, CR Jr, Leveno K, Carr BR, Hauth J, MacDonald PC. Umbilical cord plasma levels of dehydroepiandrosterone sulfate during human gestation. J Clin Endocrinol Metab 1982;54:1216–1220.
65. Parker, CR Jr, Faye-Petersen O, Stankovic AK, Mason JI, Grizzle WE. Immunohistochemical evaluation of the cellular localization and ontogeny of 3β-hydroxysteroid dehydrogenase/delta 5-4 isomerase in the human fetal adrenal. Endocr Res 1995;21:69–80.
66. Dupont E, Luu-The V, Labrie F, Pelletier G. Ontogeny of 3β-hydroxysteroid dehydrogenase/delta5-

delta4 isomerase (3βHSD) in human adrenal gland performed by immunocytochemistry. Mol Cell Endocrinol 1990;74:R7–R10.
67. Voutilainen R, Ilvesmaki V, Miettinen PJ. Low expression of 3β-hydroxy-5-ene-steroid dehydrogenase gene in human fetal adrenals in vivo; adrenocorticotropin and protein kinase c-dependent regulation in adrenocortical cultures. J Clin Endocrinol Metab 1991;72:761–767.
68. Parker CR Jr, Falany CN, Stockard CR, Stankovic AK, Grizzle WE. Immunohistochemical localization of dehyhdroepiandrosterone sulfotransferase in human fetal tissues. J Clin Endocrinol Metab 1994;78:234–236.
69. Bech K, Tygstrup I, Nerup I. The involution of the fetal adrenal cortex. A light microscopic study. Acta Path Microbiol Scand 1969;76:391–400.
70. Dhom G. The prepuberal and puberal growth of the adrenal (Adrenarche). Beitr Pathol BD 1973;150:357–377.
71. Simpson ER, Carr BR, John ME, et al. Cholesterol metabolism in the adrenals of normal and anencephalic human fetuses. In: Albrecht E, Pepe GJ, eds. Perinatal Endocrinology. Perinatology, Ithaca, NY, 1985, pp. 161–173.
72. Carr, BR, Parker CR Jr, Milewich L, Porter JC, MacDonald PC, Simpson ER. Regulation of steroid production by adrenal tissue of a human anencephalic fetus. J Clin Endocrinol Metab 1980;50:870–873.
73. Parker CR Jr, Carr BR, Winkel CA, Casey LM, Simpson ER, MacDonald PC. Hypercholesterolemia due to elevated low-density lipoprotein-cholesterol in newborns with anencephaly and adrenal atrophy. J Clin Endocrinol Metab 1983;57:37–43.
74. Parker CR Jr, Stankovic AK, Falany CN, Faye-Petersen O, Grizzle WE. Immunocytochemical analyses of dehydroepiandrosterone sulfotransferase in cultured human fetal adrenal cells. J Clin Endocrinol Metab 1995;80:1027–1031.
75. McAllister JM, Hornsby PJ. Dual regulation of 3β-hydroxysteroid dehydrogenase, 17α-hydroxylase, and dehydroepiandrosterone sulfotransferase by adenosine 3′,5′-monophosphate and activators of protein kinase c in cultured human adrenocortical cells. Endocrinology 1988;122:2012–2018.
76. Doody KM, Carr BR, Rainey WE, et al. 3β-hydroxysteroid dehydrogenase/isomerase in the fetal zone and neocortex of the human fetal adrenal gland. Endocrinology 1990;126:2487–2492.
77. Carr BR, Simpson ER. Lipoprotein utilization and cholesterol synthesis by the human fetal adrenal gland. Endocr Rev 1981;2:306–326.
78. Han VKM, Lund PK, Lee DC, D'Ercole AJ. Expression of somatomedin/insulin-like growth factor messenger ribonucleic acids in the human fetus: Identification, characterization, and tissue distribution. J Clin Endocrinol Metab 1988;66:422–429.
79. Fugeida K, Faiman C, Reyes RI, Winter JSD. The control of steroidogenesis by human fetal adrenal cells in tissue culture. IV. The effect of exposure to placental steroids. J Clin Endocrinol Metab 1982;54:89–94.
80. Mesiano S, Jaffe RB. Interaction of insulin-like growth factor-II and estradiol directs steroidogenesis in the human fetal adrenal toward dehydroepiandrosterone sulfate production. J Clin Endocrinol Metab 1993;77:754–758.
81. Parker CR Jr, Porter JC. Ontogeny of multiple molecular weight forms of immunoreactive (IR) ACTH in the human pituitary gland. Proc 7th Int Congress Endocrinol pp 1265 (Abstract 2010), 1984.
82. Sato SM, Mains RE. Posttranslational processing of proadrenocorticotropin/endorphin-derived peptides during postnatal development in the rat pituitary. Endocrinology 1985;117:773–786.
83. Carr GA, Jacobs RA, Young R. Development of adrenocorticotropin-(1–39) and precursor peptide secretory responses in the fetal sheep during the last third of gestation. Endocrinology 1995;136:5020–5027.
84. Parker CR Jr, Atkinson MW, Owen J, Andrews WW. Dynamics of the fetal adrenal, cholesterol and apolipoprotein B responses to antenatal betamethasone therapy. Am J Obstet Gynecol 1996;174:562–565.
85. Siiteri PK, MacDonald, PC. Placental estrogen biosynthesis during human pregnancy. J Clin Endocrinol Metab 1966;26:751–761.
86. Daywood MY. Hormones in amniotic fluid. Am J Obstet Gynecol 1977;128:576–583.
87. Parker CR Jr, Hankins GDV, Carr BR, Leveno KJ, Gant NF, MacDonald PC. The effect of hypertension in pregnant women on fetal adrenal function and fetal plasma lipoprotein-cholesterol metabolism. Am J Obstet Gynecol 1984;150:263–269.
88. Procianoy RS, Cecin SKG. Umbilical cord dehydroepiandrosterone sulfate and cortisol levels in preterm infants born to pre-eclamptic mothers. Acta Paediatr Scand 1986;75:279–282.

89. Turnipseed MR, Bentley K, Reynolds JW. Serum dehydroepiandrosterone sulfate in premature infants and infants with intrauterine growth retardation. J Clin Endocrinol Metab 1976;43:1219–1225.
90. Parker CR Jr, Buchina ES, Barefoot TK. Abnormal adrenal steroidogenesis in growth-retarded newborn infants. Pediatr Res 1994;35:633–636.
91. Harlin CA, Tucker JM, Winkler C, Henson B, Parker CR Jr. Altered adrenal steroid production in term infants having repiratory acidemia. Acta Endocrinol 1993;128:136–139.
92. Murphy BEP. Cortisol and cortisone levels in the cord blood at delivery of infants with and without respiratory distress syndrome. Am J Obstet Gynecol 1974;119:1112–1120.
93. Dorr HG, Versmold HT, Sippel WG, Bidlingmaier F, Knorr D. Antenatal betamethasone therapy: Effects on maternal, fetal, and neonatal mineralocorticoids, glucocorticoids, and progestins. J Pediatr 1986;10:990–993.
94. Reynolds JW. Serum total corticoid and cortisol levels in premature infants with respiratory distress syndrome. Pediatrics 1973;51:884–890.
95. Strauss A, Brakin M, Norris MK, Modanlou HD. Adrenal responsiveness in very-low-birth-weight infants treated with dexamethasone. Dev Pharmacol Ther 1992;19:147–154.
96. Rizvi ZB, Aniol HS, Myers TF, Zeller WP, Fisher SG, Anderson CL. Effects of dexamethasone on the hypothalamic–pituitary–adrenal axis in preterm infants. J Pediatr 1992;120:961–965.
97. Watterberg KL, Scott SM. Evidence of early adrenal insufficiency in babies who develop bronchopulmonary dysplasia. Pediatrics 1995;95:120–125.
98. Sippell WG, Becker H, Versmold HT, Bidlingmaier F, Knorr D. Longitudinal studies of plasma aldosterone, corticosterone, deoxycorticosterone, progesterone, 17-hydroxyprogesterone, cortisol and cortisone determined simultaneously in mother and child at birth and during the early neonatal period. I. Spontaneous delivery. J Clin Endocrinol Metab 1978;46:971–984.
99. Endoh A. Trend analysis of serum progesterone, deoxycorticosterone, deoxycorticosterone sulfate, cortisol, corticosterone, 18-hydroxydeoxycorticosterone and estradiol in early neonates. Endocrinol Japon 1989;36:851–858.
100. Metzger DL, Wright NM, Veldhuis JD, Rogol AD, Kerrigan JR. Characterization of pulsatile secretion and clearance of plasma cortisol in premature and term neonates using deconvolution analysis. J Clin Endocrinol Metab 1993;77:458–463.
101. Anand KJS, Aynsley-Green A. Measuring the severity of surgical stress in newborn infants. J Ped Surg 1988;23:297–305.
102. Milner RDG, Cser A, Goode M, Ratcliffe JG. Adrenocorticotrophin and glucocorticoid response to exchange transfusion. Acta Paediatr Scand 1976;65:439–444.
103. Francis SJ, Walker RF, Riad-Fahmy D, Hughes D, Murphy JF, Gray OP. Assessment of adrenocortical activity in term newborn infants using salivary cortisol determinations. J Pediatr 1987;111:129–133.
104. Gutai JP, Migeon CJ. Adrenal insufficiency during the neonatal period. Clin Perinatol 1975;2:163–182.
105. Sulyok E, Kovacs L, Lichardus B, et al. Late hyponatremia in premature infants: role of aldosterone and arginine vasopressin. J Pediatr 1985;106:990–994.
106. Parker CR Jr, Carr BR, Casey ML, Gant NF, MacDonald PC. Extraadrenal deoxycorticosterone (DOC) production in hypoestrogenic pregnancies: serum concentrations of progesterone and DOC in anencephalic fetuses and in women pregnant with an anencephalic fetus. Am J Obstet Gynecol 1983;147:415–23.
107. O'Rahilly R. The timing and sequence of events in the development of the human endocrine system during the embryonic period proper. Anat Embryol 1983;166:439–451.
108. Turkel SB, Itabashi, HH. The natural history of neuroblastic cells in the fetal adrenal gland. Am J Pathol 1974;76:225–244.
109. Copeland RE. The prenatal development of the abdominal para-aortic bodies in man. J Anat 1952;86:357–372.
110. Cooper MJ, Hutchins GM, Cohen PS, Helman LJ, Mennie RJ, Israel MA. Human neuroblastoma tumor cell lines correspond to the arrested differentiation of chromaffin adrenal medullary neuroblasts. Cell Growth Differ 1990;1:149–159.
111. Bohn MC, Goldstein M, Black IB. Role of glucocorticoids in expression of the adrenergic phenotype in rat embryonic adrenal gland. Dev Biol 1981;82:1–10.
112. Seidl K, Unsicker K. The determination of the adrenal medullary cell fate during embryogenesis. Dev Biol 1989;136:481–490.
113. Namnoum AB, Hutchins GM. Accelerated maturation of the adrenal medulla in anencephaly. Pediatr Pathol 1990;10:895–900.

114. Wurtman RJ, Axelrod J. Control of enzymatic synthesis of adrenaline in the adrenal medulla by adrenal cortical steroids. J Biol Chem 1966;241:2301–2304.
115. Evans CJ, Erdelyi E, Weber E, Barchas JD. Identification of proopiomelanocortin-derived peptides in the human adrenal medulla. Science 1983;221:957–960.
116. Hinson JP. Paracrine control of adrenocortical function: a new role for the medulla? J Endocrinol 1990;124:7–9.
117. Henion PD, Landis SC. Developmental regulation of leucine-enkephalin expression in adrenal chromaffin cells by glucocorticoids and innervation. J Neurosci 1992;12:3818–3827.
118. Suda T, Tomori N, Yajima F, Odagiri E, Demura H, Shizume K. Characterizaiton of immunoreactive corticotropin and corticotropin-releasing factor in human adrenal and ovarian tumors. Acta Endocrinol 1986;111:546–552.
119. Hokfelt B. Noradrenaline and adrenaline in mammalian tissue. Acta Physiol Scand 1951;25 (Suppl 92):5–134.
120. Yashiro Y, Kudo T, Kishimoto Y. Catecholamines in amniotic fluid as indicators of intrapartum fetal stress. Acta Med Okayama 1985;39:253–263.
121. Lagercrantz H, Bistoletti P. Catecholamine release in the newborn infant at birth. Pediatr Res 1977;11:889–893.
122. Holden KR, Young RB, Piland JH, Hurt GW. Plasma pressors in the normal and stressed newbord infant. Pediatrics 1972;49:495–503.
123. Greenough A, Nicolaides KH, Lagercrantz H. Human fetal sympathoadrenal responsiveness. Early Hum Dev 1990;23:9–13.
124. Quinn MW, Wild J, Dean HG, et al. Randomised double-blind controlled trial of effect of morphine on catecholamine concentrations in ventilated pre-term babies. Lancet 1993;342:324–327.
125. Anand KJS, Sippell WG, Schofield NM, Aynsley-Green A. Does halothane anesthesia decrease the metabolic and endocrine stress responses of newborn infants undergoing operation? Brit Med J 1988;296:668–672.
126. Stranek B, Lischka A, Hortnagl H, Pollak A. Sympatho-adrenal reponse to hypoglycaemia in infants. Eur J Pediatr 1988; 148:253–256.
127. Sarne DH, DeGroot LJ. Hypothalamic and neuroendocrine regulation of thyroid hormone. In: DeGroot LJ, ed. Endocrinology. WB Saunders, Philadelphia, 1989, pp. 574–589.
128. Burrow GN, Fisher DA, Larsen PR. Maternal and fetal thyroid function. N Engl J Med 1994;331:1072–1078.
129. Gorodzinsky P, Howard NU, Ginsberg J, Walfish PG. Cord serum thyroxine and thyrotropin values between twenty and thirty week's gestation. J Pediatr 1979;94:971–973.
130. Oppenheimer JH. Role of plasma proteins in the binding, distribution, and metabolism of the thyroid hormones. N Engl J Med 1968;278:1153–1162.
131. Chopra IJ, Sack J, Fisher DA. Circulating 3,3',5'-triiodothyronine (reverse T3) in the human newborn. J Clin Invest 1975;55:1137–1141.
132. Fisher DA. Thyroid disease in the neonate and in childhood. In: DeGroot LJ ed. Endocrinology. WB Saunders, Philadelphia, 1989, pp. 733–745.
133. Walfish PG, Tseng KH. Thyroid Physiology and Pathology. In: Collu R, Ducharme JR, Guyda HJ, eds. Pediatric Endocrinology, Raven, New York, 1989, pp. 367–448.

3 Growth, Development, and Critical Disease

Pamela A. Clark, MD,
and Alan D. Rogol, MD, PhD

Contents

> Normal Growth and Development
> Puberty
> Regulation of Growth and Development
> Growth in Various Disease States
> Renal Disease
> Oncologic Disease
> Pulmonary Disease
> Cardiac Disease
> Gastrointestinal Disease
> Immunologic Disease
> Metabolic Disease
> Endocrine Disease
> Conclusion
> References

NORMAL GROWTH AND DEVELOPMENT

Normal growth and development is testimony to the overall good general health of a child or adolescent. What constitutes the range of normal varies with the age, gender, and genetic background of the individual. Deviation from a previously defined pattern of growth or failure to undergo adolescent development at the appropriate time or tempo can often be the first clue to an underlying disease process.

The growth process represents the complex interaction of genetic and environmental factors. Sinclair (1) has shown that an individual's size, shape, and pattern of growth are strongly influenced by the genetic background. Although the exact contribution of heredity cannot be precisely determined, an estimate of an individual's genetic growth potential can be made by calculation of the midparental height. For females, 13 cm (~5 in.) is subtracted from the father's height, and averaged with the mother's height; for males, 13 cm is added to the mother's height and averaged with the father's height; 8.5 cm on either side of this value represents the target range for the 3rd to 97th percentiles

From *Contemporary Endocrinology: Endocrinology of Critical Disease*
Edited by K. P. Ober   Humana Press Inc., Totowa, NJ

for anticipated adult height *(2)*. For children with delayed or accelerated growth, it is helpful to adjust the child's height to the appropriate height percentile based on his/her skeletal (biological) age rather than chronologic age to determine more accurately if the child is growing appropriately for his/her genetic potential *(3)*.

Growth during the first year of life is marked by rapid increases in length and weight, averaging a gain of 25–30 cm and a tripling of birthweight *(4)*. During the second year of life, growth continues to decelerate, resulting in an average increase in size of 12 cm and 2.5 kg, as the child begins to attain a more linear habitus and becomes more muscular *(4)*. During these first 2 yr, a shift in the growth pattern is often observed as the child seeks the growth channel that has been genetically predetermined. This physiologic crossing of growth percentiles is typically accomplished by 12–18 mo in those infants experiencing "catch-up" growth, and by 18–24 mo in those shifting downward on the growth curve *(5)*. With the exception of puberty, crossing percentiles on the growth curve after this period is always of concern and warrants investigation.

After the age of 2 yr, growth during childhood is marked by a relatively constant rate averaging 5–6 cm and 2.5 kg/yr in both genders *(6)*. A wide range of normal exists for the growth velocity, however, and is dependent on which percentile a child is growing. Those children growing along the 3rd percentile average 5.1 cm/yr, whereas boys growing at the 97th percentile generally grow 6.4 cm/yr and girls 7.1 cm/yr during childhood to maintain their present trajectory *(7–9)*.

PUBERTY

Puberty is a time marked by rapid changes in body size, shape, and composition, all of which are sexually dimorphic. The sequence of events is the same within each gender, but significant individual differences exist with regard to the timing and tempo of pubertal growth and development. On average, girls enter and complete each stage of puberty earlier than boys. Just prior to the onset of the pubertal growth spurt, the height velocity slows to a nadir. The timing of the pubertal growth spurt occurs earlier in pubertal development in girls and does not reach the magnitude of that of boys. On average, girls reach their peak height velocity of 9 cm/yr at age 12 *(10)*, and boys attain a rate of 10.3 cm/yr on average 2 yr later *(11)*. The longer period of prepubertal growth in combination with a higher peak height velocity results in the average adult male being taller by 13 cm *(6)*. Growth virtually ceases when epiphyseal plate fusion occurs, typically around age 15 in girls and age 17 in boys. Adolescents (primarily boys) who enter puberty later than average appear to drift away from their previously defined growth channel, because they have not experienced an acceleration in growth typical for their chronologic age. This pattern of growth, in the absence of an underlying pathologic cause, is often familial and is associated with a delayed skeletal age. This is considered a normal variant of growth, and is referred to as constitutional delay of growth and adolescence.

Changes in body proportions are an important component of growth. During infancy the head-to-body ratio is approx 1:4, and the upper-to-lower segment ratio is about 1.7:1. Differential growth of the body and lower extremities results in a head-to-body ratio of 1:7.5 and an upper (crown to pubis) to lower (pubis to sole) segment ratio slightly <1.0 in adults *(1)*. Unusual body proportions for a child's chronologic age are a strong clue to a delay in growth and skeletal maturation secondary to an underlying illness or hormonal deficiency. At puberty, marked changes in body shape and composition occur, and result in typical female–male differences. Under the influence of gonadal steroid hormones, the typical android and gynoid patterns of body fat distribution are established; and there is differential growth of the shoulders and hips, and differences in lean tissue accrual between males and females. Fat accumulation decelerates in both genders as peak height velocity is approached, and there is an actual loss of fat in boys. As height velocity declines, fat accumulation resumes and is approximately twice as rapid in girls *(3)*. The net result is a decrease in the proportion of adipose to lean tissue in boys and an increase in girls. The increase in skeletal size, as well as muscle mass, during puberty is greater in boys, leading to increased strength. Children with pubertal delay or arrest will demonstrate a more childlike body shape and proportions, and may not accrue bone mineral normally owing to sex steroid hormone deficiency.

REGULATION OF GROWTH AND DEVELOPMENT

A variety of factors are responsible for normal growth and development. Prerequisites include: an adequate intrauterine environment, including a sufficient placenta, good maternal health and nutrition, and absence of exposure to maternal medications, substance abuse, and smoking; the absence of genetic syndromes affecting growth, such as skeletal dysplasias, the Turner syndrome, Down's syndrome, and Russell-Silver syndrome; and an adequate psychosocial environment. Nutrition, including energy intake, nutrient content, and proper gastrointestinal absorption, are paramount to normal growth and development. Finally, growth and development are regulated by several important hormones. Growth hormone (GH), its related peptide, insulin—like growth factor 1 (IGF-1), their binding proteins, and thyroid hormone are the primary hormones essential for prepubertal growth. GH promotes the synthesis of protein, inhibits the formation of fat and carbohydrate, and is necessary for cartilage proliferation at the epiphyseal plate leading to bone growth *(12)*. Thyroid hormone is essential to normal growth and development of the central nervous system, and works in concert with GH to promote cartilage and bone formation *(3)*. At puberty the gonadal steroid hormones and their interaction with the GH–IGF-1 axis are responsible for the acceleration of linear growth, sexual development, and the marked changes in body composition.

GROWTH IN VARIOUS DISEASE STATES

Abnormalities of growth and development owing to acute or chronic disease can result from a number of factors that are not mutually exclusive for any particular disease state. The mechanisms of growth retardation include those associated with:

1. The primary disease process;
2. Medical therapy, including glucocorticoids, chemotherapeutic agents, surgery, and irradiation;
3. Nutritional deprivation, including decreased intake, malabsorption, increased resting energy expenditure, or complications of restricted diets;
4. Hormonal derangements, primarily disorders of the GH, thyroid, adrenal, and gonadal axes; and
5. Psychosocial issues related to chronic illness.

Apart from organic causes of impaired growth, psychosocial dwarfism can occur in children with clinical depression or an inadequate emotional environment *(13)*. It should be noted that even seemingly inconsequential illnesses may disrupt the growth process. Children with frequent otitis media or upper respiratory tract infections may demonstrate suboptimal growth and cross percentiles on the growth curve, and even isolated bouts of influenza may transiently alter the rate of growth. Studies of short-term growth in children have shown that shrinkage may even occur during periods of catabolic stress, presumably owing to compression of nongrowing bone and cartilage and a possible shift in the balance between bone deposition and resorption during illness *(14)*. In general, such illnesses have self-limited effects, and catch-up growth is almost universally observed following resolution of symptoms. Our discussion will focus on those disease states, which have significant and enduring effects on growth and adolescent development.

RENAL DISEASE

Chronic renal insufficiency (CRI) is perhaps one of the best-studied disease states resulting in slow normal growth, but often growth failure, in children. The mechanism behind growth impairment is multifactorial, including metabolic acidosis, uremia, poor nutrition secondary to dietary restrictions and anorexia of chronic disease, anemia, calcium and phosphorus imbalance, renal osteodystrophy, and potential adverse effects on the circulating concentrations of growth factors and their binding proteins *(15)*. Additionally, the use of glucocorticoids to control the disease process has untoward effects on growth, possibly through a depressant effect on the hypothalamic–pituitary pulsatile release of GH, which contributes to an attenuated pubertal growth spurt *(16)*, as well as the action of the glucocorticoids on muscle anabolism and catabolism *(17)*.

The growth pattern of children with CRI was described by Betts and MacGrath in 1974 *(18)*. This and other studies demonstrated that more than one-half of these children have a final adult height at least 2 standard deviations (SD) below the mean *(18)*. Despite advances in medical therapy, including improved dialysis methods and renal transplantation, increases in growth velocity are not universal *(19,20)*. Rizzoni et al. *(21)* found that 62% of boys and 41% of girls undergoing therapy for end-stage renal disease (ESRD) before the age of 15 had a final adult height more than 2 SD below the mean, and a recent study of stature at the time of renal transplant has shown these children's heights to average -2.21 ± 0.004 SD *(20)*. Pubertal growth in children with CRI can be markedly retarded with a resultant decrease in final adult height *(22)*.

Despite consistent abnormalities of growth, measures of GH, IGF-1, and its primary binding protein, IGF-BP3, are typically normal in CRI, change with pubertal stage as in healthy children, and do not correlate with height SD scores *(23–25)*. Some investigators have postulated that there is partial resistance to GH in the uremic state. Reduced GH receptors in the liver, as indicated by low GH binding protein concentrations, result in decreased IGF-1 secretion *(26–28)*. The lowered receptor concentration in combination with reduced renal clearance of low-mol-wt fragments of IGF-BP3 act to decrease the availability of free, biolgically active IGF-1 *(29,30)*. The partial resistance to GH has been the rationale for the use of pharmacologic doses of recombinant human GH (rhGH) in CRI *(31)*.

The use of rhGH in CRI has now become the standard of care. Numerous studies over the past decade have confirmed a sustained increase in linear growth rate in children undergoing therapy for CRI, but especially following renal transplantation *(32–37)*. Although an accelerated growth rate has been documented with rhGH treatment among children receiving dialysis therapy, the response has generally been less robust than in those children who do not require dialysis *(31,38)*. The time required for catch-up growth varies and is probably determined mainly by the magnitude of the growth retardation at the initiation of rhGH therapy *(39)*. In addition to increases in stature, weight gain and an increase in midarm muscle circumference have been documented owing to the anabolic effects of GH *(33)*. Most studies have shown a greater response to rhGH in the first year of therapy for children with CRI as well as for most children with other conditions receiving rhGH therapy (e.g., GH deficiency and the Turner syndrome) *(38–42)*, but a persistent rise in growth velocity over baseline continues in subsequent years, resulting in an increase of 1.0–1.5 SD in final height *(43,44)*.

Potential adverse effects of rhGH therapy on the disease process have thus far not been detected. Investigators have reported no deterioration of renal disease, as indicated by creatinine clearance and glomerular filtration rate *(33,35,38,39)*, no exacerbation of the glucose intolerance of uremia *(31,32,39)*, and no aggravation of renal bone disease *(35)*. In addition, skeletal age does not advance more rapidly than chronologic age during therapy *(32,33,35,38)*, and may even mature less rapidly resulting in an increased adult height potential *(39)*. Some investigators have postulated the rhGH therapy may play a role in stimulating IGF-1 mRNA or changing the level of IGF-1 in tissues, such as kidney, bone, and muscle, where its paracrine or autocrine actions promote growth *(28)*. The interaction of nutritional state and IGF-1 transcription by the liver *(28)* has led some physicians to combine dietary therapy with rhGH treatment to optimize growth potential *(35)*.

Growth impairment in renal tubular acidosis (RTA) is distinct from CRI, since it does not result from a decline in renal function, but rather from significant acid-base disturbances. The resultant nonanion gap acidosis, likely in combination with poor nutrition, can lead to decreased GH secretion, as indicated by diminished GH secretory pulse area and pulse height *(45)*. Adequate bicarbonate therapy results in catch-up growth in the majority of children with RTA, which is often complete within 2 yr in those treated before the age of 2 yr, but frequently taking longer in older patients *(46,47)*.

ONCOLOGIC DISEASE

Growth impairment in children with malignancy has assumed greater importance with the advent of better treatment modalities that have permitted survival into adulthood. The survival rate is now >50% for children with acute lymphoblastic leukemia (ALL), especially since the introduction of CNS prophylactic irradiation *(48–50)*. The mechanism of growth impairment is typically multifactorial, and may present early during the course of the disease or many years after remission. Poor nutrition secondary to anorexia or vomiting owing to various chemotherapeutic agents is a major cause of diminished growth during the chemotherapy phase of treatment. Such effects are generally self-limited, and normal (or even catch-up) growth can be expected with the institution of proper nutrition. Additionally, chemotherapeutic agents typically do not damage the pituitary gland or the gonads, leaving pubertal development and growth undisturbed *(51)*.

A much different scenario exists for those children receiving CNS irradiation. Although short-term effects on appetite are also seen, the major concerns are those related to hypothalamic–pituitary dysfunction, gonadal damage, and injury to the growth centers of the spine. Growth failure is most commonly seen following craniospinal irradiation for brain tumors and total body irradiation in preparation for bone marrow transplantation *(51–53)*. One study noted similar decrements in linear growth with these two treatment modalities, but the time-courses differed. Diminished growth was observed in children receiving CNS irradiation in conjunction with chemotherapy at 1 yr followed by further declines at 2 and 3 yr. However, those children receiving total body irradiation plus chemotherapy did not manifest growth failure until the third year *(54)*. Cohen et al. *(52)* also reported growth impairment in children receiving either fractionated total body irradiation or cranial irradiation, and this was more marked in the latter group. The radiation dose itself is also an important factor. Rappaport and Brauner *(55)* reported that doses of 35–40 gy resulted in lower growth velocities as early as 2 yr after treatment with a mean loss of height potential of >1.0 SD by 7 yr after therapy, and doses in excess of 45 gy produced a more rapid decline in growth with 50% of those children losing 1.5 SD of height by 2 yr after therapy. Although growth is uniformly impaired following irradiation with >30 gy, more commonly employed doses of 18–24 gy have produced variable results *(56–60)*. Linear growth can also be affected by a deficiency of thyroid hormone secondary to head and neck irradiation. The threshold for thyroid damage is approx 10 gy delivered in conventional fractions, and clinically significant thyroid failure occurs with doses in excess of 20 gy (e.g, mantle field for Hodgkin's disease and craniospinal radiation for medulloblastoma) *(61)*.

Effects of therapy on growth and development extend beyond impairment of linear growth. One study has described smaller head circumferences in children treated with cranial irradiation at a dose of 24 gy, indicative of impaired brain growth *(62)*. Obesity following treatment of ALL and other tumors, especially craniopharyngiomas, is frequently observed *(62,63)*. Speculation on the etiology of the weight gain includes prior glucocorticoid therapy, stress hyperphagia, or injury to the hypothalamic satiety center secondary to surgery or irradiation. Schoenle et al. *(64)* treated a group of prepubertal children with rhGH following surgery for craniopharyngioma,and reported that although it did not influence height velocity, it decreased the body mass index and skinfold thickness, indicating a selective loss of fat tissue.

Effects on pubertal development are generally seen in those children undergoing irradiation. Direct gonadal damage is frequently seen in girls following abdominal, craniospinal, and total body irradiation, and in boys subsequent to direct testicular irradiation resulting in Leydig cell injury *(51,65)*. In such children, gonadal steroid hormone replacement will be necessary to induce sexual development. True precocious puberty may occur in very young girls receiving CNS irradiation owing to the increased sensitivity of the young hypothalamus to radiation *(66,67)*. Although initially described in children receiving >25 gy of cranial irradiation, it has more recently been observed with as low as 18 gy used for CNS prophylaxis in ALL *(68)*. Mild degrees of gonadal or hypothalamic dysfunction may also lead to early sexual maturation, primarily in girls. Although not true precocious puberty, the age of menarche in these girls is often advanced by approx 1 yr *(62,69)*. Gonadotropin-releasing hormone (GnRH) deficiency is rare following irradiation, except for very high-dose cranial irradiation (>35 gy) to the hypothalmic–pituitary region *(70)*, and these girls may have elevated levels of gonadotropins, indicative of subtle germ cell damage *(62,69)*. There appears to be no protective effect on the gonad of radiation delivered prior to the onset of puberty, and the spectrum of effect ranges from progressive damage from an early age to latent effects, which may not be evident until the onset of puberty or well into adulthood *(69)*. Some investigators have observed unexpected pubertal growth impairments in both early and normally maturing girls, leading to a diminished adolescent growth spurt and additional loss of height potential *(68,71)*.

Therapy for ALL has variable effects on the GH–IGF-1 axis. Although GH suppression secondary to dexamethasone therapy during the first 2 yr of treatment helps to explain the growth impairment early on *(72)*, no differences have been found between the GH profiles in children receiving total body irradiation or chemotherapy for bone marrow transplantation despite obvious differences in linear growth *(73)*. In contrast, cranial irradiation in doses in excess of 18 gy frequently induce GH deficiency, with the incidence and lag time correlated with the dose *(55,57)*. In many children, there is no correlation between results of GH testing and growth rate *(74–78)*, and IGF-1 levels tend to be within the normal range, even in those individuals whose height is below the 3rd percentile *(62)*. It is postulated that some children may not release sufficient amounts of GH under normal conditions despite adequate results on GH stimulation tests (i.e., GH neurosecretory defect) or a relative GH insufficiency, which becomes clinically apparent during puberty when the expected rise in GH secretion does not occur *(79)*. Conversely, in children who are growing at an age-appropriate rate, normal IGF-1 or insulin concentrations may explain adequate growth in the face of suboptimal GH levels *(74)*. The effects of radiation dose on the GH axis are not entirely clear. Some investigators have found no differences in GH secretion among children not irradiated and those receiving 18 or 24 gy *(72)*; however, others have found adverse dose-dependent effects, either related to the total radiation dose or the biologically effective dose, determined by the number of fractions, dose per fraction, and duration of therapy *(74,80,81)*. Treatment with 24 gy appears to affect GH secretion through dopaminergic pathways, implying selective damage to the hypothalamic GH-releasing neurons *(74)*.

Therapy with rhGH in children treated for neoplasms remains controversial, but studies to date have not found an increased risk of tumor recurrence or leukemia with its prudent use *(82–84)*. Therapy is generally delayed 6 mo to 1 yr after successful treatment of the underlying disease. Children with a history of spinal irradiation typically show an attenuated reponse to rhGH therapy *(85)*, and caution is warranted owing to the risk of disproportionate growth of the extremities with its use. Although rhGH treatment does not typically result in sustained catch-up growth or an increase final stature, it may prevent further loss of height in children treated with irradiation *(77,78,84)*.

PULMONARY DISEASE

The most common chronic pulmonary illness afflicting children is asthma. Growth retardation has been observed prior to the institution of glucocorticoid therapy, especially in those with poorly controlled asthma, indicating a direct effect of the disease process itself *(86–88)*. In those children and adolescents requiring frequent or continuous oral corticosteroid therapy, the inhibitory effects on growth are amplified, especially when the dose exceeds 0.35 mg/kg/d of prednisone *(89)*. Falliers et al. *(90)* found that 15% of children receiving intermittent glucocorticoid therapy and 35% on continuous oral glucocorticoid therapy had heights more than 2 SD below the mean. Alternate-day therapy of oral glucocorticoids decreases the adverse effects on growth, but many children still experience growth failure *(17,91,92)*.

The effects of regular, prophylactic doses of inhaled steroids, however, are less clear. Crowley et al. *(93)* studied 56 prepubertal children with asthma longitudinally, and found that 50% on standard doses of beclomethasone and nearly 20% on budesonide grew more slowly than controls, despite no differences in GH secretion or IGF-1 levels.

Lower growth velocities only at higher dosage levels (e.g., 800 µg/d of budesonide) have also been observed *(94)*. The method of administration may also be important, since metered dose inhalers deliver only 10–20% of the drug to the lungs and nearly 80% in the oropharynx where it is absorbed systemically *(95,96)*. The proper use of a spacer device can result in increased pulmonary delivery and lower systemic absorption *(97)*. Some investigators have documented lower growth velocities in boys, but not girls, receiving inhaled glucocorticoids, and propose that this may represent a delay in pubertal development in the boys secondary to asthma and/or typical patterns of male pubertal maturation (CDGA) rather than an adverse drug effect *(88,98)*.

Most investigators have not found any detrimental effects on growth velocity or skeletal maturation from inhaled steroids at conventional doses (e.g., up to 600 µg/d of budesonide or beclomethasone) *(94,99–101)*. Allen et al. *(102)* also found no evidence for growth suppression secondary to beclomethasone therapy, even when used in higher doses, for prolonged periods of time, or in children with more severe asthma. Individual sensitivity to glucocorticoids and simultaneous use of nasal steroids, however, may also influence their effects on growth *(103,104)*. Studies of final height attainment have generally been favorable. Although high-dose inhaled steroids may influence short-term measures of growth, there appears to be no decrease in adult stature *(105)*. Nevertheless, careful monitoring of growth is warranted in these children, especially when receiving high-dose inhaled steroid treatment chronically *(99)*. Oral calcium supplementation should also be considered owing to decreased osteocalcin, a marker of osteoblast activity and bone formation, in some children on chronic inhaled steroid therapy *(106)*. This is especially important during adolescence, a period of marked skeletal calcium accrual.

Cystic fibrosis (CF), although generally thought of as a chronic pulmonary disease, also overlaps with gastrointestinal illnesses owing to significant nutritional problems related to malabsorption. Growth retardation in children with CF is ultimately related to three factors that produce an energy deficit sufficient to limit growth or result in weight loss:

1. Poor nutritional intake;
2. Increased fecal losses through maldigestion and/or malabsorption; and
3. Increased energy requirements *(107)*.

Energy needs have been estimated at 120–150% of the RDA for age to compensate for these problems *(108–110)*, but studies of actual intake have found it to be only in the range of 80–100% when the children are relatively well and free from infection *(111–113)*. During bouts of infection, intake is typically less and is coupled with increased energy requirements. Fecal energy losses are substantial and can be equivalent to 5–20% of the gross energy intake, compared to 3–4% in healthy control children *(107)*. These losses are not simply the result of steatorrhea, since less than half of the energy within the stool has been attributed to lipid maldigestion *(107)*. Resting energy expenditure (REE) elevation appears to be related to pulmonary function, which typically worsens with age *(114)*. Infant studies utilizing doubly labeled water have detected a 25% increase in REE compared to healthy control babies *(115)*.

At birth infants with CF have a mean length close to normal, but over the first few months of life, linear growth is slow, resulting in a mean length SD of –1.3 by 3 mo of age *(116)*. Growth during childhood is largely dependent on the severity of disease, but pubertal growth is typically blunted. The adolescent growth spurt is delayed an average of 0.8 yr, and is marked by a lower height at takeoff and a decreased peak height velocity (approx 1 cm/yr slower) *(117)*. The peak height velocity is lower than expected, even for late-maturing children, especially in those with poor pulmonary function. Final height is generally diminished in patients with CF. Girls homozygous for the common δ F508 mutation are significantly more growth retarded than those with other CF mutations *(117)*, perhaps related to a greater REE associated with the mutation *(107)*.

Therapy for severe lung disease and chronic pulmonary infections can negatively impact growth. Children who are glucocorticoid-dependent have the most severe growth retardation. Alternate-day prednisone therapy should be used when possible in such children to attenuate the adverse effects on growth. Eigen et al. *(118)* demonstrated the efficacy of 1 mg/kg of prednisone given on alternate days on pulmonary function. This dose was associated with fewer abnormalities in glucose metabolism and less growth retardation than a dose of 2 mg/kg, but a decrease in height velocity was nonetheless noted after 24 mo of therapy. In children requiring chronic glucocorticoid therapy, rhGH treatment has not been efficacious *(119)*. Pancreatic insufficiency has a significant impact on nutrition and growth, especially prior to the institution of pancreatic enzyme replacement therapy. One study of infants with CF found a high incidence of fat malabsorption (up to 92% by 1 yr of age), resulting in slow weight gain, decreased body fat stores, and low serum albumin levels *(120)*. An aggressive regimen of pancreatic enzyme supplementation and high caloric intake can support normal growth in those children with mild disease *(121)*, but does not abolish steatorrhea in all children. Famotidine, a histamine receptor blocker that inhibits gastric acid secretion, has been found to be a useful adjunct to pancreatic enzyme treatment in some children to improve fat absorption, weight gain, and linear growth *(122)*. Tolbutamide, an agent that acts to augment insulin secretion and/or action, has also shown to be beneficial in some nondiabetic children with CF, resulting in a significant increase in growth velocity and lean body mass *(123)*.

CARDIAC DISEASE

Growth failure in children with congenital heart disease is primarily owing to inadequate nutrition in the setting of increased energy expenditure. A significant problem in these children is a poor appetite or refusal to eat, and investigators have found decreased weight, linear growth, and upper arm circumference measurements in those children with feeding difficulties *(124)*. Studies have consistently found that the caloric intake of children with congenital heart disease is less than that recommended for healthy children, despite their greater energy requirement *(124–126)*. Hansen and Dorup *(126)* found energy intake in children with congenital heart disease to be 88% of that recommended for actual weight, and demonstrated a significant correlation between energy intake and weight SD score. Over time, suboptimal nutrition leads to a decline in linear growth, but this tends to be less marked than the reduction in weight *(127)*. Growth retardation has been found to be greater in those children with cyanotic heart disease (tetralogy of Fallot, transposition of the great arteries) and to increase proportionately with the size of the left-to-right intracardial shunt *(127)*.

A high caloric diet is recommended for children with congenital heart disease to offset their elevated resting energy expenditure and to provide substrate for catch-up growth *(125,126)*. High-energy feedings have been shown to increase caloric intake by 31.7% and result in weight gains nearly 4.5 times those of similar children fed traditional diets *(125)*. Resting oxygen consumption, as indexed by VO_2 mL/kg/min, is comparable to that of normal formula feeds, although the respiratory quotient rises reflecting increased carbohydrate intake *(125)*. In addition to inadequate caloric intake, deficiencies of various nutrients also may contribute to the growth disturbance. Although protein intake is generally adequate in these children, even to support catch-up growth, intake of iron, zinc, calcium, and vitamins D, E, C, B_1, and B_6 typically fall below the recommended daily amounts, and should be supplemented in those children with poor growth and weight gain *(126)*.

GASTROINTESTINAL DISEASE

Celiac disease is a classic example of a chronic illness resulting in diminished growth, which can be completely reversed with proper dietary intervention. Although some investigators have found decreased weight, but not height, in children with celiac disease at the time of diagnosis *(128)*, most have observed decrements in linear growth as well. In fact, an "occult" form of the disease has been described in which short stature (mild growth failure) is the primary manifestation *(129,130)*. Hernandez et al. *(131)* found that in children diagnosed before age 2 yr, weight was most affected, but in those greater than age 2 yr, the decrease in height velocity was more pronounced than that in weight velocity. Retrospective studies have noted decreasing growth rate in the year prior to diagnosis, with a progressive decline in the mean weight-for-height 12–18 mo before diagnosis *(132)*. Radzikowski et al. *(133)* observed a lowered weight-for-age and height-for-age, and a delayed skeletal age for height prior to diagnosis. These were attributed to the children's progressive decline in nutritional status. Although no consistent endocrine abnormalities are found in these children, lower serum IGF-BP3 levels and increased somatostatin concentrations in the jejunal mucosa during active disease have been noted and return to normal with therapy *(131)*.

With the institution of a gluten-free diet, a marked acceleration in linear growth and weight gain is typically observed. The increase in weight-for-height is most dramatic during the first year of treatment and is generally within the normal range after 15 mo of therapy *(132)*. Linear catch-up growth is typically complete in 2–3 yr *(132,134)*. Damen et al. *(132)* found that children who were treated prior to age 9 yr had complete catch-up growth and a final height prognosis appropriate for genetic potential, independent of the degree of wasting, diagnostic delay, and strictness of the gluten-free diet.

Growth impairment in inflammatory bowel disease (Crohn's disease and ulcerative colitis) is typically multifactorial. Decreased appetite, malabsorption, frequent or continuous use of glucocorticoids, surgery, and extraintestinal complications act to hinder linear growth and weight gain. However, other yet undefined factors also influence linear growth velocity. Growth failure is common in Crohn's disease and may precede weight loss, thus, being the earliest manifestation of the disease in some children *(135)*. Serum IGF-1 levels are lower in those children with growth failure *(136)*, although it is unclear whether this reflects a poorer nutritional state or a specific manifestation of the disease process itself. Therapy in inflammatory bowel disease should be aimed at early and intensive nutritional support, and the use of steroid-sparing agents, such as 6-mercaptopurine, as well as the induction and maintenance of remission prior to and during adolescence to preserve the pubertal growth spurt *(137)*. The use of rhGH in children with inflammatory bowel disease is not recommended, since it does not overcome growth problems during active disease. Instead, adequate therapy of the underlying illness and an intense effort at proper nutrition result in an acceleration of weight gain and catch-up growth, without a need for rhGH treatment *(119)*.

IMMUNOLOGIC DISEASE

Disorders afflecting the immune system reflect a spectrum of illnesses from IgA deficiency to severe combined immunodeficiency syndome (SCID) to AIDS. Growth disorders in these conditions are primarily owing to the nutritional and metabolic effects of chronic infection and their treatment. AIDS is somewhat distinctive because of the associated wasting syndrome. In the most acutely ill patients with AIDS and secondary infection, a catabolic state exists characterized by hypermetabolism and depletion of lean body mass. The adaptive mechanisms that normally act to decrease energy expenditure and preserve lean body mass appear to be overridden or not operative *(138)*. This scenario is distinctly different from starvation in which fat tissue is preferentially depleted. Instead patients with AIDS may lose muscle protein along with fat in the early stages of the wasting syndrome *(139)*. Other causes of growth failure in children with AIDS include hypofunction of endocrine organs secondary to severe illness (e.g., adrenal insufficiency, thyroid abnormalities), endocrine side effects of treatment modalities, and in rare cases, infiltration of endocrine tissue by a secondary malignant process leading to hormonal insufficiency *(139,140)*. Hypogonadotropic hypogonadism, although infrequently seen, can contribute to a diminished growth velocity at the time of adolescence and failure to undergo spontaneous pubertal development *(140)*. Primary testicular involvement has also been observed in men with AIDS *(141)*, but the incidence in adolescents is unknown.

METABOLIC DISEASE

The most common metabolic disorder affecting children is insulin-dependent (type 1 diabetes) diabetes mellitus (IDDM). Although the Mauriac syndrome, that is, severe growth retardation in children with poorly controlled IDDM *(142)*, is now rare, more subtle growth disturbances are a source of continuing controversy. Malone et al. *(143)* observed that the distribution of heights in children with IDDM were skewed to the left with 61% less than the 50th percentile and 11% were shorter than expected for the normal distribution. Penfold et al. *(144)* found the mean adult height SD score of a group of individuals with IDDM to be -0.22 ± 1.15, which was reduced compared to the general population and to the subjects' parents and siblings. Several investigators have found the duration of IDDM to have a great influence on stature, with small decrements in height noted by 3–4 yr after diagnosis, but became statistically significant only at 7 yr *(143,145,146)*. Differences in adult stature have been found by some to depend on the age at diagnosis. Brown et al. *(147)* observed that those children aged 5–10 yr at diagnosis tended to be taller than control children initially, but subsequently had the greatest loss of height (final height SDS 0.0 ± 1.26). Children older than age 10 at diagnosis tended to be similar in height to control children and appeared to have the greatest final adult height (height SDS 0.09 ± 1.10); however, those <5 yr of age at diagnosis were initially much shorter than controls and remained so as adults (height SDS -0.74 ± 0.96) *(147)*. Price and Burden *(148)* reported that the loss of height between diagnosis and the onset of puberty averaged 0.06 SD/yr, resulting in a stunting of final height in those children who developed IDDM before puberty.

More optimistic findings of adult height attainment in children with IDDM have been reported by other investigators. Clarke et al. *(149)* and Vanelli et al. *(150)* found no overall decrease in height, either during childhood or as adults, in those children receiving standard insulin therapy. Delayed pubertal development and a blunting of the pubertal growth spurt were frequently reported in early studies of children with IDDM *(145,147,151)*, but these now appear to be uncommon *(149,152)*.

One of the factors frequently cited as influencing growth in children with IDDM is level of metabolic control. Although this relationship has been frequently studied, it remains controversial. Although several investigators have reported greater height velocity in children with good metabolic control *(143,153)*, others have found no relationship between glycosylated hemoglobin level and growth *(146,149,151,154–156)*. In addition, Wise et al. *(157)* reported a significant relationship between growth velocity and degree of metabolic control prepubertally, but this was overridden by the hormonal changes of puberty.

Batch and Werther *(158)* and Clark et al. *(159)* found patterns of GH secretion and levels of IGF-1 and binding proteins in children and adolescents with IDDM paralleling those of healthy controls. However, dysregulation of the GH–IGF-1 axis in children with IDDM has been frequently described, and characterized by elevated circulating levels of GH and lower concentrations of IGF-1 and IGF-BP3, the primary circulating binding protein for IGF-1 *(160–164)*. The mechanism in such cases is not entirely clear, but may represent "intracellular starvation" owing to inadequate metabolic control, akin to the GH–IGF-1 alterations seen in malnutrition and starvation *(165–168)*. Despite these abnormalities, no consistent relationship to linear growth velocity has been established, and the enhancement in GH secretion that occurs during puberty may be robust enough to override or reverse them *(157,159)*.

Weight is also an important issue in children with IDDM. At diagnosis, weight tends to be lower than age-matched children, with an average SD score reported by Thon et al. *(146)* as -0.26 ± 0.10, although by 2 yr after diagnosis, the children were heavier than controls; and at 3 yr, a dramatic increase in the weight-for-height ratio was detected. Weight during ongoing therapy, however, generally depends on the level of metabolic control, especially when the glycosylated hemoglobin level is at either extreme. Children in very poor control lose a substantial number of calories in urine and tend to be thin, whereas those who maintain very good control at the expense of additional insulin injections to compensate for food intake or frequent snacks to treat hypoglycemia are often overweight-for-height. This underscores the importance of proper nutritional counseling for these children and adolescents to provide a balance between adequate calorie intake and appropriate insulin dosage.

ENDOCRINE DISEASE

During childhood, the most common endocrine causes of growth impairment include hypopituitarism, isolated GH deficiency, hypothyroidism, cortisol excess (Cushing's disease or syndrome), and metabolic bone disease. In its most severe form, GH insufficiency is represented by the Laron syndrome, a hereditary insensitivity to GH owing to a receptor or postreceptor defect leading to the inability to generate IGF-1 *(169)*. Affected individuals exibit marked growth retardation from birth, and adult height typically ranges from 119–143 cm in males and 100–136 cm in females *(170)*. Treatment with rhGH is ineffective, but biosynthetic IGF-1 results in acceleration of linear growth velocity and a reduction in body fat content *(169)*.

More commonly found is isolated GH deficiency or GH deficiency associated with panhypopituitarism, both of which may be congenital or acquired. The clinical presentation in complete GH deficiency is age-dependent. Infants frequently have hypoglycemia in the newborn period and males may have microphallus *(171)*. Children experience marked growth failure, truncal fat deposition, an increased weight-for-height ratio, and a significant delay in skeletal maturation *(172)*. Growth impairment in the congenital form is evident shortly after birth. Wit and van Unen *(173)* found the mean length of infants with complete GH deficiency at age 4 mo to be –3.3 SD, which increased to –4.9 SD by 9 mo of age without intervention. Mean height in children with complete GH deficiency has been reported to be > –4 SD at the time of diagnosis *(172,174,175)*.

In children with complete GH deficiency, levels of circulating GH are low, but the diagnosis of GH deficiency cannot simply be made by measurement of random GH concentrations because of the pulsatile fashion in which GH is secreted. The use of 12- or 24-h measures of spontaneous GH secretion or provocative GH testing has not proven to be as helpful as once believed in discriminating idiopathic short stature from GH deficiency *(172)*. Children with complete GH deficiency do not have a significant rise of GH levels with pharmacologic stimulation, but the definition of a subnormal response is arbitrary and remains controversial *(176)*. Low levels of IGF-1 and IGF-BP3 are helpful in the diagnosis of GH deficiency and help to distinguish it from slow growth owing to inadequate nutrition (i.e., low IGF-1 with normal IGF-BP3). The response to rhGH therapy has also been proposed as one criterion for the diagnosis of growth hormone deficiency in children whose evaluation is not completely clear. A doubling or tripling of the growth velocity can be anticipated during the first year of therapy in children who are truly GH-deficient.

Therapy with rhGH results in a dramatic acceleration of growth velocity and catch-up growth, as well as favorable effects on body composition. Shih et al. *(175)* reported an increase in height velocity from 3.4 ± 0.7 to 11.3 ± 2.0 cm/yr during the first year of treatment, increasing the height SD score from -4.0 ± 0.5 to -2.7 ± 0.7. Zantleifer et al. *(177)* observed an increase in height of 1.3 SD during the first year of therapy, with a continued but smaller gain of 0.5 SD during the subsequent year. GH also results in a redistribution of abdominal fat to more peripheral sites *(178)* and increases bone mineralization *(179)*. Skeletal age tends to advance commensurate with chronological age during therapy, resulting in an increased final height prediction *(174,175)*.

Adult height of GH-deficient children treated with rhGH may depend on the growth deficit at the time of therapy. Boersma et al. *(174)* found that catch-up growth was nearly complete in those children with a height between –2 and –4 SD at the initiation of therapy, but those who were below –4 SD did not experience full catch-up growth during the first 4 yr of treatment. Pubertal maturation may also influence the reponse to rhGH therapy. Stanhope et al. *(180)* suggested that progression through puberty may be accelerated in children receiving rhGH treatment, which may act to counterbalance the gain in height prepubertally. Wit et al. *(172)* studied children with either isolated GH deficiency or panhypopituitarism who received rhGH therapy. Those children with isolated GH deficiency, who underwent spontaneous pubertal development, had an increase in height SD score from –4.7 to –2.8; however, those with hypogonadotropic hypogonadism who required gonadal steroid hormone replacement during adolescence had an increase in height SD score from –4.7 to –1.6. The greater final height in the hypogonadotropic group was attributed to a later onset of puberty and a relatively small dose of gonadal steroid hormone replacement, resulting in longer periods of prepubertal and pubertal growth.

Hypothyroidism is a well-recognized cause of growth failure in children. Since the majority of infants with congenital hypothyroidism appear normal at birth, thyroid screening during the newborn period was introduced in 1974 *(181)* and is now routine in North America, western Europe, Japan, New Zealand, Australia, and Israel *(182)*. The prognosis for normal growth and development is excellent in most infants in whom therapy is begun in the first weeks of life and in whom the serum thyroxine level is maintained in the upper portion of the normal range during the first year *(183–185)*.

Currently children with unrecognized acquired thyroid disease are those most likely to have significant growth retardation, especially when the diagnosis is delayed. Ozer et al. *(186)* studied a large cohort of children with hypothyroidism and found that with advancing age, the incidence of height below the 5th percentile increased from 44–80%. Skeletal age is significantly delayed, and may reflect the age of onset of hypothryroidism in those children with long-standing disease. Most children with untreated hypothyroidism will experience pubertal delay, but occasionally precocious puberty is observed and negatively influences the final height prognosis *(187)*. Therapy with l-thyroxine results in a significant acceleration of growth velocity and a period of rapid catch-up growth. Despite adequate treatment, however, some children have incomplete catch-up growth and do not achieve their target height *(188)*. This condition may occur in children with long-standing disease; skeletal maturation may occur more rapidly than normal when replacement therapy is instituted and the growth period becomes truncated.

Cushing's disease (pituitary adenoma) and Cushing's syndrome (adrenal tumor, ectopic ACTH production, or exogenous glucocorticoid excess) result in growth failure by a mechanism similar to that discussed in children with severe asthma *(189)*. Growth failure may occur long before the appearance of obesity or other symptoms, making it the presenting sign for some children *(190,191)*. Skeletal age and pubertal development are typically retarded owing to the inhibitory effects of glucocorticoids *(192)*, but may be normal or even advanced if an excess of adrenal androgens is also present *(193)*. Treatment is surgical in most cases and results in a rapid restoration of normal growth and development, often with catch-up growth to the original growth percentile, and a dramatic change in body habitus. Children and adolescents treated with irradiation typically experience a lag period of 6–12 mo before such effects become apparent *(194)*.

Metabolic bone disease resulting in rickets can produce profound growth retardation. Vitamin D-deficient rickets is now an uncommon disorder in industrialized countries, but can be seen among exclusively breast-fed toddlers or in children who do not consume dairy products. In children with hypophosphatemic rickets, an X-linked dominant disorder of renal tubular phosphate reabsorption, growth failure is the dominant feature *(195)*. Treatment with a combination of phosphate salts and calcitriol results in increased growth velocity *(196–198)*. The use of rhGH has also been suggested as an adjunct to improve growth and phosphate balance *(199)*.

In summary, most endocrine disorders result in a decrease in linear growth. However, unlike many of the illnesses discussed earlier, nutrition and weight are not adversely affected, and an increase in the weight-for-height ratio is commonly seen. In conditions accompanied by a delay in skeletal maturation, this, in part, reflects more infantile body proportions. Appropriate hormonal replacement or correction of hormonal excesses results in a period of rapid catch-up growth, which may be complete, although children with long-standing illness may not reach their genetically determined height potential.

CONCLUSION

One of the major consequences of systemic illness is an alteration of normal growth and pubertal maturation. The degree of influence ranges from mild delay in growth and adolescent development to profound growth retardation and failure to undergo spontaneous sexual maturation. Many of the adverse effects on growth and development are secondary to inadequate nutrition or side effects of therapy, particularly glucocorticoid administration, rather than the disease process itself. The aims of therapy should focus on adequate treatment of the underlying illness and optimal energy and nutrient intake. When feasible, therapies that adversely affect growth should be avoided or minimized. Currently, the use of rhGH therapy has documented benefit in only a few disorders, GH deficiency, CRI, and the Turner syndrome. Its use in other conditions is under investigation, but it has not been shown to be efficacious in disorders requiring chronic or frequent oral glucocorticoid therapy.

REFERENCES

1. Sinclair D. Human Growth After Birth, 3rd ed. Oxford University Press, London, 1978.
2. Tanner JM, Goldstein H, Whitehouse RH. Standards for children's heights at ages 2–9 years allowing for height of parents. Arch Dis Child 1970;45:755–762.
3. Rallison ML. Growth Disorders in Infants, Children, and Adolescents. John Wiley, New York, 1986.
4. Vaughan VC III. Growth and development. In: Vaughan VC, McKay RJ, Behrman RE, eds. Nelson's Textbook of Pediatrics, Saunders, Philadelphia, 1979;13–28.
5. Smith DW, Truog W, Rogers JE, Greitzer LJ, Skinner AL, McCann JJ, Harvey MA. Shifting linear growth during infancy: illustration of genetic factors in growth from fetal life through infancy. J Pediatr 1976;89:225–230.
6. Tanner JM. Fetus into Man; Physical Growth from Conception to Maturity. Harvard University Press, Cambridge, MA, 1978.
7. Roche AF, Himes JH. Incremental growth charts. Am J Clin Nutr 1980;33:2042–2052.
8. Baumgartner RN, Roche AF, Himes JH. Incremental growth tables. Am J Clin Nutr 1986;43:711–722.
9. World Health Organization. Measuring change in nutritional status. Geneva, 1983.
10. Marshall WA, Tanner JM. Variations in patterns of pubertal changes in girls. Arch Dis Child 1969;44:291–303.
11. Marshall WA, Tanner JM. Variations in patterns of pubertal changes in boys. Arch Dis Child 1970;45:13–23.
12. Zapf J, Schmid CH, Froesch ER. Biological and immunological properties of insulin-like growth factors (IGF) I and II. Clin Endocrinol Metab 1984;13:3–30.
13. Blizzard RM. Psychosocial short stature. In: Lifshitz, F, ed. Pediatric Endocrinology, 2nd ed. Dekker, New York, 1990, pp. 77–92.
14. Wales JKH, Gibson AT. Short term growth: rhythms, chaos, or noise? Arch Dis Child 1994;71:84–89.
15. Kaiser BA, Polinsky MS, Stover J, Morgenstern BZ, Baluarte HJ. Growth of children following the initiation of dialysis: a comparison of three dialysis modalities. Pediatr Nephrol 1994;8:733–738.
16. Rees L, Rigden SP, Chantler C. The influence of steroid therapy and recombinant human erythropoietin on the growth of children with renal disease. Pediatr Nephrol 1991;5:556–558.
17. Allen DB, Goldberg BD. Stimulation of collagen synthesis and linear growth by growth hormone in glucocorticoid-treated children. Pediatrics 1992;89:416–421.
18. Betts PR, MacGrath G. Growth patterns and dietary intake of children with chronic renal insufficiency. Br Med J 1974;2:189–193.
19. Fine RN. Growth after renal transplantation in children. Journal of Pediatrics 1987;110:414–416.
20. Stablein DM. Annual report 1992: North American Pediatric Renal Transplant Cooperative Study (NAPRTCS). Presented at the Annual NAPRTCS Meeting, Vancouver, Canada, October 1992.
21. Rizzoni G, Broyer M, Brunner FP, et al. Combined report on regular dialysis and transplantation of children in Europe. Proc Eur Dial Transplant Assoc—Eur Renal Assoc 1985;21:66–95.
22. Schafer F, Seidel C, Binding A, Gasser T, Largo RH, Prader A, Scharer K. Pubertal growth in chronic renal failure. Pediatr Res 1990;28:5–10.

23. Hodson EM, Brown AS, Roy LP, Rosenberg AR. Insulin-like growth factor-1, growth hormone-dependent insulin-like growth factor-binding protein and growth in children with chronic renal failure. Pediatr Nephrol 1992;6:433–438.
24. Jasper HG, Ferraris JR. Insulin-like growth factor 1 (IGF-1) and growth in children undergoing henodialysis or after successful renal transplantation. Medicina 1991;51:127–132.
25. Samaan NA, Freeman RM. Growth hormone levels in severe renal failure. Metab Clin Exp 1970;19:102–113.
26. Postel-Vinay MC, Tar A, Crosnier H, Broyer M, Rappaport R, Tonshoff B, Mehls O. Plasma growth hormone-binding activity is low in uraemic serum. Pediatr Nephrol 1991;5:545–547.
27. Blum WF. Insulin-like growth factors (IGFs) and IGF binding proteins in chronic renal failure: evidence for reduced secretion of IGFs. Acta Paediatr Scand 1991;379:S24–31.
28. Chan W, Valerie KC, Chan JCM. Expression of insulin-like growth factor-1 in uremic rats: growth hormone resistance and nutritional intake. Kidney Int 1993;43:790–795.
29. Powell DR, Liu F, Baker B, Lee PD, Belsha CW, Brewer ED, Hintz RL. Characterization of insulin-like growth factor binding protein 3 in chronic renal failure serum. Pediatr Res 1993;33:136–143.
30. Valentini RP, Mudge NA, Bunchman TE. Dialysis modality comparison of insulin-like growth factor binding protein-3 removal in children: could this have a potential growth benefit? Adv Peritoneal Dial 1994;10:327–330.
31. Hammerli I, Neuhaus T, Leumann E, Nussli R, Vischer D, Zachmann M. Therapy with growth hormone in pediatric patients with chronic kidney insufficiency. J Suisse Med 1994;124:1575–1580.
32. Fine RN, Pyke-Grimm K, Nelson PA, Boechat MI, Lippe BM, Yadin O, Kamil E. Recombinant human growth hormone treatment of children with chronic renal failure: long-term (1- to 3-year) outcome. Pediatr Nephrol 1991;5:477–481.
33. Fine RN, Yadin O, Moulton L, Nelson PA, Boechat MI, Lippe BM. Five years experience with recombinant human growth hormone treatment of children with chronic renal failure. J Pediatr Endocrinol 1994;7:1–12.
34. Lippe B, Yadin O, Fine RN, Moulton L, Nelson PA. Use of recombinant human growth hormone in children with chronic renal insufficiency: an update. Horm Res 1993;40:102–108.
35. Van Renen MJ, Hogg RJ, Sweeney AL, Henning PH, Penfold JL, Jureidini KF. Accelerated growth in short children with chronic renal failure treated with both strict dietary therapy and recombinant growth hormone. Pediatr Nephrol 1992;6:451–458.
36. Johansson G, Sietneiks A, Janssens F, et al. Recombinant human growth hormone treatment in children with chronic renal disease, before transplantation or with functioning renal transplants: An interim report on five European studies. Acta Paediatr Scand 1990;370:36–42.
37. Rees L, Rigden S, Ward G, Preece MA. Treatment of short stature in renal disease with recombinant human growth hormone. Arch Dis Child 1990;65:856–860.
38. Mehls O, Broyer M. Growth response to recombinant human growth hormone in short prepubertal children with chronic renal failure with or without dialysis. The European/Australian Study Group. Acta Paediatr Suppl 1994;399:81–87.
39. Fine RN, Kohault EC, Brown D, Perlman AJ. Growth after recombinant human growth hormone treatment in children with chronic renal failure: a report of a multicenter randomized double-blind placebo-controlled study. Genentech Cooperative Study Group. J Pediatr 1994;124:374–382.
40. Rongen-Westerlaken C, van Es A, Wit J-M, et al. Growth hormone therapy in Turner's syndrome: impact of injection frequency and initial bone age. Am J Dis Child 1992;146:817–820.
41. Rosenfeld RG, Frane J, Attie KM, et al. Six-year results of a randomized, prospective trial of human growth hormone and oxandrolone in Turner syndrome. J Pediatr 1992;121:49–55.
42. Furlanetto RW, et al. Guidelines for the use of growth hormone in children with short stature. A report by the Drug and Therapeutics Committee of the Lawson Wilkins Pediatric Endocrine Society. J Pediatr 1995;127:857–867.
43. Tonshoff B, Dietz M, Haffner D, Tonshoff C, Stover B, Mehls O. Effects of two years of growth hormone treatment in short children with renal disease. The German Study Group for Growth Hormone Treatment in Chronic Renal Failure. Acta Paediatr Scand 1991;379:S33–41.
44. Van Es A. Growth hormone treatment in short children with chronic renal failure after renal transplantation: combined data from European clinical trials. Acta Paediatr Scand 1991;379:S42–48.
45. Challa A, Krieg RJ, Thabet MA, Veldhuis JD, Chan JCM. Metabolic acidosis inhibits growth hormone secretion in rats: mechanism of growth retardation. Am J Physiol 1993;265:E547–553.

46. Caldas A, Broyer M, Dechaux M, Kleinknecht C. Primary distal tubular acidosis in childhood: clinical study and long-term follow-up of 28 patients. J Pediatr 1992;121:233–241.
47. Tsau YK, Chen CH, Tsai WS, Chiou YM. Renal tubular acidosis in childhood. Acta Paediatr Sinica 1990;31:205–213.
48. Pinkel D. Curing children of leukemia. Cancer 1987;59:1683–1691.
49. Morris-Jones PH, Craft AW. Childhood cancer at what cost? Arch Dis Child 1990;65:638–640.
50. Goldman JM. Prospects for cure in leukemia. J Clin Pathol 1987;40:985–994.
51. Sklar CA. Growth and pubertal development in survivors of childhood cancer. Pediatrician 1991;18:53–60.
52. Cohen A, van Lint MT, Uderzo C, Rovelli A, Lavagetto A, Vitale V, Morchio A, Locasciulli A, Bacigalupo A, Romano C. Growth in patients after allogenic bone marrow transplant for hematological diseases in childhood. Bone Marrow Transplant 1995;15:343–348.
53. Avizonis VN, Fuller DB, Thomson JW, Walker MJ, Nilsson DE, Menlove RL. Late effects following central nervous system radiation in a pediatric population. Neuropediatrics 1992;23:228–234.
54. Bozzola M, Giorgiani G, Locatelli F, Cisternino M, Gambarana D, Zecca M, Torcetta F, Severi F. Growth in children after bone marrow transplantation. Horm Res 1993;39:122–126.
55. Rappaport R, Brauner R. Growth and endocrine disorders secondary to cranial irradiation. Pediatr Res 1989;25:561–567.
56. Clayton PE, Shalet SM, Morris-Jones PH, Price DA. Growth in children treated for acute lymphoblastic leukemia. Lancet 1988;1:490–462.
57. Shalet SM, Clayton PE, Price DA. Growth and pituitary function in children treated for brain tumors or acute lymphoblastic leukemia. Horm Res 1988;30:53–61.
58. Kirk JA, Raghupathy P, Stevens MM, Cowell CT, Menser MA, Bergin M, Tink A, Vines RH, Silink M. Growth failure and growth hormone deficiency after treatment for acute lymphoblastic leukemia. Lancet 1987;1:190–193.
59. Wells RJ, Foster MB, D'Ercole J, McMillan CW. The impact of cranial irradiation on the growth of children with acute lymphoblastic leukemia. Am J Dis Child 1988;137:37–39.
60. Robinson LL, Nesbit ME, Sather HN, Meadows AT, Ortega JA, Hammond GD. Height of children treated for acute lymphoblastic leukemia: a report from the Late Effects Study Committee of Childrens Cancer Study Group. Med Pediatr Oncol 1985;13:14–21.
61. Schimpff SG, Diggs GH, Wiswell JG, Salvatore PC, Wiernik PH. Radiation related thyroid dysfunction: implications for the treatment of Hodgkin's disease. Ann Intern Med 1980;92:91–98.
62. Dacou-Voutetakis C, Kitra V, Grafakos S, Polychronopoulou S, Drakopoulou M, Haidas S. Auxologic data and hormonal profile in long-term survivors of childhood acute lymphoid leukemia. Amer J Pediatr Hematol Oncol 1993;15:277–283.
63. Sainsbury CPQ, Newcombe RG, Hughes IA. Weight gain and height velocity during prolonged first remission from acute lymphoblastic leukemia. Arch Dis Child 1985;60:832–836.
64. Schoenle EJ, Zapf J, Prader A, Torresani T, Werder EA, Zachmann M. Replacement of growth hormone (GH) in normally growing GH-deficient patients operated for craniopharyngioma. J Clin Endocrinol Metab 1995;80:374–378.
65. Shalet SM. Gonadal function following radiation and cytotoxic chemotherapy in children. Ergeb Inn Med Kinderheilkd 1989;58:1–21.
66. Shalet SM, Crowne EC, Didi MA, Ogilvy-Stuart AL, Wallace WH. Irradiation-induced growth failure. Bailliere's Clin Endocrinol Metab 1992;6:513–526.
67. Brauner R. Hypothalamic–hypophyseal function after treatment of cancers. Ann Endocrinol 1995;56:127–131.
68. Leiper AD, Stanhope R, Kitching P, Chessells JM. Precocious and premature puberty associated with treatment of acute lymphoblastic leukemia. Arch Dis Child 1987;62:1107–1112.
69. Quigley C, Cowell C, Jimenez M, Burger H, Kirk J, Bergin M, Stevens M, Simpson J, Silink M. Normal or early development of puberty despite gonadal damage in children treated for acute lymphoblastic leukemia. N Engl J Med 1989;321:143–151.
70. Rappaport R, Brauner R, Czernichow P, Thibaud E, Renier D, Zucker JM, Lemerle J. Effect of hypothalamic and pituitary irradiation on pubertal development in children with cranial tumors. J Clin Endocrinol Metab 1982;54:1164–1168.
71. Oberfield SE, Allen JC, Pollack J, New MI, Levine LS. Long-term endocrine sequelae after treatment of medulloblastoma: prospective study of growth and thyroid function. J Pediatr 1986;108:219–223.

72. Marky I, Mellander L, Lannering B, Albertsson-Wikland K. A longitudinal study of growth and growth hormone secretion in children during treatment for acute lymphoblastic leukemia. Med Pediatr Oncol 1991;19:258–264.
73. Brauner R, Fontoura M, Zucker JM, Devergie A, Souberbbielle JC, Prevot-Saucet C, Michon J, Gluckman E, Griscelli C, Fischer A, et al. Growth and growth hormone secretion after bone marrow transplantation. Arch Dis Child 1993;68:58–463.
74. Cicognani A, Emanuele C, Vecchi V, Cau M, Balsamo A, Pirazzoli P, Tosi M, Rosito P, Paolucci G. Differential effects of 18- and 24-Gy cranial irradiation on growth rate and growth hormone release in children with prolonged survival after acute lymphocytic leukemia. Am J Dis Child 1988;142:1199–1202.
75. Shalet SM, Price DA, Beardwell CG, Jones PH, Pearson D. Normal growth despite abnormalities of growth hormone secretion in children treated for acute leukemia. J Pediatr 1979;4:719–722.
76. Blatt J, Bercu BB, Gillin JC, Mendelson WB, Poplack DG. Reduced pulsatile growth hormone secretion in children after therapy for acute leukemia. J Pediatr 1984;108:182–186.
77. Brauner R, Prevot C, Roy MP, Rappaport R. Growth, growth hormone secretion and somatomedin C after cranial irradiation for acute lymphoblastic leukemia. Acta Endocrinol 1986;279:178–182.
78. Cowell CT, Quigley CA, Moore B, Kirk JA, Bergin M, Jimenez M, Stevens MM, Howard NJ, Menser MA, Silink M. Growth and growth hormone therapy in children treated for leukemia. Acta Paediatr Scand 1988;343:152–161.
79. Moell C, Garwicz S, Westgren U, Wiebe T, Albertsson-Wikland K. Suppressed spontaneous secretion of growth hormone in girls after treatment for acute lymphoblastic leukemia. Arch Dis Child 1989;64:258–262.
80. Ellis F. Dose, time and fractionation: a clinical hypothesis. Radiology 1969;20:1–7.
81. Shalet SM, Beardwell CG, Pearson D, Jones PH. The effect of various doses of cerebral irradiation on growth hormone production in childhood. Clin Endocrinol 1976;5:287–290.
82. Arslanian SA, Becker DJ, Lee PA, Drash AL, Foley TP Jr.. Growth hormone therapy and tumor recurrence. Findings in children with brain neoplasms and hypopituitarism. Am J Dis Child 1985;139:347–350.
83. Clayton PE, Shalet SM, Gattamaneni HR, Price DA. Does growth hormone therapy cause relapse of brain tumors? Lancet 1987;1:711–713.
84. Livesey EA, Hindmarsh PC, Brook CGD, Whitton AC, Bloom HJ, Tobias JS, Godlea TN, Britton J. Endocrine disorders following treatment of childhood brain tumors. B J Cancer 1990;61:622–625.
85. Clayton PE, Shalet SM, Price DA. Growth response to growth hormone therapy following craniospinal irradiation. Eur J Pediatr 1988;147:597–601.
86. Nasiff E, Weinberger M, Sherman B, Brown K. Extrapulmonary effects of maintenance corticosteroid therapy with alternate day prednisolone and inhaled beclomethasone in children with chronic asthma. J Allergy Clin Immunol 1987;80:518–528.
87. Ninan TK, Russell G. Asthma, inhaled corticosteroid treatment, and growth. Arch Dis Child 1992;67:703–705.
88. Balfour-Lynn L. Growth and childhood asthma. Arch Dis Child 1986;61:1049–1055.
89. Rivkees SA, Danon M, Herrin J. Prednisone dose limitation of growth hormone treatment of steroid-induced growth failure. J Pediatr 1994;125:322–325.
90. Falliers CJ, Tan LS, Szentivanyi J, Jorgensen JR, Bukantz SC. Childhood asthma and steroid therapy as influences on growth. Am J Dis Child 1963;105:127–137.
91. Reimer LG, Morris HG, Ellis FE. Growth of asthmatic children during treatment with alternate-day steroids. J Allergy Clin Immunol 1975;55:224–231.
92. Avioli LV. Glucocorticoid effects on statural growth. Br J Rheumatol 1993;32:27–30.
93. Crowley S, Hindmarsh PC, Matthews DR, Brook CG. Growth and the growth hormone axis in prepubertal children with asthma. J Pediatr 1995;126:297–303.
94. Wolthers OD, Pedersen S. Controlled study of linear growth in asthmatic children during treatment with inhaled glucocorticosteroids. Pediatr 1992;89:839–842.
95. Toogood JH, Frankish CW, Jennings BH, Baskerville JC, Borga O, Lefcoe NM, Johansson SA. A study of the mechanism of the anti-asthmatic action of inhaled budesonide. J Allergy Clin Immunol 1990;85:872–880.
96. Newman SP, Pavia D, Morer F. Deposition of pressurised aerosols in the human respiratory tract. Thorax 1981;36:52–55.
97. Newman SP, Miller AB, Lennard-Jones TR. Improvement of pressurised aerosol/deposition with Nebuhaler spacer device. Thorax 1984;39:935–941.

98. Merkus PJ, van Essen-Zandvliet EE, Duiverman EJ, van Houwelingen HC, Kerrebijn KF, Quanjer PH. Long-term effects of inhaled corticosteroids on growth rate in adolescents with asthma. Pediatrics 1993;91:1121–1126.
99. Price JF. Asthma, growth and inhaled corticosteroids. Resp Med 1993;87:23–26.
100. Ruiz RG, Price JF. Growth and adrenal responsiveness with budesonide in young asthmatics. Resp Med 1994;88:17–20.
101. Volovitz B, Amir J, Malik H, Kauschansky A, Varsano I. Growth and pituitary-adrenal function in children with severe asthma treated with inhaled budesonide. N Eng J Med 1993;329:1703–1708.
102. Allen DB, Mullen M, Mullen B. A meta-analysis of the effect of oral and inhaled corticosteroids on growth. J Allergy Clin Immunol 1994;93:967–976.
103. Wales JKH, Barnes MD, Swift PGP. Growth retardation in children on steroids for asthma. Lancet 1991;338:1535.
104. Hollman GA, Allen DB. Overt glucocorticoid excess due to inhaled corticosteroid therapy. Pediatrics 1988;81:452–455.
105. Barnes NC. Safety of high-dose inhaled corticosteroids. Resp Med 1993;87:27–31.
106. Boner AL, Piacentini GL. Inhaled corticosteroids in children. Is there a "safe" dosage? Drug Safety 1993;9:9–20.
107. Wooton SA, Murphy JL, Bond SA, Ellis JE, Jackson AA. Energy balance and growth in cystic fibrosis. J R Soc Med 1991;84:22–27.
108. Littlewood JM, MacDonald A. Rationale of modern dietary recommendations in cystic fibrosis. J R Soc Med 1987;80:16–24.
109. Hubbard VS. Nutritional considerations in cystic fibrosis. Semin Resp Med 1985;6:308–313.
110. Roy CC, Darling P, Weber AM. A rational approach to meeting the macro-and micronutrient needs in cystic fibrosis. J Paediatr Gastroenterol Nutr 1984;3:S154–162.
111. Bell L, Linton W, Corey ML, Durie P, Forstner GG. Nutrient intakes of adolescents with cystic fibrosis. J Can Diet Assoc 1981;42:62–71.
112. Buchdahl RM, Fully Lare C, Marchant JL, Warner JO, Brueton MJ. Energy and nutrient intakes in cystic fibrosis. Arch Dis Child 1989;64:373–378.
113. Chase HP, Long MA, Lavin MH. Cystic fibrosis and malnutrition. J Pediatr 1979;95:337–347.
114. Vaisman N, Pencharz PB, Corey M, Canny GJ, Hahn E. Energy expenditure in patients with cystic fibrosis. J Pediatr 1987;111:496–500.
115. Shepherd RH, Holt TL, Vasques-Velasquez L, Coward WA, Prentice A, Lucas A. Increased energy expenditure in young children with cystic fibrosis. Lancet 1988;1:1300–1303.
116. Karlberg J, Kjellmer I, Kristiansson B. Linear growth in children with cystic fibrosis. Acta Paediatr Scand 1991;80:508–514.
117. Byard PJ. The adolescent growth spurt in children with cystic fibrosis. Ann Hum Biol 1994;21:229–240.
118. Eigen H, Rosenstein BJ, FitzSimmons S, Schidlow DV. A multicenter study of alternate-day prednisone therapy in patients with cystic fibrosis. Cystic Fibrosis Foundation Prednisone Trial Group. J Pediatr 1995;126:515–523.
119. Allen DB, Brook CGD, Bridges NA, Hindmarsh PC, Guyda HJ, Frazier D. Therapeutic controversies: Growth hormone (GH) treatment of non-GH deficient subjects. J Clin Endocrinol Metab 1994;79:1239–1248.
120. Bronstein MN, Sokol RJ, Abman SH, Chatfield BA, Hammond KB, Hambidge KM, Stall CD, Accurso FJ. Pancreatic insufficiency, growth, and nutrition in infants identified by newborn screening as having cystic fibrosis. J Pediatr 1992;120:533–540.
121. Tomezsko JL, Stallings VA, Scanlin TF. Dietary intake of healthy children with cystic fibrosis compared with normal control children. Pediatr. 1992;90:547–553.
122. Carroccio A, Pardo F, Montalto G, Iapichino L, Soresi M, Averna MR, Iacono G, Notarbartolo A. Use of famotidine in severe exocrine pancreatic insufficiency with persistent maldigestion on enzymatic replacement therapy. A long-term study in cystic fibrosis. Dig Dis Sci 1992;37:1441–1446.
123. Zipf WB, Kien CL, Horswill CA, McCoy KS, O'Dorisio T, Pinyerd BL. Effects of tolbutamide on growth and body composition of nondiabetic children with cystic fibrosis. Pediatr Res 1991;30:309–314.
124. Thommessen M, Heiberg A, Kase BF. Feeding problems in children with congenital heart disease: the impact on energy intake and growth outcome. Eur J Clin Nutr 1992;46:457–464.
125. Jackson M, Poskitt EM. The effects of high-energy feeding on energy balance and growth in infants with congenital heart disease and failure to thrive. Br J Nutr 1991;65:131–143.

126. Hansen SR, Dorup I. Energy and nutrient intakes in congenital heart disease. Acta Paediatr 1993;82:166–172.
127. Tambic-Bukovac L, Malcic I. Growth and development in children with congenital heart defects. Lijecnicki Vjesnik 1993;115:79–84.
128. Bode SH, Bachman EH, Gudmand-Hoyer E, Jensen GB. Stature of adult coeliac patients: no evidence for decreased attained height. Eur J Clin Nutr 1991;45:145–149.
129. Groll A, Candy DCA, Preece MA, Tanner JM, Harries JT. Short stature as the primary manifestation of coeliac disease. Lancet 1980;2:1097–1099.
130. Rosenbach Y, Dinari G, Zahavi I, Nitzan M. Short stature as the major manifestation of celiac disease in older children. Clin Pediatr 1986;25:13–16.
131. Hernandez M, Argente J, Navarro A, Caballo N, Barrios V, Hervas F, Polanco I. Growth in malnutrition related to gastrointestinal diseases: coeliac disease. Horm Res 1992;38:79–84.
132. Damen GM, Boersma B, Wit JM, Heymans HS. Catch-up growth in 60 children with celiac disease. J Pediatr Gastroenterol Nutr 1994;19:394–400.
133. Radzikowski A, Kulus M, Krauze A, Wojnar M, Koczynski A. Growth, bone age and nutritional status in neglected coeliac disease. Materia Medica Polona 1991;23:146–150.
134. Boersma B, Wynne HJ, Wit JM. A mathematical model describing catch-up growth in celiac disease. Acta Paediatr 1994;83:1097–1099.
135. Kanof ME, Lake AM, Bayless TM. Decreased height velocity in children and adolescents before the diagnosis of Crohn's disease. Gastroenterology 1988;95:1523–1527.
136. Kirschner BS, Sretton MM. Somatomedin-C levels in growth impaired children and adolescents with chronic inflammatory bowel disease. Gastroenterology 1986;91:830–836.
137. Brain CE, Savage MO. Growth and puberty in chronic inflammatory bowel disease. Baillieres Clin Gastroenterol 1994;8:83–100.
138. Grinspoon SK, Donovan DS, Bilezikian JP. Aetiology and pathogenesis of hormonal and metabolic disorders in HIV infection. Baillieres Clin Endocrinol Metab 1994;8:735–755.
139. Grinspoon SK, Bilezikian JP. HIV disease and the endocrine system. N Engl J Med 1992;327:1360–1364.
140. Strauss KW. Endocrine complications of the acquired immunodeficiency syndrome. Arch Int Med 1991;151:1441–1444.
141. Masharani U, Schambelan M. The endocrine complications of acquired immunodeficiency syndrome. Adv Int Med 1993;38:323–336.
142. Mauras N, Merimee T, Rogol AD. Function of the growth hormone—insulin-like growth factor I axis in the profoundly growth-retarded diabetic child: evidence for defective target organ responsiveness in the Mauriac syndrome. Metabolism 1991;40:1106–1111.
143. Malone JI, Lowitt S, Duncan JA, Shah SC, Vargas A, Root AW. Hypercalciuria, hyperphosphaturia, and growth retardation in children with diabetes mellitus. Pediatrics 1986;78:298–304.
144. Penfold J, Chase HP, Marshall G, Walravens CF, Walravens PA, Garg SK. Final adult height and its relationship to blood glucose control and microvascular complications in IDDM. Diabetic Med 1995;12:129–133.
145. Lee TJ, Stewart-Brown S, Wadsworth J, Savage DCL. Growth in children with diabetes. In: Borms J, ed. Human Growth and Development Plenum, New York, 1984, pp 613–618.
146. Thon A, Heinze E, Feilen K-D, Holl RW, Schmidt H, Koletzko S, Wendel U, Nothjunge J. Development of height and weight in children with diabetes mellitus: report on two prospective multicentre studies, one cross-sectional, one longitudinal. Eur J Pediatr 1992;151:258–262.
147. Brown M, Ahmed ML, Clayton KL, Dunger DB. Growth during childhood and final height in type 1 diabetes. Diabetic Med 1994;11:182–187.
148. Price D, Burden A. Growth of children before onset of diabetes. Diabetes Care 1992;15:1393–1395.
149. Clarke WL, Vance ML, Rogol AD. Growth and the child with diabetes mellitus. Diabetes Care 1993;16:101–106.
150. Vanelli M, de Fanti A, Adinolfi B, Ghizzoni L. Clinical data regarding the growth of diabetic children. Horm Res 1992;37:65–69.
151. Salardi S, Tonoili S, Tassoni P, Tellarini M, Mazzanti L, Cacciari E. Growth and growth factors in diabetes mellitus. Arch Dis Child 1987;62:57–62.
152. Dunger DB, Edge JAE, Ahmed ML. Diabetes mellitus and growth. Unpublished.
153. Jackson R, Holland E, Chatman T, Guthrie D, Hewett J. Growth and maturation of children with insulin dependent diabetes mellitus. Diabetes Care 1978;1:94–107.

154. Hjelt K, Braendholt V, Kamper J, Vestermark S. Growth in children with diabetes mellitus. Dan Med Bull 1983;30:28–33.
155. Herber SM, Dunsmore IR. Does control affect growth in diabetes mellitus? Acta Paediatr Scand 1988;77:303–305.
156. Clarson C, Daneman D, Ehrlich RM. The relationship of metabolic control to growth and pubertal development in children with insulin-dependent diabetes. Diabetes Res 1988;2:237–241.
157. Wise JE, Kolb EL, Sauder SE. Effect of glycemic control on growth velocity in children with IDDM. Diabetes Care 1992;15:826–830.
158. Batch JA, Werther GA. Changes in growth hormone concentrations during puberty in adolescents with insulin dependent diabetes. Clin Endocrinol 1992;36:411–416.
159. Clark PA, Clarke WL, Peddada S, Reiss A, Langlois C, Nieves-Rivera F, Rogol AD, unpublished. The effect of pubertal status on the growth hormone–IGF-1 axis in boys with diabetes mellitus.
160. Edge JA, Dunger DB, Matthews DR, Gilbert JP, Smith CP. Increased overnight growth hormone concentrations in diabetic compared to normal adolescents. J Clin Endocrinol Metab 1990;71:1356–1362.
161. Holl RW, Siegler B, Scherbaum WA, Heinze E. The serum growth hormone-binding protein is reduced in young patients with insulin-dependent diabetes mellitus. J Clin Endocrinol Metab 1993;76:165–167.
162. Batch JA, Baxter RC, Werther G. Abnormal regulation of insulin-like growth factor binding proteins in adolescents with insulin-dependent diabetes. J Clin Endocrinol Metab 1991;73:964–968.
163. Clayton KL, Holly JMP, Carlsson LMS, Jones J, Cheetham TD, Taylor AM, Dunger DB. Loss of the normal relationships between growth hormone, growth hormone-binding protein and insulin-like growth factor-1 in adolescents with insulin-dependent diabetes mellitus. Clin Endocrinol 1994;41:517–524.
164. Nieves-Rivera F, Rogol AD, Veldhuis JD, Branscom DK, Martha PM Jr, Clarke WL. Alterations in growth hormone secretion and clearance in adolescent boys with insulin-dependent diabetes mellitus. J Clin Endocrinol Metab 1993;77:638–643.
165. Oster MH, Fielder PJ, Levin N, Cronin MJ. Adaption of the growth hormone and insulin-like growth factor-I axis to chronic and severe calorie or protein malnutrition. J Clin Invest 1995;95:2258–2265.
166. Abdenur JE, Pugliese MT, Cervantes C, Fort P, Lifshitz F. Alterations in spontaneous growth hormone (GH) secretion and the response to GH-releasing hormone in children with nonorganic nutritional dwarfing. J Clin Endocrinol Metab 1992;75:930–934.
167. Hochberg Z, Hertz P, Colin V, Ish-Shalom S, Yeshurun D, Youdim M, Amit T. The distal axis of growth hormone (GH) in nutritional disorders: GH-binding protein, insulin-like growth factor-1, and IGF-1 receptors in obesity and anorexia nervosa. Metabolism 1992;41:106–112.
168. Smith WJ, Underwood LE, Clemmons DR. Effects of calorie or protein restriction on insulin-like growth factor-1 (IGF-1) and IGF-binding proteins in children and adults. J Clin Endocrinol Metab 1995;80:443–449.
169. Laron Z, Klinger B. Laron syndrome: clinical features, molecular pathology and treatment. Horm Res 1994;42:198–202.
170. Laron Z. Laron type dwarfism (hereditary somatomedin deficiency): a review. Adv Int Med Pediatr Idlebey, Springer-Verlag, 1984, p. 118.
171. Lovinger RD, Kaplan SL, Grumbach MM. Congenital hypopituitarism associated with neonatal hypoglycemia and microphallus: four cases secondary to hypothalamic hormone deficiencies. J Pediatr 1975;87:1171–1181.
172. Wit JM, Kamp GA, Rikken B. Spontaneous growth and response to growth hormone treatment in children with growth hormone deficiency and idiopathic short stature. Pediatr Res 1996;39:295–302.
173. Wit JM, van Unen H. Growth of infants with neonatal growth hormone deficiency. Arch Dis Child 1992;67:920–924.
174. Boersma B, Rikken B, Wit JM. Catch-up growth in early treated patients with growth hormone deficiency. Dutch Growth Hormone Working Group. Arch Dis Child 1995;72:427–431.
175. Shih KC, Ho LT, Kuo HF, Chang TC, Liu PC, Chen CK, Tiu CM. Linear growth response to recombinant human growth hormone in children with growth hormone deficiency. Chinese Med J 1994;54:7–13.
176. Rosenfeld RG, Albertsson-Wikland K, Cassorla F, et al. Diagnostic controversy: the diagnosis of childhood growth hormone deficiency revisited. J Clin Endocrinol Metab 1995;80:1532–1540.
177. Zantleifer D, Awadalla S, Brauner R. Growth response to growth hormone during the first year as a diagnosis criterion of growth hormone deficiency. Horm Res 1993;40:123–127.

178. Rosenbaum M, Gertner JM, Gidfar N, Hirsh J, Leibe R. Effects of systemic growth hormone (GH) administration on regional adipose tissue in children with non-GH deficient short stature. J Clin Endocrinol Metab 1992;75:151–156.
179. Saggesse G, Baroncelli GI, Bertelloni S, Cinquanta L, Di Nero G. Effects of long-term treatment with growth hormone on bone and mineral metabolism in children with growth hormone deficiency. J Pediatr 1993;122:37–45.
180. Stanhope R, Albanese A, Hindmarsh P, Brook CG. The effects of growth hormone therapy on spontaneous sexual development. Horm Res 1992;38:9–13.
181. Dussault JH, Coulombe P, Laberge C, Letarte J, Guyda H, Khoury K. Preliminary report on a mass screening program for neonatal hypothyroidism. J Pediatr 1975;86:670–674.
182. LaFranchi S. Congenital hypothyroidism: a newborn screening success story? Endocrinologist 1994;4:477–486.
183. Grant DB. Growth in early treated congenital hypothyroidism. Arch Dis Child 1994;70:464–468.
184. Glorieux J, Dussault JH, Morissette J, Desjardins M, Letarte J, Guyda H. Follow-up at ages 5 and 7 years on mental development in children with hypothyroidism detected by Quebec Screening Program. J Pediatr 1985;107:913–915.
185. Fisher DA, Foley BL. Early treatment of congenital hypothyroidism. Pediatrics 1989;83:785–789.
186. Ozer G, Yuksel B, Kozanoglu M, Serbest M, Turgut C. Growth and development of 280 hypothyroidic patients at diagnosis. Acta Paediatr Japonica 1995;37:145–149.
187. Van Wyk JJ, Grumbach MM. Syndrome of precocious menstruation and galactorrhea in juvenile hypothyroidism: an example of hormonal overlap in pituitary feedback. J Pediatr 1960;57:416.
188. Rivkees SA, Bode HH, Crawford JD. Long-term growth in juvenile acquired hypothyroidism: the failure to achieve normal adult stature. N Engl J Med 1988;318:599–602.
189. Strickland AL, Underwood LE, Voina SJ, French FS, Van Wyk JJ. Growth retardation in Cushing's syndrome. Am J Dis Child 1972;123:207–213.
190. Lee PA, Weldon VV, Migeon CJ. Short stature as the only sign of Cushing's syndrome. J Pediatr 1975;86:89–91.
191. Streeten DHP, Faas FH, Elders MJ, Dalakos TG, Voorhess M. Hypercortisolism in childhood: shortcomings of conventional diagnostic criteria. Pediatrics 1975;56:797–803.
192. McArthur RG, Cloutier MD, Hayles AB, Sprague RE. Cushing's disease in children. Findings in 13 cases. Mayo Clin Proc 1972;47:318–326.
193. Magiakou MA, Mastorakos G, Oldfield EH, Gomez MT, Doppman JL, Cutler GB, Nieman LK, Chrousos GP. Cushing's syndrome in children and adolescents: presentation, diagnosis, and therapy. N Engl J Med 1994;331:629–636.
194. Jennings AS, Liddle GW, Orth DN. Results of treating childhood Cushings's disease with pituitary irradiation. N Engl J Med 1977;297:957–962.
195. Chan JC, Alon U, Hirschman GM. Renal hypophosphatemic rickets. J Pediatr 1985;106:533–544.
196. Chesney RW, Mazess RB, Rose P, Hanstra AJ, DeLuca HF, Breed AL. Long-term influence of calcitriol (1,25-dihydroxyvitamin D) and supplemental phosphate in X-linked hypophosphatemic rickets. Pediatr. 1983;71:559–567.
197. Tsuru N, Chan JCM, Chinchilli V. Renal hypophosphatemic rickets: growth and mineral metabolism after treatment with calcitriol (1,25-dihydroxyvitamin D3) and phosphate supplementation. Am J Dis Child 1987;141:108–110.
198. Pronicka E, Rowinska E, Buczen K, Lorenc R, Gradzka I. Growth rate in children with vitamin-D-dependent rickets in relation to 1-alpha-hydroxyvitamin D3 dosage. Endokrynologia Polska 1992;43:145–152.
199. Wilson DM, Lee PD, Morris AH, Reiter EO, Gertner JM, Marcus R, Quarmby VE, Rosenfeld RG. Growth hormone therapy in hypophosphatemic rickets. Am J Dis Child 1991;145:1165–1170.

4 Pituitary Response to Stress
Growth Hormone and Prolactin

Mark E. Molitch, MD

CONTENTS

    NEUROENDOCRINE REGULATION OF PROLACTIN SECRETION
    NEUROENDOCRINE REGULATION OF GROWTH
       HORMONE SECRETION
    CHANGES IN PROLACTIN SECRETION WITH STRESS
    CHANGES IN GROWTH HORMONE SECRETION WITH STRESS
    EFFECT OF PROLACTIN ON CARBOHYDRATE METABOLISM
    EFFECT OF PROLACTIN ON THE IMMUNE SYSTEM
    EFFECT OF GROWTH HORMONE ON INTERMEDIARY METABOLISM
    EFFECT OF GROWTH HORMONE ON THE IMMUNE SYSTEM
    CONCLUSIONS
    REFERENCES

NEUROENDOCRINE REGULATION OF PROLACTIN (PRL) SECRETION

The hypothalamus exerts a predominantly inhibitory influence on PRL secretion through one or more PRL inhibitory factors (PIF) that reach the pituitary via the hypothalamic–pituitary portal vessels (Fig. 1). There are PRL-releasing factors (PRF's) as well. Disruption of the pituitary stalk leads to a moderate increase in PRL secretion as well as to decreased secretion of the other pituitary hormones.

Dopamine (DA) is the predominant, physiologic PIF. Stimuli that result in an acute release of PRL usually also result in an acute decrease in portal vessel DA levels *(1,2)*. Studies with low-dose DA infusions in humans have shown that DA blood concentrations similar to those found in rat and monkey hypothalamic–pituitary portal blood *(3)* are able to suppress PRL secretion *(4)*. Blockade of endogenous DA receptors by a variety of drugs, including phenothiazines and butyrophenones, causes a rise in PRL *(5)*. The axons responsible for the release of DA into the median eminence originate in perikarya in the arcuate ventromedial nuclei of the hypothalamus *(6,7)*. The DA that traverses this pathway binds to the class of DA receptors referred to as D_2 receptors on the lactotroph cell membrane *(8)*.

Considerable PIF activity is found in rat hypothalamic extracts in which DA had been removed, however. A 56 amino acid polypeptide that is present in the carboxy-terminal region of the precursor to gonadotropin-releasing hormone (GnRH), termed gonadotropin-

From *Contemporary Endocrinology: Endocrinology of Critical Disease*
Edited by K. P. Ober   Humana Press Inc., Totowa, NJ

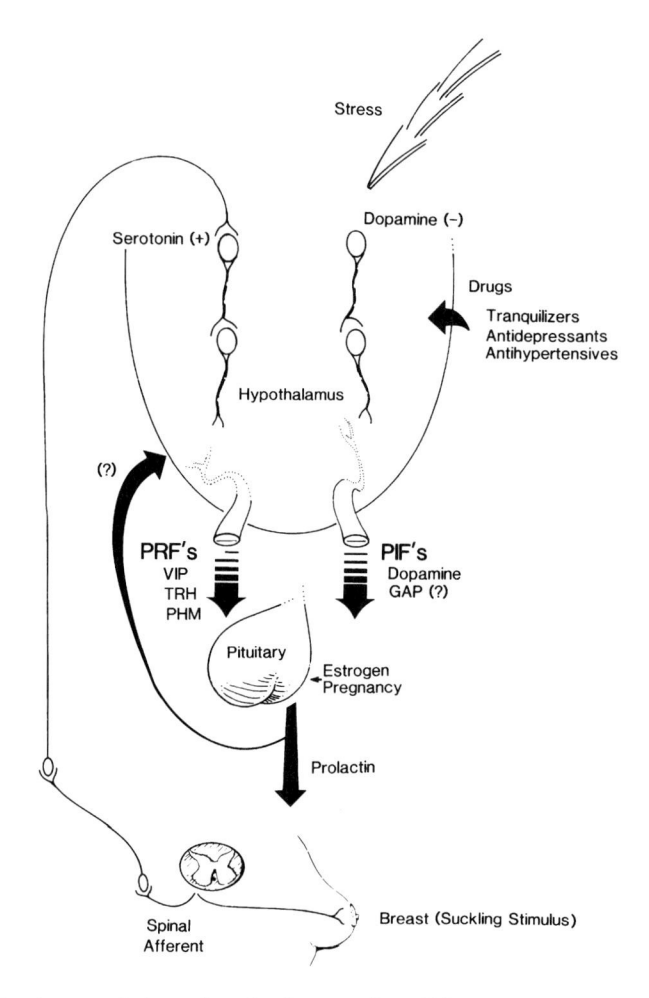

Fig. 1. Neuroendocrine regulation of prolactin secretion. GAP, gonadotropin-releasing hormone-associated peptide; PHM, peptide histidine methionine; PIF, prolactin inhibitory factor; PRF, prolactin-releasing factor; TRH, thyrotropin-releasing hormone; VIP, vasoactive intestinal peptide. (Reproduced with permission from Molitch ME. Pathological hyperprolactinemia. Endocr Metab Clin North Am 1992;21:877.)

associated peptide (GAP), inhibits PRL secretion at much lower concentrations than DA in rats *(9)*. Passive immunization of rabbits against GAP resulted in marked elevations of endogenous PRL levels *(9)*. However, subsequent experiments have been less conclusive. At this point the physiologic significance of GAP as a PIF vis-à-vis DA, especially in humans, is still not clear. The neurotransmitter γ-amino butyric acid (GABA) has also been found to inhibit PRL secretion in various animal and human studies *(10)*, but its physiologic significance is also not clear.

Thyrotropin-releasing hormone (TRH) causes a rapid release of PRL from pituitary cell cultures *(11)* and in humans after iv injection *(12)*. A number of different experimental approaches have failed to clarify the physiologic role of TRH as a PRF, however. The smallest dose of TRH that releases TSH also releases PRL in humans *(13)*. Immunoneutralization of endogenous TRH with TRH antisera causes a suppression of basal PRL levels in rats in some studies *(14)*, but not in others *(15,16)*. Such immunization also did not affect the PRL response to electrical stimulation of the paraventricular nucleus or suckling *(16)*. Suckling causes an increase in hypothalamic and portal vessel TRH levels as well as a decrease in DA levels *(1)*. If TRH mediates the PRL response to suckling, even in part, it ought to be accompanied by an increase in TSH, but this is not the case, at least in humans *(17)*. The above conflicting data from passive immunization studies, observation of TSH levels during lactation, and examination of PRL levels in various thyroid states support a role for TRH as a physiologic PRF, although not the primary one or even one of major importance.

Vasoactive intestinal peptide (VIP) has stimulatory effects that are selective for PRL and additive to TRH in causing PRL release *(18)* at concentrations found in hypothalamic–pituitary portal blood *(19)*. Both TRH and VIP neuronal perikarya are present in the parvicellular region of the paraventricular nucleus with axons terminating in the external zone of the median eminence *(3)*. Passive immunoneutralization with anti-VIP antisera partially inhibits the PRL responses to suckling, stress, and other stimuli *(20,21)*. Part of the 170 amino acid VIP precursor is another similarly sized peptide known as peptide histidine methionine (PHM—the analogous porcine structure is called PHI) *(22)*. PHI is of similar potency to VIP in releasing PRL from rat pituitaries in vitro and in vivo *(23)*. Furthermore, passive immunoneutralization with anti-PHI plus anti-VIP antisera causes a greater suppression of the PRL responses to various stimuli than either anti-PHI or anti-VIP antisera alone *(21)*. PHM given to humans has caused a PRL increment in some experiments *(24)* and not others *(25)*.

Further complicating the role of VIP as a PRF is the finding that VIP is actually synthesized by anterior pituitary tissue *(26)*. Antisera to VIP inhibit basal PRL secretion from dispersed pituitary cells in vitro *(27)*, suggesting a local "autocrine" role for VIP in PRL regulation within the pituitary. The physiologic role of VIP as a PRF appears to be warranted by the experimental data. The precise roles of VIP vs PHM, hypothalamic VIP vs pituitary VIP, and VIP/PHM vs other PRFs, such as TRH, are not clear.

Other peptides have been shown to have PRL-releasing properties in a variety of experimental studies, including opioid peptides, cholecystokinin, substance P, neurotensin, growth hormone-releasing hormone, GnRH, oxytocin, vasopressin, galanin, and many others *(10)*. Their physiologic significance, especially in humans, is not clear. Other central bioaminergic systems are probably also important in PRL regulation in addition to DA and GABA *(10)*. Serotonin generally has been found to be a physiologically important stimulator of PRL secretion and histamine may also be important, mediated through H_1 receptors. Acetylcholine generally is inhibitory, acting through muscarinic receptors.

NEUROENDOCRINE REGULATION OF GROWTH HORMONE (GH) SECRETION

There is a dual regulatory mechanism for GH secretion, GH-releasing hormone (GHRH) serving as the stimulatory input, and somatostatin serving as the inhibitory input (Fig. 2). In addition, there is a negative feedback regulatory mechanism exerted by insulin-like growth factor I (IGF-1, also known as somatomedin C).

GHRH exists in 40 and 44 amino acid forms, both of which being present in roughly equal quantities in the human hypothalamus *(28–30)*. GHRH causes a dose-dependent increase in GH secretion, GHRH 1–40 being equipotent to GHRH 1–44 in vivo *(31)*.

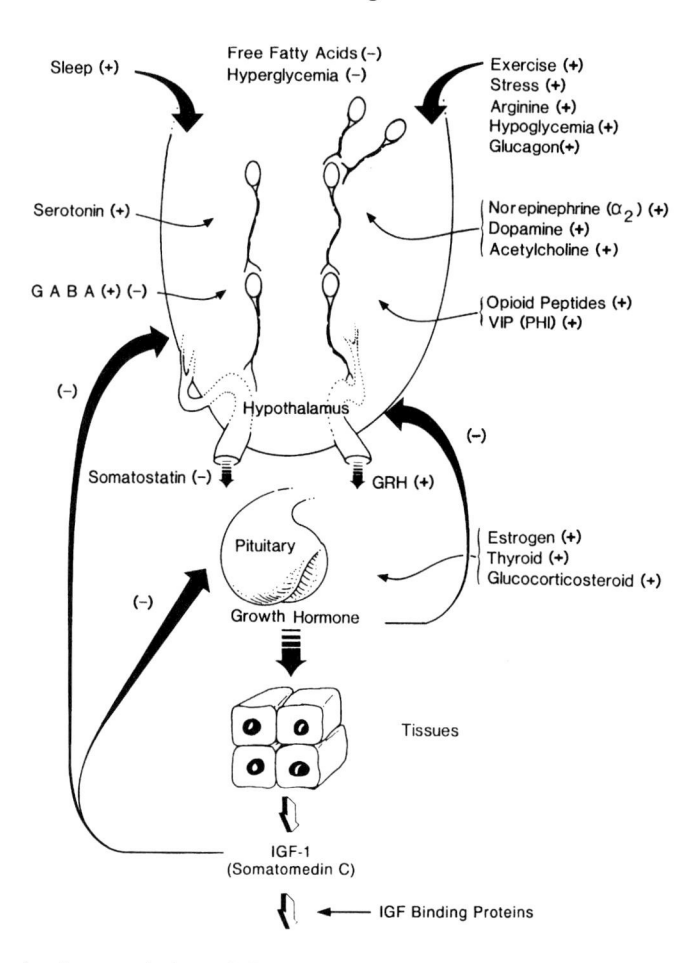

Fig. 2. Neuroendocrine regulation of GH secretion. GRH, growth hormone-releasing hormone; GABA, γ-aminobutyric acid; VIP, vasoactive intestinal peptide.

GHRH stimulates GH mRNA transcription, as well as GH release with no effects on PRL mRNA transcription *(32)*. The GHRH receptor is coupled to a guanine nucleotide binding protein, which activates adenyl cyclase, generating intracellular cAMP *(33,34)*. The biologic necessity of GHRH for normal growth was demonstrated by the finding that passive immunization of rats with antibodies to rat GHRH results in a decrease in somatic growth *(35)*. Both GHRH 1–40 and 1–44 are active in humans in stimulating GH release, GH levels increasing within 5 min and peaking between 30 and 60 min *(36,37)*. In some studies, GHRH has been shown to have PRL-releasing properties *(38)*, but the physiologic significance of this has not been established. The GHRH neuronal perikarya are located in the arcuate-ventromedial area with projections to the median eminence, terminating on portal vessels *(39)*.

Somatostatin similarly exists in two forms, somatostatin-14 and somatostatin-18, both forms having bioactivity and being present in the hypothalamus *(40–43)*. The administration of antisomatostatin antiserum to rats results in an elevation of trough GH levels *(44)*. Antisomatostatin antiserum also prevents the inhibition of GH secretion in the rat that occurs in response to stress *(45)*. In humans, somatostatin inhibits the GH response to a wide range of stimuli, including L-DOPA, arginine, sleep, and hypoglycemia *(46,47)*. The tuberoinfundibular somatostatinergic fibers originate in the anterior periventricular nucleus and the medial division of the paraventricular nucleus. Five subtypes of the somatostatin receptor have been characterized and cloned, and are identical in 42–60% of their amino acid sequences *(48,49)*. The receptors belong to the receptor class that has seven transmembrane domains and are linked to adenylyl cyclase through guanine nucleotide binding proteins *(48,49)*. Subtypes 2 and 5 are the primary somatostatin receptors in the normal pituitary *(48,49)*.

The interaction of somatostatin and GHRH on GH secretion is complex. Both somatostatin and GHRH are secreted episodically into the portal system in rats and sheep in an independent manner in which the secretory bursts are often asynchronous. Thus, GH secretory episodes are associated with increased GHRH secretion accompanied by low somatostatin levels and the basal or trough GH levels with low GHRH levels and more elevated somatostatin levels *(50–52)*. Furthermore, somatostatin may also partially inhibit GHRH secretion, and somatostatin receptors have been found on GHRH neuronal perikarya in the arcuate nucleus *(53,54)*. Conversely GHRH may stimulate somatostatin release *(55)*. Because GH responses to exogenous GHRH are variable, it is possible that hypothalamic somatostatin secretion in humans may also be intermittent *(56)*.

Studies of bioaminergic regulation have shown that stimulatory adrenergic effects are mediated by α_2-receptors causing both GHRH release *(57)* and somatostatin suppression *(58,59)*, and that α_1 and β_2 stimulation are inhibitory to GH secretion *(60)*. DA has a stimulatory effect centrally which overrides a direct pituitary inhibitory effect, possibly by decreasing somatostatin secretion *(61)*. Cholinergic pathways are stimulatory possibly by both decreasing somatostatin secretion *(62)* and increasing GHRH *(63)*.

CHANGES IN PRL SECRETION WITH STRESS

PRL has long been known to be one of the pituitary hormones released by stress, along with ACTH and GH. Neill initially demonstrated the release of PRL from rats with ether stress *(64)*, and Noel et al. demonstrated the release of PRL in response to physical stress in humans (Fig. 3) *(65)*. Although stress may decrease PRL secretion in rats under some circumstances *(66)*, this has not been documented in humans. The teleologic significance for this stress-induced release of PRL is not clear, although there may be some beneficial effects on the immune system *(66)* and in maintaining blood glucose levels *(see below)*. The stress-induced rise in PRL generally consists of a doubling or tripling of PRL levels and lasts <1 h. This rise in PRL may be limited by the concomitant release of cortisol, which suppresses further PRL release, as evidenced by the fact that stress applied to adrenalectomized rats results in a PRL increase that is sustained for as long as the stressful stimulus is applied *(67,68)*.

The neuroendocrine mediation of the stress response is probably multifactorial, but does not include a decrease in DA *(66)*. Corenblum and Taylor *(69)* attempted to dissect out the neurotransmitter regulation of the PRL stress response in humans by administering various blocking agents immediately prior to surgery. Blockade of histamine H_1 receptors using chlorpheniramine, serotonin receptors using cyproheptadine, and DA receptors using pimozide had little effect on the peak PRL level reached during surgery. Blockade of opi-

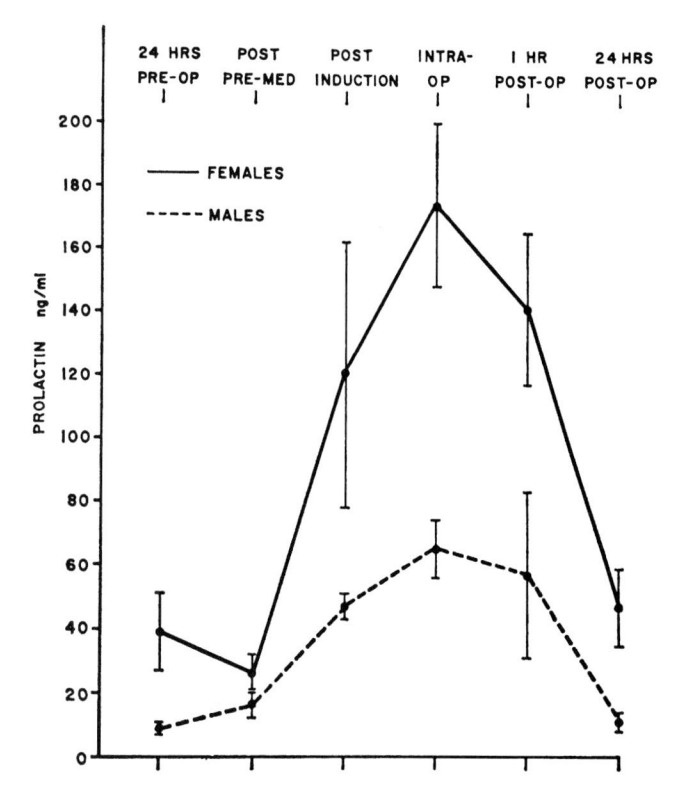

Fig. 3. PRL concentrations during surgery with general anesthesia in 19 women and 7 men. Vertical lines indicate SEM. (Reproduced with permission of The Endocrine Society from ref. 65.)

ate receptors with high-dose naloxone resulted in a significant blunting, but not complete inhibition of the PRL response. These studies imply that the endogenous opiate-like peptidergic pathways may play a role in the PRL stress response. On the other hand, in humans, naloxone has generally not been found to be able to block the PRL response to hypoglycemia (70). We found that VIP antisera inhibited the ether-induced PRL rise in rats (20), and Kaji et al. (21) found that antisera to VIP and PHI were additive in this regard. Other factors, including serotonin, oxytocin, and possibly unidentified posterior pituitary PRL-releasing substances, may also be involved, but their relative roles are still obscure (66).

Hypoglycemia has been regarded as a form of stress, but whether it acts as a nonspecific stressor or has more specific effects is not clear. Among their tests of various types of stress, Noel et al. (65) showed that PRL did indeed rise with hypoglycemia. Woolf et al. (71) evaluated this effect systematically in normal men and women, finding that PRL levels increased by at least 10 ng/mL with a doubling of baseline levels in 2/3 of normal subjects, the maximal rise occurring between 40 and 90 min after the injection of IV insulin. 2-Deoxy-D-glucose, which causes intracellular glucopenia, also causes a rise in PRL levels (72). Studies using combinations of inhibitors of DA, histamine, and serotonin suggest that at least some of the PRL response to hypoglycemia may be mediated by serotoninergic pathways (73).

Acute exercise has also been regarded as a form of stress and results in an acute, transient increase in PRL levels (65,74). Although chronic, high-level exercise often results in menstrual disturbance, it is not associated with sustained hyperprolactinemia (74, 75).

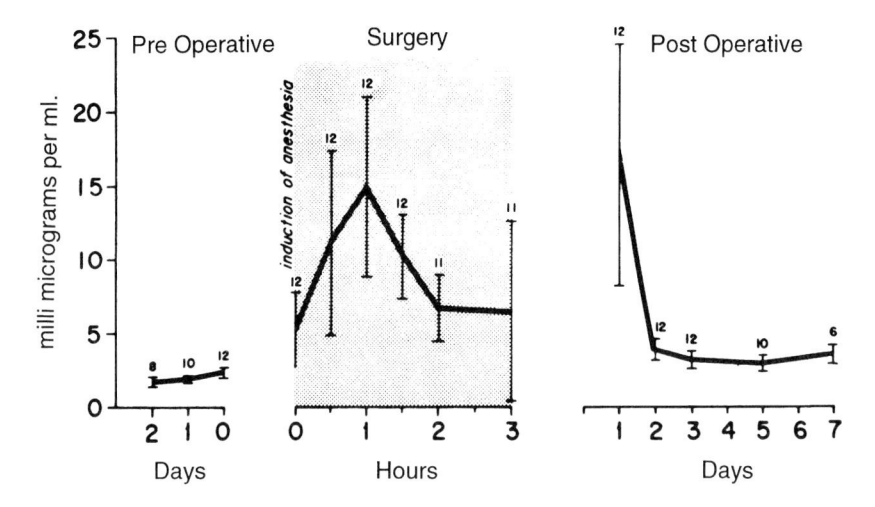

Fig. 4. GH secretion during and following surgical stress. A transient increase occurred during operation. The vertical bars represent standard error of the mean and the number of subjects is indicated. (Reproduced with permission of The Endocrine Society from ref. 78.)

CHANGES IN GH SECRETION WITH STRESS

A variety of physical stresses elicit the acute release of GH. Minimal pain or discomfort associated with artery or vein puncture, gastroscopy, or proctoscopy results in a variable GH response *(65,76,77)*. Major bodily trauma and surgery cause 5- to 10-fold increases in GH levels that last for several hours with a return to normal by the first postoperative day in most individuals (Fig. 4) *(65,77–81)*. During operations, the induction of anesthesia is not associated with an increase in GH; skin incision has to take place before GH levels increase *(65,80)*. The GH response to operations is mediated by afferent neural pathways, as evidenced by lack of such a GH increase with spinal or epidural anesthesia compared with that occurring during operations with general, inhalational anesthesia *(80,81)*.

Exogenous pyrogen also increases GH levels acutely *(82,83)*. Clinically, GH levels are markedly elevated with acute, severe illness, such as trauma with hemorrhagic shock *(79)* or bacterial sepsis *(84)*. However, less severe acute illness, such as acute respiratory insufficiency, does not cause an increase in GH levels, although such illness causes an increase in cortisol *(85)*. Chronic illness, such as cancer, uncommonly causes elevations in basal GH levels *(86)*, although GH may respond to TRH in up to two-thirds of such patients *(86)*.

It is likely that the acute stress-induced rise in GH is mediated by an increase in GHRH and not a decrease in somatostatin, since TSH levels are not increased by or are decreased in stress *(87)*. This stress-induced release of GHRH is probably owing to stimulation by noradrenergic pathways, since the stress-induced rise in GH may be inhibited by α-adrenergic antagonism *(88,89)*. In humans, the opiate-like peptidergic pathways appear to have at most a modulatory role in regulating the acute stress-induced GH release *(70)*.

Acute hypoglycemia causes an abrupt release of GH *(90–95)*, and insulin-induced hypoglycemia has long been used as a test of GH secretory ability. However, the late decrease in blood glucose levels following oral glucose ingestion from elevated to still normal glucose levels similarly causes an increase in GH levels in most normal individuals *(94)*, suggesting that this may be a specific effect of falling glucose and not a nonspecific "stress" effect.

Acute exercise results in GH release in most individuals in proportion to the degree of exertion *(65,77,95)*. Whether the GH release with exercise is due simply to the "stress" effect or is specific to exercise is not known.

EFFECT OF PRL ON CARBOHYDRATE METABOLISM

PRL receptors have been found in islet cells *(96)*, but the role of PRL in normal carbohydrate homeostasis is not known. Patients with hyperprolactinemia with or without evidence of prolactinoma have mildly increased (still within the normal range) blood glucose levels during glucose tolerance tests compared with normal controls *(97,98)*. Insulin levels are also increased in these patients, indicating mild insulin resistance *(97,98)*. The insulin resistance is due to a decrease in the number of receptors rather than a decrease in receptor affinity *(99)*. Treatment with bromocriptine causes a return to normal of both glucose and insulin levels *(97)*. However, in normoprolactinemic subjects with insulin-dependent diabetes, suppression of PRL levels with bromocriptine had no effect on glucose control *(100)*.

EFFECTS OF PRL ON THE IMMUNE SYSTEM

Normal PRL levels appear to be essential for normal immune function in rats, although the precise role of PRL in humans in this regard is not clear (Table 1). Hypophysectomized rats have decreased antibody production against sheep red blood cells, skin responses to dinitrochlorobenzene, and rejection of skin grafts *(101)*. These immune responses can be restored with treatment of the hypophysectomized rats with rPRL, rGH, bPRL, bGH, hPL, and hGH *(102)*. Other studies have shown that PRL increases mitogenesis and the expression of lymphocyte gene products *(103)*. Lymphocytes and thymic epithelial cells have PRL receptors *(104,105)*. Hypoprolactinemia induced with bromocriptine results in impaired lymphocyte proliferation and decreased production of macrophage-activating factors by lymphocytes, as well as decreased tumoricidal activation of macrophages after infections; these effects could be reversed with ovine PRL administration to the rats *(106)*. Hypoprolactinemia similarly induced with bromocriptine in humans causes a decrease in antinuclear autoantibody levels in sera of patients with uveitis *(107)*. In more detailed studies, PRL was found to be necessary for interleukin-2 (IL-2) stimulated proliferation of T-lymphocytes *(108)* and to regulate T-cell proliferation by enhancing the expression of genes necessary for entry into S-phase *(109)*.

Neutralization of PRL with anti-PRL antibodies inhibits the in vitro lymphocyte proliferative response to T- and B-cell mitogens in both rat and human preparations, but neutralization with antibodies to other pituitary hormones has no effect *(110)*. However, when lymphocytes are cultured in serum-free medium, anti-PRL antibodies similarly inhibit lymphocyte proliferation, implying the presence of a necessary, lymphocyte-produced PRL-like protein *(110)*. In other studies, in response to stimulation with conconavalin A, a PRL-like substance has been found to be produced from murine splenic mononuclear cells that reacts with anti-PRL antibodies and is mitogenic in the Nb_2 node lymphoma bioassay *(111)*. mRNA obtained from such lymphocytes hybridizes with PRL and GH cDNA probes

Table 1
Immune Functions Requiring Normal PRL Levels

Function	Species	Refs.
Antibody production to RBCs	Rat	101
Skin responses to Dintrochlorobenzene	Rat	101
Rejection of skin grafts	Rat	101
Lymphocyte proliferation	Rat	106
Antinucelar antibody production with uveitis	Human	107
IL-2 stimulation of T-lymphocyte proliferation	Rat	108
Lymphocyte proliferative response to T- and B-cell mitogens in vitro	Rat, human	110

(112). Furthermore, the immunosuppressive drug cyclosporin A has been found to compete with PRL for a common binding site on rat lymphocytes, and stimulation of PRL secretion reverses the immunosuppression induced by cyclosporin *(112)*. Presumably, this rat lymphocytic PRL-like substance is analogous to lymphoblastoid PRL produced by human IM-9 lymphocytes *(113)*. A prolactin-like molecule produced by concanavalin A or phytohemagglutinin stimulated human peripheral blood mononuclear cells has also been found to cause lymphoproliferation, a phenomenon blocked by antihuman PRL antibodies *(114)*. Human T-lymphocytes contain the genes for hPRL and the PRL receptor, but the lymphocyte hPRL gene has an extra 5′-noncoding exon similar to that found for decidual PRL *(115)*. PRL mRNA has been localized to a variety of human immune tissues, including thymus, spleen, tonsils, and lymph nodes using *in situ* hybridization; within these tissues, the mRNA was detected in lymphocytes, epithelial cells, and vascular cells *(116)*.

A variety of cytokines affect pituitary PRL secretion and may be mediators, in part, of the PRL response to stress. In various experimental paradigms, IL-2 and IL-6 have been found to increase PRL secretion, and IL-1 and interferon-γ inhibit PRL secretion *(117–119)*. However, in vivo these substances have little effect on PRL secretion in rats *(119)*.

Prolactin may have some clinically relevant effects on the immune system as well. Hyperprolactinemia caused by injections of ovine PRL into mice caused an increase in phagocytosis, intracellular killing of salmonella typhimurium, chemotaxis, and overall survival *(120)*. Moreover, hyperprolactinemia caused by implanting pituitaries under the renal capsule caused increased autoimmune phenomena in the b/w mouse model *(121)*. In human patients with prolactinomas, polymorphonuclear cells show reduced chemotaxis *(122,123)*, but monocytes display significantly increased bactericidal activity against *Mycobacterium avium (124)*. However, other studies have shown that hyperprolactinemic patients display decreased natural killer T-cell function, and this effect is reversed with bromocriptine treatment *(125)*.

Data on PRL levels in patients with various autoimmune disorders are conflicting. Nagy et al. *(126)* found a low PRL bioactivity to immunoreactivity ratio in patients with rheumatoid arthritis owing to serum factors capable of inhibiting PRL bioactivity. In other studies, hyperprolactinemia has been found in substantial portions of men and women with systemic lupus erythematosus *(127–132)*, and in some of these studies, PRL levels correlated with the extent of clinical disease and antinuclear antibody activity *(129,131)*. However, in most of these studies, no information is given regarding renal function, CNS involvement, or medication use so that whether the hyperprolactinemia is truly related to autoimmune disease or other factors known to elevate PRL levels is not clear. In the studies by Pauzner et al. *(130)* and Neidhart *(131)*, lupus nephritis, hypothyroidism, and other known causes of hyperprolactinemia were specifically excluded. In one study of lupus in children, 3 of 33 had elevated PRL levels, but all 3 had evidence of CNS lupus *(132)*. In studies of another inflammatory condition, Jara et al. *(133)* found PRL levels to be elevated in 36% of patients with Reiter's syndrome. Furthermore, Bravo et al. found that four patients with Reiter's syndrome had dramatic clinical improvement when treated with bromocriptine *(134)*.

The clinical relevance of lymphoblastoid PRL and changes in immune function in normal individuals and those with hyperprolactinemia is still unclear. Although there is strong evidence in rodents that PRL is important in this regard, the evidence in humans is still very preliminary, and what does exist is often contradictory and suggests that these effects of PRL are relatively minor compared to those of other immune regulators *(135)*. The transient, mild elevation of PRL occurring with acute or chronic stress is unlikely to play a significant role in the overall immune response to stress.

EFFECT OF GH ON INTERMEDIARY METABOLISM

The precise roles of GH and IGF-1 in intermediary metabolism have become less clear now that it has been shown that IGF-1 can be generated locally from a number of tissues in response to GH *(136)*. GH has been shown to have early (1–3 h after administration) direct, insulin-like, activities, such as stimulation of glucose uptake and oxidation and inhibition of lipolysis *(137–139)*. Whether these early insulin-like effects of GH are physiologic or pharmacologic has been debated *(137)*, and these effects have little relevance to the increases in GH seen with stress. Of more importance clinically are the direct effects of GH to stimulate amino acid uptake and protein synthesis, as well as to increase insulin resistance and to increase lipolysis *(137,140–145)*.

The more chronic stimulatory effects of GH on protein synthesis and growth, including stimulation of RNA and DNA synthesis, glucose uptake and oxidation or incorporation into glycogen, and mitogenic activity are mediated by IGF-1 *(136)*. Elevations of GH during sleep contribute to morning insulin resistance, known as the "dawn phenomenon" *(146)*. Elevated levels of GH, such as those seen in acromegaly, cause insulin resistance *(143,147–149)*. It is also likely that the increased levels of GH may play a role in the insulin resistance of acute trauma and stress with resultant hyperglycemia and lipolysis *(143,147,150)*, but is likely to be a relatively minor effect compared to the effects of the increase in plasma levels of the other stress hormones, epinephrine, cortisol, and glucagon *(151,152)*.

Despite the increase of GH levels that occurs with stress, plasma IGF-1 levels decrease, and this may be important in the protein catabolism that occurs with severe physical stress *(153,154)*. In the later catabolic "flow" phase of injury, GH levels are actually decreased *(155)*.

These findings of decreased GH levels in later periods following stress combined with decreased IGF-1 levels during the entire poststress time have led to the use of recombinant human GH (hGH) as a potential therapeutic modality in the poststress period to reduce catabolism and promote recovery. Preliminary studies have shown that although such treatment results in some insulin resistance that does not appear to be clinically significant, protein catabolism is significantly improved *(156–160)*. Currently, a large number of trials are ongoing to assess the role of short-term GH and IGF-1 treatment of physically stressed patients.

EFFECT OF GH ON THE IMMUNE SYSTEM

As discussed above for PRL, early studies also showed requirement for GH in the normal functioning of the immune system in rats (Table 2) *(101,102)*. The situation for GH is more complex, however, in that multiple components of the axis, GH itself, IGF-1, GHRH, and even somatostatin may each have actions on the immune system.

Mice deficient in GH and PRL have decreased spleen and thymus weights with decreased numbers of lymphocytes in these organs, and these defects can be reversed with injections of GH *(161)*, with an increase in the number of CD4+/CD8+ progenitor T-cells *(162)*. Similar effects can be seen with administration of IGF-1 *(163)*. Receptors for GH *(164,165)*, IGF-1 *(166)*, and somatostatin *(167)* have been found on human monocytes, B-lymphocytes, and T-lymphocytes. Human GH and IGF-1 can stimulate human B-cells to proliferate and produce immunoglobulins, effects that can be blocked by specific anti-GH and anti-IGF-1 antibodies, respectively *(168)*. Although both GH and IGF-1 simulate the growth and maturation of marrow granulocyte precursors, this effect is blocked by anti-IGF-1 antibodies for both hormones, suggesting that it is the IGF-1 that mediates this effect *(169)*. Somatostatin has been found to have both stimulatory and inhibitory effects on lymphocyte proliferation *(170)*.

Specific functions of these white cell populations have also been found to be stimulated. GH and IGF-1 cause activation of human macrophages *(171)* and activation of monocytes for superoxide production *(172)*. Although GHRH has also been found to stimulate various aspects of lymphocyte function in some studies, the results in general have been variable *(173)*. Somatostatin suppresses immunoglobulin synthesis, but enhances human natural killer cell activity *(174,175)*.

GH itself is produced by human lymphocytes *(176–179)* as are IGF-1 *(180)* and GHRH *(181)*. The lymphocyte-produced GH is not affected by either GHRH or somatostatin *(178)*. The interrelationship of these lymphocyte-produced hormones with each other and with their counterparts in the normal GH axis remains to be determined.

The interrelationships of various cytokines with GHRH, somatostatin, and GH regulation is very complex. IL-1, IL-6, and tumor necrosis factor (TNF)-α all stimulate somatostatin release, but IL-1 also stimulates GHRH *(119)*. At the pituitary level, IL-6 stimulates and IL-2 inhibits GH secretion, whereas IL-1 and TNF-α have variable effects *(118,119)*. When these substances are given systemically to rats, variable responses have been reported *(119)*. Because many of these substances are made not only by lymphoid cells, but also by central nervous system and neuroendocrine tissues, and there are various effects of certain cytokines on the production of other cytokines by these tissues, it is extremely difficult to dissect out precise roles of the various substances involved, and their roles in the regulation of GH secretion in the human remain to be defined.

In clinical studies, GH-deficient children *(182,183)* and adults *(184)* have generally not been found to have significant deficiencies of lymphocyte or natural killer cell numbers or function, or significant changes in these functions with GH treatment. A few studies have, however, shown some increase in response to GH treatment of the lym-

Table 2
Immune Functions Requiring Normal GH Levels

Function	Species	Refs.
Antibody production to RBCs	Rat	101
Skin responses to Dintrochlorobenzene	Rat	101
Rejection of skin grafts	Rat	101
No. of spleen and thymus lymphocytes	Mouse	161
No. of CD4+/CD8+ progenitor T-cells	Mouse	162

phocytic mitogenic response *(184)* and in natural killer cell activity *(185)*. In general, hGH-deficient children and adults do not appear to be clinically immunodeficient *(117,185)*. In patients at the opposite extreme with acromegaly, B-cell differentiation in response to pokeweed mitogen is defective *(186)*, as is neutrophil chemotaxis *(123)*. As with PRL, it is unlikely that the transient elevation of GH seen with stress plays a significant role in immunomodulation.

CONCLUSIONS

Both PRL and GH are released with acute stress. Although the bioaminergic and hypophysiotropic pathways involved in the release of these hormones during stress have been reasonably well delineated over the years, recent information regarding the release of various cytokines involved in infectious and other forms of stress has yet to be fully integrated into this neuroendocrine framework. In general, the duration of elevation of these hormones following stress ranges from minutes to hours. These elevated levels of PRL and GH may well contribute to the insulin resistance that occurs with stress, although it is likely that this effect is minor compared to the effects of catecholamine and glucocorticoids. The later suppression of GH and IGF-1 that occurs with more prolonged stress may contribute significantly to the catabolic state associated with such conditions, and this hypothesis is currently being tested by a number of studies in which GH and IGF-1 are being given in an attempt to reverse this catabolism. Although animal studies suggest that PRL and GH are critical for normal immune function, data in humans to this effect are less impressive. Neither states of hormone deficiency nor those of gross excess (prolactinomas, acromegaly) are associated with clinically significant immune morbidity. Again, the effects of prolonged stress with prolonged suppression of GH and IGF-1 on the immune system are being evaluated by studies of GH and IGF-1 supplementation. I expect that the results of these studies will help to define the role of GH and IGF-1 in the human stress response more clearly over the next few years.

REFERENCES

1. De Greef WJ, Visser TJ. Evidence for the involvement of hypothalamic dopamine and thyrotrophin-releasing hormone in suckling-induced release of prolactin. J Endocrinol 1981;91:213–223.
2. Plotsky PM, Neill JD. Interactions of dopamine and thyrotropin-releasing hormone in the regulation of prolactin release in lactating rats. Endocrinology 1982;111:168–173.
3. Gibbs DM, Neill JD. Dopamine levels in hypophysial stalk blood in the rat are sufficient to inhibit prolactin secretion *in vivo*. Endocrinology 1978;102:1895–1900.
4. Leblanc H, Lachelin CL, Abu-Fadil S, Yen SSC. Effects of dopamine infusion on pituitary hormone secretion in humans. J Clin Endocrinol Metab 1976;43:668–674.

5. De Rivera JL, Lal S, Ettigi P, et al. Effect of acute and chronic neuroleptic therapy on serum prolactin levels in men and women of different age groups. Clin Endocrinol 1976;5:273–278.
6. Fuxe K. Cellular localization of monoamines in the median eminence and in the infundibular stem of some mammals. Acta Physiol Scan 1963;58:383–384.
7. Lechan RM. Neuroendocrinology of pituitary hormone regulation. Endocrinol Metab Clinics North Am 1987;16:475–501.
8. Foord SM, Peters JR, Dieguez C, Scanlon MF, Hall R. Dopamine receptors on intact anterior pituitary cells in culture: Functional association with the inhibition of prolactin and thyrotropin. Endocrinology 1983;112:1567–1577.
9. Nikolics K, Mason AJ, Szonyi E, Ramachandran J, Seeburg PH. A prolactin-inhibiting factor within the precursor for human gonadotropin-releasing hormone. Nature 1985;316:511–517.
10. Molitch ME. Prolactin. In: Melmed S, ed. The Pituitary. Blackwell Science, Cambridge, MA, 1995, pp. 136–186.
11. Tashjian AH Jr, Barowsky NJ, Jensen DK. Thyrotropin releasing hormone: direct evidence for stimulation of prolactin production by pituitary cells in culture. Biochem Biophys Res Commun 1971;43:516–523.
12. Jacobs LS, Snyder PJ, Wilber JF, Utiger RD, Daughaday WH. Increased serum prolactin after administration of synthetic thyrotropin releasing hormone (TRH) in man. J Clin Endocrinol Metab 1971;33:996–998.
13. Noel GL, Dimond RC, Wartofsky L, Earll JM, Grantz AG. Studies of prolactin and TSH secretion by continuous infusion of small amounts of thyrotropin-releasing hormone (TRH). J Clin Endocrinol Metab 1974;39:6–17.
14. Koch Y, Goldhaber G, Fireman I, Zor U, Shani J, Tal E. Suppression of prolactin and thyrotropin secretion in the rat by anti-serum to thyrotropin-releasing hormone. Endocrinology 1977;100:1476–1478.
15. Harris ARC, Christianson D, Smith MS, Fang SL, et al. The physiological role of thyrotropin-releasing hormone in the regulation of thyroid-stimulating hormone and prolactin secretion in the rat. J Clin Invest 1978;61:441–448.
16. Sheward WJ, Fraser HM, Fink G. Effect of immunoneutralization of thyrotrophin-releasing hormone on the release of thyrotrophin and prolactin during suckling or in response to electrical stimulation of the hypothalamus in the anaesthetized rat. J Endocrinol 1985;106:113–119.
17. Gautvik KM, Tashjian AH Jr, Kourides IA, et al. Thyrotropin-releasing hormone is not the sole physiologic mediator of prolactin release during suckling. N Engl J Med 1974;290:1162–1165.
18. Kato Y, Iwasaki Y, Iwasaki J, Abe H, Yanaihara N, Imura H. Prolactin release by vasoactive intestinal polypeptide in rats. Endocrinology 1978;103:554–558.
19. Said S, Porter JC. Vasoactive intestinal polypeptide. Release into hypophyseal portal blood. Life Sci 1979;24:227–230.
20. Abe H, Engler D, Molitch ME, Bollinger-Gruber J, Reichlin. Vasoactive intestinal peptide is a physiological mediator of prolactin release in the rat. Endocrinology 1985;116:1383–1390.
21. Kaji H, Chihara C, Abe H, Kita T. Effect of passive immunization with antisera to vasoactive intestinal polypeptide and peptide histidine isoleucine amide on 5-hydroxy-l-tryptophan-induced prolactin release in rats. Endocrinology 1985;117:1914–1919.
22. Itoh N, Obata K, Yanaihara N, Okamoto H. Human preprovasoactive intestinal polypeptide contains a novel PHI-27-like peptide, PHM-27. Nature 1983;304:547–549.
23. Ohta H, Kato Y, Tojo H. Further evidence that peptide histidine isoleucine (PHI) may function as a prolactin releasing factor in rats. Peptides 1985;6:709–712.
24. Sasaki At, Sato S, Go M, et al. Distribution, plasma concentration, and in vivo prolactin-releasing activity of peptide histidine methionine in humans. J Clin Endocrinol Metab 1987;65:683–688.
25. Yiangou Y, Gill JS, Chrysanthou BJ, Burrin J, Bloom SB. Infusion of prepro-VIP derived peptides in man: Effect on secretion of prolactin. Neuroendocrinology 1988;48:615–618.
26. Arnaout MA, Garthwaite TL, Martinson DR. Vasoactive intestinal polypeptide is synthesized in anterior pituitary tissue. Endocrinology 119:5:2052–2057.
27. Hagen TC, Arnaout MA, Scherzer Wj, Martinson DR. Antisera to vasoactive intestinal polypeptide inhibit basal prolactin release from dispersed anterior pituitary cells. Neuroendocrinol 1986;43:641–645.
28. Rivier J, Spiess J, Thorner M, Vale W. characterization of a growth hormone-releasing factor from a human pancreatic islet tumour. Nature 1982;300:276–278.
29. Guillemin R, Brazeau P, Bohlen P, Esch F, Ling N, Wehrenberg WB. Growth hormone-releasing factor from a human pancreatic tumor that caused acromegaly. Science 1982;218:585–587.

30. Bohlen P, Brazeau P, Bloch B, Ling N, Gaillard R, Guillemin R. Human hypothalamic growth hormone releasing factor (GRF): Evidence for two forms identical to tumor derived GRF-44-NH2 and GRF-40. Biochem Biophys Res Commun 1983;114:930–936.
31. Wehrenberg WB, Ling N, Brazeau P, et al. somatocrinin, growth hormone releasing factor, stimulates secretion of growth hormone in anesthetized rats. Biochem Biophys Res Commun 1982;109:382–387.
32. Barinaga M, Yamomoto G, Rivier C, Vale W, Evans R, Rosenfeld MG. Transcriptional regulation of growth hormone gene expression by growth hormone-releasing factor. Nature 1983;306:74,75.
33. Bilizikjian IM, Vale WW. Stimulation of adenosine 3′-5′-monophosphate production by growth hormone-releasing factor and its inhibition by somatostatin in anterior pituitary cells in vitro. Endocrinology 1983;113:1726–1731.
34. Spada A, Vallar L, Giannattasio G. Presence of an adenylate cyclase dually regulated by somatostatin and human pancreatic growth hormone (GH)-releasing factor in GH-secreting cells. Endocrinology 1984;115:1203–1209.
35. Wehrenberg WB, Block B, Phillips BJ. Antibodies to growth hormone-releasing factor inhibit somatic growth. Endocrinology 1984;115:1218–1220.
36. Thorner MO, Spiess J, Vance ML, et al. Human pancreatic growth-hormone-releasing factor selectively stimulates growth hormone secretion in man. Lancet 1983;1:24–28.
37. Rosenthal Sm, Schirock EA, Kaplan SL, Guillemin R, Grumbach MM. Synthetic human pancreas growth hormone-releasing factor stimulates growth hormone secretion in normal men. J Clin Endocrinol Metab 1983;57:677–679.
38. Goldman JA, Molitch M, Thorner M, Vale W, Rivier J, Reichlin S. Growth hormone and prolactin response to bolus and sustained infusions of GHRH-1-40-OH in man. J Endocrinol Invest.
39. Lechan RM, Lin HD, Ling N, Jackson IMD, Jacobson S, Reichlin S. Distribution of immunoreactive growth hormone releasing factor (1-44) NH2 in the tuberoinfundibular system of the rhesus monkey. Brain Res 1984;309:55–61.
40. Shen L-P, Rutter JW. Sequence of the human somatostatin gene. Science 1984;224:168–170.
41. Charpenet G, Patel YC. Characterization of tissue and releasable molecular forms of somatostatin-$28_{[1-12]}$ like immunoreactivity in rat median eminence. Endocrinology 1985;116:1868–1868.
42. Millar RP, Klaff LJ, Barron JL, Levitt NS, Ling N. Somatostatin-28 and somatostatin-14 suppression of arginine, insulin-, and TRH-stimulated GH and PRL secretion in man. Clin Endocrinol 1983;18:277–285.
43. Abe H, Kato Y, Chiba T, Taminato T, Fujita T. Plasma immunoreactive somatostatin levels in rat hypophysial portal blood: effect of glucagon administration. Life Sci 1978;23:1647–1654.
44. Terry LC, Martin JB. The effects of lateral hypothalamic-medial forebrain stimulation and somatostatin antiserum on pulsatile growth hormone secretion in freely behaving rats: evidence for a dual regulatory mechanism. Endocrinology 1981;109:622–627.
45. Terry LC, Willoughby JO, Brazeau P, Martin JB. Antiserum to somatostatin prevents stress-induced inhibition of growth hormone secretion in the rat. Science 1976;192:565–567.
46. Siler TM, VandenBerg G, Yen SSC, Brazeau P, Vale W, Guillemin R. Inhibition of growth hormone release in humans by somatostatin. J Clin Endocrinol 1973;37:632–634.
47. Copinschi G, Vitasoro E, Vanhaelst L, Leclercq R, Golstein J, L'Hermite M. Specific inhibition by somatostatin of growth hormone release after hypoglycemia in normal man. Clin Endocrinol 1974;3:441–445.
48. Lamberts SWJ, van der Lely A-J, de Herder WW, Hofland LJ. Octreotide. N Engl J Med 1996;334:246–254.
49. James RA, Weightman DR. Somatostatin receptors: types and classification in the pituitary. The Endocrinologist 1995;5:55–60.
50. Plotsky PM, Vale W. Patterns of growth hormone-releasing factor and somatostatin secretion into the hypophysial-portal circulation of the rat. Science 1985;230:461.
51. Tannenbaum GS, Ling N. The interrelationship of growth hormone (GH)-releasing factor and somatostatin in generation of the ultradian rhythm of GH secretion. Endocrinology 1984;115:1952.
52. Frohman LA, Downs TR, Clarke IJ, Thomas GB: Measurement of growth hormone-releasing hormone and somatostatin in hypothalamic-portal plasma of unanesthetized sheep. J Clin Invest 1990;86:17.
53. Katakami H, Downs TR, Frohman LA. Inhibitory effect of hypothalamic medial preoptic area somatostatin on growth hormone-releasing factor in the rat. Endocrinology 1988;123:1103.
54. Epelbaum J, Moyse E, Tannenbaum GS, Kordon C, Beaudet A. Combined autoradiographic and immunohistochemical evidence for an association of somatostatin binding sites with growth hormone-releasing factor-containing nerve cell bodies in the rat arcuate nucleus. J Neuroendocrinol 1989;1:109.

55. Aguila MC, McCann. Evidence that growth hormone-releasing factor stimulates somatostatin release *in vitro* via β-endorphin. Endocrinology 1987;120:341.
56. Martha PM Jr., Blizzard RM, McDonald JA, Thorner MO, Rogol AD. A persistent pattern of varying pituitary responsivity to exogenous growth hormone (GH)-releasing hormone in GH-deficient children: evidence supporting periodic somatostatin secretion. J Clin Endocrinol Metab 1988;67:449.
57. Miki N, Ono M, Shizume K. Evidence that opiatergic and α-aerenergic mechanisms stimulate rat growth hormone release via growth hormone-releasing factor (GRF). Endocrinology 1984;114:1950–1952.
58. Torres I, Guaza C, Fernandez-Durango R, Borrell J, Charo AL. Evidence for modulatory role of catecholamine on hypothalamic somatostatin in the rat. Neuroendocrinology 1982;35:159–162.
59. Chihara K, Minamitani N, Kaji H, Kodama H, Kita T, Fujita T. Noradrenegic modulation of human pancreatic growth hormone-releasing factor (hpGHRF1-44)-induced growth hormone release in conscious male rabbits: involvement of endogenous somatostatin. Endocrinology 1984;114:1402–1406.
60. Krulich L, Mayfield MA, Steele MK, McMillen BA, McCann SM, Koenig JI. Differential effects of pharmacological manipulations of central α1 and α2-adrenergic receptors on the secretion of thyrotropin and growth hormone in male rats. Endocrinology 1982;110:796–804.
61. Vance ML, Kaiser DL, Frohman LA, Rivier J, Vale WW, Thorner MO. Role of dopamine and bromocriptine augment growth hormone (GH)-releasing hormone-stimulated GH secretion in normal man. J Clin Endocrinol Metab 1987;64:1136–1141.
62. Casanueva FF, Villanueva L, Dieguez C, et al. Atropine blockade of GHRH-induced GH secretion in man is not exerted at pituitary level. J Clin Endocrinol Metab 1986;64:186–191.
63. Jaffe CA, DeMott-Friberg R, Barkan AL. Endogenous growth hormone (GH)-releasing hormone is required for GH responses to pharmacological stimuli. J Clin Invest 1996;97:934–940.
64. Neill JD. Effect of "stress" on serum prolactin and luteinizing hormone levels during the estrous cycle of the rat. Endocrinology 1970;87:1192–1197.
65. Noel GL, Suh HK, Stone SJG, Frantz AE. Human prolactin and growth hormone release during surgery and other conditions of stress. J Clin Endocrinol Metab 1972;35:840–851.
66. Gala RR. The physiology and mechanisms of the stress induced changes in prolactin secretion in the rat. Life Sci 1990;46:1407–1420.
67. Harms PG, Langlier P, McCann SM. Modification of stress-induced prolactin release by dexamethasone or adrenalectomy. Endocrinology 1975;96:475–478.
68. Subramanian MG, Gala RR. The influence of adrenalectomy and of corticosterone administration on the ether-induced increase in plasma prolactin in ovariectomized estrogen-treated rats. Proc Soc Exp Biol Med 1978;157:415–417.
69. Corenblum B, Taylor PJ. Mechanisms of control of prolactin release in response to apprehension stress and anesthesia-surgery success. Fertil Steril 1981;36:712–715.
70. Spiler IJ, Molitch ME. Lack of modulation of pituitary hormone stress response by neural pathways involving opiate receptors. J Clin Endocrinol Metab 1980;50:516–520.
71. Woolf PD, Lee LA, Leebaw WF. Hypoglycemia as a provocative test of prolactin release. Metabolism 1978;27:869–877.
72. Woolf PD, Lee LA, Leebaw W, Thompson D. Intracellular glucopenia causes prolactin release in man. J Clinic Endocrinol Metab 1977;45:377–382.
73. Whitaker MB, Corenblum B, Taylor PJ. Control of the hypoglycemia release of prolactin. Prog Reprod Biol 1980;6:77–82.
74. Chang FE, Dodds WG, Sullivan M, Kim MH. The acute effects of exercise on prolactin and growth hormone secretion: Comparison between sedentary women and women runners with normal and abnormal menstrual cycles. J Clin Endocrinol Metab 1986;62:551–556.
75. Chang FE, Richards SR, Kim MII, Malarkey WB. Twenty-four hour prolactin profiles and prolactin responses to dopamine in long distance running women. J Clin Endocrinol Metab 1984;58:631–635.
76. Copinschi G, Hartog M, Earll JM, Havel RJ. Effect of various blood sampling procedures on serum levels of immunoreactive human growth hormone. Metabolism 1967;16:402–409.
77. Schalch DS. The influence of physical stress and exercise on growth hormone and insulin secretion in man. J Lab Clin Med 1967;69:256–269.
78. Charters AC, Odell WD, Thompson JC. Anterior pituitary function during surgical stress and convalescence. Radioimmunoassay measurement of blood TSH, LH, FSH and growth hormone. J Clin Endocrinol 1969;29:63–71.
79. Carey LC, Cloutier CT, Lowery BD. Growth hormone and adrenal cortical response to shock and trauma in the human. Ann Surg 1971;174:451–460.

80. Newsome HH, Rose JC. The response of human adrenocorticotrophic hormone and growth hormone to surgical stress. J Clin Endocrinol 1971;33:481–487.
81. Hagen C, Brandt MR, Kehlet H. Prolactin, LH, FSH, GH and cortisol response to surgery and the effect of epidural analgesia. Acta Endocrinol 1980;94:151–154.
82. Frohman LA, Horton ES, Lebovitz HE. Growth hormone releasing action of a pseudomonas endotoxin (Piromen). Metabolism 1967;16:57–67.
83. Kohler PO, O'Malley BW, Rayford PL, Lipsett MB, Odell WD. Effect of pyrogen on blood levels of pituitary trophic hormones. Observations of the usefulness of the growth hormone response in the detection of pituitary disease. J Clin Endocrinol Metab 1967;27:219–226.
84. Sibbald WJ, Short A, Cohen MP, Wilson RF. Variations in adrenocortical responsiveness during severe bacterial infections. Ann Surg 1966;186:29–33.
85. Cornil A, Glinoer D, Leclercq R, Copinschi G. Adrenocortical and somatotropic secretions in acute and chronic respiratory insufficiency. Am Rev Respir Dis 1975;112:77–81.
86. Kamijo K, Saito A, Yachi A, Wada T. Growth hormone response to thryotrophin-releasing hormone in cancer patients. Endocrinol Japon 1980;27:451–455.
87. Richmand DA, Molitch ME, O'Donnell T. Altered thyroid hormone levels in bacterial sepsis: the role of nutritional adequacy. Metabolism 1980;29:936–942.
88. Vigas M, Malatinsky J, Nemeth S, Jurcovicova J. Alpha-adrenergic control of growth hormone release during surgical stress in man. Metabolism 1977;26:399–402.
89. Martin JB. Functions of central nervous system neurotransmitters in regulation of growth hormone secretion. Fed Proc 1980;39:2902–2906.
90. Roth J, Glick SM, Yalow RS, Berson SA. Hypoglycemia: a potent stimulus to secretion of growth hormone. Science 1963;140:987–988.
91. Frantz AG, Rabkin MT. Human growth hormone. Clinical measurement: response to hypoglycemia and suppression by corticosteroids. N Engl J Med 1964;271:1375–1381.
92. Schalch DS, Parker ML. A sensitive double antibody immunoassay for human growth hormone in plasma. Nature 1964;203:1141–1142.
93. Greenwood FC, Landon J, Stamp TCB. The plasma sugar, free fatty acid, cortisol, and growth hormone response to insulin. I. In control subjects. J Clin Invest 1966;45:429–436.
94. Glick SM. Hypoglycemic threshold for human growth hormone release. J Clin Endocrinol Metab 1970;30:619–623.
95. Lin T, Tucci JR. Provocative tests of growth hormone release. A comparison of results with seven stimuli. Ann Intern Med 1974;80:464–469.
96. Tesone M, Filho-Oliveira RM, Charreau EH. Prolactin binding in rat Langerhans islets. J Receptor Res 1980;1:355–372.
97. Landgraf R, Leurs-Landgraf MMC, Weissmann A, Hörl R, von Werder K, Scriba PC. Prolactin: A diabetogenic hormone. Diabetologia 1977;13:99–104.
98. Gustafson AB, Banasiak MF, Kalkhoff RK, Hagen TC, Kim H-J. Correlation of hyperprolactinemia with altered plasma insulin and glucagon: Similarity to effects of late human pregnancy. J Clin Endocrinol Metab 1980;51:242–246.
99. Schernthaner G, Prager R, Punzengruber C, Luger A. Severe hyperprolactinaemia is associated with decreased insulin binding in vitro and insulin resistance in vivo. Diabetologia 1985;28:138–142.
100. Scobie IN, Kesson CM, Ratcliffe JG, MacCuish AC. The effects of prolonged bromocriptine administration on PRL secretion, GH and glycaemic control in stable insulin-dependent diabetes mellitus. Clin Endocrinol 1983;18:179–185.
101. Nagy E, Berczi I. Immunodeficiency in hypophysectomized rats. Acta Endocrinol 1978;89:530–537.
102. Nagy E, Berczi I, Friesen HG. Regulation of immunity in rats by lactogenic and growth hormones. Acta Endocrinol 1983;102:351–357.
103. Russel DM, Kibler R, Matrisian L, Larsen DF, Poulos B, Magun BE. Prolactin receptor on rat lymphoid tissues and on human T- and B-lymphocytes Antagonism of prolactin binding by cyclosporine. J Immunol 1985;134:3027–3031.
104. O'Neal KD, Schwarz LA, Yu-Lee L-Y. Prolactin receptor gene expression in lymphoid cells. Mol Cell Endocrinol 1991;82:127–135.
105. Dardenne M, Kelly PA, Bach J-F, Savino W. Identification and functional activity of prolactin receptors in thymic epithelial cells. Proc Natl Acad Sci USA 1991;88:9700–9704.
106. Bernton EW, Meltzer MS, Holaday JW. Suppression of macrophage activation and t-lymphocyte function in hypoprolactinemic mice. Science 1988;239:401–404.

107. Blank M, Palestine A, Nussenblatt R, Shoenfeld Y: Down-regulation of autoantibody levels of cyclosporine and bromocriptine treatment in patients with uremia. Clin Immunol Immunopathol 1990;54:87–97.
108. Clevenger CV, Altmann SW, Prystowsky MB. Requirement of nuclear prolactin for interleukin-2-stimulated proliferation of T lymphocytes. Science 1991;253:77–79.
109. Clevenger CV, Sillman AL, Hanley-Hyde J, Prystowsky MB. Requirement for prolactin during cell cycle regulated gene expression in cloned T-lymphocytes. Endocrinology 1992;1309:3216–3222.
110. Hartman DP, Holaday JW, Bernton EW. Inhibition of lymphocyte proliferation by antibodies to prolactin. FASEB 1989;3:2194–2202.
111. Montgomery DW, Zukoski CF, Shah GN. Concanavalin A-stimulated murine splenocytes produce a factor with prolactin-like bioactivity and immunoreactivity. J Biochem Biophys 1987;145(2):692–698.
112. Hiestand PC, Mekler P, Nordmann R. Prolactin as a modulator of lymphocyte responsiveness provides a possible mechanism of action for cyclosporine. Proc. Natl Acad Sci USA 1986;83:2599–2603.
113. DiMattia GE, Gellersen B, Bohnet HG, Friesen HG. A Human B-lymphoblastoid cell line produces prolactin. Endocrinology 1988;122:2508–2517.
114. Sabharwal P, Glaser R, Lafuse W, Varma S, Liu Q, Arkins S, Kooijman R, Kutz L, Kelley KW, Malarkey WB. Prolactin synthesized and secreted by human peripheral blood mononuclear cells: an autocrine growth factor for lymphoproliferation. Proc Natl Aced Sci USA 1992;89:7713–7716.
115. Pelligrini K, Lebrun J-J, Ali S, Kelly PA. Expression of prolactin and its receptor in human lymphoid cells. Mol Endocrinol 1992;6:1023–1031.
116. Wu H, Devi R, Malarkey WB. Expression and localization of prolactin messenger ribonucleic acid in the human immune system. Endocrinology 1996;137:349–353.
117. Azad N, Agrawal L, Emanuele MA, Kelley MR, Mohagheghpour N, Lawrence AM, Emanuele NV. Neuroimmunoendocrinology. Am J Reprod Immunol 1991;26:160–172.
118. Smith EM. Hormonal activities of cytokines. In: Blalock JE, ed. Neuroimmunoendocrinology, 2nd ed., S. Karger, Basel, 1992, pp. 154–169.
119. Mandrup-Poulsen T, Nerup J, Reimers JI, Pociot F, Anderson HU, Karlsen A, Bjerre U, Bergholdt R. Cytokines and the endocrine system. I. The immunoendocrine network. Eur J Endocrinol 1995;133:660–671.
120. Di Carlo R, Meli R, Galdiero M, Nuzzo I, Bentivoglio C, Romano Carratelli C. Prolactin protection against lethal effects of salmonella typhimurium. Life Sci 1993;53:981–989.
121. McMurray R, Keisler D, Kanuckel K, Izui S, Walker SE. Prolactin influences autoimmune disease activity in the female B/W mouse. J Immunol 1991;147:3780–3787.
122. Harris RD, Kay NE, Seljeskog EL, Murray KJ, Douglas SD. Prolactin suppression of leukocyte chemotaxis *in vitro*. J Neurosurg 1979;50:462–465.
123. Fornari MC, Palacios MF, Diez RA, Intebi AD. Decreased chemotaxis of neutrophils in acromegaly and hyperprolactinemia. Eur J Endocrinol 1994;130:463–468.
124. Sabharwal P, Zwilling B, Glaser R, Malarkey WB. Cellular immunity in patients with acromegaly and prolactinomas. Prog Neuroendocrinimmunology 1992;5:120–125.
125. Vidaller A, Guadarrama F, Llorente L, Méndez JP, Larrea F, Villa AR, Alarcón-Segovia D. Hyperprolactinemia inhibits natural killer (NK) cell function *in vivo* and its bromocriptine treatment not only corrects it but makes it more efficient. J Clin Immunol 1992;12:210–215.
126. Nagy E, Chalmers IM, Baragar FD, Friesen HG, Berczi I. Prolactin deficiency in rheumatoid arthritis. J Rheumatol 1991;18:1662–1668.
127. Lavalle C, Loyo E, Paniagua R, Bermudez JA, Herrera J, Graef A, Gonzalez-Barcena D, Fraga A. Correlation study between prolactin and androgens in male patients with systemic lupus erythematosus. J Rheumatol 1987;14:268–272.
128. Polomeev M, Prokaeva T, Nassonova V, Nassonova E, Masenko V, Ovtraht N. Prolactin levels in men with SLE and RA: J Rheumatol 1990;17:1569–1570.
129. Jara LJ, Gomez-Sanchez C, Silveira LH, Martinez-Osuna P, Vasey FB, Espinoza LR. Hyperprolactinemia in systemic lupus erythematosus: association with disease activity. Am J Med Sci 1992;303:222–226.
130. Pauzner R, Urowitz MB, Gladman DD, Gough JM. Prolactin in systemic lupus erythematosus. J Rheumatol 1994;21:2064–2067.
131. Neidhart M. Elevated serum prolactin or elevated prolatin/cortisol ratio are associated with autoimmune processes in systemic lupus erythematosus and other connective tissue diseases. J Rheumatol 1996;23:476–481.

132. El-Garf A, Salah S, Shaarawy M, Zaki S, Anwer S. Prolactin hormone in juvenile systemic lupus erythematosus: a possible relationship to disease activity and CNS manifestations. J Rheumatol 1996;23:374–377.
133. Jara LJ, Silveira LH, Cuellar ML, Pineda CJ, Scopelitis E, Espinoz LR. Hyperprolactinemia in Reiter's syndrome. J Rheumatol 1994;21:1292–1297.
134. Bravo G, Zazueta B, Lavalle C. An acute remission of Reiter's syndrome in male patients treated with bromocriptine. J Rheumatol 1992;19:747–750.
135. Murphy WJ, Rui H, Longo DL. Effects of growth hormone and prolactin immune development and function. Life Sci 1995;57:1–14.
136. Jones JI, Clemmons DR. Insulin-like growth factors and their binding proteins: biological actions. Endocr Rev 1995;16:3–34.
137. Merimee TJ, Rabin D. A survey of growth hormone secretion and action. Metabolism 1973;22:1235–1251.
138. Fix JA, Moore WV. Growth hormone stimulation of glucose transport in isolated rat hepatocyte suspensions and primary cultures. Endocrinology 1981;108:239–246.
139. Goodman HM. Biological activity of bacterial derived human growth hormone in adipose tissue of hypophysectomized rats. Endocrinology 1984;114:131–135.
140. Albertsson-Wikland K, Isaksson O. Time course of the effect of growth hormone in vitro on amino acid and monosaccharide transport and on protein synthesis in diaphragm of young normal rats. Endocrinology 1978;102:1445–1451.
141. Schwartz J. Rapid modulation of protein synthesis in normal rats by specific neutralization and repolacement of growth hormone. Endocrinology 1982;111:2087–2090.
142. Rabinowitz D, Klassen GA, Zierler KL. Effect of human growth hormone on muscle and adipose tissue metabolism in the forearm of man. J Clin Invest 1965;44:51–61.
143. Rizza RA, Mandarino LJ, Gerich JE. Effects of growth hormone on insulin action in man. Mechanisms of insulin resistance, impaired suppression of glucose production, and impaired stimulation of glucose utilization. Diabetes 1982;31:663–669.
144. Schoenle E, Zapf J, Froesch ER. Regulation of rat adipocyte glucose transport by growth hormone: no mediation by insulin-like growth factors. Endocrinology 1983;112:384–386.
145. Gerich JE, Lorenzi M, Bier DM, et al. Effects of physiologic levels of glucagon and growth hormone on human carbohydrate and lipid metabolism. J Clin Invest 1976;57:875–884.
146. Bolli GB, Gerich JE. The "dawn phenomenon"—a common occurrence in both non-insulin-dependent and insulin-dependent diabetes mellitus. N Engl J Med 1984;310:746–750.
147. Bratusch-Marrain P, Gasic S, Waldhaus WK, Nowotny P. Effect of growth hormone on splanchnic glucose and substrate metabolism following oral glucose loading in healthy man. Diabetes 1984;33:19–25.
148. Fowelin J, Attvall S, von Schenk H, Smith U, Lager I. Characterization of the insulin-antagonistic effect of growth hormone in man. Diabetologia 1991;34:500–506.
149. Fowelin J, Attvall S, von Schenck H, Smith U, Lager I. Characterization of the insulin-antagonistic effect of growth hormone in insulin-dependent diabetes mellitus. Diabetic Med 1995;12:990–996.
150. Keller V, Schnell H, Girard J, Stauffacher W. Effect of physiological elevation of plasma growth hormone levels on ketone body kinetics and lipolysis in normal acutely insulin deficient man. Diabetologia 1984;26:103–108.
151. Weissman C. The metabolic response to stress: an overview and update. Anesthesiology 1990;73:308–327.
152. Mizock BA. Alterations in carbohydrate metabolism during stress: a review of the literature. Am J Med 1995;98:75–84.
153. Frayn KN, Price DA, Maycock PF, Carroll SM. Plasma somatomedin activity after injury in man and its relationship to other hormonal and metabolic changes. Clin Endocrinol 1984;20:179–187.
154. Dahn MS, Lange P, Jacobs LA. Insulin-like growth factor I production is inhibited in human sepsis. Arch Surg 1988;123:1409–1414.
155. Jeevanandam M, Ramias L, Shamos RF, Schiller WR. Decreased growth hormone levels in the catabolic phase of severe injury. Surgery 1992;111:495–502.
156. Wilmore DW, Moylan JA, Breistow BF, Mason AD, Pruitt BA. Anabolic effects of human growth hormone and high caloric feedings following thermal injury. Surg Gynecol Obstet 1974;138:875–884.
157. Gore DC, Honeycutt D, Jahoor F, Wolfe RR, Herndon DN. Effect of exogenous growth hormone on whole-body and isolated-limb protein kinetics in burned patients. Arch Surg 1991;126:38–43.

158. Gore DC, Honeycutt D, Jahoor F, Rutan T, Wolfe RR, Herndon DN. Effect of exogenous growth hormone on glucose utilization in burn patients. J Surg Res 1991;51:518–523.
159. Ziegler TR, Rombeau JL, Young LS, Fong Y, Marano M, Lowry SF, Wilmore DW. Recombinant human growth hormone enhances the metabolic efficacy of parenteral nutrition: a double-blind, randomized controlled study. J Clin Endocrinol Metab 1992;74:865–863.
160. Voerman HJ, Strack van Schijndel RJM, Groeneveld ABJ, de Boer H, Nauta JP, van der Veen EA, Thijs LG. Effects of recombinant human growth hormone in patients with severe sepsis. Ann Surg 1992;216:648–655.
161. Villanua MA, Szary A, Bartke A, Esquifino AI. Changes in lymphoid organs of Ames dwarf mice after treatment with growth hormone, prolactin, or ectopic pituitary transplants. J Endocrinol Invest 1992;15:587–592.
162. Murphy WJ, Durum SK, Longo DL. Differential effects of growth hormone and prolactin on murine T cell development and function. J Exp Med 1993;178:231–236.
163. Clark R, Strasser J, McCabe S, Robbins K, Jardieu P. Insulin-like growth factor-I stimulation of lymphopoiesis. J Clin Invest 1993;92:540–548.
164. Lesniak MA, Gorden P, Roth J, Gavin JR. Binding of 125I-human growth hormone to specific receptors in human cultured lymphocytes. J Biol Chem 1974;249:1661–1667.
165. Badolato R, Bond HM, Valerio G, Petrella A, Morrone G, Waters MJ, et al. Differential expression of surface membrane growth hormone receptor on human peripheral blood lymphocytes by dual fluorochrome flow cytometry. J Clin Endocrinol Metab 1994;79:984–990.
166. Kooijman R, Willems M, De Haas CJ, Rijkers GT, Schuurmans AI, Buul-Offers SC, et al. Expression of type I insulin-like factor receptors on human peripheral blood mononuclear cells. Endocrinology 1992;131:2244–2250.
167. Bathena SJ, Louie J, Schechter GP, Redmond RS, Wahl L, Recant L. Identification of human mononuclear leucocytes bearing receptors for somatostatin and glucagon. Diabetes 1981;30:127–131.
168. Kimata H, Yoshida A. Effect of growth hormone and insulin-like growth factor-I on immunoglobulin production by and growth of B-cells. J Clin Endocrinol Metab 1994;78:635–641.
169. Merchav S, Tatarsky H, Hochberg Z. Enhancement of human granulopoiesis in vitro by biosynthetic insulin-like growth factor I/Somatomedin C and human growth hormone. J Clin Invest 1988;81:791–797.
170. Pawlikowski M, Stepien H, Kunert-Radek J, Zelazowski P, Schally AV. Immunomodulatory action of somatostatin. Ann NY Aced Sci 1987;496:233–239.
171. Edwards CK III, Arkins S, Yunger LM, Blum A, Dantzer R, Kelley KW. The macrophage-activating properties of growth hormone. Cell Mol Neurobiol 1992;12:499–510.
172. Warwick-Davies J, Lowrie DB, Cole PJ. Growth hormone activation of human monocytes for superoxide production but not tumor necrosis factor production, cell adherence or action against *Mycobacterium tuberculosis*. Infect Immun 1995;4312–4136, 1995.
173. Auernhammer CJ, Strasburger CJ. Effects of growth hormone and insulin-like growth factor I on the immune system. Eur J Endocrinol 1995;133:635–645.
174. Payon DA, Levin JD, Goetzl EJ. Modulation of immunity and hypersensitivity by sensory neuropeptides. J Immunol 1984;132:1601–1604.
175. Pawlikowski M, Zelazowski P, Stepine H. Enhancement of human lymphocyte natural killer activity by somatostatin. Neuropeptides 1989;13:75–77.
176. Hattori N, Shimatsu A, Sugita M, Kumagai S, Imura H. Immunoreactive growth hormone (GH) secretion by human lymphocytes: augmented release by exogenous GH. Biochem Biophys Res Commun 1990;168:396–401.
177. Varma S, Sabharwal P, Sheridan JF, Malarkey WB. Growth hormone secretion by human peripheral blood mononuclear cells detected by an enzyme-linked immunoplaque assay. J Clin Endocrinol Metab 1993;76:49–53.
178. Hattori N, Ikekubo K, Ishihara T, Moridera K, Hino M, Kurahachi H. Spontaneous growth hormone (GH) secretion by unstimulated human lymphocytes and the effects of GH-releasing hormone and somatostatin. J Clin Endocrinol Metab 1994;79:1678–1680.
179. Wu H, Devi R, Malarkey WB. Localization of growth hormone messenger ribonucleic acid in the human immune system—A Clinical Research Center study. J Clin Endocrinol Metab 1996;81:127888–1282.
180. Geffner ME, Bersch N, Lippe BM, Rosenfeld RG, Hintz RL, Golde DW. Growth hormone mediates the growth of T-lymphoblast cell lines via locally generated insulin-like growth factor I. J Clin Endocrinol Metab 1990;71:464–469.

181. Stephanou A, Knight RA, Lightman SL. Production of a growth hormone-releasing hormone-like peptide and its mRNA by human lymphocytes. Neuroendocrinology 1991;53:628–631.
182. Peterson BH, Rapaport R, Henry DP, Huseman C, Moore WV. Effect of treatment with biosynthetic human growth hormone (GH) on peripheral blood lymphocyte populations and function in growth hormone-deficient children. J Clin Endocrinol Metab 1990;70:1756–1760.
183. Spadoni GL, Rossi P, Ragno W, Galli E, Cianfarani S, Galasso C, et al. Immune function in growth hormone-deficient children treated with biosynthetic growth hormone. Acta Paediatr Scand 1991;80:76–79.
184. Abbassi V, Bellanti JA. Humoral and cell-mediated immunity in growth hormone-deficient children: effect of therapy with human growth hormone. Pediatr Res 1985;19:299–301.
185. Crist DM, Kraner JC. Supplemental growth hormone increases the tumor cytotoxic activity of natural killer cells in healthy adults with normal growth hormone secretion. Metabolism 1990;39:1320–1324.
186. Intebi AD, Palacios MF, Sen L, Diez RA. Defective B-cell differentiation under PWM induction in acromegaly. Prog Neuroendocrinimmunol 1992;5:62–69.

5 The Sympathoadrenomedullary Response to Critical Illness

Otto Kuchel, MD

CONTENTS

    INTRODUCTION
    SYMPATHOADRENOMEDULLARY RESPONSES TO STRESS
      AND THEIR BIOLOGICAL ROLE
    ASSESSMENT OF SYMPATHOADRENOMEDULLARY ACTIVITY
      IN RESPONSE TO STRESS
    THE SURVIVAL VALUE VS THE POTENTIALLY DAMAGING ROLE
      OF STRESS-INDUCED CATECHOLAMINE MOBILIZATION
    ROLE OF SYMPATHOADRENAL STRESS RESPONSES IN SEVERAL
      DISEASES AND CONDITIONS
    LIFESTYLE AND PHARMACOLOGICAL INTERVENTIONS
      IMPROVING COPING WITH STRESS-INDUCED
      SYMPATHOADRENAL ACTIVATION
    ACKNOWLEDGMENTS
    REFERENCES

INTRODUCTION

Any illness, particularly a critical one, is a major threat to the integrity of the human organism and endangers its survival. Approximately a century ago, Claude Bernard theorized that the "milieu interne" must be maintained to preserve life. At about the same time, Walter Cannon introduced the term homeostasis to characterize "the coordinated physiological reactions that maintain the steady state of body" via the integrated cooperative activity of a wide range of organs (1). He was the first to recognize that physical and emotional disturbances could elicit sympathoadrenomedullary responses, which are typical of physiological change seen in preparation for "fight or flight." He also demonstrated that physical and emotional upsets trigger the same responses and that there are limits to the ability to compensate. The cardiovascular, renal, visceral, cutaneous, pulmonary, and metabolic components of these responses may have survival value in preparing the body for action. However, their biochemistry remained unknown even though adrenaline was already discovered through the pioneering work of Abel and Loewi.

Selye's *(2)* concept of the general adaptation syndrome shifted attention to adrenal steroids by pinpointing the three stages of adaptation. In the late 1940s, new biochemical methods confirmed Selye's hypothesis on the role of adrenal steroids in stress. However, a better understanding of the involvement of catecholamines in stress was only developed in the 1950s and 1960s, after von Euler et al. *(3)* demonstrated in 1948 that norepinephrine (NE) was released from sympathetic nerve endings. On the basis of regional localization and pharmacologic alterations of NE levels in the hypothalamus and mesencephalon, Marthe Voght suggested that NE and epinephrine (E) might be neurotransmitters in the central nervous system. The development of spectrofluorometry, followed by radiolabelling techniques, high-performance liquid chromatography (HPLC), and more recently, measurements of neuronal activity, tracer-kinetic, nuclear scanning and molecular biology techniques provided a strong impetus for the investigation of catecholamines in stress between the 1970s and 1990s. Axelrod and Weinshilboum *(4)* and Kopin *(5)* made significant contributions by their definition of catecholamine synthesis, metabolism, and disposition. The development of radioenzymatic methods of measuring catecholamines, their metabolites, and enzymes involved in their biosynthesis as well as the discovery of catecholaminergic neuronal pathways in the brain by fluorescent histologic techniques *(6)* added new tools for the exploration of catecholamines in stress. The availability of new drugs inhibiting the biosynthetic enzymes of catecholamines, interfering with their storage, inactivation, and particularly with their receptor action, improved our understanding of their biological role. Goldstein *(7)* provided evidence that each stressor has a neurochemical "signature" with the quantitatively, if not qualitatively, distinct central and peripheral mechanisms as determined by adrenocorticotropic hormone (ACTH), NE (sampled in blood and paraventricular nucleus), and E. Another dimension emerged with the demonstration that dopamine (DA), which had been regarded as a precursor of NE, is probably a neurotransmitter of equal importance (for review, *see 8*).

The cloning and chromosome location of enzymes involved in catecholamine synthesis, metabolism, neuronal uptake (for review, *see 9*), and most receptor actions (for review, *see 10*) added a genetic dimension to the role of catecholamines in adaptation to stress. The genetic make-up of this "first-line" stress-responsive homeostatic system may affect its coping ability with endogenous and exogenous stressors. Several identified enzymatic defects may explain a breakdown of this defense line; occasionally not only defects, but a hyperresponsiveness to stressors may occur when a catecholamine metabolism or neuronal reuptake enzyme is deficient.

The neurochemical specificity of stressors is inconsistent with Selye's "nonspecificity" doctrine of the body's response to any challenge. This new concept *(7)* puts the role of endogenous catecholamines (NE, E, and DA) into the framework of a coordinated activation of the body's several stress systems in primitively specific patterns during exposure to various stressors. The impact of the autonomic nervous system in response to stress is further integrated, rather than isolated, by close interactions between catecholamines and neuropeptides *(11)*. Hypothalamic corticotrophin-releasing hormone (CRH) neurons stimulate both pituitary ACTH secretion and the central autonomic-arousal, locus cerulus (LC) norepinephrine (LC-NE) system leading, respectively, to glucocorticoid and NE secretion *(12)* (Fig. 1). On the other hand, hypothalamic CRH neurons, particularly the paraventricular nucleus, receive positive noradrenergic input from the central LC-NE limbic system, cholinergic and serotoninergic stimulation, and inhibition by opioid peptidergic and GABAergic fibers.

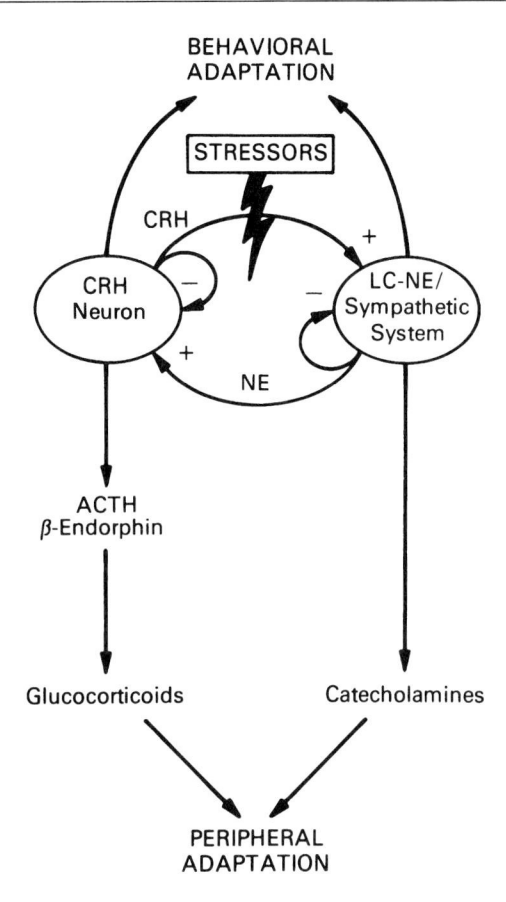

Fig. 1. The stress system and neurotransmitter as well as neurohormonal control mechanisms modulating glucocorticoid and catecholamine secretion. Hypothalamic CRH neurons stimulate both pituitary ACTH secretion and the central autonomic-arousal systems (LC-NE) leading, respectively, to glucocorticoid and catecholamine NE secretion. The positive reverberating loop between the CRH neuron and the autonomic-arousal centers is under ultrashort loop feedback control, by CRH and noradrenergic presynaptic inhibition, respectively. Plus signs represent stimulation, and minus signs represent inhibition (with permission from ref. *12*).

Eventually, other neuropeptides interacting with the neuronal activity and steroids affecting some steps in catecholamine synthesis and metabolism are involved in the final pathway in which the response to stress materializes in an individual and neurochemical specificity. The adrenergic receptor responsiveness as well as several intrinsic feedback systems add another dimension to the complexity of actions of the individual catecholamine response to stress.

SYMPATHOADRENOMEDULLARY RESPONSES TO STRESS AND THEIR BIOLOGICAL ROLE

Lack of precision and insufficient inclusiveness in the definition of the popular term "stress" make its precise scientific definition difficult. Some psychologically oriented subjective definitions (such as "stress is pressure outside that makes you feel tense inside") may well reflect competitive situations, deadlines, anticipation of an exciting event, disasters, and so forth, but exclude many biological or environmental stressors. In general terms, stressors are referred to as "forces or stimuli which tend to disturb a steady state." These include destabilization of the internal environment (e.g., anoxia, hypoglycemia), environmental extremes (e.g., heat, cold, weightlessness), psychological disturbances (e.g. fear, anger, surprise), and distress of various types (e.g., pain, depression). In the final balance, the actions of these stressors, which are usually combined (e.g., pain and trauma), have to be evaluated in relation to the degree of the threat and, not less importantly, its perception, which often determines the gravity of the homeostatic disturbance *(13)*.

The responses to stressors fall into two general categories. In the first are homeostatic responses specific to the stimulus and serving useful adaptive functions. They are generally mediated by the autonomic nervous system and are relatively predictable with small individual variations. They require energy, but usually remain functional in nature without inducing structural or anatomical changes.

In the second category are the more generalized responses, which follow when the disturbances are severe, persistent, and/or not corrected adequately by homeostatic mechanisms. These responses include sympathoadrenomedullary and adrenocortical activation. They exhibit wide individual, genetically determined differences in the threshold disturbances-evoking intensity. When persistent, generalized responses result in drastic structural changes (from hypertrophy through dysfunction to tissue damage), these cellular changes are apparently the price paid by exceeding the simple energy utilization, which characterizes homeostatic responses. The links between generalized responses and tissue damage are metabolic disturbances that threaten life (e.g., anoxia, hemorrhage, circulatory collapse, hypoglycemia). These disturbances are either mediated or compensated by adrenomedullary discharge, predominantly of E. This hormonal response increases glycemia, has a stimulatory β-adrenergic receptor-mediated effect on the heart, but increases or decreases blood pressure, enhances pulmonary ventilation, activates platelets, and so forth. In contrast to this massive and usually uniform E response, the sympathetic neuronal system reactions reflected by NE and mostly α-adrenergic receptor-mediated are highly variable. The role of a third peripheral autocrine-paracrine system reflected by DA sulfate increase during stress *(8,14)* still remains controversial.

Psychological stressors are also highly variable, but frequently elicit generalized responses. Alerting reactions progress to alarm or irritation, and then to fear or anger and aggression. On failure to escape, avoid, or reverse a disturbance, progressively more intense attendant physiological and biochemical responses can lead to extremes of panic or rage. These responses represent a continuum between a relaxed state and the extremes of "fight or flight" *(1)*.

Studies of adrenergic responses to stress require the selection of experimental or naturally occurring situations believed to be stressful, and appropriate methods must be available to measure the sympathoadrenomedullary reactions. For this purpose, several animal models have been chosen. In animals, the intensity of stress can be graded from slight disturbances (opening the cage, turning on the lights, transfer of cage to another room, gentle handling of the animal) to major physical (shock, immobilization, heat, cold, hemorrhage, hypoxia, fracture), pharmacological (e.g., ether), or psychological threats (e.g., exposure to predators) *(15)*. In humans, the choice of stress is more complex and difficult, ranging from interview, games *(16)*, and shocking experiences to job stress (e.g., air traffic controllers) or opportunistic situations (exposure to surgery or other stressful conditions).

Mechanisms of Sympathoadrenomedullary Responses to Stress

The final common pathway for initial homeostatic responses to various stressors is the regional activation of sympathetic neurons followed, in more generalized reactions, by adrenomedullary discharge *(15)*. The pattern of response depends on nerve impulses that originate from preganglionic cholinergic neurons located in the intermediolateral gray matter of the thoracic and upper lumbar segments of the spinal cord. Activity of these preganglionic neurons is regulated by fibers descending from the medulla and brainstem as well as by local spinal innervation. These pathways are under the modulatory and integrating control of the cerebral cortex, limbic system, hypothalamus, brainstem, and medulla.

The mechanisms underlying increased catecholamine release and decreased degradation under the influence of stress are becoming recognized thanks to recent investigations into enzymatic steps in catecholamine biosynthesis and metabolism and their genetics.

Eventually, the final pathway of the catecholamine responses to stress is determined by the responsiveness of α, β and dopaminergic receptors of catecholamine action, which were recently identified as several subgroups (for review, *see 10*). This identification started from pharmacological studies, and progressed through cloning and chromosomal location to one of the most prolific new horizons of catecholamine involvement in homeostatic responses. Adrenergic receptors and postreceptor events following chronic stress are thus another important determinant of the stress-related catecholamine action. An example of such a condition is the change in β-adrenergically stimulated cyclic AMP (cAMP) synthesis and adenylate cyclase activity in lymphocytes and platelets of patients with post traumatic stress disorders *(17)*. Such alterations are interpreted as a downregulation of cAMP signal amplification as a consequence of chronic stress.

As outlined in Fig. 2 *(18)*, tyrosine conversion to dihydroxyphenylalanine (DOPA) is catalyzed by the enzyme tyrosine hydroxylase (TH), which is believed to be the rate-limiting step in the synthesis of catecholamines. High levels of the relatively nonspecific aromatic L-amino acid decarboxylase (AADC) rapidly decarboxylate DOPA to DA, which enters the chromaffin granules of the sympathetic nerves and adrenal medulla where it is converted to NE by the enzyme dopamine-β-hydroxylase (DβH). Conversion of NE to E by phenylethanolamine-*N*-methyl transferase (PNMT), the final step in biosynthesis, occurs mainly in the adrenal medulla. This latter step in catecholamine synthesis has a relationship to the adrenal cortex, since PNMT activity within the medulla is regulated by glucocorticoids produced in the cortex *(4)*. The chromaffin cells of the medulla thus represent a "target organ" for glucocorticoids. The complexity of catecholamine responses to stress is further underlined by factors, such as adrenocortical or pituitary insufficiency, altering the synthesis of glucocorticoids that may exert some of their effects as a result of changes in the availability of E.

The pioneering work of Kopin *(5)* and his group has demonstrated that the main cause of activation of the sympathoadrenomedullary system by stress is the approximately threefold increase in TH activity, while DβH doubles and PNMT is augmented by about 50%. Comparison of innervated and denervated adrenals has shown that innervation

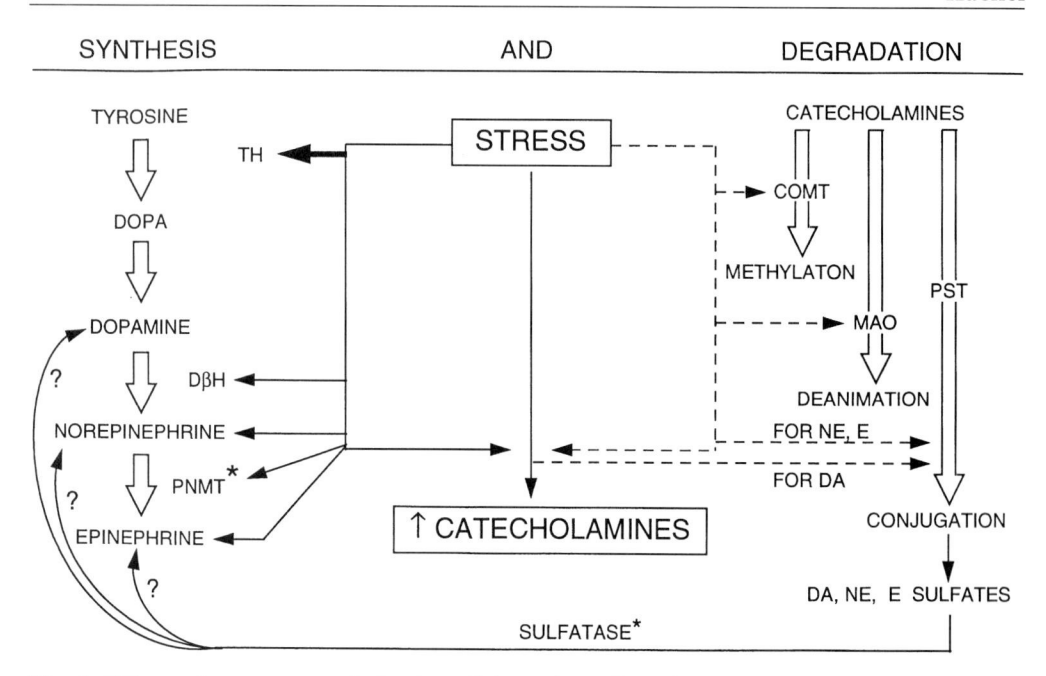

Fig. 2. Effects of stress on catecholamines. Schematic outline of catecholamine metabolism during stress. Stress increases the synthesis of catecholamines, predominantly by stimulating rate-limiting tyrosine hydroxylase TH activity. There is, at the same time, an inhibition of enzymes involved in the degradation of catecholamines, possibly resulting in a decreased catecholamine metabolism. The sulfoconjugation of NE and E appears to be reduced during acute stress, but that of DA remains unaffected. COMT, catechol-*O*-methyltransferase; DβH, dopamine-β-hydroxylase; MAO, monoamine oxidase; PNMT, phenylethanolamine-*N*-methyltransferase; PST, phenolsulfo-transferase. Sulfatase stimulation by stress (glucocorticoid-stimulated) may limit or even reverse the stress-induced rise in DA, NE, and E sulfates. Catecholamine sulfates represent a potential precursor of free catecholamines, which may be in short supply during stress. *, Glucocorticoid-stimulated. ⟶, Increase or Stimulation. --▶, decrease or inhibition.

affects stress-induced TH and DβH activity, but nerve impulses are not necessary to increase PNMT, which is under hormonal control. As evidence of this control, the adrenomedullary PNMT activity decrease in hypophysectomized animals is prevented or reversed by ACTH or glucocorticoid treatment. In contrast to this glucocorticoid dependency of PNMT, TH activity (mostly under neural control) appears to be partly ACTH-dependent, mediated by cAMP stimulation. In addition, some other neuropeptides from the secretin-glucagon family, such as secretin and vasoactive intestinal peptide (VIP) were found to stimulate TH activity *(19)* in the superior cervical ganglia. Medullary neurons activated by angiotensin II are located within the solitary tract, neurolateral medulla and include catecholamine (TH-positive) neurons *(20)*.

Although most stress-related catecholamine release studies concentrated on NE and E, recent investigations indicate that, to a point, DA release may be predominant in temporarily transforming an adrenergic into a dopaminergic terminal *(8)*. DA release may predominate when DβH activation does not keep pace with rate-limiting TH activation or when the autocrine-paracrine generation of DA *(14)* predominates. For example, immobilization produces a decrease of NE with an increase of DA content in the hamster heart *(21)*.

From an evolutionary viewpoint, DA release in excess of NE may represent regression to an archaic regulatory response. DA is the most prevalent catecholamine in invertebrates and some fish, whereas NE and E are latter acquisitions in the animal kingdom *(22)*. It is well known that stress responses represent a certain return to archaic homeostatic (i.e., "fight or flight") reactions under different modern life circumstances *(23)*. DA release during stress may be one such return to ancient reaction patterns in the catecholamine cascade.

Different activation patterns of catecholamine-synthesizing enzymes may at least partially account for the very distinct effects of individual stressors with their different intensities in releasing NE, E, and possibly, DA. Although TH activity predominantly dependent on nervous impulses determines overall catecholamine synthesis, DβH activity influenced by both nervous and pituitary-adrenal systems (as well as PNMT activity mostly dependent on the latter) modulates the ratio between NE and DA release and between NE and E release. Humans exposed to stress apparently undergo changes in catecholamine-synthesizing enzyme levels similar to those observed in animals. One part of the stress-induced increase in catecholamines may be owing not only to their enhanced synthesis and release, but also to their decreased degradation. Stressful stimuli have been demonstrated to exert an inhibiting action on some enzymes, such as catechol-*O*-methyltransferase (COMT), monoamine oxidase (MAO), and phenolsulfotransferase (PST), involved in the degradation of catecholamines. On the other hand, stress-induced glucocorticoid increase may activate sulfatase and so facilitate the free catecholamine generation from its sulfate *(9)*.

Such a mechanism of free catecholamine release in glucocorticoid-treated humans can be observed by determining free and sulfated catecholamines following dexamethasome administration, which results in an increased free NE and DA and decrease of NE and DA sulfate (Fig. 3). This adds a potential explanation to a previous observation of increased plasma-free DA following dexamethasone *(24)*.

It can be assumed that the stress-related and parallel glucocortical increase-mediated free catecholamine may serve as a mechanism making free catecholamines more rapidly available under emergency conditions than by the multistep process of synthesis, release, and reuptake. An example of such a possible contributory source to NE + E increase is the comparison of a catecholamine sampling without any stress by an indwelling catheter and by direct punction (Fig. 4). The minor stress of direct puncture compared with sampling from an indwelling catheter resulted in a plasma-free NE + E increase associated by a decrease in NE + E sulfate.

The above-described catecholamine synthesis and metabolism changes, mostly studied in peripheral neuronal tissue, probably also apply to the brain where DA and NE particularly, found in the LC-NE system, are important neurotransmitters. Stress increased the TH activity and NE synthesis, and release in LC-NE neurons. This could be alleviated by antidepressant drugs *(25)*. Thus, the LC-NE system plays a role in mediating neuroendocrine responses to stress, and these effects may be partly attenuated by antidepressants.

Molecular Biological, Macrobiological, Environmental, and Pathological Modulation of the Sympathoadrenal Response to Stress

Molecular biological techniques and their use in a novel approach to understanding cellular stress mechanisms revolutionized and further increased the complexity of the role of catecholamines in homeostatic regulations. All major enzymes in catecholamine

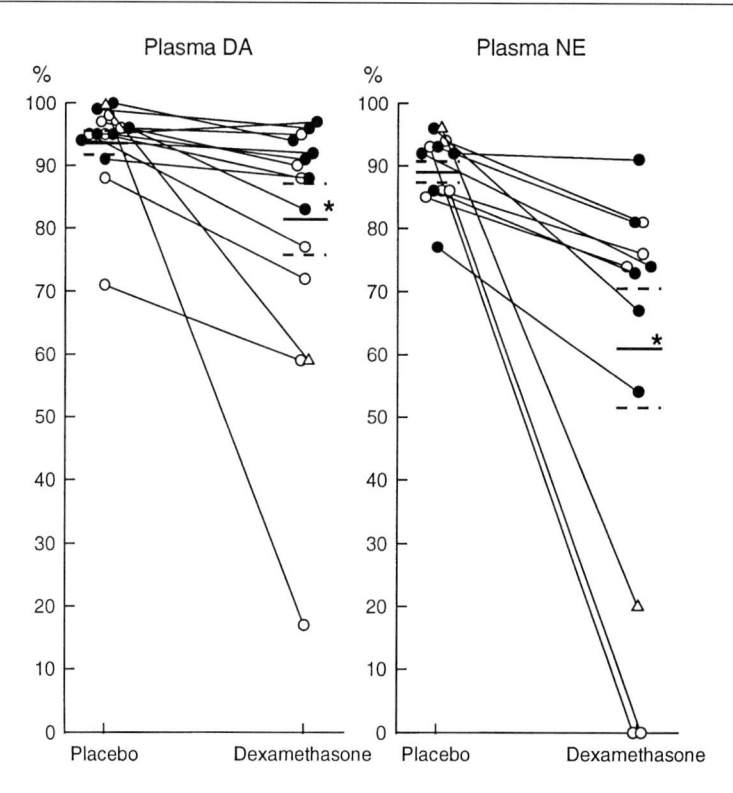

Fig. 3. The degree (%) of conjugation on placebo and dexamethasone of plasma DA and Plasma NE. The effect of dexamethasone (0.5 mg each 6 h for 24 h) compared to a control placebo period under same conditions (recumbency, diet) in three subjects. Dexamethasone administration resulted in a mean increase of plasma-free DA from 66–865 pg/mL, and free NE from 45–142 pg/mL. DA sulfate decreased from 4310–2280 pg/mL and NE sulfate from 850–373 pg/mL. This shift is best reflected by a dexamethasone-induced significant decrease in the degree (%) of plasma DA and NE sulfoconjugation (unpublished observations) *p < 0.05. ○, T.T; ●, N.D.; △, D.M.

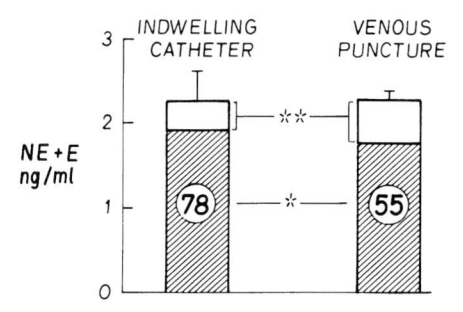

Fig. 4. Technique of blood sampling: effect on free and conjugated catecholamines in essential hypertension. Comparison of plasma-free (open area) and conjugated (hatched area) NE + E mean ± SE in 24 essential hypertensive patients (having blood sampled by an indwelling catheter or by direct venous puncture). Patients having direct puncture had more free NE + E and less (78 ± 3 vs 55 ± 13%) conjugated plasma NE + E. *p < 0.05, **p < 0.01.

synthesis, metabolism, and uptake have been cloned and their chromosal sites mostly located (for review, *see 91*). The same also applies to the rapidly progressing cloning and location of the adrenergic receptors and their subgroups *(10)*.

From the point of view of stress, the main determinant of the stress response, TH activation, exemplifies molecular biological mechanisms regulating TH responsiveness. TH gene expression is modulated by several cofactors, one of them being the concentration of tetrahydrobioptin (BH_4). BH_4 is synthesized from guanosine triphosphate (GTP) partly by GTP cyclohydrolase I (GCH_1). Thus, the activity of GCH_1 indirectly regulates TH activity via BH_4 concentration. The cloning of the cDNA of human GCH_1 *(26)* allowed the identification of the rate at which GCH_1 may regulate catecholamine biosynthesis under stress and BH_4 levels, and their disturbance in hereditary progressive dystonia *(27)*. In the immobilization stress model, stress elicited an increase in the transcription of genes for catecholamine biosynthetic enzymes, particularly TH, preproneuropeptide Y, preproenkephalin in rat adrenal medulla, and several sympathetic ganglia. TH mRNA levels were also elevated by immobilization, even after splanchnicotomy and repeated stress required maximal elevation of the DβH gene expression. It is postulated that distinct mechanisms and interactions of different transcription factors for immobilization-elicited changes in expression of these genes exist. Posttranscriptional calcium-mediated mechanisms were also postulated to be involved in establishing final levels of TH mRNA and, hence, TH protein in adrenomedullary chromaffin cells *(28)*.

The DβH rat gene is also dependent on a DβH promoter. In a final analysis, this promoter interacts with cellular second messengers. This convergence of extracellular and intracellular signals ultimately leads to the regulation and expression of the catecholamine biosynthetic gene at a certain number of defined sites *(29)*.

Macrobiological factors determining catecholamines and their responses to stress have been studied for many years. Gender does not appear to influence sympathetic neural reactivity to stress in healthy humans *(30)*. Blacks have higher E, altered NE kinetics, adrenergic receptor sensitivity, and greater stress- and menstrual cycle-dependent vascular and E responses than white subjects *(31)*. There are well-established differences dependent on diurnal rhythm of catecholamines and particularly their age-dependent changes (for review, *see 32*). There is an age-dependent increase in circulating NE partly associated with its increased responsiveness to stress. E changes are less dependent on age, and DA responses tend to decrease with age. The personality-dependent concentrations of catecholamines and their responsiveness to stress are controversial. Nevertheless, the genetic dependence of catecholamines concomitant with genetic influences on personality makes such a relationship very probable.

Environmental influences on catecholamine responses to stress also represent a widely studied and controversial subject. They distinctively affect individual catecholamines. Therefore, in descending order, NE will be most responsive to treadmill exercise, orthostatism, caffeine, cold pressure, and dietary salt restriction; E, in the same order, will be most responsive to caffeine, treadmill, cold pressure; and handgrip *(33)*, whereas DA increases in response to cold, hypoglycemia *(34)*, and high salt intake *(8)*. A physiological decrease with age of the natriuretic and antihypertensive DA *(32)* may explain why blood pressure physiologically increases with age (as a consequence of DA decrease) only in societies with high salt intake and not in those where salt intake is low *(9)*. Mental stress (Stroop's color-word compact test) was found to increase the renal veinous NE and DA overflow in healthy volunteers (in parallel with increased renal vascular resistence), whereas E increase correlated with an enhanced (β-adrenergic stimulation-mediated) renin release *(35)*.

Eventually, pathological conditions affecting any level of the integrated neurohormonal response to stress may result in an inadequate (or exceptionally excessive) response to stress. Most affected are patients with autonomic dysfunction of either central or peripheral origin. Any additional adrenal defect, whether cortical or adrenomedullary, as well as cardiac, renal, vascular, and particularly brain diseases may further compromise the ability to respond to stress adequately.

Stress-Related Interactions Among Catecholamines, Neuropeptides, Steroids, Neurosteroids, and Other Hormones

The close interaction between catecholamines and peptides at central and peripheral catecholaminergic and peptidergic neural sites represents an integrated control system activated in response to stress *(36)*. Opioid peptides are synthesized, stored and secreted by the adrenal medulla, and by the adenohypophysis in response to stress. Often, β-endorphin activity runs parallel to ACTH. Opioid receptors play a significant role in different types of stress by modulating the synthesis and release of adrenergic neurotransmitters *(37)*. Endorphins produce dose-dependent, naloxone-reversible increases in plasma NE, E, and DA by enhancing sympathetic outflow. All these findings suggest that the stress-related functions of β-endorphin, acting at opioid receptor sites, mediate an increase in sympathetic outflow. The morphine-induced stimulation of adrenal medullary DA release *(8)* is compatible with the presence of adrenomedullary opioid receptors. Other recently recognized peptides under morphinomimetic control, such as atrial natriuretic factor (ANF) *(38)*, may also be involved in the stress-related activation of the catecholamine-peptidergic cascade. This may be of particular interest, since ANF has been demonstrated to be a neurotransmitter in physiological concentrations *(39)* and an inhibitory neuromodulator of peripheral neurotransmission *(40)* in pharmacological settings. Closer to the periphery, catecholamines act directly on adrenergic receptors in a close interplay with peripheral peptides, steroids, and other hormones. Such a combined action affects vascular reactivity, renal sodium excreting mechanisms, and other target actions of homeostatic nature. Multiple other neuropeptides appear to be involved as modulators or cotransmitters of the sympathoadrenomedullary response to stress.

Neuropeptide Y (NPY) is a vasoconstrictor adrenergic cotransmitter abundant in the central and peripheral nervous system and the adrenal medula. It had been demonstrated that chronic and intense stress promotes NPY release, whereas catecholamines induce vascular hypersensitivity to NPY and promote NPY-mediated vasospasms and hypertrophy, leading to the development of cardiovascular disease *(41)*. The regional vasoconstrictor response to NPY is biphasic; the hypertensive response *(42)* is followed by a depressor action dependent on histamine release from mast cells probably contributing to flushing seen under some stressful conditions.

Chromogranin A (CGA), a heritable neuropeptide, costored and coreleased with catecholamines by exocytosis, has been shown to be a precursor of peptides that exert feedback regulatory control on catecholamine secretion. It is a useful marker of exocytotic sympathoadrenomedullary activity. Its elevation in established hypertension is associated with evidence of increased vesicular stores and adrenergic hyperactivity *(43)*. A physiological condition with massive corelease of CGA and NE can be demonstrated in the fetus' response to the stress of birth *(44)*.

Adrenomedullin is a novel hypotensive vasodilating peptide; its mRNA can be demonstrated in adrenal medulla and many other organs. Its increase in several conditions associated with sympathetic discharge *(45)* suggests a yet unclear relationship to catecholamine release, possibly opposing their vasoconstrictor action.

There are several other neuropeptides with relationship to sympathetic activity, such as substance P, secretin, angiotensin II, neurotensin, vasoactive intestinal peptide (VIP), and atrial natriuretic peptide, which may be potentially involved as modulators of the stress response. Concomitant neuropeptide response (e.g., of substance P) may be essential for maintaining adrenal catecholamine secretion in response to stress induced by hypoglycemia, cold, and histamine *(46)*.

Steroids, and more recently neurosteroids, represent another group of sympathoadrenomedullary modulators. Glucocorticoids, the most copious stress hormones, are known to be involved in the transcriptional and posttranscriptional regulation of the PNMT expression, and so indirectly in E synthesis *(47)*. They have an effect on the gene expression of enzymes involved in biosynthesis of other catecholamines during stress as well as on their release, reuptake, and metabolism *(48)*. In addition, they are involved in the feedback regulation restraining stress-induced increases in CRH and arginin-vasopression (AVP), as well as TH activity in the LC. The observation that the glucocorticoid receptor mRNA levels at these feedback sites is downregulated in response to chronic stress *(49)* suggests that during stress, there is a reduced glucocorticoid negative feedback resulting in the enhancement of stress-induced stimulation of these areas.

Recent observations point to a link between the stress-induced hypothalamo-sympathoadrenal activation and neurosteroids, one of them being the ouabain-like compound (OLC). In response to a swim stress, the plasma catecholamine increase was paralleled by an OLC increase, suggesting its function as a stress hormone *(50)*.

Close interaction at several levels exists also between catecholamines and thyroid hormones. In hypothyroidism, catecholamines increase, whereas in hyperthyroidism, an opposite, apparently compensatory, decrease occurs. This interaction may occur at several levels, be it catecholamine synthesis *(51)* or conjugation *(52)*, but probably mainly their receptor action. An influence of this interaction on the impact of the catecholamine response to stress is apparent.

Cardiovascular, Metabolic, and Other Consequences of Stress-Induced Catecholamine Changes

Table 1 summarizes the stress-induced increments in plasma catecholamine levels after exposure to several representative stressors. The elevations in NE levels during standing, hyperthermia, cold, moderate exercise, and cigaret smoking are relatively greater than those of E. These conditions require compensatory changes in the distribution of cardiac output, and NE release serves a homeostatic purpose. The same purpose is apparently served by hypoglycemia-induced E release, which balances hypoglycemia by accelerating glycogenolysis and glucose release.

The increment of E exceeding NE during public speaking probably represents an alerting reaction. With myocardial infarction, shock, and hemorrhage, associated anxiety may shift the balance further toward an E excess. Dorsal spinal column stimulation in humans is an example of a stimulus in which increased DA release exceeds NE and E

Table 1
Stress-Induced Increments in Human Plasma Catecholamines (% Basal)

Stimulus	NE	E	DA
Standing	+110	+10	+23
Public speaking	+60	+140	
Cigaret smoking	+120	+35	+25
Cold pressor test	+250	+60	+25
Hyperthermia (41.5°C)	+350	+30	
Mild hypoglycemia (60 mg%)	+50	+550	+25
Severe hypoglycemia	+280	+2,000	
Moderate exercise	+500	+200	+61
Strenuous exercise	+700	+1,800	+150
Diabetic ketosis	+500	+1,000	
Myocardial infarction	+1,000	+2,000	
Shock, hemorrhage	+1,500	+3,000	+1,200
Surgery	+100	+100	+100
Dorsal column stimulation	+70	+70	+150

secretion (8). It probably operates by activating specific neural pathways resulting in DA release, possibly because TH activation exceeds that of DβH.

Augmented arterial plasma catecholamine levels are not necessarily followed by equal increments in venous levels. There are thus multiple patterns of sympathoadrenomedullary activation that vary with the nature and severity of stress, with the differentiation of the region from which catecholamine outflow occurs, with the metabolic patterns of the respective catecholamine, and with hemodynamics (53). Some adrenomedullary secretory responses to stress may depend on temperature, and this may be important under conditions, such as hypothermia and shock (54). Changes in catecholamine responses to stress develop during ontogenesis, beginning with fetal life, and followed by the first stress of extrauterine life, the survival of the birth (55).

The metabolic responses to E and NE release are characterized by three main components: mobilization of fat, glycogenolysis, and gluconeogenesis. Lipomobilization yields free fatty acids and promotes ketogenesis as an efficient source of energy for muscle contraction. Psychosocial stressors were found to be capable of inhibiting the rate-limiting steps of essential fatty acid metabolism in rats (56). Glycogenolysis is the source of glucose for many other tissues, particularly for the brain, which becomes very dependent on it during stress. Hepatic gluconeogenesis using lactate liberated from muscle is another source of glucose. The availability of glucose to the brain during stress is also supported by an inhibitory action of E on glucose utilization in muscles and by its suppressive influence on insulin secretion. The latter effect decreases glucose utilization in peripheral tissues. The main metabolic actions of catecholamines mobilized during stress are summarized in Fig. 5.

Adaptive (e.g., Training) Adjustment to Prolonged or Repeated Stress

When stress is prolonged or repeated, there are considerable adaptive changes (57). These alterations also affect adrenergic receptors, and usually downregulation occurs in some adrenergic receptors. There is also a reduction of catecholamine biosynthetic

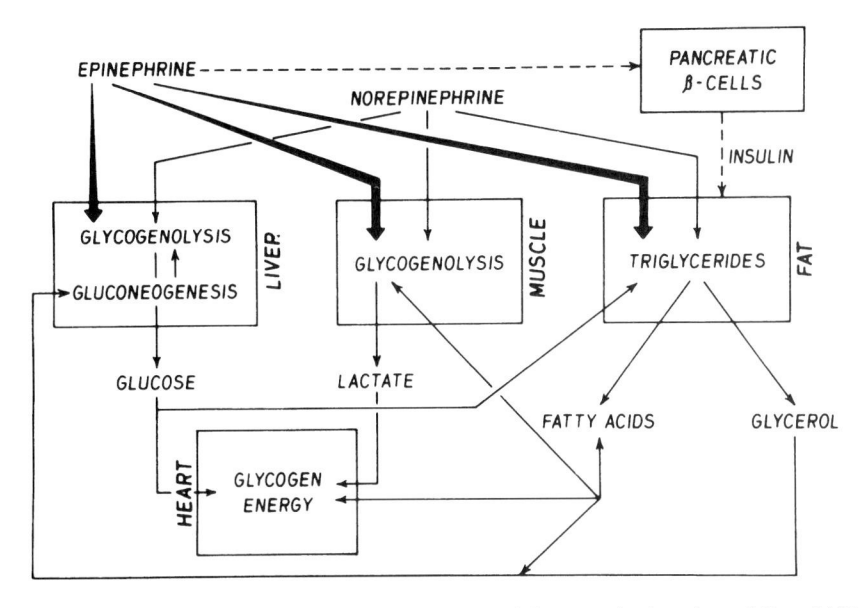

Fig. 5. Schematic outline of the main mechanisms by which excessively released E and NE during stress affect metabolic pathways in the liver, muscle, and fat to make metabolism better adapted to the energy of the muscles, heart and brain: --▶, inhibitory action; ⟶▶, stimulatory pathways. The strength of the arrows indicates the relative potency of the metabolic actions of E and NE.

enzymes in the adrenal medulla and sympathetic nerves. It appears that repeated stress can affect the release of catecholamines and their metabolism in different directions. Comparisons of experienced and inexperienced pilots have shown that those repeatedly subjected to stress have less NE and E release than inexperienced pilots. However, the excretion rate of NE and E metabolites presents an opposite difference between both groups *(58)*, suggesting that differences may be accounted for by changes in metabolic enzyme activities. Some processes that alter organ structure (e.g., of the heart and vascular smooth muscle) may be initiated. Such effects may be important in influencing cardiovascular, gastrointestinal, and immunological functions. It is therefore necessary to define better mechanisms that are involved in disorders related to chronic or repeated stress.

The adaptive process needed to develop resistance to severe stress requires functional and metabolic changes in the myocardium protecting the heart. Such a protection implies opposing actions of toxic levels of catecholamines causing myocardial ischemia and others, such as ouabain. Stress induces the adenylate cyclase-cAMP stimulation, the latter triggering some key enzymes, such as Na^+/K^+ ATPase and phosphodiesterase (PDE). This "delayed cardioprotection" *(59)* appears to be based on excessive hydrolysis of cAMP carried out by an enhanced PDE activity. This results in attenuation of responses to β-adrenergic stimuli and electrophysiological changes, such as prolongation of the effective refractory period and action potential duration, both moderating arrhythmias owing to ischemia and reperfusion.

Adaptation to cold had been shown in rats to prolong their survival time at high altitude *(60)*. However, great variability exists dependent on the species and type of stress. Particular distinction has to be made between psychosocial and physical stress in men and take into account their motivation to tolerate the latter. Physical stress of an ambitious sportsman cannot be compared with the same stress of a prisoner. The adrenomedullary response to psychosocial stress may induce an adaptive response *(61)*; enhanced cardiovascular fitness may be characterized by an attenuated plasma NE response to a vigilance task with sustained cognitive performance subsequent to the task *(62)*. On the other hand, physical training *(63)* and religious winter austerity in a Buddhist sect consisting of cold water bathing, hunger, and sleep deprivation *(64)* enhanced the NE and E release or excretion.

ASSESSMENT OF SYMPATHOADRENOMEDULLARY ACTIVITY IN RESPONSE TO STRESS

Overall Biological Indices

The changes associated with sympathoadrenomedullary activation in response to stress are numerous, with only some of them (heart rate, blood pressure, skin conductivity, and sweating) being quantifiable. They can be used as they have been prior to the development of more sophisticated measurements as a rough index of autonomic responses.

In relationship to the role of adrenergic nerve activity in human hypertension, some pharmacologic tools proved to be useful in establishing increased adrenergic activity in patients with borderline hypertension contrasting with vascular hyperreactivity to adrenergic stimulation in established hypertension *(65)*. The interaction of genetics and stress has to be taken into account when evaluating these overall indices in relationship to others, such as sodium and potassium excretion *(66)*.

Biochemical Measurement of Catecholamines

The development of new techniques, particularly HPLC with electrochemical detection, has permitted rapid and convenient measurements of *O*-methylated and deaminated metabolites in addition to catecholamines in plasma and urine.

The assessment of sympathoadrenomedullary activation in response to stress is complicated by an internal circle of catecholamine release and inactivation best illustrated by NE. Released from sympathetic nerve terminals into the synaptic cleft of neuroeffector junctions, NE is mainly reuptaken (uptake I) into the nerve terminals where it is either inactivated by MAO to form dihydroxyphenylglycol (DHPG) or taken up to synaptic vesicles to be reused. NE, which escapes reuptake into the nerve terminals, is taken up (uptake 2) into extraneuronal cells or diffuses into the circulation. It is estimated that only 2–10% of released NE reaches effluent blood. A large portion (80%) of NE released into the portal venous blood is removed during a single passage through the liver. This vastly underestimates the visceral component of NE released at peripheral sympathetic nerve terminals. Further modifications of plasma NE levels occur as blood passes through the lungs and peripheral tissues.

The best way to assess regional differences in the release of NE into the circulation is the measurement of total body and regional NE spillover calculated from the rate of infusion of labeled NE and the specific activity of arterial NE; regional NE release can be estimated for these vascular beds from which effluent venous blood is sampled *(67)*. Plasma NE levels in blood obtained from the antecubital vein have limited value in assessing regional changes in sympathetic activity, since they may only reflect alterations in generalized sympathetic activity. In general, plasma NE concentrations parallel the known level of sympathetic tone in a variety of experimental and clinical circumstances, and to a certain degree reflect the stress-induced activation of the sympathetic nervous system usually parallel to the total body NE spillover rate. Regional organ NE spillover into plasma represents approx 30% of the total NE spillover rate for the lung, 25% for the kidney, and 20% for skeletal muscle, with the rest (between 2 and 6%) being contributed by the hepato-mesenteric regions, skin, heart, adrenals, and brain *(68)*. These organ spillover rates depend partly on the stress-related sympathetic nerve firing rate into the respective organ and on other factors (sympathetic nerve density, organ mass, synaptic cleft width, capacity for NE uptake, for *O*-methylation, conjugation, capillary permeability to NE, and blood flow). Stress-related changes in regional NE spillover rates have not yet been systematically studied. Despite some of the above-mentioned limitations in their interpretation, they may advance our understanding of the role of catecholamines in defense reactions *(69)* characterized by increased sympathetic outflow to the heart and kidney in the presence of normal skeletal muscle sympathetic activity *(70)*. It is probably no coincidence that young essential hypertensive patients who have hemodynamic changes compatible with the "fight or flight" defense reaction and/or behavior patterns of suppressed hostility particularly exhibit exactly these regional NE spillover patterns, i.e., an increased kidney and heart NE spillover rate contributing to their elevated total NE spillover rate *(68)*. This is the mechanism partially underlying the elevated plasma NE levels found in young hypertensive patients in response to mental stress *(71)*.

Another recently used principle in evaluating sympathetic nerve activity is the determination of catecholamine metabolites, which are metabolized more slowly than released catecholamines. This means that, with rapidly changing neuronal firing rates and NE release in response to stress, these measurements reflect an overall means of sympathetic activation during a certain period of time (hours rather than minutes), but are less sensitive indices of rapid, minute-to-minute changes in sympathetic activity and catecholamine release.

An example of this approach is the use of DHPG and monohydroxyphenylglycol (MHPG) as adjuncts to assessing sympathetic activation *(72)*. NE taken up by the nerves is largely metabolized to DHPG and MHPG. Measurements of these metabolites in conjunction with the total body NE spillover rate, arterial E, NE, and pressor responses to a mental challenge (playing a video game) give a more complex image than an isolated assessment of any of these indices alone *(72)*. Plasma metadrenalines provide supplementary information in addition to being most useful in detecting pheochromocytoma *(73)*.

Another potential, but controversial aspect of measurements of catecholamine metabolites in response to stress is the evaluation of catecholamine conjugates. In surgical stress, a distinct stress-induced response of NE and E conjugates (decrease) and DA conjugates (increase) is evident, particularly in arterial blood, and of NE and E in venous blood *(74)*. This increase of DA conjugate (sulfate in this case) originates in the adrenal medulla, as suggested by arteriovenous differences and findings of DA sulfate within the granular fraction of the medulla. During exercise in humans, NE and E sulfate also decrease, whereas free NE and E increase *(75)*. It thus appears that NE and E conjugates tend to respond to sympathoadrenomedullary activation with a decrease, whereas DA sulfate reacts in several experimental and clinical situations in the opposite direction, with an increase, possibly depending on the acuteness of the stressor. There is also a dependence on the type and intensity of stress, type of conjugation in different species, and so forth. The main reason is apparently a difference between NE and E conjugation on the one hand and DA conjugation on the other, in the way they are generated and possibly also hydrolyzed. DA is avidly sulfoconjugated owing to its high affinity for PST, so that DA release results in high DA sulfate levels, which appear to be relatively stable and is considered to be the main product of the autocrine-paracrine third catecholamine system *(14)*. NE and E sulfoconjugation, on the other hand, is a low-affinity process, and the stability of NE and E sulfates appears to be much lower *(9)*. Conversion of plasma NE from conjugated form into free form can be demonstrated during exercice in patients with cardiac disease *(76)*. DA sulfates seem to be a good marker of stress-related increased free DA and possibly also DOPA *(8)*. On the other hand NE and E release is not necessarily reflected by NE and E sulfates. However, hypertensive patients with low NE + E conjugates may be hyperreactors to stimuli by excessive free NE + E increase owing to its insufficient "buffering" by sulfoconjugation when compared with patients with normal NE + E conjugates. Those are the patients contributing in randomly selected hypertensives to the free NE + E hyperresponsiveness to a minor stress of direct venous puncture (Fig. 4) and having hyperadrenergic features imitating pheochromocytoma *(77)* (Fig. 6).

There are many unknown facts about the site of catecholamine sulfoconjugation and their potential biological role (reserve form, buffers of catecholamine excess[?], weak agonists[?]). Some findings, such as stimulation of PST activity by dexamethasone in the presence or absence of the adrenals *(78)*, suggest that corticoids control conjugation (and deconjugation, *see* Fig. 3) during stress similarly to the effect of cortisol on PNMT *(4)*. Studies on the metabolic fate of DA glucuronide in rats *(79)* also indicate that catecholamine conjugates other than sulfates may be potential precursors of free amines. Catecholamine conjugation (and deconjugation [9]) during stress may thus play a regulatory role and can become a contributory determinant of the availability of free catecholamines.

In contrast to NE, E is almost entirely derived from the adrenal medulla and secreted directly into the circulation; hence, its plasma antecubital vein levels appear to reflect adrenal medullary activity adequately. A considerable portion of E is removed during the passage of blood through tissues (particularly the lung). Basal E levels are low (50 pg/mL), but even small increments (100 pg/mL or more) can elicit physiological responses. Such increases occur on exposure to moderate stimuli (cigaret smoking, moderate hypoglycemia, or exercise) *(80)*, in contrast to NE whose basal levels (about 250 pg/mL) have to rise at least five- to sixfold to exert a biological action. This may be owing to the gradient of NE concentration between plasma and the synaptic clefts. Such increases in plasma NE are known to occur only after strenuous exercise, shock or hemorrhage, myocardial infarction, or in pheochromocytoma. In addition to plasma catecholamines and their metabolites, platelet catecholamines, free and sulfates, were found to provide a useful cumulative index of chronic sympathoadrenal activity *(81)*.

The serum DβH is a concomitant marker of the synaptic NE release, and the longer DβH half-life than that of NE qualifies plasma DβH as an index of NE exocytosis during stress *(4)*. More recently, it appears that CGA coreleased with catecholamines into the bloodstream is an even better marker of NE exocytosis *(82)*.

Determination of Peripheral Sympathetic Neural Activity

This represents an alternative approach to evaluating sympathetic activation by stress. It had been demonstrated under various conditions that there is a systematic relationship between muscle sympathetic activity and venous plasma NE concentrations

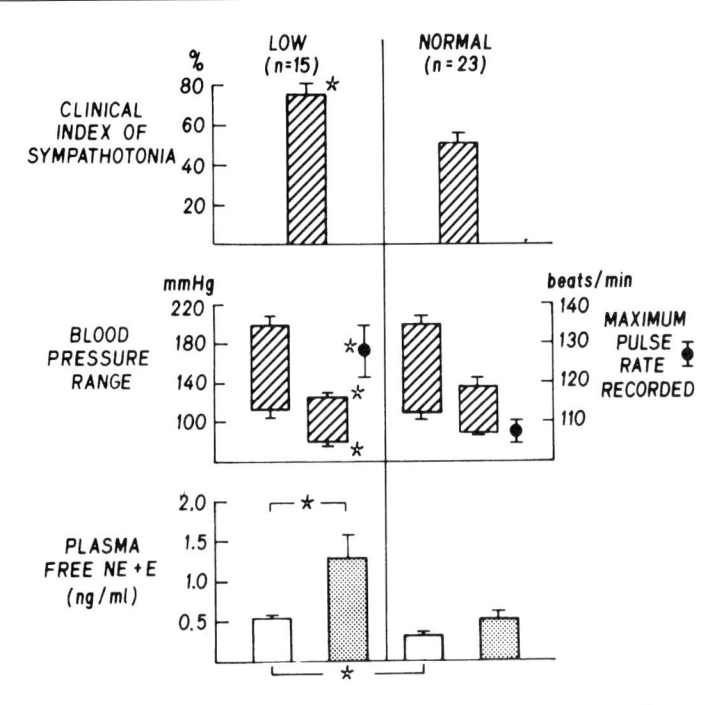

Fig. 6. Essential hypertension with low plasma conjugated NE + E. Some differences between two subgroups of essential hypertensive patients with low (<0.23 ng/mL) and normal plasma-conjugated NE + E. The clinical index of sympathotonia is based on 10 main symptoms in descending order of weighing (10 points attributed to first, 1 to last): palpitations, sweating, anxiety, weakness, loss of weight, dyspnea, headache, nausea, abdominal or lumbar pain, and tremor. The final individual score was expressed as a percentage of the maximum possible score of 55. The middle panel demonstrates the higher range between maximum and minimum blood pressure and the higher pulse rate in patients with low conjugated NE + E. In the bottom panel are results of free NE + E sampling by indwelling catheter avoiding the stress of the immediate venous puncture (open columns) compared with sampling by direct venous puncture (dotted columns). Mean ± SE, *$p < 0.05$ or less (data from ref. 77).

(83). This procedure, requiring considerable technical expertise, has been used mainly in humans (84) and does not necessarily provide an index of overall sympathoadrenomedullary activity. The neural and hormonal responses to stress are not necessarily parallel. Insulin-induced hypoglycemia increases muscle sympathetic neural outflow in insulin-dependent diabetes and controls. There is however a lack of correlation between neural activity and E increase, indicating that the adrenomedullary and peripheral sympathetic responses to hypoglycemia are independently mediated (85).

Recording of sympathetic activity has also been possible in anesthetized small animals, but this method has apparent limitations in the study of stress.

THE SURVIVAL VALUE VS THE POTENTIALLY DAMAGING ROLE OF STRESS-INDUCED CATECHOLAMINE MOBILIZATION

The role of catecholamines in stress must be viewed from three different, but closely related perspectives:

1. The survival value of catecholamine mobilization probably applies to situations in which an adaptive homeostatic release of catecholamines occurs. Adaptation to any stress-induced

swing in homeostasis depends on the efficient and rapid stimulation of catecholamine secretion. This holds true for conditions inducing hypovolemia (hemorrhage, shock, orthostatism) or hypoglycemia (e.g., insulin shock), which have to be corrected by catecholamine release. Adrenergic stimulation maintains cerebral and coronary arterial perfusion. It also promotes increased glucose production and decreased glucose utilization, thus ensuring supplies of this critical metabolic fuel to the central nervous system. The inability to counter these catastrophic threats to survival by catecholamine release in patients with autonomic insufficiency or after extensive sympathectomy may prove to be fatal. Catecholamines released by the adrenal medulla during birth play a key role in the adaptation of the newborn to extrauterine life. Respiratory, metabolic, and cardiovascular adaptations to the hypoxia and other stresses associated with delivery are dependent on a profound surge of adrenomedullary activity, which occurs despite the immaturity of connections between the central nervous system and the adrenal (*86*). The positive survival value of E in older population is suggested by the finding that 70-yr-old men with high plasma E had the best survival rate during the 7-yr follow-up period, probably because they also had the best physical working capacity (*87*). High plasma NE values were, however, associated with a reduced survival rate. In addition, E increase in response to acute swim stress was associated with a considerable improvement of the spatial deficit recovery of aged rats (*88*).

2. On the other hand, even some initially beneficial homeostatic responses of catecholamines have a tendency to "overshoot" with a continuing action of the stressor and defy their initial purpose. An example is the continuing E-induced hypoglycemia following extenuating physical exercise, which is certainly not in accordance with the initial purpose of E release and the metabolic need of the organism under such circumstances (*89*). The negative evolutionary connotation of stress-induced catecholamine release outliving their initial purpose is particularly applicable to several so-called civilization disorders (*23*). Phylogenetically older primitive homeostatic stereotypes continue to be activated in response to stress irrespectively of different conditions of life in modern society. The "fight or flight" reaction requires a massive mobilization of catecholamines in order to increase cardiac output, divert blood from the immediately less vital organs (kidney, viscera) to muscles by regional splanchnic vasoconstriction and make energy rapidly available by E-induced glycogenolysis. Stress in modern life is usually not physical, but symbolic, mediated by the central nervous system and originating in anxiety, insecurity, and feelings of being threatened. The phylogenetically old homeostatic stereotypes, however, remain identical (increased cardiac output, renal vasoconstriction) and inappropriate to living conditions in modern society. Accelerated heart activity, renal vasoconstriction, hyperglycemia, and ketoacidosis combined can all precipitate the phenotype based on the genetic disposition to typical diseases of modern civilization: hypertension, coronary heart disease, diabetes, and others. These reactivity patterns can be compounded by sedentary living with inadequate muscular activity, overeating with excess fat and salt, smoking, pollution, noise, and multiple other stressful stimuli of our modern lifestyle.

3. Beyond the survival value of catecholamines, their *release*, particularly if excessive and prolonged, may become highly detrimental to the organism. If the underlying condition that led to catecholamine release is not corrected and massive adrenergic discharge continues unabated, the initial "compensatory" response can critically compromise the perfusion of other organs and lead to death. There is apparently a critical threshold of increase of plasma E, the most important response to stress, further exacerbated by the parallel release of NE. In an intensive care unit, an acute maximal stress, such as cardiac arrest, resulted in a >300-fold increase in plasma E (compared to 32-fold increase in plasma NE). Successfully resuscitated patients can achieve a further up to 25-fold peak increase in

plasma E and NE, possibly the limit or survivability of stress (90). Both catecholamines and DβH levels were significantly higher in nonsurviving than surviving animals exposed to neurologic shock; these extremely high levels probably reflect the stage of irreversibility of the shock (91). The concentrations of plasma E seen during acute myocardial infarction are particularly detrimental, being both arrhythmogenic and proischemic (92).

ROLE OF SYMPATHOADRENAL STRESS RESPONSES IN SEVERAL DISEASES AND CONDITIONS

Cardiovascular and Pulmonary Diseases

The dual role of stress-induced catecholamine stimulation (i.e., its beneficial homeostatic vs potential pathogenetic role in the disease) is most evident in cardiovascular and pulmonary diseases. Virtually every cardiopulmonary disease and most of their medications affect catecholaminergic functions in some way (93). However, the distinction between catecholamine increase becoming a healthy defense reaction and such an increase becoming pathogenetic is very difficult.

Congestive heart failure, a condition occasionally likened to a "heart crying for help," is probably benefiting at least temporarily from adrenergic stimulation. Heart failure depletes NE stores by a not yet fully understood mechanism. It is not clear to what degree the compensatory sympathoneuronal recruitment reflected by increased NE spillover helps to maintain cardiac contractility. The additional increase of E adds to the sympathetic discharge and may reflect a component of emotional distress. Since the E increase appears to be nonneuronal and extra-adrenal (94), alternative sources of free catecholamines, such as their liberation from catecholamine sulfates, suspected to occur in heart failure (76,95), have to be considered. All these sources of catecholamine release, particularly that of E, may be superimposed on painful and emotional distress causing condition, such as coronary insufficiency and precipitate cardiac necrosis, myocardial infarction, arrythmias, or sudden death (92). In addition, the β-adrenergic receptor density was found to be lower, whereas plasma catecholamines increased in cardiac failure (96), suggesting a dynamic relationship between catecholamines and their site of action.

HYPERTENSION, HYPOTENSION, AND PULMONARY DISEASE

Despite extensive literature on the role of stress-induced mobilization of catecholamines in hypertension, the role of catecholamines in hypertension is not yet clear. The reason may be that research continues to focus on single effector systems and less on the overall complex neurohormonal pathways. Increased NE and E baselines in response to stimulation were found in young borderline hypertensive patients (97), but only in association with tasks that elicit active behavioral coping responses. When progressing into stable hypertension, these sympathetic indices became normal. The intricate relationship among personality, environment, perceived stress, and cardiovascular response, including hypertension (98), is outlined in Fig. 7. There is a mutual relationship between those entities with retrograde influences. As an example, the simple awareness that the blood pressure has been found to be elevated resulted in an exaggerated blood pressure and heart rate response during a cold pressor test and plasma E and blood pressure hyperresponsiveness to mental stress (99).

Hypertension is thus a complex disorder. The balance within the autonomic nervous system may also be related to the salt balance. Since excessive salt retention is a focal

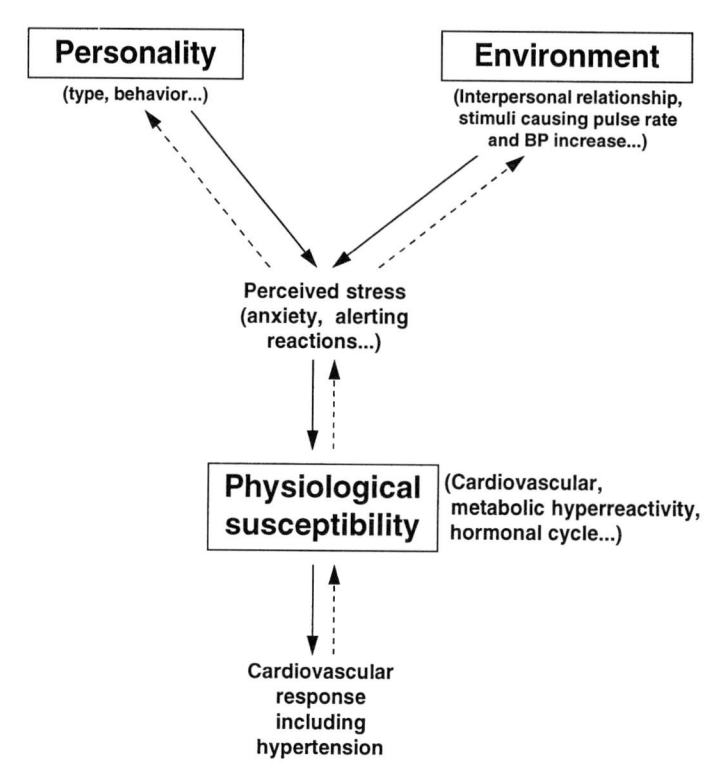

Fig. 7. Hypothetical interactions of three major factors determining the effect of stress on cardiovascular diseases *(98)* and their retrograde (--▶) repercussions.

point by which stress may precipitate the development of hypertension in genetically susceptible individuals, catecholamines exemplify hypertension as an evolutionary "hangover" *(23)* that may explain some observed phenomena. As previously outlined, the main catecholamine in fish is not NE, but rather its precursor DA. Homeostatic systems are more prone to protect the salt balance, in the case of fish living in salty environment, by expelling excess salt from the organism by natriuretic substances (in addition to DA, others, such as ANF), which are highly developed in fish. When life enters the earth, where salt becomes a rare commodity, these hormones are overshadowed by potent antinatriuretic factors, such as NE and renin-angiotensin-aldosterone. The predominance of these factors is such that humans can survive on minimal amounts of environmental salt, although they are unable to survive on salty sea water like fish because natriuretic factors became suppressed to such a degree by adaptation to terrestrial life.

In terms of catecholamines, the excessive release of NE and E continues to dominate homeostatic responses. DA, DOPA, and other sideline metabolic products, such as octopamine *(100)*, going back to lower animals, continue to express themselves as markers of sympathetic activation *(101)*. In this respect, the neuronal origin of DOPA *(102)* and its correlation with NE are particularly interesting. The biological purpose of these substances, which are underdeveloped in humans when compared to NE, escapes us at present. They may be simple markers of sympathetic discharge, parallel to NE and E, occasionally elevated during stress even without elevation of NE and E. The existence of such a condition in hyperadrenergic episodic hypertension is demonstrated by

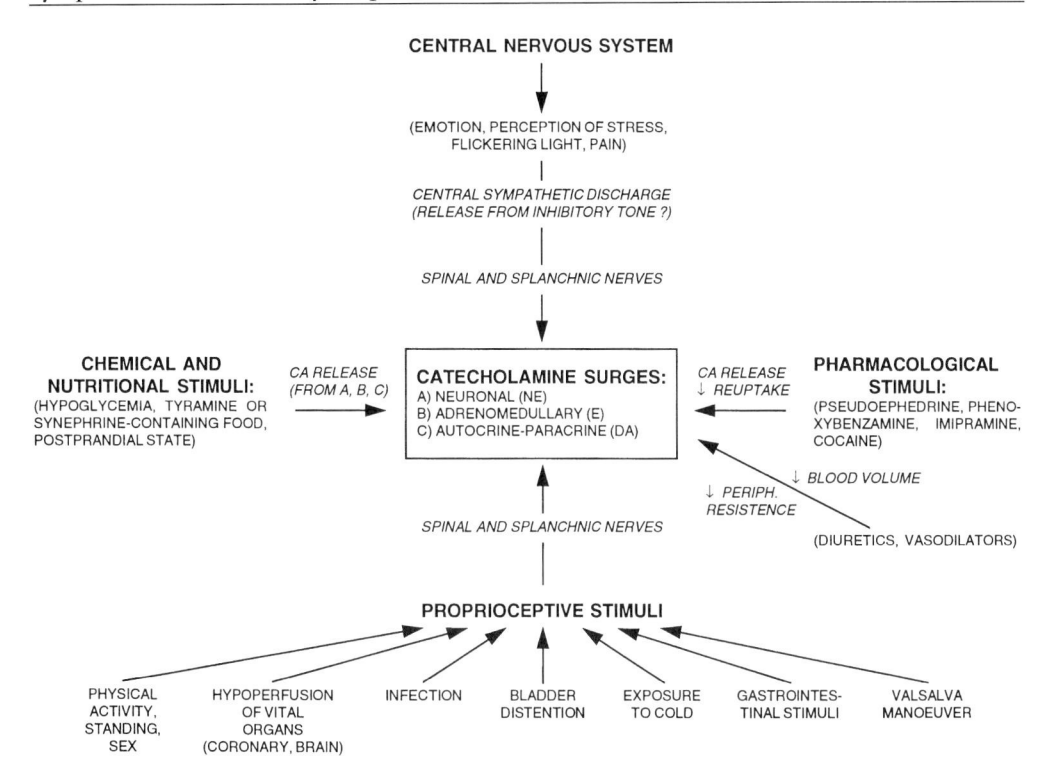

Fig. 8. The multiplicity of observed *(77,103)* stimuli triggering catecholamine surges in hyperadrenergic hyperkinetic hypertensive patients in whom pheochromocytoma had been eliminated. The supposed pathways of their provocative action are indicated by italics. The ratio of NE, E, and DA discharge depends on multiple factors, including genetics *(9)*.

surges of DA becoming the main outlet of the sympathetic discharge *(8)* in the absence of an increase in NE and E *(103)*. Alternatively, other hypertensive patients may have an episodic predominantly free NE and E release exemplified by patients with low conjugated NE + E *(77)*. Both types of episodic hyperadrenergic hypertension have an extreme hyperreactivity to minor stimuli in common, which led to their labeling as "hyperreactors." In addition, because of clinical similarity to pheochromocytoma and increased catecholamines as well as frequent nonfunctional incidental adrenal adenoma in hypertension, they were occasionally exposed to unjustified adrenal surgery. When all the observed provoking stimuli of hyperadrenergic episodes with catecholamine discharge, whether it is free NE + E *(77)* or DA sulfate *(103)* in paroxysmal (nonpheochromocytoma) hypertensive patients, are summarized (Fig. 8), it is evident how minor and variable can be the so-called stress trigger provoking hypertensive episodes in a predisposed hyperreactive patient.

Considering their biological activity, the prohypertensive and antinatriuretic action of NE may be the opposite of DA, an intrinsic natriuretic and vasodilatory factor. Placed into a wider framework of pro- and antinatriuretic factors (reflected by the balance between renin-angiotensin-aldosterone and ANF on one hand and other natriuretic hormones on the other), the NE–DA balance represents a key interplay within the autonomic nervous system, necessary for understanding of sodium-retaining pathologies (hypertension, cardiac failure, ascitic cirrhosis, edema).

As monitored by the pulse rate response, hypertension can be separated by the sympathetic discharge following assuming upright position into the hypo- and hyperadrenergic variety. Since orthostatism represents a special form of stress, coping with the gravity-induced pooling of part of the circulating blood in the lower extremities, the adequacy of the sympathetic response is a factor determining whether hypotension, particularly orthostatic, has its origin within or outside the autonomic nervous system; hypoadrenergic responses characterize the first case, and hyperadrenergic responses represent an adequate adjustment to other causes of hypotension beyond the autonomic nervous system, such as hypovolemia. Severe orthostatic intolerance following weightlessness represents one of the main medical problems during prolonged space travel *(104)*. It is a typical example of a suppressed autonomic nervous system owing to the absence of stimulus for the autonomic nervous system—the gravitational stress, an essential part of life on this planet. It also demonstrates the relativity of the term "stress" in relationship to the environment; instead of gravity being a stress, its absence threatens human survival during space travel. Only long-term weightlessness may result in a homeostatic adaptation to extraterrestrial life, but this is an extremely long evolutionary process.

Similar examples of sympathoadrenomedullary adjustments induced by cardiorespiratory changes are hypoxia-induced changes by living in (or going up to) high altitudes, resulting in changes in cardiac output and blood pressure *(105)*. Physical activity, distressful when one is forced to do it, but becoming a beneficial stress under motivated conditions, is also a potent sympathoadrenomedullary stimulant. Its extent depends on the level of training and psychosocial circumstances under which it is executed. Therefore, exercise-induced catecholamine changes are extremely variable. Aerobic exercise reduces blood pressure, which is at least partially mediated by changes in plasma catecholamine levels *(106)*.

Some conditions, such as an asthmatic attack, can be exercise-induced, although repetitive exercise may prevent it. Since repetitive exercise in asthmatic subjects increased the NE and E release *(107)*, progressive bronchodilation (by β-adrenergic stimulation), airway hyperemia, and edema reduction (by α-adrenergic stimulation) may occur in the asthmatic at the end of the workload, thus decreasing the apparent magnitude of the obstructive response.

Metabolic Diseases

The closely interrelated cardiovascular and metabolic changes under distress are linked to the catecholamine responses in both ways. The main metabolism-related catecholamine is E. Any metabolic emergency, such as hypoglycemia, is a potent stimulus for a corrective E release. Although E release protects against fatal hypoglycemia, an uncontrolled continuous E release may cause considerable catabolism, lead to diabetes, or cause a clinical hypermetabolic state similar to hyperthyroidism.

The counterregulatory E release is of particular importance in insulin-dependent diabetes mellitus (IDDM). It represents a balancing act to counter the stress of insulin-induced hypoglycemia. The adrenomedullary E response to hypoglycemia was found to be decreased in IDDM, whereas other catecholamine responses were normal *(108)*. It is thus a very selective and specifically hypoglycemia-associated autonomic failure. This decreased sympathochromaffin activity may be a component of diabetic neuropathy. Its recognition is important to avoid occasionally fatal hypoglycemia. Children *(109)* and pregnant women *(110)* with IDDM appear to be particularly susceptible to E and other counterregulatory hormone deficiencies.

E release not only has a protective effect against insulin-induced hypoglycemia, but increased E and NE reduce insulin-mediated glucose disposal (i.e., induce insulin resistance). The mental stress-induced increase in NE and E, blood pressure, and heart rate was, however, not found to be associated with an increased glucose concentration *(111)*. This suggests that there is a much more complex relationship among insulin action, glycemia, and mental stress-stimulated catecholamine release; a possible increase in skeletal muscle blood flow during mental stress with increased substrate delivery to the metabolically active muscle cells is a possible explanation. Responses to mental stress are, in addition, distinct in high and low reactors based on the NE and E change from the mean rest and task conditions with high reactors having less favorable lipid profiles than low reactors *(112)*.

A role of sympathomedullary responses in weight control is suggested by the finding that fasting decreases, whereas eating or overeating increases, the activity of the sympathetic nervous system. Thus, a catecholamine-mediated increase in the thermic response during the absorptive phase of the meal, or its absence, could determine the rates of degradation and synthesis of fuel stores, and affect weight control *(113)*. In the relationship of sympathoadrenal activity to obesity, there are indications that, in obesity, there is an impaired plasma catecholamine response to stress, such as submaximal treadmill exercise *(114)*. Although the possibilities that a reduced ability of catecholamines to increase the rate of substrate cycling and thermic response *(115)* or a faulty integration between catecholamine and insulin are attractive, the role of catecholamine suppression in obesity is not yet clear.

Another interaction that may determine the eventual impact of sympathoadrenal activation on metabolism concerns the role of catecholamines and thyroid hormones. This interaction is most evident at the adrenergic receptor level, but may also relate to catecholamine release and metabolism. Hyperthyroid patients exposed to dynamic exercise were found to have decreased sympathetic neuronal, but increased adrenomedullary responses. These abnormalities normalized when patients were controlled by antithyroid therapy *(116)*.

Neuropsychological Disorders

As a consequence of neurological pathways in the sympathetic outflow regulation, many neurological lesions are responsible for abnormal sympathetic discharge in response to any intrinsic or extrinsic signalization. Starting from afferent information, baroreceptor dysfunction is the best-defined syndrome of erratic catecholamine and cardiovascular responsiveness, often manifested by episodic hypertension *(117)*. These patients usually have a history of surgical or traumatic lesions around the neck, and many may be extremely responsive to banal stimuli, such as assuming upright posture or minor emotion *(118)*. Tetraplegic patients with spinal cord transsections have plasma NE extremely hyperresponsive to minor stimuli, such as fullness of the bladder *(119)*. On the other hand, patients with multiple-system atrophy or pure autonomic failure exhibit decreased catecholamine responses to stimulation *(120)*. The autonomic failure is also present in Parkinson patients, but not in the early stage *(121)*. Patients with neurocardiogenic (vasovagal) syncope exposed to head-up tilt testing were found to have a diminished NE (neuronal sympathetic), but enhanced E (adrenomedullary) response *(122)*.

Psychological effects on adrenergic responses are widely recognized. The anticipation of stress is so evident that the psychological effect prior to anesthetic administration before surgery was found to be as great as or greater than the changes seen after anesthetic administration and surgery *(123)*. Anticipation of stress or verbal stimulation appears to be occasionally more effective in precipitating crises in patients with baroreceptor dysfunction than stress itself *(117,118)*. Panic disorder patients exhibit cardiorespiratory features during crises very suggestive of an autonomic hyperresponsiveness to even a minor stress. However, closer studies did not find any abnormality in the autonomic responses, suggesting the integrity of autonomic nervous system *(124)*. Therefore, it appears that the problem resides more in the excessive or aberrant perception of the threat or distress to which the autonomic nervous system adequately responds.

Immune, Inflammatory, Infectious, and Neoplastic Diseases

One of the most stressful life experience, the death of a spouse, is associated with an elevated mortality rate in bereaved spouses *(125)*. This is suspected to be owing to stress-induced autonomic nervous system-mediated immunosuppression, a lower resistance to infection, and a higher incidence of cancer *(126)*. Experimental and clinical data implicate catecholamines in the decreased immune responses following stress. Immune cytokines not only activate immune function, but also recruit central stress-responsive neurotransmitters systems in the modulation of the immune response and in the activation of behaviors that may be adaptive during injury or inflammation *(12)*. The central link in the response to cytokines appears to be the hypothalamic CRH activating not only the pituitary–adrenal axis, but interacting with the LC-NE system (*see* Fig. 1). The main effector in the neuroendocrine-immune system response is the anti-inflammatory action of hypercortisolemia. Increased cortisol has not only anti-inflammatory, but also behavioral effects, additive to the arousal of CRH and associated with the LC-NE activation. The latter is associated with melancholic depression and increased CSF content of NE metabolism, such as MHPG *(127)*. These data suggest that the concomitant activation of two principal effectors of the stress response (CRH and LC-NE), each stimulating the other's functional activity, results in clinical and biochemical manifestation of melancholic depression. The concept of melancholic depression as a disease of the stress response is also supported by the finding that the administration of tricyclic antidepressants is associated with a decreased expression of the hypothalamic CRH and LC tyrosine hydroxylase gene *(128)*. The central nervous system may also communicate with the immune system by direct interaction of lymphoid organs and changes in neurotransmitter release; exposure of volunteers to cold resulted in an increase of plasma NE associated with a reduction of the lymphoproliferative response to phytohemagglutinin *(129)*. Physical stress-exposed healthy subjects were found to have an increased plasma E associated with a decreased T-helper to T-suppressor cells ratio *(130)*.

The immune suppression of critical illness is thus characterized by "anergy" that is a failure of the delayed hypersensitivity response, primarily documented by abnormalities in neurotrophic chemotaxis and T-lymphocyte function *(131)*. Dehydroepiandrosterone sulfate (DHEAS), a newly recognized potent modulator of the human immune response, has been found to be suppressed by DA infusion *(132)* widely used as a first-choice drug in intensive care units because of its superior inotropic, renal, and splanchnic vasodilatory properties. A bona fide cardiovascular use of a catecholamine drug may thus inadvertently suppress DHEAS (in addition to prolactin), both apparently essential cofactors to recovery from the anergic state of critical illness.

There are indications that catecholamines reflecting sympathoadrenomedullary stress responses are closely linked to immunity, inflammatory, infectious, and neoplastic diseases in both directions. Behavioral syndrome, such as depression, may result from the immunitary and inflammatory neurohormonal response, on one hand, and the increased NE and E release may be operative in suppressing some immune responses, on the other hand. Therefore, it is not surprising that psychological stress becomes a cofactor of AIDS, a condition in which the immune system is already suppressed, as well as in widespread infections, such as the common cold *(133)*.

Surgical, Traumatic, and Thermal Stress, Anesthesia, Resuscitation, and Transplantation

Surgical stress evokes considerable NE and E increase, which may reflect an adrenergic response to afferent pain stimuli, which are not blocked by anesthesia *(134)*. This release is associated with increased pulse rate, cardiac output, and systolic blood pressure as exemplified in locally anesthesized patients undergoing dental surgery *(135)*. Concomitant increases of plasma E and cAMP can be found with a peak in the early postoperative phase; after termination of anesthesia *(136)*, the surgical stress-induced impaired insulin secretion has been partly attributed to the sympathetic nervous system activation *(137)*.

An earthquake is one of the most devastating combinations of psychological and traumatic shock. The violent January 1994 California earthquake not only resulted in traumatic deaths, but also triggered an unusually large number of sudden deaths from atherosclerotic cardiovascular disease *(138)*. There is no doubt that one of the triggers of these events is the centrally mediated catecholamine release acting mostly via ventricular fibrillation *(139)* and coronary vasoconstriction during or immediately after stress *(140)* in addition to other mechanisms, such as disruption of a vulnerable atherosclerotic plaque. Stress-induced catecholamine increases may also result in increased platelet aggregability *(141)*. Even in the long run, a stress experience in an earthquake can result in patients with "white coat" hypertension to develop at least temporarily sustained hypertension *(142)*.

The most violent thermal stress combining pain, tissue damage, infection, cardiovascular, and electrolyte disturbance is extensive burns. Catecholamine mobilization is probably the main mediator of many other hormonal and metabolic responses *(143)*. A severe stress is exposure to heat, particularly when accompanied by humidity limiting the body's heat losses. The primary stimulus to catecholamine release in the occasionally fatal heat stroke is probably volume depletion caused by dehydration. A role of catecholamines in the opposite exposure to cold is less probable, since under that condition, the body's metabolism and catecholamine release decrease (to levels seen under artificial hibernation), and the real damage occurs at the vital tissue levels (brain, heart, kidney).

Anesthesia can influence the stress response by afferent blockade (local anesthesia), central modulation (general anesthesia), or peripheral interactions with the endocrine system *(144)*. With regard to reduction of endocrine stress response, inhalation anesthesia with volatile anesthetics and nitrous oxide may be less effective than neuroleptic, spinal, or epidural anesthesia. The tracheal intubation alone is followed by an increase in NE and blood pressure *(145)*. In addition to central modulation of pain and stress, both halothane and enflurane inhibit catecholamine release from adrenal medulla. Neuroleptic and total IV anesthesia are potent central inhibitors of NE discharge even during major surgery.

Spinal and epidural anesthesia alone, as well as in combination with general anesthesia, can excessively reduce stress responses owing to sympathetic blockade. A rapid increase of NE, but particularly E, can be observed immediately after extubation *(144)*.

Cardiopulmonary resuscitation (CPR) following a cardiac arrest is the critical condition between life and death. Heart arrest is associated with extremely high, prevalently E increases (approx 3000- to 12,000-fold), but the survival apparently does not depend on the catecholamine levels alone *(146)*. It depends also on the viability of β-adrenergic receptors, which may be further stimulated by E administration. Despite very high plasma E concentrations during cardiac arrest, further E increases still elicit biological responses. This provides physiological support for large E doses to be administered during the course of CPR.

The survivability to shock in critically ill patients (following trauma, surgery, or sepsis) is dependent on a high level of oxygen delivery to meet high oxygen consumption. The action of catecholamines mobilized under these conditions is beneficial (inotropic to maintain cardiac output, vasoconstrictor to sustain blood pressure), but also detrimental (increased metabolism and tissue oxygen consumption). Agressive treatment using catecholamine-like drugs may also duplicate these occasionally detrimental actions. Instead, recent studies emphasize the importance of adequate volume replacement first to help maintain blood pressure and the use of moderate doses of inotropic drugs to maintain a normal cardiac output *(147)* with definitive treatment directed to the primary disease.

Tissue and organ transplantation: Including all previous considerations, the viability of the transplant is a decisive determinant of success. It is remarkable that even brain-dead organ donors studied during surgery had a prompt increase in plasma catecholamines *(148)*. Surgical stress can thus evoke an excessive rise of plasma NE and E even under those unexpected conditions, and this could impair allograft function. Studies on human ventricular myocardium obtained from patients transplanted for congestive heart failure have indicated that positive inotropy and automaticity can be achieved by potentiation of actions of catecholamines by caffeine *(149)*.

LIFESTYLE AND PHARMACOLOGICAL INTERVENTIONS IMPROVING COPING WITH STRESS-INDUCED SYMPATHOADRENAL ACTIVATION

Despite limited knowledge of the role of catecholamines in stress and the very arbitrary limits between beneficial and potentially damaging catecholamine stimulation, there are several lifestyle and therapeutic approaches that may limit the inconvenience, and possible injury, resulting from excessive catecholamine release without compromising their survival value.

Lifestyle changes are probably preventing the manifestations of some sympathoadrenomedullary stress-related conditions; they should usually precede pharmacologic interventions when stress-related diseases become apparent. Toxic (smoking, pollution) and drug (e.g., cocaine) abuse-induced catecholamine stimulating actions are probably the best-known factors to be avoided in order to diminish the impact of stress-induced catecholamine activation. It had been recently demonstrated that cross-sensitization between stress and drugs of abuse implicates alterations in DA transmission *(150)*. This neurochemical substrate of stress is apparently responsible for the psychostimulant-induced sensitization, which predisposes an individual exposed to stressful life events to cocaine abuse in particular.

Nutritional factors can be operative in both directions. On one hand, vitamin A depletion may cause an inadequate response to immobilization stress in animals *(151)*. Ascorbic acid deficiency may also decrease NE secretion, since it is an important cofactor for NE synthesis from DA *(152)*. Excessive salt intake may, on the other hand, facilitate NE and E release and increase vascular reactivity to adrenergic stimulation. Pyridoxin deficiency may cause an almost threefold increase in NE and E, overcompensating the defect of aromatic acid decarboxylase for which pyridoxin is an important cofactor *(153)*. The resistance to insulin-mediated glucose disposal in obesity and associated hypertension results in hyperinsulinemia stimulating the sympathetic nervous system *(154)*. This underlines the importance of obesity prevention. Whether obesity itself decreases the survivability of stress still remains unclear.

Behavioral therapies (biofeedback and relaxation) appear to have a beneficial effect, creating a resting state of plasma NE, DβH, and E release *(155)*. Since the autonomic nervous system can be modulated by conditioning, the simplest form involves "teaching" the patients to recognize their blood pressure level by rewarding them when they lower it. Relaxation therapy teaches patients to relax, either in an overall sense by methods, such as transcendental meditation *(156)*, or relaxation of specific muscle cells. Both these methods have been demonstrated to produce small declines in blood pressure while keeping plasma catecholamines at a resting state. Stress reduction through listening to meditative music is a particular form of relaxation resulting in NE and E concentration decrease *(157)*. Experienced clinicians know that an important factor determining the survival of the even most critical illness-induced autonomic alarm reaction is the patient's will to survive!

Physical activity appears to be a good antidote against consequences of stress particularly the emotional one. As outlined in Fig. 9, emotional stress, whether active and aggressive stimulating predominantly NE or passive, and anxious stimulating E *(158)*, results in free fatty acid mobilization. The long-term impact of this stress may be moderated when exercise contributes to utilization of free fatty acid in active muscles. In the absence of muscle activity, however, free fatty acids are converted to triglycerides and cholesterol, incorporated into atheroma, and contribute to myocardial ischemia. It is not yet clear, however, whether this benefit of exercise is also applicable in the short run, particularly in trained individuals in whom exercise induces an enhanced NE and E release *(63)*. Immediate consequences of the NE and particularly E release [arrhythmia *(139)*, angina *(140)*] may be deleterious. Subjects who are already suffering from coronary atherosclerosis, even clinically silent, may thus be threatened by exercise instead of enjoying its benefits.

In real-life stress situations (i.e. third molar extraction), there is a clear participation of the sympathetic nervous system in producing the circulatory responses to dental surgery. Diazepam-induced sedation eliminates the sympathetic recruitment, but there is no concomitant reduction in heart rate or systolic pressure *(135)*, suggesting that other systems besides the sympathetic nervous system influence the circulatory response to a real-life stressor. Cholinergic, serotoninergic, γ-aminobutyric acid- (GABAergic), renin-angiotensin-, NPY-, or endothelin-mediated changes are the most probable candidates of such alternative patterns. Opiates appear to be "silent modulators" of stress-induced catecholamine release *(159)*. Alpraxolone was also shown to diminish plasma E responses to stress induced by hypoglycemia *(160)* and exercise *(161)*.

Other possible drug interference with stress-induced catecholamine release, tested experimentally or clinically, has been conducted with agents affecting catecholamine

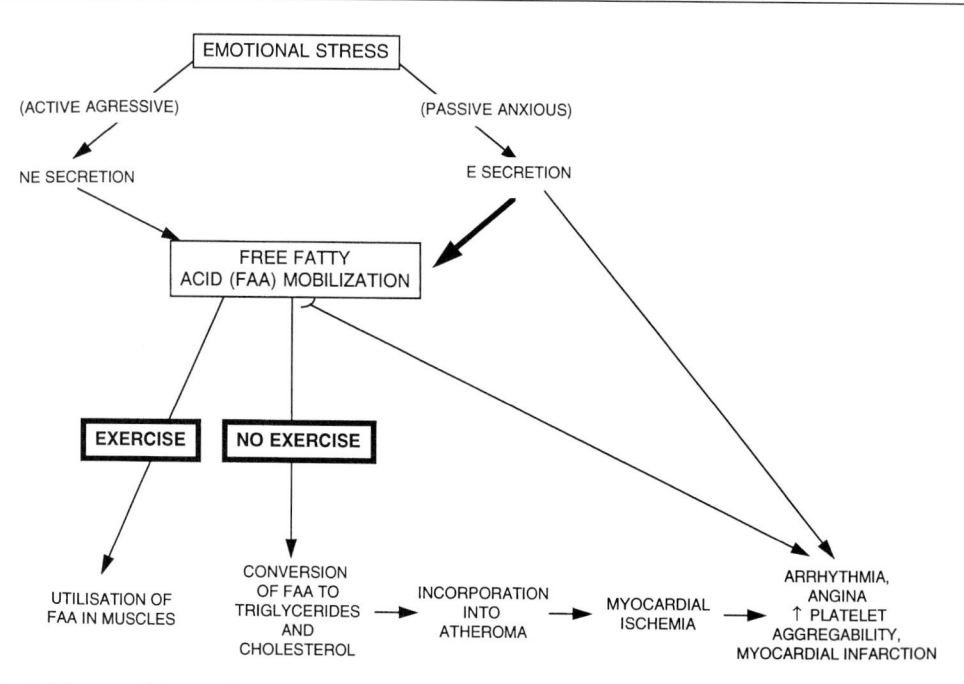

Fig. 9. The possible benefit of physical exercise as moderating the impact of emotional stress on catecholamine release-induced abnormalities.

synthesis (such as the rate-limiting TH inhibitor metyrosine), gangioplegic drugs, and sympatho-inhibitory substances (reserpine, α-methyl dopa, clonidine). Of particular interest are recent studies showing the benefits of suppression by clonidine (owing to its central α_2-agonism) of the stress-induced NE and NPY release *(162)*. Such a suppression of the congestive heart failure- and dyspnea-induced NE release proved to be beneficial by reducing preload, heart rate, and arterial pressure, all conducive to decreased myocardial energy and oxygen demand *(163)*.

It appears that most effective and potentially useful are α- and β-adrenergic receptor inhibitors. Particularly β-blockers, which penetrate the brain (e.g., propranolol) *(164)*, have an anxiolytic action, and are a useful addition to treatment of stress-related cardiovascular hyperkinesis, especially in hyper-β-adrenergic state patients (e.g., labile hypertension, hyperthyroidism). This effect does not, however, apply to all β-blockers, because it could not be reproduced by others, such as atenolol and bopindolol *(165)*. The selectivity and nonselectivity of β-blockers may explain some differences *(166)*. The combined α- and β-blocker labetalol prevented the tracheal intubation-induced NE and blood pressure increase *(145)*. The α-blockade by doxazosin reduced the response to stress (mental and isometric) more the higher the baseline plasma NE in hypertensive patients was *(167)*.

Other alternatives used to inhibit the stress-induced catecholamine release are neurotropic drugs, such as haloperidol and pimozide. Central α_2-adrenoreceptor stimulation by a new imidazole derivative (mivazerol) was found to inhibit the immobilization-stress-induced release of catecholamines in the hippocampus, attenuating the central focal source of stress-induced catecholamine discharge *(168)*. In response to surgical stress, the blockade of neural afferents (via spinal anesthesia) from the site of tissue injury suppressed the stress-induced catecholamine increase *(169)*. Some drugs promoting myocardial adaptation to repeated stress-induced catecholamine release, such as 7-oxo prostacyclin, successfully tested in dogs *(59)* may hold a future potential in stress-exposed humans.

ACKNOWLEDGMENTS

Original studies in this chapter have been supported by grants from the Medical Research Council of Canada and the Quebec Heart Foundation.

REFERENCES

1. Cannon WB. The emergency function of the adrenal medulla in pain and the major emotions. Am J Physiol 1914;33:356–372.
2. Selye H. The evolution of the stress concept. Am Scientist 1973;61:692–699.
3. von Euler US, Gemzell CA, Levi L, Ström G. Cortical and medullary adrenal activity in emotional stress. Acta Endocrinol 1959;30:567–573.
4. Axelrod J, Weinshilboum K. Catecholamines. N Engl J Med 1972;287:237–242.
5. Kopin IJ. Catecholamines, adrenal hormones, and stress. In: Krieger DT, Hughes JC, eds. Neuroendocrinology. Sunderland, Sinauer, 1980, pp. 159–166.
6. Hökfelt T, Goldstein M, Fuxe K. Characterization and tissue localization of catecholamine synthesizing enzymes. Pharmacol Rev 1972;24:293–309.
7. Goldstein DS. Stress, Catecholamines, and Cardiovascular Disease. Oxford University Press, 1995, p. 528.
8. Snider SR, Kuchel O. Dopamine: an important neurohormone of the sympathoadrenal system. Significance of increased peripheral dopamine release for the human stress response and hypertension. Endocr Rev 1983;4:291–309.
9. Kuchel O. Clinical implications of genetic and acquired defects in catecholamine synthesis and metabolism. Clin Invest Med 1994;17;4:369–388.
10. Strasser RH, Ihl-Vahl R, Marquetant R. Molecular biology of adrenergic receptors. J Hypertens 1992;10:501–506.
11. Axelrod J, Reisine TD. Stress hormones: their interaction and regulation. Science 1984;224:452–459.
12. Sternberg EM, Chrousos GP, Wilder RL, Gold PW. The stress response and the regulation of inflammatory disease. NIH Conference. Ann Intern Med 1992;117:854–866.
13. Kopin IJ. Definitions of stress and sympathetic neuronal responses. Ann NY Acad Sci 1995;771:19–30.
14. Goldstein DS, Mezey E, Yamamoto T, Aneman A, Friberg P, Eisenhofer G. Is there a third peripheral catecholaminergic system? Endogenous dopamine as an autocrine/paracrine substance derived from plasma DOPA and inactivated by conjugation. Hypertens Res 1995;18;(Suppl I):S93–S99.
15. Kopin IJ, Eisenhofer G, Goldstein D. Adrenergic response following recognition of stress. In: Breznitz S, Zinder O, eds. Molecular Biology of Stress, Liss, New York, 1989, pp. 123–132.
16. Goldstein DS, Eisenhofer G, Garty M, Sax FL, Keiser HR, Kopin IJ. Pharmacologic and tracer methods to study sympathetic function in primary hypertension. Clin Exp Hyper-Theory Pract All 1989;(Suppl I):173–189.
17. Lerer B, Ebstein RP. Alterations in cyclic adenosine monophosphate signal amplification as a consequence of chronic stress. In: Progress in catecholamine Research, part C: Clinical Aspects, Liss, New York, 1988, pp. 409–412.
18. Kvetnansky R. Recent progress in catecholamines under stress. In: Usdin E, Kvetnansky R, Kopin IJ, eds. Catecholamines and Stress: Recent Advances, Elsevier, Amsterdam, 1980, pp. 7–18.
19. Schwarzschild MA, Zigmond RE. Secretin and vasoactive intestinal peptide activate tyrosine hydroxylase and sympathetic nerve endings. J Neurosc 1989;9:160–166.
20. Hirooka Y, Head GA, Potts PD, Godwin SJ, Bendle RD, Dampney RAL. Medullary neurons activated by angiotensin II in the conscious rabbit. Hypertension 1996;27:287–296.
21. Sole MJ, Helke CF, Jacobowitz DM. Increased dopamine in the failing hamster heart: transvesicular transport of dopamine limits the rate of norepinephrine synthesis. Am J Cardiol 1982;49:1682.
22. Schwartz J. The dopaminergic system in the periphery. J Pharmacol 1984;15:401–414.
23. Charvat JP, Dell P, Folkow B. Mental factors and cardiovascular diseases. Cardiologia 1964;44:124–141.

24. Rothschild AJ, Langlais PJ, Schatzberg AF, Walsh FX, Cole JO, Bird ED. Dexamethasone increases plasma free dopamine in man. J Psychiat Res 1984;18:217–223.
25. Abercrombie ED, Page ME. Stress-induced modification of the locus coeruleus norepinephrine system: functional significance and clinical implications. Sixth symposium on catecholamines and other neurotransmitters in stress. Smolenice, June 19–24, 1995.
26. Togari A, Ichinose H, Matsumoto S, Fugita K, Nagatsu T. Multiple mRNA forms of human GTP cyclohydrolase 1. Biochem Biophys Res Commun 1992;187:359–365.
27. Ichinose H, Ohye T, Takahashi E, Seki N, Hori T, Segawa M, Nomura Y, Endo K, Tonaka H, Tsuji S. Hereditary progressive dystonia with marked diurnal fluctuation caused by mutations in the GTP cyclohydrolase I gene. Nature Gene 1994;8:236–242.
28. Craviso GL, Hemelt VB, Waymire JC, Moore R. Stress-induced alterations in tyrosine hydroxylase gene expression in adrenal medullary chromaffin cells may involve both transcriptional and post-transcriptional mechanisms. Sixth symposium on catecholamines and other neurotransmitters in stress. Smolenice June 19–24, 1995.
29. Lewis EJ, Zellmer E, Shang Z. Genetic regulatory elements of the dopamine β-hydroxylase gene. Sixth Symposium on catecholamines and other neurotransmitters in stress. Smolenice June 19–24, 1995.
30. Parker Jones P, Spraul M, Matt KS, Seals DR, Skinner JS, Ravussin E. Gender does not influence sympathetic neural reactivity to stress in healthy humans. Am J Physiol 1996;270:H350–H357.
31. Mills PJ, Nelesen RA, Ziegler MG, Parry BL, Berry CC, Dillon E, Dimsdale JE. Menstrual cycle effects on catecholamine and cardiovascular responses to acute stress in black but not white normotensive women. Hypertension 1996;27:962–967.
32. Kuchel O, Kuchel G. Circulating catecholamines and aging. In: Amenta F, ed. Aging of the Autonomic Nervous System. CRC, Boca Raton, FL, 1993, pp. 71–93.
33. Robertson D, Johnson GA, Robertson RM, Nies AS, Shand DG, Oates JA. Comparative assessment of stimuli that release neuronal and adrenomedullary catecholamines in man. Circulation 1979;59:637–643.
34. Woolf PD, Akowuah ES, Lee L, Kelly M, Feibel J. Evaluation of the dopamine response to stress in man. J Clin Endocrinol Metab 1983;56:246–250.
35. Tidgren B, Hjemdahl P. Renal responses to mental stress and epinephrine in humans. Am J Physiol 1989;257:F682–F689.
36. Padbury JF, Martinez AM, Thio SL, Burnett E. Integrated neuroendocrine stress responses in fetal sheep. In: Breznitz S, Zinder O, eds. Progress in Catecholamine Research, part C: Clinical Aspects. Liss, New York, 1989, pp. 469–474.
37. Rhee HM, Hendrix DW. Effects of stress intensity and modality on cardiovascular system: An involvement of opioid systen. In: Breznitz S, Zinder O, eds. Molecular Biology of Stress. Liss, New York, 1989, pp. 87–96.
38. Horky K, Gutkowska J, Garcia R, Thibault G, Genest J, Cantin M. Effect of different anesthetics on immunoreactive atrial natriuretic factor concentration in rat plasma. Biochem Biophys Res Commun 1985;129:651–657.
39. Debinski W, Kuchel O, Buu NT. Atrial natriuretic factor is a new neuromodulatory peptide. Neuroscience 1990;36:15–20.
40. Debinski W, Kuchel O, Buu NT, Cantin M, Genest J. Atrial natriuretic factor partially inhibits the stimulated catecholamine synthesis in superior cervical ganglia of the rat. Neurosci Lett 1987;77:92–96.
41. Zukowska-Grojec Z, Lewandowski J, Pruszczyk P, Wocial B, Sabban E. Neuropeptide Y: a major regulator of cardiovascular responses to stress. Sixth symposium on catecholamines and other neurotransmitters in stress. Smolenice June 19–24, 1995.
42. Zukowska-Grojec Z. Neuropeptide Y. A novel sympathetic stress hormone and more. Ann NY Acad Sci 1995;771:219–233.
43. Takiyyuddin MA, Parmer RJ, Kailasam MT, Cervenka JH, Kennedy B, Ziegler MG, Lin MC, Li J, Grim CE, Wright FA, O'Connor DT. Chromogranin A in human hypertension. Influence of heredity. Hypertension 1995;26:213–220.
44. Moftaquir-Handaj A, Barbe F, Barbarino-Monnier P, Aunis D, Boutroy MJ. Circulating chromogranin A and catecholamines in human fetuses at uneventful birth. Pediatr Res 1995;37(1):101–105.
45. Tanaka M, Kitaimura K, Ishizaka Y, Ishiyama Y, Kato J, Kangawa K, Eto T. Plasma adrenomedullin in various diseases and exercise-induced change in adrenomedullin in healthy subjects. Intern Med 1995;34(8):728–733.

46. Livett BTG, Zhou XF, Khalil Z, Wan DCC, Bunn SJ, Marley PD. Endogenous neuropeptides maintain adrenal catecholamine output during stress. In: Breznitz S, Zinder O, eds. Molecular Biology of Stress. Liss, New York, 1989, pp. 179–190.
47. Kvetnansky R, Pacak K, Nankova B, Fukuhara K, Goldstein D, Sabban EL, Kopin IJ. Peripheral catecholamine synthesis, release and metabolism during stress: effect of glucocorticoids. Sixth symposium on catecholamines and other neurotransmitters in stress, Smolenice June 19–24, 1995.
48. Wong DL, Morita K. Glucocorticoid control of phenylethanolamine N-methyltransferase gene expression: implications for stress and disorders of the stress axis. Sixth symposium on catecholamines and other neurotransmitters in stress, Smolenice June 19–24, 1995.
49. Makino S, Smith MA, Gold PW. Decreased capacity of glucocorticoids to inhibit locus coeruleus–HPA axis responsiveness during repeated stress. Sixth symposium on catecholamines and other neurotransmitters in stress, Smolenice June 19–24, 1995.
50. Goto A, Yamada K, Nagoshi H, Terano Y, Omata M. Stress-induced elevation of ouabainlike compound in rat plasma and adrenal. Hypertension 1995;2:1173–1176.
51. Premel-Cabic A, Gétin F, Turcant A, Rohmer V, Bigorgne JC, Allain P. Noradrénaline plasmatique dans l'hyperthyroïdie et l'hypothyroïdie. La Presse Médicale 1986;15:1625–1627.
52. Kuchel O, Buu NT, Hamet P, Larochelle P. Hypertension in hyperthyroidism: is there an epinephrine connection? Life Sci 1982;30:603–609.
53. Hjemdahl P. Plasma catecholamines—analytical challenges and physiological limitations. Baillière's Clin Endocrinol Metab 1993;7:307–353.
54. Zinder O, Greenberg A, Maer H, Hiram Y, Nir A. The adrenal medulla secretory response to stress. In: Breznitz S, Zinder O, eds. Molecular Biology of Stress. Liss, New York, 1989, pp. 167–178.
55. Slotkin TA, Seidler FJ. Catecholamines and stress in the newborn. In: Breznitz S, Zinder O, eds. Molecular Biology of Stress. Liss, New York, 1989, pp. 133–142.
56. Mills DE, Huang YS, Narce M, Poisson JP. Psychosocial stress, catecholamines and essential fatty acid metabolism in rats. PSEBM 1994;205:56–61.
57. Kvetnansky R, Torda T. Changes of heart catecholamine levels, metabolism and adrenergic receptors in acutely and repeatedly stressed rats. In: Jacob R, Gulch RW, Kissling G, eds. Cardiac Adaptation to Hemodynamic Overload, Training and Stress. 1983, pp. 265–266.
58. Krahenbuhl GS, Harris J. Biochemical measurements of the human stress response. Air Force Systems Command Technical Report AFHRL-TR-83-40. Brooks Air Force Base, Air Force Systems Command 40–46, 1984.
59. Szekeres L. On the mechanism and possible therapeutic application of delayed cardiac adaptation to stress. Can J Cardiol 1996;12:177–185.
60. LeBlanc J. The role of catecholamines in adaptation to chronic and acute stress. In: Usdin E, Kvetnansky R, Kopin IJ, eds. Catecholamines and Stress. International Symposium on Catecholamines and Stress, Bratislava, 1976, pp. 409–417.
61. Harris J, Krahenbuhl GS. Biogenic amine/metabolite patterns of stress response in normal subjects: implications in psychiatric disorders. Prog Catecholamine Res Part C: Clin Aspects, 1988;243–248.
62. Sothmann MS, Horn TS, Hart BA, Gustafson AB. Comparison of discrete cardiovascular fitness groups on plasma catecholamine and selected behavioral responses to psychological stress. Psychophysiology 1987;24–47.
63. Premel-Cabic A, Turcant A, Chaleil D, Allain P, Victor J, Tadei A. Concentration plasmatique de catécholamines á l'effort chez le sujet non entraîné et chez le sportif. Path Biol 1984;32:702–704.
64. Hashimoto K, Aizawa Y, Mori K. Changes in blood pressure, body weight and urinary catecholamines during austerities. Eur J Appl Physiol 1987;56:38–42.
65. Ibsen H, Julius S. Pharmacologic tools for assessment of adrenergic nerve activity in human hypertension. Fed Proc 1984;43:67–71.
66. Parfrey PS, Wright P, Ledingham JM. Effect of inheritance and stress on the diurnal excretion of sodium and potassium in young people with and without a family history of hypertension. Clin Sci 1980;59:161s–164s.
67. Goldstein DS. Clinical assessment of sympathetic responses to stress. Ann NY Acad Sci 1995;771:570–593.
68. Esler M, Jennings G, Leonard P, Sacharias N, Burke F, Johns J, Blombery P. Contribution of individual organs to total noradrenaline release in humans. Acta Physiol Scand 1984;527:11–16.
69. Folkow B. Nervous integration of cardiovascular function. Proc R Soc Med 1968;61:1317–1318.

70. Esler M, Lambert G, Jennings G. Regional Norepinephrine turnover in human hypertension. Clin Exp Hypertension-Theory Pract 1989;A11:75–89.
71. Lenders JWM, Willemsen JJ, Boo T, Lemmens WAJ, Thien T. Disparate effects of mental stress on plasma noradrenaline in young normotensive and hypertensive subjects. J Hypertens 1989; 7:317–323.
72. Goldstein DS, Eisenhofer G, Garty M, Sax FL, Keiser HR, Kopin IJ. Pharmacologic and tracer methods to study sympathetic function in primary hypertension. Clin Exp Hypertension-Theory Pract 1989;A11:173–189.
73. Eisenhofer G, Friberg P, Pacak K, Goldstein DS, Murphy DL, Tsigos C, Quyyumi AA, runner HG, Lenders JW. Plasma metadrenalines: do they provide useful information about sympatho-adrenal function and catecholamine metabolism? Clin Sci 1995;88(5):533–542.
74. Unger T, Buu NT, Kuchel O. Renal handling of free and conjugated catecholamines following surgical stress in the dog. Am J Physiol 1978;235:F542–F547.
75. Joyce DA, Beilin IJ, Vandongen R, Davidson I. Plasma free and sulfate conjugated catecholamines during acute physiological stimulation in man. Life Sci 1982;30:447–454.
76. Minatoguchi S, Ito H, Suzuki T, Koshiji M, Kakami M, Uno Y, Asano K, Yamashita K, Hirakawa S, Fujiwara H. Conversion of plasma noradrenaline from conjugated form into free form in the heart and its physiological significance in patients with cardiac diseases—a comaprison between at rest and during exercise. Biogenic Amines 1995;22:417–432.
77. Kuchel O, Buu NT, Hamet P, Larochelle P, Bourque M, Genest J. Essential hypertension with low conjugated catecholamines imitates pheochromocytoma. Hypertension 1981;3:347–355.
78. Maus TP, Anderson RJ, Weinshilboum RM. effect of dexamethasone on rat phenol-sulfotransferase (PST) activity. Pharmacologist 1980;22:301.
79. Claustre J, Debinski W, Buu NT, Savard C, Peyrin L, Kuchel O. Catecholamine conjugates as potential precursors for free amines: Metabolic fate of DA glucoronide in the rat. In: Van Loon GR, Kvetnansky R, McCarty R, Axelrod J, eds. Stress: Neurochemical and Humoral Mechanisms. Gordon and Breach, New York, 1989, pp. 713–720.
80. Cryer PE. Physiology and pathophysiology of the human sympathoadrenal neuroendocrine system. N Engl J Med 1980;303:436–444.
81. Chamberlain KG, Pestell RG, Best JD. Platelet catecholamine contents are cumulative indexes of sympathoadrenal activity. Am J Physiol 1990;259:E141–E147.
82. O'Connor DT, Bernstein KN. Radioimmunoassay of chromogranin A in plasma as a measure of exocytotic sympathoadrenal activity in normal subjects and patients with pheochromocytoma. New Engl J Med 1984;311(12):764–770.
83. Wallin BG. Relationship between sympathetic nerve traffic and plasma concentrations of noradrenaline in man. Pharmacol Toxicol 1988;(Suppl 1):9–11.
84. Wallin BG. Human sympathetic nerve activity and blood pressure regulation. Clin Exp Hypertension-Theory Pract All 1989;(Suppl 1):91–101.
85. Hoffman RP, Sinkey CA, Anderson EA. Hypoglycemia increases muscle sympathetic nerve activity in IDDM and control subjects. Diabetes Care 1994;17(7):673–680.
86. Slotkin TA, Seidler FJ. Adrenomedullary catecholamine release in the fetus and newborn: secretory mechanisms and their role in stress and survival. J Dev Physiol 1988;10(1):1–16.
87. Christensen NJ, Schultz-Larsen K. Resting venous plasma adrenalin in 70-year-old men correlated positively to survival in a population study: the significance of the physical working capacity. J Intern Med 1994;235:229–232.
88. McCarty R, Mabry TR, Foster TC, Gold PE. Sixth symposium on catecholamines and other neurotransmitters in stress. Smolenice June 19–24, 1995.
89. Felig P, Cherif A, Minagawa A, Wahrem J. Hypoglycemia during prolonged exercise in normal men. N Engl J Med 1982;306-895-900.
90. Wortsman J, Frank S, Cryer PE. Adrenomedullary response to maximal stress in humans. Am J Med 1984;77:779–84.
91. Tarnoky K, Nagy S. Relationship to survival of catecholamine levels and dopamine-β-hydroxylase activity in experimental haemorrhagic schock. Acta Physiologica Hungarica 1983;61:59–68.
92. McCance AJ, Forfar JC. Myocardial ischaemia and ventricular arrhythmias precipitated by physiological concentrations of adrenaline in patients with coronary heart disease. B. Heart J 1991; 66:316–319.
93. Goldstein DS. Stress, catecholamines and cardiovascular disease. Sixth symposium on catecholamines and other neurotransmitters in stress, Smolenice June 19–24, 1995.

94. Kaye DM, Lefkovits J, Cox H, Lambert G, Jennings G, Turner A, Esler MD. Regional epinephrine kinetics in human heart failure—evident for extra-adrenal, nonneural release. Am J Physiol—Heart & Circ. Physiol 1995;38:H182–H188.
95. Yoshizumi M, Nakaya Y, Hibino T, Nomura M, Minakuchi K, Kitagawa T, Katoh I, Ohuchi T, Oka M. Changes in plasma free and sulfoconjugated catecholamines before and after acute physical exercise: experimental and clinical studies. Life Sci 1992;51:227–234.
96. Lehmann M, Ruhle K, Schmid P, Klein H, Matthys K, Keul J. Hemodynamics, plasma catecholamine behavior and beta-adrenergic receptor density in trained and untrained subjects and cardiac insufficiency patients. Zeitschrift für Kardiologie 1983;72:529–536.
97. Sherwood A, Hinderliter AL, Light KC. Physiological Determinants of hyperreactivity to stress in borderline hypertension. Hypertension 1995;25:384–390.
98. Pickering TC. Does psychological stress contribute to the development of hypertension and coronary heart disease? Eur J Clin Pharmacol 1990;39:51–57.
99. Rostrup M, Mundal HH, Westheim A, Eide I. Awareness of high blood pressure increases arterial plasma catecholamines, platelet noradrenaline and adrenergic responses to mental stress. J Hypertens 1991;9:159–166.
100. Evens R. Octopamine: from metabolic mistake to modulator. Trends Neural Sci 1978;12:154–157.
101. Kuchel O, Racz K. Dopamine in the adrenal medulla and its possible role in stress. In: Amenta F, ed. Peripheral Dopamine Pathophysiology. CRC, Boca Raton, FL, 1990, pp. 185–202.
102. Eisenhofer G, Brush JE, Cannon RO III, Kopin IJ, Goldstein D. Plasma dihydroxyphenylalanine and total body and regional noradrenergic activity in humans. J Clin Endocrinol Metab 1989;68:247–255.
103. Kuchel O, Buu NT, Larochelle P, Hamet P, Genest Jr J. Episodic dopamine discharge in paroxysmal hypertension. Page's syndrome revisited. Arch Intern Med 1986;146:1315–1320.
104. Ludwig DA, Convertino VA. Predicting orthostatic intolerance: physics or physiology? Aviat Space Environ Med 1994;65:404–411.
105. Mazzeo RS, Brooks GA, Butterfield GE, Podolin DA. Wolfel EE, Reeves JT. Acclimatization to high altitude increase muscle sympathetic activity both at rest and during exercise. Am J Physiol 1995;269:R201–R207.
106. Duncan JJ, Farr JE, Upton SJ, Hagan RD, Oglesby ME, Blair SN. The effects of aerobic exercise on plasma catecholamines and blood pressure in patients with mild essential hypertension. JAMA 1985;254-2609–2613.
107. Gilbert IA, Lenner KA, McFadden ER Jr. Sympathoadrenal response to repetitive exercise in normal and asthmatic subjects. J Appl Physiol 1988;64:2667–2674.
108. Rattarasarn C, Dagogo-Jack S, Zachwieja JJ, Cryer PE. Hypoglycemia-induced autonomic failure in IDDM is specific for stimulus of hypoglycemia and is not attributable to prior autonomic activation. Diabetes 1994;43:809–818.
109. Hoffman RP, Arslanian S, Drash AL, Becker DJ. Impaired counterregulatory hormone responses to hypoglycemia in children and adolescents with new onset IDDM. J Pediatr Endocrinol 1994;7:235–244.
110. Diamond MP, Reece EA, Caprio S, Jones TW, Amiel S, DeGennaro N, Laudano A, Addabbo M, Sherwin RS, Tamborlane WV. Impairment of counterregulatory hormone responses to hypoglycemia in pregnant women with insulin-dependent diabetes mellitus. Am J Obstet Gyn 1992;166:70–77.
111. Moan A, Hoieggen A, Nordby G, Os I, Eide I, Kjeldsen SE. Mental stress increases glucose uptake during hyperinsulinemia: associations with sympathetic and cardiovascular responsiveness. Metabolism 1995;44:1303–1307.
112. Burker EJ, Fredrikson M, Rifai N, Siegel W, Blumenthal JA. Serum lipids, neuroendocrine, and cardiovascular responses to stress in men and women with mild hypertension. Behav Med 1994;19:155–161.
113. Young JB, Macdonald IA. Sympathoadrenal activity in human obesity: heterogeneity of findings since 1980. Int J Obes Related Metab Disord 1992;16:959–967.
114. Gustafson AB, Farrrell PA, Kalkhoff RK. Impaired plasma catecholamine response to submaximal treadmill exercise in obese women. Metabolism: Clin Exp 1990;39:410–417.
115. Newsholme EA. A possible metabolic basis for the control of body weight. New Engl J Med 1980;302:400–404.
116. Kitamura H, Kinugawa T, Miyakoda H, Ogino K, Tomokuni A, Saito M, Hasegawa J, Kotake H, Mashiba H. Cardiac and plasma catecholamine response to dynamic exercise in hyperthyroidism. J Cardiol 1992;22:219–225.
117. Robertson D, Hollister AS, Biaggioni I, Netterville JL, Mossqueda-Garcia R, Robertson RM. The diagnosis and treatment of baroreflex failure. N Engl J Med 1993;329:1449–1455.

118. Kuchel O, Cusson JR, Larochelle P, Buu NT, Genest J. Posture- and emotion-induced severe hypertensive paroxysms with baroreceptor dysfunction. J Hypertens 1987;5:277–283.
119. Mathias CJ, Christensen NJ, Frankel HL, Spalding JM. Cardiovascular control in recently injured tetraplegics in spinal shock. Quart J Med 1979;48:273–287.
120. Polinsky RJ, Brown RT, Curras MT, Baser SM, Baucom CE, Hooper DR, Marini AM. Central and peripheral effects of arecoline in patients with autonomic failure. J Neurol, Neurosurg & Psychiatry 1991;54:807–812.
121. Durrieu G, Senard JM, Rascol O, Tran MA, Lataste X, Rascol A, Montastruc JL. Blood pressure and plasma catecholamines in never-treated parkinsonian patients: effect of a selective D1 agonist (CY 208–243). Neurology 1990;40:707–709.
122. Sra JS, Murthy V, Natale A, Jazayeri MR, Dhala A, Deshpande S, Sheth M, Akhtar M. Circulatory and catecholamine changes during head-up tilt testing in neurocardiogenic (vasovagal) syncope. Am J Cardiol 1994;73:33–37.
123. Moss J, Donlon JV, McGoldrick KE, Lichtor JL. Perioperative anxiety: difference in the adrenergic responses to local and general anesthesia. In: Progress in Catecholamine Research, part C. Clinical Aspects. Liss, New York, 1988, 469–474.
124. Stein MB, Asmundson GJ. Autonomic function in panic disorder: cardiorespiratory and plasma catecholamine responsivity to multiple challenges of the autonomic nervous system. Biol Psychiatry 1994;36:548–558.
125. Osterweis M, Solomon F, Green F. Bereavement reactions, consequences and care. National Academy Press, Washington, DC, 1984.
126. Irwin M. Stress-induced immune suppression. Role of the autonomic nervous system. Ann NY Acad Sci 1993;697:203–218.
127. Gold PW, Goodwin FK, Chrousos GP. Clinical and biochemical manifestations of depression: relation to the neurobiology of stress. N Engl J Med 1988;319:413–420.
128. Brady LS, Whitfield HJ Jr, Fox RJ, Gold PW, Herkenham M. Long term antidepressant administration alters corticotropin-releasing hormone, tyrosine hydroxylase and mineralocorticoid receptor gene expression in the brain. J Clin Invest 1991;87:831–837.
129. Jurankova E, Jezova D, Vigas M. Central stimulation of hormone release and the proliferative response of lymphocytes in humans. Mol Chem Neuropathol 1995;25:213–223.
130. Landmann RM, Muller FB, Perini C, Wesp M, Erne P, Buhler FR. Changes of immunoregulatory cells induced by psychological and physical stress: relationship to plasma catecholamines. Clin Exp Immunol 1984;58:127–135.
131. McRitchie DI, Girotti MJ, Rotstein OD, Teodorczyk-Injeyan JA. Impaired antibody production in blunt trauma: Possible role for T cell dysfunction. Arch Surg 1990;125:91–96.
132. Van den Berghe G, de Zegher F, Wouters P, Schetz M, Verwaest C, Ferdinande P, Lauwers P. Dehydroepiandrosterone sulphate in critical illness: effect of dopamine. Clin Endocrinol 1995;43:457–463.
133. Cohen S, Tyrell DA, Smith AP. Psychological stress and susceptibility to the common cold. N Engl J Med 1991;325:606–612.
134. Halter JB, Pflug AE, Porte D. Mechanism of plasma catecholamine increases during surgical stress in man. J Clin Endocrinol Metal 1977;45:936–944.
135. Goldstein DS, Dionne R, Sweet J, Gracely R, Brewer BH, Gregg R, Keiser HR. Circulatory, plasma catecholamine, cortisol, lipid, and psychological responses to a real-life stress (third molar extractions): effects of diazepam sedation and of inclusion of epinephrine with the local anesthetic. Psychosom Med 1982;44:259–272.
136. Madsen SN, Fog-Moller F, Christiansen C, Vester-Andersen T, Engquist A. Cyclic AMP, adrenaline and noradrenaline in plasma during surgery. Br J Surg 1978;65:191–193.
137. Halter JB, Pflug AE. Relationship of impaired insulin secretion during surgical stress to anesthesia and catecholamine release. J Clin Endocrinol Met 1980;51:1093–1098.
138. Muller JE, Verrier RL. Triggering of sudden death—lessons from an earthquake. N Engl J Med 1996;334:460–461.
139. Schwartz PJ, La Rovere MT, Vanoli E. Autonomic nervous system and sudden cardiac death: experimental basis and clinical observation for post myocardial risk stratification. Circulation 1992;85:I-77–I-79.
140. Verrier RL, Dickerson LW. Autonomic nervous system and coronary blood flow changes related to emotional activation and sleep. Circulation 1991;83:II-81–II-89.

141. Kjeldsen SE, Eide I, Aakesson I, Oian P, Maltau JM, Lande K, Gjesdal K. Increased arterial adrenaline is highly correlated to blood pressure and in vivo platelet function in pre-eclampsia. J Hypertens 1985;3:S93–S95.
142. Kario K, Matsuo T, Shimada K. Follow-up of white-coat hypertension in the Hanshin-Awaji earthquake. Lancet 1996;347:626–627.
143. Wilmore DW, Long JM, Masson AD Jr, Skreen RW, Pruitt BA Jr. Catecholamines: mediator of the hypermetabolic response to thermal injury. Ann Surg 1974;180:653–669.
144. Adams HA, Hempelmann G. The endocrine stress reaction in anesthesia and surgery—origin and significance. Anasthesiologie, Intensivmedizin, Notfallmedizin, Schmerztherapie 1991;26:294–305.
145. Lavies NG, Meiklejohn BH, May AE, Achola KJ, Fell D. Hypertensive and catecholamine response to tracheal intubation in patients with pregnancy-induced hypertension. Br J Anaesth 1989;63:429–434.
146. Wortsman J, Paradis NA, Martin GB, Rivers EP, Goetting MG, Nowak RM, Cryer PE. Functional responses to extremely high plasma epinephrine concentrations in cardiac arrest. Crit Care Med 1993;21:692–697.
147. Gattinoni L, Brazzi L, Peolsi P. A trial of goal-oriented hemodynamic therapy in critically ill patients. N Engl J Med 1995;333:1025–1032.
148. Fitzgerald RD, Dechtyar I, Templ E, Fridrich P, Lackner FX. Cardiovascular and catecholamine response to surgery in brain-dead organ donors. Anaesthesia 1995;50:388–392.
149. Chang CY, Yeh TC, Chiu HC, Huang JH, Lin CI. Electromechanical effects of caffeine in failing human ventricular myocardium. Int J Cardiol 1995;50:43–50.
150. Prasad BM, Sorg BA, Ulibarri C, Kalivas PW. Sensitization to stress and psychostimulants. Ann NY Acad Sci 1995;771:617–625.
151. Mizutani R, Nakano K. Effect of vitamin A depletion on stress-induced change in urinary output of catecholamines. J Nutr 1982;112:2205–2211.
152. Levine M, Hartzell W, Dhriwal K, Washko P, Bergsten P. Ascorbic acid regulation of norepinephrine biosynthesis *in situ*. In: Breznitz S, Zinder O, eds. Molecular Biology of Stress, vol 97. Liss, New York, 1989, pp. 191–201.
153. Paulose CS, Dakshinamurti K, Packer S, Stephens NL. Sympathetic stimulation and hypertension in the pyridoxine-deficient adult rat. Hypertension 1988;11:387–391.
154. Reaven GM, Lithell H, Landsberg L. Hypertension and associated metabolic abnormalities—the role of insulin resistance and the sympathoadrenal system. N Engl J Med 1996;334:374–381.
155. Abboud FM. Relaxation, autonomic control and hypertension. N Engl J Med 1976;294:107–109.
156. Michaels RR, Huber MJ, McCann DS. Evaluation of transcendental meditation as a method of reducing stress. Science 1976;192:1242–1244.
157. Mockel M, Stork T, Vollert J, Rocker L, Danne O, Hochrein H, Eichstadt H, Frei U. Stress reduction through listening to music: effects on stress hormones, hemodynamics and mental state in patients with arterial hypertension and in healthy persons. Deutsche Medizinische Wochenschrift 1995;120:745–752.
158. Taggart P, Carruthers M. Behaviour patterns and emotional stress in the etiology of coronary heart disease: Cardiological and biochemical correlates. In: Wheastley D, ed. Stress and the Heart. Raven, New York, 1981, pp. 25–37.
159. Epple A, Nibbio B, Horak P, Specter S, Dores RM. Codeine, morphine and met-enkephalin: endogenous regulators of catecholamine release. Sixth Symposium on catecholamines and other neurotransmitters in stress, Smolenice June 19–24, 1995.
160. Breier A, Davis O, Buchanan R, Listwak SJ, Holmes C, Pickar D, Goldstein DS. Effects of alprazolam on pituitary-adrenal and catecholaminergic responses to metabolic stress in humans. Biol Psychiatry 1992;32:80–890.
161. Stratton JR, Halter JB. Effect of a benzodiazepine (alprazolam) on plasma epinephrine and norepinephrine levels during exercise stress. Am J Cardiol 1985;56:136–139.
162. Puybasset L, Lacolley P, Laurent S, Mignon F, Billaud E, Cuche J-L, Comoy E, Safar M. Effects of clonidine on plasma catecholamines and neuropeptide Y in hypertensive patients at rest and during stress. J Cardiovasc Pharmacol 1993;21:912–919.
163. Manolis AJ, Olympios C, Sifaki M, Handanis S, Bresnahan M, Gavras I, Gavras H. Suppressing sympathetic activation in congestive heart failure—a new therapeutic strategy. Hypertension 1995;26:719–724.
164. Greenwood DT, Murray RJ. Stress-catecholamines and β-adrenoceptor blockade. In: Progress in Catecholamine Research Part C: Clinical Aspects. 1988, pp. 125–129.

165. Paran E, Neumann L, Cristal N. Effects of mental and physical stress on plasma catecholamine levels before and after beta-adrenoceptor blocker treatment. Eur J Clin Pharmacol 1992;43:11–15.
166. Neftel KA, Käser HE, Vorkauf H. Different effects of selective and nonselective beta adrenoceptor blockade on urinary catecholamine and creatinine excretion in stress. Int J Clin Pharmacol, Ther Toxicol 1984;22:118–119.
167. Lee D, Lu ZW, DeQuattro V. Neural mechanisms in primary hypertension—Efficacy of α-blockade with doxazosin during stress. Am J Hypertens 1996;9:47–53.
168. Zhang X, Kindel GH, Wülfert E, Hanin I. Effects of immobilization stress on hippocampal monoamine release: modification by mivazerol, a new α_2-adrenoceptor agonist. Neuropharmacology 1995;34:1661–1672.
169. Pflug AE, Halter JB. Effect of spinal anesthesia on adrenergic tone and the neuroendocrine responses to surgical stress in humans. Anesthesiology 1981;55:120–126.

6 The Adrenocortical Response to Critical Illness
The CRH–ACTH–Cortisol Axis

*Jay Watsky, MD
and Matthew C. Leinung, MD*

CONTENTS
INTRODUCTION
PHYSIOLOGY OF CRH–ACTH–CORTISOL AXIS
CLINICAL RESPONSE OF CRH–ACTH–CORTISOL AXIS
　TO ILLNESS
CRH–ACTH–CORTISOL INSUFFICIENCY
THERAPEUTIC USE OF GLUCOCORTICOIDS
SUMMARY
REFERENCES

INTRODUCTION

The maintenance of normal, coordinated physiologic functioning of various organ systems of the body is the primary role of the endocrine system *(1)*. Although the endocrine response to many forms of stress is relatively uniform, it is nevertheless complicated and comprehensive in scope. The adrenal cortex is a critical player in the endocrine response to major stress. Cortisol, the primary glucocorticoid secreted from the human adrenal gland, has long been recognized as a requirement for survival in critical illness. Although the physiologic effects of cortisol are widespread and complex, it may be reasonable to summarize its role in critical illness by stating that it prevents an overexuberant response of the potentially self-destructive immune system *(2)*.

PHYSIOLOGY OF CRH–ACTH–CORTISOL AXIS

Regulation of Cortisol Production

The production of glucocorticoids by the adrenal cortex is regulated predominantly by adrenocorticotropic hormone (ACTH). The corticotrophs of the anterior pituitary secrete ACTH under the regulatory influence of hypothalamic corticotropin-releasing hormone (CRH) and arginine vasopressin, which are in turn under direct feedback inhi-

*From Contemporary Endocrinology: Endocrinology of Critical Disease
Edited by K. P. Ober Humana Press Inc., Totowa, NJ*

bition from cortisol. Secretion of these hypothalamic hormones is also regulated by numerous neurochemicals that modulate the central nervous system (CNS) response to stress *(3)* (*see* Chapter 1).

Production of cortisol in adrenocortical cells in response to ACTH occurs within minutes and begins with enzymatic cleavage of the side chain of cholesterol to generate pregnenolone. Although this first step is known to be rate-limiting, it has become apparent that it is not the P-450$_{scc}$ (side chain cleavage enzyme) *per se* that is rate-determining, but rather transfer of cholesterol to the inner mitochondrial membrane (where the enzyme resides) *(4)*. This in turn is dependent on the amount of cholesterol within the cytosol and its transport into the mitochondria by a family of proteins called steroidogenic acute regulatory (StAR) proteins. Cholesterol can be manufactured in adrenal cells *de novo*, but most is supplied via lipoproteins (LDL). When delivery of cholesterol to adrenocortical cells is impaired, endogenous adrenal production increases, though it may not be enough to supply needs during prolonged requirements *(5)*.

Pregnenolone is acted on by four additional enzyme systems to generate cortisol. These enzymatic steps require NADPH and oxygen. In addition to the rapid (minutes) effects on pregnenolone production mentioned above, ACTH stimulation will cause an increase in adrenocortical cell growth, DNA transcription, and protein translation over a matter of hours to days. This includes increased production of the steroidogenic enzymes *(6)*. Further enhancement of glucocorticoid production may occur during acute illness by a shift of adrenal steroid production away from the other products of the adrenal cortex (androgens and mineralocorticoids) to cortisol *(7)*.

Normal daily production of cortisol is approx 15–20 mg daily *(8)*. During major surgery, production rates increase to 75–150 mg/d *(9)*, and the maximal output from the adrenals has been estimated at no more than 200 mg/d *(10)*. This level of production leads to mean cortisol values ranging from 30–50 mg/dL during sepsis and major surgery *(11,12)*.

Immune Endocrine Interactions

Acute stress activates the CRH–ACTH–cortisol axis. Stimuli from centers in the brainstem cause the release of CRH and arginine vasopressin (AVP), which in turn leads to increased ACTH and cortisol secretion. The type and severity of stress influence the degree of activation. Elevated cortisol levels will block the pituitary–adrenal response to minor stress (feedback inhibition), but may not alter the response to major stress *(13)*. The increased circulating cortisol restrains the immune system, and helps maintain cardiovascular and metabolic integrity of the organism.

Although this classic description is conceptually very useful, it is a gross simplification of a complicated and poorly understood process. The interactions between the immune system and the cortisol axis are intricate and profound. Although the immunosuppressive effects of cortisol have been known for years, it has recently become apparent that immune–endocrine interactions are bidirectional *(14–16)*. Cytokines, polypeptides produced by activated immune cells, have recently been shown to affect both endocrine and metabolic functions *(17)*. Cytokines appear to be able to modulate the CRH–ACTH–cortisol axis at each level: the hypothalamus, pituitary, and adrenal *(18)*. However, the exact role these peptides play is far from clear. Interleukin I (IL-I), IL-2, IL-6, tumor necrosis factor (TNF) α, and γ-interferon are perhaps the best studied in terms of their endocrine effects, but the data are confusing. Some of this is owing to species differences, but also to the difficulty of studying effects in vivo and the fact that agents such as catecholamines, prostaglandins, and nitric oxide, can function as cytokine mediators *(18)*.

An additional level of complexity in the endocrine–immune interactions is also becoming apparent. Receptors for pituitary hormones, hypothalamic hypophysiotropic hormones, gastrointestinal peptides, and other neuropeptides have been demonstrated on lymphoid and accessory cells *(9)*. These substances can stimulate or depress immune responses. In addition, many hormones and neuropeptides can be produced by immune cells, and they appear to be regulated by hypothalamic stimulatory or inhibitory factors as well as by hormones involved in negative feedback *(16)*. Although the amounts produced appear small, this does not preclude an important paracrine or autocrine role. Once again, their precise role in this regard is unclear, but one is struck by a case report of Cushing's syndrome resulting from granulomatous production of ACTH *(20)*. It has been suggested that immune cells could be considered as a diffuse, sensorial receptor organ *(16)*. Information processed by the immune system is transmitted to the brain or brain-controlled structures (via cytokines and other products), where it plays a role in the integrated response of the organism to stress.

Cortisol in the Circulation and in Tissues

Cortisol circulates bound in large measure to plasma proteins, predominantly cortisol binding globulin (CBG). The free hormone hypothesis holds that only the unbound, or "free" hormone, is able to interact with receptor and is thus biologically active *(21)*. In its simplest form, this hypothesis ascribes to CBG the minor role of carrier protein and reservoir of cortisol. However, there is evidence that CBG has additional functions. The molecule is a member of the serpin (serine proteinase inhibitor) superfamily. Based on the characteristics of other family members, it was predicted that cleavage of CBG by a serine proteinase could disrupt its steroid binding site and result in the local release of cortisol at sites of inflammation *(22)*. This concept has been confirmed in vivo and in vitro *(23)*.

The glucocorticoid receptor (GR) belongs to a superfamily of nuclear hormone receptors, which includes receptors for mineralocorticoids, androgens, progestins, estrogens, vitamin D, thyroid hormone, and retinoic acid. In the unliganded state, GR is part of a multiprotein complex that includes, among other proteins, heat-shock proteins. These attached proteins may play a role in shuttling of the complex between the cytosol and the nucleus *(24)*. The main function of the complex appears to be to keep the receptor in an inactive, yet receptive state. When ligand (cortisol) is bound, conformational changes take place leading to dissociation of heat-shock proteins, increased receptor protein phosphorylation, and unmasking of nuclear localization signals. The activated receptor–ligand complex can then act in two ways. It can bind directly to specific sites in the promoter region of glucocorticoid response genes (called a glucocorticoid response element, or GRE), or it can interact with transcription factors, such as c-jun *(24)*. The latter mechanism allows for glucocorticoid regulation of many genes that do not have specific GREs.

Thus, the response of a cell to cortisol depends on a number of factors: the intracellular availability of free hormone, the amount and affinity of the glucocorticoid receptor complex, and the ability of the liganded receptor to bind to DNA and stimulate or repress transcription. Numerous regulatory agents have been found at all these steps (*see* Fig. 1). For example, intracellular cortisol levels can be regulated by 11 β-hydroxysteroid dehy-

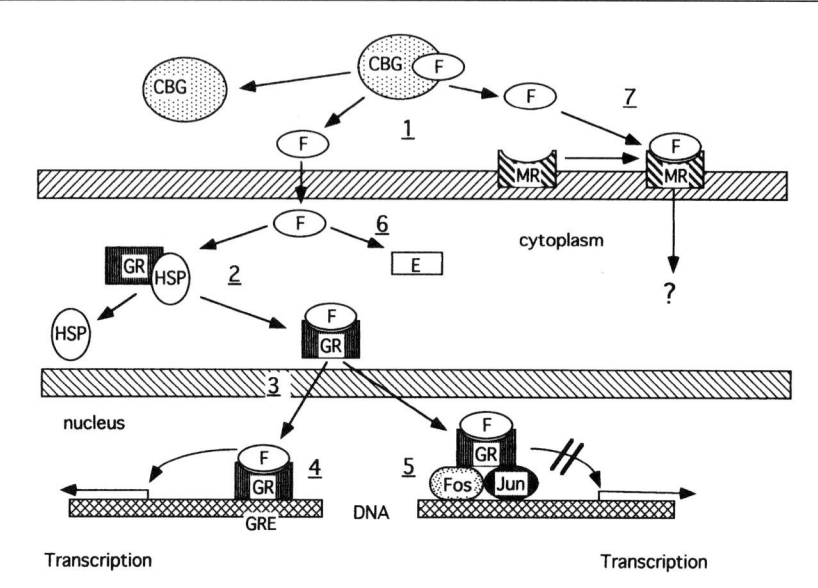

Fig. 1. Simplified model of cellular mechanisms of glucocorticoid actions. Cortisol (F) dissociates from CBG 1, making it available within the cytoplasm for binding to the GR-heat-shock protein (HSP) complex 2. After translocation to the nucleus 3, the receptor–ligand complex can affect transcription in one of two ways: by binding to a GRE and initiating transcription 4, or by interacting with transcription factors, such as c-jun 5 (which is generally inhibitory for transcription). Cortisol can be inactivated by conversion to cortisone (E) or other metabolites 6. Evidence exists that cortisol may also act through nongenomic actions, such as by interaction with membrane receptors (MR) on the cell surface 7. Adapted from Bamberger et al. (24) (see text).

drogenase, which converts cortisol to cortisone and renders it inactive. Glucocorticoids are able to downregulate the number of GRs (25), and GR transcription and expression can be affected by second messenger systems, neurotransmitters, and other factors (26–28). There is evidence that some of these regulators may play roles in gene expression in both GR and immune cells (29,30). The effect of critical illness on these mediators is currently not known.

There is accumulating evidence that glucocorticoids may work through nongenomic actions as well (31). Steroid effects that occur more rapidly than could be expected from the generation of protein products are candidates for nongenomic mechanisms. Membrane binding sites for steroid hormones have been described, though the physiologic significance is uncertain (31,32).

Physiologic Actions of Glucocorticoids

Glucocorticoids play an important role in the metabolism of carbohydrates, lipids, and proteins, and have profound regulatory effects on immune and circulatory function (33). The primary action on carbohydrate metabolism is to increase glucose production via effects on gluconeogenesis and antagonism of insulin action. Lipolysis is stimulated by glucocorticoids, leading to increases in circulating free fatty acids. Excess cortisol will stimulate proteolysis in fat, skeletal muscle, bone, lymphoid, and connective tissue, making amino acid substrates available for gluconeogenesis. Cardiac muscle and the diaphragm are spared from this catabolic action.

Some of the immune effects of cortisol have already been mentioned. As a general rule, glucocorticoids inhibit most immunologic and inflammatory responses *(33,34)*. In response to excess cortisol secretion, lymphopenia, eosinophilia, and monocytopenia occur. There is an increase in polymorphonuclear cell release from bone marrow, but the activity of these cells is depressed, and they are unable to mount a normal immune response. Glucocorticoids have also been found to prevent activation of the complement cascade, prevent prostaglandin generation, and inhibit nitric oxide synthesis *(33,35)*. In addition, glucocorticoids have a positive inotropic influence on the heart, a permissive effect on the actions of epinephrine and norepinephrine, and at high doses, they interact with the mineralocorticoid receptor to induce actions normally associated with mineralocorticoid hormones. Thus, in addition to immune modulation, the increases in cortisol production in critical illness are believed to enhance survival via increased cardiac contractility, cardiac output, sensitivity to catecholamines, work capacity of skeletal muscles, and capacity to mobilize energy sources through gluconeogenesis, proteolysis, and lipolysis *(33)*.

Although glucocorticoids are required for survival, excessive amounts can be life-threatening, as exemplified by the mortality and morbidity associated with untreated Cushing's syndrome. Suppressed immune function results in susceptibility to infections *(36)*. Psychiatric effects, including depression and frank psychosis, can be profound. Exogenous glucocorticoid use has also been associated with pancreatitis, vasculitis, and intracranial hypertension *(36)*. Acute metabolic abnormalities include poor wound healing, diabetes mellitus, and hyperlipidemia. Chronic metabolic abnormalities can lead to myopathy, atherosclerosis, avascular necrosis, and osteoporosis.

CLINICAL RESPONSE OF CRH–ACTH–CORTISOL AXIS TO ILLNESS

Surgery has long been known as a potent stimulator of the CRH–ACTH–cortisol axis *(37)*. The degree of activation is dependent on the type of surgery *(11)* and anesthesia *(13)*. During a major surgical procedure, CRH, ACTH, and cortisol levels rise significantly *(38)*. The rise in ACTH and cortisol can be abolished by interrupting the neural connections from the operative site *(8)*. Reversal of anesthesia is also a potent stimulator of ACTH secretion *(39)*. However, by the first postoperative day, ACTH and CRH levels have been found to drop below presurgical levels, whereas cortisol levels remain high, although lower than during surgery *(38)*. Over the next few days, cortisol levels continue to fall while ACTH levels remain suppressed before returning to normal by days 5–7. Cortisol elevation after surgery is not owing to altered half-life *(40)*, but rather is a reflection of increased sensitivity of the adrenals to ACTH stimulation *(38)*. This increased sensitivity may begin during surgery and be the result of release of cytokines in response to surgical trauma *(38,39)*. TNF and IL-6 have been found to be elevated intraoperatively and for the ensuing 48–72 h in pancreatoduodenectomy patients, corresponding to the period of increased levels of cortisol *(41)*. The suppressed ACTH level shortly after surgery represents a return of normal feedback sensitivity. In summary, in response to major surgery, there is an initial phase of stimulation of the entire CRH–ACTH–cortisol axis, followed by a return of cortisol feedback inhibition, but continued increased cortisol production, and subsequent gradual return to basal activity.

Patients who suffer cardiac arrest experience significant increases in serum cortisol levels *(42)*. In patients surviving the acute event, this elevation peaks within a few hours and continues for 24–48 h *(43)*. ACTH levels peak in the first few hours and fall toward normal by the second day *(43)*.

Bacterial sepsis is another potent stimulator of the CRH–ACTH–cortisol axis *(44)*. Unlike the response to major surgery, the loss of feedback inhibition by elevated cortisol levels may last for days *(45,46)*, perhaps owing to continued stressful stimulus. During this time, the pituitary is hyperresponsive to stimulation by CRH *(47)*. A number of explanations have been offered for this, including diminished glucocorticoid receptor affinity, direct cytokine effects on the pituitary, and prolonged half-life of ACTH *(46,47)*. However, it appears that elevated ACTH levels cannot be sustained indefinitely. For example, the persistently elevated cortisol levels seen in the chronic severe illness of late-stage HIV disease are accompanied by suppressed ACTH values *(48)*.

The continued secretion of increased amounts of cortisol in the presence of subnormal levels of ACTH, whether postoperatively, with bacterial sepsis, or trauma, indicates heightened sensitivity of the adrenals to ACTH and/or the presence of non-ACTH stimulators of cortisol synthesis. As mentioned above, cytokines, such as IL-1 and α–interferon, have been suggested to play such a role *(48)*. It also appears that "priming" of the adrenals by the earlier elevation of ACTH plays a role *(38)*.

Another adaptive response to critical illness is the shift of steroid production in the adrenals from mineralocorticoid and androgens to cortisol *(7,49)* . The mechanism for this is unknown, though cytokines once again appear a likely candidate. The benefits of such a shift are obvious in terms of ensuring cholesterol is not directed away from cortisol production.

CRH–ACTH–CORTISOL INSUFFICIENCY

Etiology

Although it has long been appreciated for over a century that the Addisonian patient succumbs readily to stress, it is unknown how often an insufficient response of the CRH–ACTH–cortisol axis in the non-Addisonian patient may cause or contribute to poor clinical outcome in critical illness. Many authors have concluded that adrenal insufficiency is rare in the setting of critical illness, finding only sporadic cases in prospective series *(12,50,51)*. However, the methods commonly used to make the diagnosis of adrenal insufficiency are not necessarily applicable in the critically ill patient. There is no validated method for diagnosing relative adrenal insufficiency during stress.

Some authors have reported significantly higher rates of insufficient adrenal response in critical illness. Soni et al. reported that 5 of 21 patients (23.8%) with septic shock had insufficient response to ACTH stimulation (serum cortisol <18 mg/dL) *(52)*. Three of these patients received steroid supplementation with rapid improvement in hemodynamic parameters. An earlier study in septic patients by Sibbald et al. found insufficient response to ACTH in 19.2% *(53)*. Rothwell et al. *(54)* found 13 of 32 patients in septic shock had insufficient response to ACTH, all of whom died (compared to 6 deaths among the 19 with adequate responses) *(55)*. Thus, relative adrenal insufficiency may be common in certain critical illnesses.

Adrenal insufficiency can be classified as primary or secondary (*see* Table 1). Although all causes of adrenal insufficiency are relatively rare, certain etiologies are more likely to be seen in the setting of critical illness. For example, bilateral adrenal hemorrhage, initially considered a rare cause of death *(55)*, is being recognized with

Table 1
Etiologies of Adrenal Insufficiency

Primary adrenal insufficiency
  Autoimmune
    infections:
      Mycobacterial
      Fungal: histoplasmosis, blastomycosis, coccidiomycosis, cryptococcosis
      Viral: CMV, HIV
  Adrenal hemorrhage:
    Waterhouse-Friderichsen syndrome, Lupus anticoagulant, ITP, anticoagulation
  Metastatic disease
    Lung, gastric, breast, melanoma, lymphoma
  Genetic
    Adrenoleukodystrophy, adrenomyeloneuropathy, familial glucocorticoid deficiency

Secondary adrenal insufficiency
  Administration of glucocorticoids or agents with glucocorticoid activity
  Pituitary or hypothalamic tumors:
    Pituitary adenoma, craniopharyngioma
  Isolated ACTH deficiency
  Surgery
  Infiltrative diseases:
    Sarcoid, hemochromatosis, autoimmune, hemorrhage
  Trauma
  Cranial irradiation

increasing frequency in acutely ill patients *(56)*. Risk factors include heart disease, infection, coagulopathy (spontaneous or iatrogenic), and surgery *(57)*. The clinical presentation of adrenal hemorrhage is often vague and indolent, with the exception of the Waterhouse-Friderichsen syndrome *(56)*. Pain in the abdomen, flank, back, or chest is often reported, followed in decreasing frequency by fever, hypotension, anorexia, nausea, vomiting, psychiatric symptoms, and abdominal rigidity or rebound *(57)*. Laboratory findings can include a sharp drop in hemoglobin, hyponatremia, hyperkalemia, leukocytosis, azotemia, and acidosis *(56)*. The increased susceptibility of the adrenal to hemorrhage in critical illness may be owing in part to ACTH-induced increase in adrenal blood flow. This accelerated blood flow may exceed the limited venous drainage from the adrenal, leading to stasis and hemorrhagic necrosis *(56)*.

The most common cause of secondary adrenal insufficiency is therapeutic use of glucocorticoids. Unfortunately, the degree of suppression cannot be reliably predicted based on the dose or duration of glucocorticoid use *(58)*. Recently, the suppressive effects of some progestational agents have been recognized *(59)*. For example, the progestational agent megestrol acetate (Megace), used for treatment of AIDS cachexia, breast cancer, and prostate cancer, has been found to induce adrenal insufficiency when withdrawn after chronic use *(60)*.

Kidess et al. *(61)* recently reported on three cases of apparent transient corticotropin deficiency in critical illness. Cortisol levels perioperatively were not elevated, but did respond to cortrosyn stimulation. In addition, the patients responded dramatically to the addition of hydrocortisone to their iv fluids. ACTH levels were not measured, but were presumed low. One of their hypotheses was that TNF may have been inhibiting ACTH secretion *(61)*. It is reasonable to speculate that an imbalance of cytokine production (ACTH/CRH inhibitors vs stimulators) may have occurred for some reason in these patients. Another possibility would be production of a substance that impairs sensitivity of the adrenals to ACTH. A family of such peptides (called corticostatins) has been described, one of which (HP4) has been isolated from human neutrophils *(67)*. A response to the supraphysiologic doses of ACTH given in the cortrosyn stimulation test does not rule this possibility out. Patients such as these may be common, though there is some evidence to refute this *(63)*.

Speculation has arisen that some people may have a defective hypothalamic response to immune and inflammatory stimuli, and an inadequate production of cortisol *(64)*. The animal model for this is the Lewis rat, which is unable to produce CRH in response to inflammation *(18)*. These rats are readily susceptible to arthritis. Similarly, humans with rheumatoid arthritis have been found to fail to increase cortisol secretion appropriately following surgery, but to respond normally to CRH *(64)*.

Testing of the CRH–ACTH–Cortisol Axis

The evaluation of patients for adrenal insufficiency often requires the use of dynamic testing. Symptoms may be nonspecific, and baseline cortisol values are not accurate for the diagnosis. Blevins demonstrated this nicely in an unstressed population with suspected impairment of ACTH reserve *(65)*. A cortisol level of <18 mg/dL provided 100% sensitivity for adrenal insufficiency, but only 14% specificity. Changing criteria to improve the specificity to 97% causes the sensitivity to drop to only 10%.

Though mean values for cortisol are elevated during critical illness, the range is extremely wide. Some studies have found a tendency for lower basal values to be correlated with poorer outcome, perhaps a reflection of adrenal insufficiency *(52,53)*. Conversely, it is clear that some critically ill patients may have basal levels in the normal range for unstressed patients, and yet have an adequate response to ACTH stimulation and a good clinical outcome *(50,51)*. In addition, a level above which adrenal insufficiency can be excluded in critical illness has not been determined. For example, Streeten et al. recently reported a postoperative patient with signs and symptoms of adrenal insufficiency and a basal cortisol of 21.7 mg/dL *(66)*. This patient had a dramatic response to glucocorticoid therapy, and after recovery, an abnormal response to metyrapone was observed. Thus, basal cortisol determinations suffer from the same lack of reliability during critical illness as they do in ambulatory, unstressed populations.

For years, the rapid ACTH stimulation test has been accepted as a completely reliable method for establishing the integrity of the hypothalamic–pituitary–adrenal (HPA) axis *(67)*. However, reports have surfaced showing that some patients may have defects in ACTH release in response to hypoglycemic stress or metyrapone stimulation despite having normal responses to the rapid ACTH test *(66,68–72)*. Thus, the reliability of the rapid ACTH test in diagnosing secondary adrenal insufficiency is questionable. The longer 8-h ACTH infusion still appears to be reliable *(66)*, but is more cumbersome and seldom used. The tests against which the rapid ACTH test have been compared, the insulin tolerance test and the metyrapone stimulation test, are of course not feasible during acute illness.

In the hope of finding a way to improve the reliability of rapid ACTH testing, some authors have been investigating using lower doses of ACTH, with good results *(73,74)*. Tordjman et al. *(75)* administered 1 µg (vs the usual 250 mcg) to three groups of patients: one with pituitary disease and proven impairment of HPA function, another with similar pituitary pathology, but adequate HPA function, and normal controls. None of the patients in the first group had a normal response to the low dose of ACTH, though 9 of 10 passed the standard 250-mcg test. Two of nine patients with pituitary disease, but normal response to insulin tolerance testing failed the low-dose ACTH test. Whether this indicated some subtle abnormalities not detected by insulin tolerance testing or represented false-positive results is unknown *(75)*. Further studies are needed.

Testing the HPA axis with CRH may prove to be useful. When CRH is given to patients who have been receiving glucocorticoids, there is a blunted cortisol response *(76)*. Though currently unavailable, this agent's status may change by the time this is published. However, some have expressed skepticism about the utility of CRH testing since this would fail to determine if hypothalamic function is intact *(66,77)*. Nevertheless, data so far indicate it may become the best method for evaluating corticotroph function *(58)*.

Another agent receiving some attention, as a surrogate for CRH, is naloxone. Administration of this agent produces a rise in ACTH and cortisol similar to stimulation by CRH *(77)*. However, experience with this agent is limited.

Given the above shortcomings of ACTH stimulation testing, the lack of experience with low-dose ACTH testing and CRH, and the lack of a meaningful measure of relative adrenocortical deficiency during critical illness, the diagnosis must often rest on clinical parameters and judgment. Suspicion is the key, and consideration should be given to the diagnosis of adrenal insufficiency when the patient's clinical course is not improving and is accompanied by findings, such as hypotension, hyponatremia, hyperkalemia, or abdominal complaints.

THERAPEUTIC USE OF GLUCOCORTICOIDS

Severe Illness

The dramatic response of cardiovascular status in Addisonian patients to glucocorticoids, the high levels of cortisol seen in acute illness, and the anti-inflammatory properties of glucocorticoids have led to speculation that pharmacologic administration of glucocorticoids might be beneficial in severe illness, such as septic shock. Indeed, prior to the publication in 1987 of two large-scale, placebo-controlled, double-blind studies that showed high-dose steroids were of no benefit, patients were often treated with high-dose steroids in this setting *(78,79)*. Two recent meta-analyses on the use of steroids in sepsis reached similar conclusions *(80,81)*. In one analysis, there was a trend toward higher mortality associated with secondary infections in the treated groups *(81)*. High-dose corticosteroid use has also been found not to be beneficial in adult respiratory distress syndrome resulting from a variety of causes *(82)*. An exception to this is severe *Pneumocystis carinii* pneumonia (PCP) in patients with AIDS, where administration of pharmacologic doses of prednisone have been found to improve pulmonary function and survival *(83)*.

The anti-inflammatory properties of corticosteroids have led to their use in critical illness involving the CNS. Corticosteroid use after acute CNS trauma has been advocated by many *(84,85)*, but beneficial effects have not been demonstrated consistently *(86,87)*. Efficacy has been demonstrated in *Haemophilus influenzae* meningitis in children *(88)*.

However, the vast majority of studies evaluating the use of corticosteroids in critical illness have used doses more than 10-fold greater than the maximum secretory capacity of the adrenal. Doses in this range may induce reponses that overide specific beneficial actions present at lower doses *(89)*. Given the difficulty in determining the true incidence of adrenal insufficiency in critical illness (including relative insufficiency) and the dramatic role corticosteroids play in survival in Addisonian patients, it is reasonable to think that corticosteroid administration in physiologic doses might be beneficial *(54)*. In the absence of further data, it is reasonable to treat patients suspected clinically of having partial or relative adrenal insufficiency with physiologic stress doses of corticosteroids.

Adrenal Insufficiency

In patients known to have adrenal insufficiency who are acutely ill, corticosteroid therapy can be life-saving. Intravenous hydrocortisone is the drug of choice and is given in doses of 100 mg every 6–8 h. The dose should be tapered to standard replacement doses as rapidly as the patient's condition permits (12–15 mg hydrocortisone/m^2 d) *(56)*. Treatment is the same whether the adrenal insufficiency is primary or secondary.

In patients suspected of having adrenal insufficiency, blood can be drawn for cortisol and ACTH levels, and dexamethasone (4–5 mg) given. This allows for ACTH stimulation testing if desired, since dexamethasone will not interfere with the measurement of cortisol. Hydrocortisone is subsequently administered as outlined above.

Rates of cortisol secretion during and after surgery have been studied and allow for rational guidelines regarding corticosteroid therapy in patients with adrenal insufficiency *(9)*. For minor surgical stress (hand surgery, hemorrhoidectomy, inguinal herniorrhapy, and so on), 50 mg/d hydrocortisone equivalent for 1–2 d are sufficient *(56)*. For major surgical stress (chest surgery, upper abdominal surgery), 100 mg hydrocortisone equivalent every 8 h starting prior to surgery and continuing for 2–3 d are recommended *(67)*. In the absence of complications, the dose is then tapered over the next 2–3 d toward maintenance levels. Although these recommended doses may be less than is commonly prescribed, there is no evidence that they need to be exceeded *(67,90)*.

SUMMARY

Corticosteroids are necessary for survival during periods of critical illness. Their beneficial cardiovascular and metabolic effects are well known. Recently, an appreciation of the profound complexity of the role of corticosteroids in stress has been developing. As a result, the traditional view of interactions between the CRH–ACTH–cortisol axis and the immune system is undergoing modification. During stress, the systems interact at multiple levels in an attempt to provide a coordinated response that meets the challenge to homeostasis with minimal damage to the organism as a whole. Although it is clear that an organism's response may not always be appropriate, determining how and when to intervene is problematic. Simply gauging what is an adequate response of the adrenal glands to critical illness is fraught with difficulties, and defining the role of therapeutic use of corticosteroids has been difficult. Further research is needed to enhance our understanding and ability to intervene appropriately.

Despite the incomplete nature of our understanding of the role of the CRH–ACTH–cortisol axis in critical illness, the astute clinician can provide benefit to acutely ill patients. Recognition of adrenal insufficiency and thoughtful use of corticosteroids can improve patient outcome and be life-saving.

REFERENCES

1. Rolih C, Ober K. The endocrine response to critical illness. Med Clin North Am 1995;79:211–224.
2. Munck A, Guyre PM, Holbrook NJ. Physiological functions of glucocorticoids in stress and their relation to pharmacological actions. Endocr Rev 1984;5:25–44.
3. Chrousos GP, Gold PW. The concepts of stress and stress system disorders. JAMA 1992;267:1244–1252.
4. Stocco DM, Clark BJ. Regulation of the acute production of steroids in steroidogenic cells. Endocr Rev 1996;17:221–244.
5. Illingworth DR, Kenny TA, Orwoll ES. Adrenal function in heterozygous and homozygous hypobelalipoproteinemia. J Clin Endocrinol Metab 1982;54:27–33.
6. Simpson ER, Waterman MR. Regulation of the synthesis of steroidogenic enzymes in adrenal cortical cells by ACTH. Annu Rev Physiol 1988;50:427–440.
7. Parker LN, Levin ER, Lifrak ET. Evidence for adrenocortical adaptation to severe illness. J Clin Endocrinol Metab 1985;60:947–952.
8. Orth DN, Kovacs WJ, Debold CR. The adrenal cortex. In: Wilson JD, Foster DW, eds. Williams Textbook of Endocrinology, 8th ed. Philadephia, Saunders 1992, pp. 489–620.
9. Kehlet H. A rational approach to dosage and preparation of parenteral glucocorticoid substitution therapy during surgical procedure. Acta Anaesth Scand 1975;19:260–264.
10. Loriaux DL. Adrenocortical insufficiency. In: Becker KL, ed. Principles and Practice of Endocrinology and Metablosim, 8th ed. J Lippincott, Philadelphia, 1995, pp. 682–695.
11. Chernow B, Alexamder HR, Smallridge RC, Thompson WR, Cook D, Beardsley D, Fink MP, Lake R, Fletcher JR. Hormonal responses to graded surgical stress. Arch Intern Med 1987;147:1273–1278.
12. Schein RM, Sprung CL, Marcial E, Napolitano L, Chernow B. Plasma cortisol levels in patients with septic shock. Crit Care Med 1990;18:259–263.
13. Raff H, Norton AJ, Flemma RJ, Findling JW. Inhibition of the adrenocorticotropin response to surgery in humans: interaction between dexamethasone and fentanyl. J Clin Endocrinol Metab 1987;65:295–298.
14. Spangelo BL, Macleod RM. The role of immunopeptides in the regulation of anterior pituitary hormone release. Trends Endocrinol Metab 1990;1:408–412.
15. Blalock JE. A molecular basis for bidirectional communication between the immune and neuroendocrine systems. Physiol Rev 1989;69:1–32.
16. Besedovsky HO, Del Rey A. Immune-neuro-endocrine interactions: facts and hypotheses. Endocr Rev 1996;17:64–102.
17. Besedovsky HO, Del Rey A. Immune-neuroendocrine circuits: integrative role of cytokines. Front Neuroendocrinol 1992;13:61–94.
18. Gaillard RC. Neuroendocrine-immune system interactions. Trends in Endocrinol Metab 1994;5:303–309.
19. Weigent DA, Blalock JE. Interaction between the neuroendocrine and immune systems: common hormones and receptors. Immunol Rev 1987;100:79–108.
20. Dupont AG, Somers G, Van Steirteghem AC, Warson F, Vanhaelst L. Ectopic adrenocorticotropin production: disappearance after removal of inflammatory tissue. J Clin Endocrinol Metab 1984;58:654–658.
21. Mendel CM. The free hormone hypothesis: a physiologically based mathematical model. Endocr Rev 1989;10:232–274.
22. Rosner W. Plasma steroid-binding proteins. Endocrinol Metab Clin North Am 1991;20:697–720.
23. Hammond GL. Potential functions of plasma steroid-binding proteins. Trends Endocrinol Metab 1995;6:298–304.
24. Bamberger CM, Schulte HN, Chrousos GP. Molecular determinants of glucocorticoid receptor function and tissue sensitivity to glucocorticoids. Endocr Rev 1996;17:245–268.
25. Burnstein KL, Bellingham DL, Jewell CM, Powell-Oliver FE, Cidlowski JA. Autoregulation of glucocorticoid receptor gene expression. Steroids 1991;56:52–58.
26. Antakly T, Mercille S, Cote JP. Tissue-specific dopaminergic regulation of the glucocorticoid receptor in the rat pituitary. Endocrinology 1987;120:1558–1562.
27. Peiffer A, Bardin N. Estrogen-induced decrease of glucocorticoid receptor messenger ribonucleic acid concentration in the anterior pituitary gland. Mol Endocrinol 1987;1:435–440.
28. Moyer ML, Borror KC, Bona BJ, DeFranco DB, Nordeen SK. Modulation of cell signaling pathways can enhance or impair glucocorticoid-induced gene expression without altering the state of receptor phosphorylation. J Biol Chem 1993;22:933–940.
29. Renoir JM, Mercier-Bodard C, Hoffmann K. LeBihan S, Ning YM, Sanchez ER, Handschumacher RE, Baulieu EE. Cyclosprorin A potentiates the dexamethasone-induced mouse mammary tumor virus-

chloramphenical acetyltransferase activity in LMCAT cells: a possible role for different heat shock protein-binding immunophilins in glucocorticoid receptor-mediated gene expression. Proc Natl Acad Sci USA 1995;92:4977–4981.
30. Liu J, Farmer JC, Lane WE, Friedman J, Weissman I, Schreiber SL. Calicineurin is a common target of cyclophilin-cyclosporin A and FKBP-FK506 complexes. Cell 1991;66:807–815.
31. Wehling M. Nongenomic actions of steroid hormones. Trends Endocrinol Metab 1994;5:347–353.
32. Suyemitsu, T, Terayama H. Specific binding sites for natural glucocorticoids in plasma membranes of rat liver. Endocrinology 1975;96:1499–1508.
33. White PC, Pescovitz OH, Cutler GB. Synthesis and metabolism of corticosteroids. In: Becker KL, ed. Principles and Practice of Endocrinology and Metabolism, 2nd ed. Philadelphia, Lippincott, 1995, pp. 647–662.
34. Parrillo JE, Fauci AS. Mechanisms of glucocorticoid action on immune processes. Annu Rev Pharmacol Toxicol 1979;19:179.
35. Moncada S, Higgs A. The L-arginine-nitric oxide pathway. N Engl J Med 1993;329:2002–2012.
36. Tyrrell JB. Glucocorticoid therapy. In: Felig P, Baxter JD, Frohman LA eds. Endocrinology and Metabloism, 3rd ed. McGraw Hill, New York, 1995, 855–882.
37. Hume DM, Bell CC, Bartter F. Direct measurement of adrenal secretion during operative trauma and convalescence. Surgery 1962;52:174.
38. Naito Y, Fukuta J, Tamai S, Seo N, Nakai Y, Mori K, Imura H. Biphasic changes in hypothalamo-pituitary-adrenal function during the early recovery period after major abdominal surgery. J Clin Endocrinol Metab 1991;73:111–117.
39. Udelsman R, Norton JA, Jelenich SE, Goldstein DS, Linehan WM, Loriaux DL, Chrousos GP. Responses of the hypothalamic–pituitary–adrenal and renin-angiotensin axes and the sympathetic system during controlled surgical and anesthetic stress. J Clin Endocrinol Metab 1987;64:986–994.
40. Kehlet H, Binder CHR. Alterations in distribution volume and biological half-life of cortisol during major surgery. J Clin Endocrinol Metab 1972;36:330–333.
41. Naito Y, Tamai S, Shingu K, Shindo K, Matsui T, Segawa H, NakaiY, Mori K. Responses of plasma adrenocorticotropic hor-mone, cortisol, and cytokines during and after upper abdominal surgery. Anesthesiology 1992;77: 426–431.
42. Wortsman J, Wehrenberg WB, Petra PH, Murphy JE. Melanocyte-stimulating hormone immunoreactivity is a component of the neuroendocrine response to maximal stress (cardiac arrest). J Clin Endocrinol Metab 1985;61:355–360.
43. Schultz CH, Rivers EP, Feldkamp CS, Goad EG, Smithline HA, Martin GC, Fath JJ,Wortsman J, Nowak RM. A characterization of hypothalamic–pituitary–adrenal axis function during and after human cardiac arrest. Crit Care Med 1993;21:1339–1347.
44. Melby JC, Spink WW. Comparative studies on adrenal cortical function and cortisol metabolism in healthy adults and in patients with shock due to infection. J Clin Invest 1958;37:1791–1798.
45. Vermes I, Beishuizen A, Hampsink RM, Haanen C. Dissociation of plasma adrenocortioctropin and cortisol levels in criticaly ill patients: possible role of endothelin and atrial natriuretic hormone. J Clin Endocrinol Metab 1995;80:1238–1242.
46. Siegel LM, Grinspoon SK, Garvey GJ, Bilezekian JP. Sepsis and adrenal function. Trends Endocrinol Metab 1994;5:324–328.
47. Reincke M, Allolio B, Wurth G, Winkelmann W. The hypothalamic-pituitary-adrenal axis in critical illness: response to dexamethasone and corticotropin-releasing hormone. J Clin Endocrinol Metab 1993;77:151–156.
48. Lortholary O, Christeff N, Casassus P, Thobein N, Veyssier P, Trogoff B, Tocci O, Brauner M, Nunez CA, Guillouin L. Hypothamo-pituitary-adrenal function in human immunodeficiency virus infected men. J Clin Endocrinol Metab 1996;81:791–796.
49. Drucker D, McLaughlin J. Adrenocortical dysfunction in acute medical illness. Crit Care Med 1986;14:789–791.
50. Jurney TH, Cockrell JL, Lindberg JS, Lamiell JM, Wade CE. Spectrum of serum cortisol response to ACTH in ICU patients. Chest 1987;92:292–295.
51. Drucker D, shandling M. Variable adrenocortical function in acute medical illness. Crit Care Med 1985;13:477–479.
52. Soni A, Pepper GM, Wyrwinski PM, Ramirez NE, Simon R, Pina T, Gruenspan H, Vaca CE. Adrenal insufficiency occurring during septic shock: incidence, outcome, and relationship to peripheral cytokine levels. Am J Med 1995;98:266–271.

53. Sibbald WJ, Short A, Cohen MP, Wilson RF. Variations in adrenocortical responsiveness during severe bacterial infections. Ann Surg 1977;186:29–33.
54. Rothwell PM, Udwadia ZF, Lawler PC. Cortisol response to corticotropin and survival in septic shock. Lancet 1991;337:582–583.
55. Xarli VP, Steele AA, Davis PJ, Buescher ES, Rios CN, Carcia-Bunuel R. Adrenal hemorrhage in the adult. Medicine 1978;57:211–221.
56. Werbel SS, Ober KP. Acute adrenal insufficiency. Endocrinol Metab Clin North Am 1993;22:303–328.
57. Rao RH, Bagnucci AH, Amico JA. Bilateral massive adrenal hemorrhage: early recognition and treatment. Ann Intern Med 1989;110:227–235.
58. Schlaghecke R, Kornely E, Santen RH, Ridderskamp. The effect of long-term glucocorticoid therapy on pituitary-adrenal responses to exogenous cortictropin-releasing hormone. N Engl J Med 1992;326:226–230.
59. Mann M, Malozowski S, Murgo A, Bacsanyi J, Breen L, Koller E. 1996 The glucocorticoid activity of megestrol acetate: report on 56 cases. Program of the 10th International Congress of Endocrinology, San Francisco, P3-604 (Abstract).
60. Leinung MC, Liporace R, Miller CH. Induction of adrenal suppression by megestrol acetate in patients with AIDS. Ann Intern Med 1995;122:843–845.
61. Kidess AJ, Caplan RH, Reynertson RH, Wickus GG, Goodnough DE. Transient corticotropin deficiency in critical illness. Mayo Clin Proc 1993;68:435–441.
62. Solomon S. Corticostatins. Trends Endocrinol Metab 1993;4:260.
63. Mohler JL, Michael KA, Freedman AM, McRoberts JW, Gerferr WO Jr. The evaluation of postoperative function of the adrenal gland. Surg Gynecol Obstet 1985;161:551–556.
64. Chikanza IC, Petrou P, Kingsley G, Chrousos G, Panayi GS. Defective hypothalamic response to immune and inflammatory stimuli in patients with rheumatoid arthritis. Arthritis Rheum 1992;35:1281–1288.
65. Blevins LS. Serum cortisol is not an accurate predictor of the integrity of the hypothalamic-pituitary-adrenocortical axis. Clin Endocrinol 1995;42:101–102.
66. Streeten DHP, Anderson GH, Bonaventura MM. The potential for serious consequences from misinterpreting normal responses to the rapid adrencorticotropin test. J Clin Endocrinol Metab 1996;81:285–290.
67. Salem M, Tainsh RE, Bromberg J, Loriaux DL, Chernow B. Perioperative glucocorticoid coverage. Ann Surg 1994;219:416–425.
68. Borst GC, Michenfelder HJ, O'Brian JT. Discordant cortisol response to exogenous ACTH and insulin-induced hypoglycemia in patients with pituitary disease. N Engl J Med 1982;306:1462–1464.
69. Resclini E, Cartana A, Giustina G. Plasma cortisol response to ACTH does not accurately indicate the state of the hypothalamic–pituitary–adrenal axis. J Endocrinol Invest 1982;5:259–261.
70. Cunningham SK, Moore A, McKenna TJ. Normal cortisol response to corticotropin in patients with secondary adrenal failure. Arch Intern Med 1982;143:2276–2279.
71. Lindholm J, Kehlet H. Re-evaluation of the clinical value of the 30 minute ACTH test in assessing the hypothalamic-pituitary-adrenocortical function. Clin Endocrinol (Oxford) 1987;26:53–59.
72. Fiad TM, Kirby JM, Cunningham SK, McKenna TJ. The overnight single-dose metyrapone test is a simple and reliable index of the hypothalamic–pituitary–adrenal axis. Clin Endocrinol (Oxford) 1994;40:603–609.
73. Dickstein G, Shechner C, Nicholson WE, Rosner I, Shen-Orr Z, Adawi F, Lahav M. Adrenocorticotropin stimulaiton test: effects of basal cortisol level, time of day, and suggested new sensitive low dose test. J Clin Endocrinol Metab 1991;72:773–778.
74. Broide J, Soferman R, Kivity S, Golander A, Dickstein G, Spirer Z, Weisman Y. Low-dose adrenocorticotropin test reveals impaired adrenal function in patients taking inhaled corticosteroids. J Clin Endocrinol Metab 1995;80:1243–1246.
75. Tordjman K, Jaffe A, Grazas N, Apter C, Stern N. The role of the low dose (1 mcg) adrenocorticotropin test in the evaluation of patients with pituitary diseases. J Clin Endocrinol Metab 1995;80:1301–1305.
76. Watson AC, Rosenfield RL, Fang VS. Recovery from glucocorticoid inhibition of the responses to corticotropin-releasing hormone. Clin Endocrinol 1988;28:471–477.
77. Orth DN. Corticotropin-releasing hormone in humans. Endocr Rev 1992;13:164–190.
78. Bone RC, Fisher CJ, Clemmer TP, et al. A controlled clinical trial of high-dose methylprednisolone in the treatment of severe sepsis and septic shock. N Engl J Med 1987;317:653–658.
79. The Veterans Administration Systemic Sepsis Cooperative Study Group. Effect of high-dose glucocorticoid therapy on mortality in patients with clinical signs of sepsis. N Engl J Med 1987;317:659–665.

80. Lefering R, Neugebauer EA. Steroid controversy in sepsis and septic shock: a meta-analysis. Crit Care Med 1995;23:1294–1303.
81. Cronin L, Cook DJ, Carlet J, Heyland OK, King D, Lansang MAD, Fisher CJ. Corticosteroid treatment for sepsis: a critical appraisal and meta-analysis of the literature. Crit Care Med 1995;23:1403–1409.
82. Bernard GR, Luce JM, Sprung CL, Rinaldo JE, Tate RM, Sibbald WJ, Kariman K, Higgins S, Brodley R, Metz CA, Harris TR, Brigham K. High-dose corticosteroids in patients with the adult respiratory distress syndrome. N Engl J Med 1987;317:1565–70.
83. Masur H. Prevention and treatment of pneumocystis pneumonia. N Engl J Med 1992;327:1853–1860.
84. Olshaker JS, Whye DW. Head trauma. Emerg Med Clin North Am 1993;11:165–183.
85. Bracken M, Shepard M, Collins W, et al. A randomized, controlled trial of methylprednisolone or naloxone in the treatment of acute spinal-cord injury. N Engl J Med 1990; 322:1405–1411.
86. Galandiuk S, Raque G, Appel S, Polk HC. The two-edged sword of large-dose steroids for spinal cord trauma. Ann Surg 1993;218:419–427.
87. George ER, Scholten DJ, Buechler CM, Jordan-Tibbs J, et al. Failure of methylprednisolone to improve the outcome of spinal cord injuries, An Surg 1995;61(8):659–664.
88. Bell WE. Bacterial meningitis in children. Pediatr Clin North Am 1992;39:651–660.
89. Hall ED. Lipid antioxidants in acute central nervous system injury. Ann Emerg Med 1993;22:1022–1027.
90. Friedman RJ, Schiff CF, Bromberg JS. Use of supplemental steroids in patients having orthopaedic operations. J Bone Joint Sur 1995;77(12):1801–1806.

7 Adrenocortical Response to Critical Illness
The Renin-Aldosterone Axis

Paul I. Jagger, MD

CONTENTS

INTRODUCTION
RENIN
ANGIOTENSINOGEN
ANGIOTENSIN
ALDOSTERONE
PRIMARY VS SECONDARY ALDOSTERONISM
SECONDARY ALDOSTERONISM OWING TO EXTRARENAL SODIUM
 AND VOLUME LOSS
SECONDARY ALDOSTERONISM OWING TO RENAL SODIUM
 AND VOLUME LOSS
SECONDARY ALDOSTERONISM OWING TO SODIUM AND VOLUME
 REDISTRIBUTION
SECONDARY ALDOSTERONISM IN HYPERTENSION
SECONDARY ALDOSTERONISM IN PREGNANCY
RECOGNITION AND TREATMENT OF SECONDARY
 ALDOSTERONISM
HYPOALDOSTERONISM
HYPORENINEMIC HYPOALDOSTERONISM
HYPERRENINEMIC HYPOALDOSTERONISM
HYPOALDOSTERONISM IN CRITICAL ILLNESS
RECOGNITION AND TREATMENT OF HYPOALDOSTERONISM
ACKNOWLEDGMENT
REFERENCES

INTRODUCTION

Maintainence of the appropriate volume of extracellular body fluid and, particularly, of that 25% of extracellular fluid that is within the vascular tree is a critical survival mechanism. The three hormones that have been identified as being most important in

From *Contemporary Endocrinology: Endocrinology of Critical Disease*
Edited by K. P. Ober   Humana Press Inc., Totowa, NJ

maintaining this volume homeostasis are aldosterone, antidiuretic hormone, and atrial natriuretic peptide *(1)*. This chapter focuses on the first of these, aldosterone. The purpose is to review the steps in the renin–angiotensin–aldosterone (RAA) pathway, to discuss the participation of angiotensin and aldosterone in the regulation of volume status and blood pressure, and then to explore the response of the RAA axis to critical illness. It should be emphasized at the start, however, that in the conditions to be discussed, angiotensin and aldosterone usually act in concert with antidiuretic hormone and atrial natriuretic peptide, as well as with other body defense mechanisms.

Critical illness of a variety of types usually results in stimulation as opposed to suppression of the RAA axis. When the critical illness involves true volume loss, this stimulation should help to repair the deficit and is appropriate. In other illnesses, however, especially when the major problem involves volume redistribution rather than true loss, the response may not help to correct the problem and, in fact, may lead to further complications *(2)*.

RENIN

It is appropriate first to describe the components of the RAA axis and to discuss their interrelationships. The reader is referred to recent detailed and extensively referenced textbook presentations for additional information *(3,4)*. The first component usually listed is renin, a protease enzyme synthesized mainly by the juxtaglomerular (JG) cells of the afferent arterioles of the kidney *(5)*. There is, however, a precursor, prorenin. The conversion of prorenin to renin in the kidney is regulated by a number of factors, not all of which are understood. Prostaglandin I_2 does appear to play a role *(6,7)*. Kallikreins may be involved, but recent data have brought this involvement into question *(8)*. There is a nonregulated constitutive pathway for prorenin that does not involve conversion, and therefore, both prorenin and renin are released from JG cells and circulate in plasma *(9)*. Although the kidney appears to be the major source for prorenin and renin, there is evidence that there are other sources as well, and there is growing evidence that local renin–angiotensin systems may subserve important functions *(10,11)*. The possible significance of the cardiac renin–angiotensin system will be discussed later.

The stimuli to renin synthesis and release are listed in Table 1. Extrinsic stimuli to renin release are delivered to the kidney both by sympathetic nerve terminals and by circulating catecholamines. Renal sympathetic nerves terminate in smooth muscle cells of renal afferent arterioles and in the JG cells. Activation of these renal sympathetics can affect renal hemodynamics and stimulate renin release, but the two effects can be separated. There are α- and β-receptors in the area of the JG cells; α stimulation inhibits renin release, whereas β stimulation enhances release *(12–14)*. Other circulating factors also modulate renin release. These include vasopressin, atrial natriuretic peptide, and angiotensin II itself, with increasing concentrations of each inhibiting release *(12,15,16)*. Prostaglandin I_2 may play a role in renin release as well as in the conversion of prorenin to renin *(6,7)*.

The JG cells also receive signals from immediately adjacent structures. Baroreceptors in the afferent arterioles respond to changes in renal perfusion pressure. The mechanism may actually involve changes in stretch in the JG cells. Decreased perfusion pressure enhances renin release, whereas increased pressure inhibits release *(12)*.

Changes in sodium delivery to the distal renal tubule also affect renin release. These changes are sensed by the macula densa, the specialized segment of the distal renal tubule that contacts the afferent arteriole before it enters the glomerulus. These cells synthesize

Table 1
Factors Controlling Renin Synthesis and Release

Prostaglandins
Kallikreins (?)
Renal sympathetic nerves
Catecholamines
Vasopressin
Atrial natriuretic peptide
Angiotensin II
Renal afferent arteriole baroreceptors
Sodium concentration at the macula densa

adenosine in direct proportion to sodium transport, and the adenosine acts on the neighboring JG cells to inhibit renin release; therefore, increasing sodium concentration inhibits renin release, and decreasing sodium concentration enhances release *(13,17,18)*.

ANGIOTENSINOGEN

Renin acts on a circulating glycoprotein angiotensinogen (renin substrate) to catalyze its cleavage to the decapeptide angiotensin I. Angiotensinogen is synthesized predominantly in the liver. Circulating levels of angiotensinogen are regulated in part by estrogens, and so are increased in pregnancy and in women taking birth control pills *(19)*. The relationship between circulating angiotensinogen levels and angiotensin I generation has not been completely resolved; however, there is sufficient angiotensinogen available for the generation of high levels of angiotensin I even in patients with severe liver disease.

ANGIOTENSIN

Angiotensin I is not biologically active. When it is converted to the octapeptide angiotensin II, however, a potent vasoconstrictor and a stimulator of aldosterone synthesis and secretion is produced. This cleavage of the two carboxy-terminal amino acids is catalyzed by angiotensin-converting enzyme (ACE), a glycoprotein found primarily in the lungs and blood vessels *(20,21)*. This same enzyme also inactivates bradykinin *(8,22)*.

Two types of angiotensin II receptors have been identified, AT_1 and AT_2; however, the physiological actions of angiotensin II identified thus far appear to involve the AT_1 receptor *(21,23)*. Angiotensin II causes vasoconstriction through its direct action on vascular smooth muscle, and this action occurs within seconds. Thus, when the initial insult to body homeostasis involves a drop in effective blood pressure, this action of angiotensin II provides rapid counteraction. This is amplified further by its action to stimulate the sympathetic nervous system *(23)*. Angiotensin II also has selective effects on intrarenal vasculature, and in fact, there is evidence for a specific intrarenal renin–angiotensin system *(24,25)*. This may be a particularly important adjustment mechanism when renal function is compromised. Further discussion of this aspect is beyond the scope of this chapter.

ALDOSTERONE

Angiotensin II stimulates the synthesis and secretion of aldosterone in the zona glomerulosa of the adrenal cortex. Secretion occurs within minutes. Though angiotensin

Table 2
Factors Controlling Aldosterone Synthesis and Release

Angiotensin II
Potassium ion concentration
Sodium ion concentration
ACTH
Vasopressin
Atrial natriuretic peptide
Dopamine

II would appear to be the most significant physiologic stimulus to aldosterone synthesis and secretion, there also are other important controls *(26)*. These are listed in Table 2 and discussed below.

An increase in potassium ion concentration, produced either by dietary manipulation or iv infusion, stimulates aldosterone production *(26,27)*. Furthermore, increased potassium concentration potentiates the response to angiotensin II *(28,29)*. Serum sodium concentration, perhaps through the concomitant change in serum osmolality, can be shown to have a direct effect on aldosterone secretion *(30)*. In most clinical situations, however, it is the effect of sodium intake on intravascular volume, rather than an effect on serum sodium concentration, that is important.

Adrenocorticotropic hormone (ACTH) acutely increases aldosterone secretion in humans, but this effect lasts less than 24 h in spite of continued administration *(31,32)*. Even so, this may be an important component of the response to acute stress *(33)*. There also is some evidence that ACTH may be required for the maximum response of aldosterone to angiotensin II, since hyponatremia has been reported in patients with panhypopituitarism, and a blunted response of aldosterone to sodium restriction also has been demonstrated *(34,35)*; the hyponatremia of thyroid hormone deficiency and glucocorticoid deficiency (both of which contribute to the hyponatremia of hypopituitarism) are discussed further in Chapter 12. Vasopressin also stimulates aldosterone secretion and can be demonstrated to be as potent as angiotensin II *(36)*. The significance of this observation has not been established, but it would seem appropriate to mobilize sodium-retaining mechanisms in many of those situations where enhanced water reabsorption is indicated.

As noted above, atrial natriuretic peptide suppresses renin release. It also has been demonstrated to inhibit aldosterone synthesis *(16,37)*. Dopamine also inhibits synthesis *(38)*.

About 60% of aldosterone released into the circulation is weakly bound to proteins, including albumin and cortisol binding globulin *(39)*. There also is binding to red cells *(40)*. Aldosterone turnover in plasma is rapid, with a half-life of 15 min or less. It is almost completely removed by one passage through the liver *(41)*. As discussed later, this may have implications in patients with abnormal liver function.

Aldosterone exerts its action by first binding to specific mineralocorticoid receptors present in the cytosol of mineralocorticoid-responsive tissues *(23,42)*. Renal tubular cells are the most important sites for mineralocorticoid binding and action. The target cells in the kidney are located in the connecting segments and the cortical and medullary collecting tubules *(23,42)*. There is a latent period of 1–2 h between exposure to aldosterone and evident renal effect *(43)*. Aldosterone acts in the kidney to promote the reabsorption of sodium and the secretion of potassium and hydrogen. Though only a fraction of sodium filtered by the glomerulus reaches the distal portions of the renal tubule, the action of aldosterone on this fraction can have major effects on sodium, potassium, and hydrogen balance.

Aldosterone acts to promote sodium reabsorption by increasing the cellular permeability to sodium in the apical membrane of the renal tubular cell and by stimulating the Na^+, K^+-dependent ATPase pump on the serosal side of the cell *(42,43)*. Less is known regarding the exact mechanisms by which aldosterone stimulates potassium ion secretion. It does seem evident that there is an exchange of potassium for sodium via the Na^+, K^+-dependent ATPase pump action at the serosal surface of the renal tubule cell. There also is passive diffusion of potassium into the collecting tubule secondary to the electronegativity generated by sodium reabsorption *(43,44)*. Aldosterone's action to promote hydrogen ion secretion appears to take place in the medullary collecting tubules. As in the case of potassium, part of the hydrogen movement appears to be related to electronegativity resulting from sodium reabsorption; however, the linkage between sodium reabsorption and hydrogen secretion is even looser than that for sodium reabsorption and potassium secretion, and, therefore, other mechanisms must be involved *(42–45)*.

Aldosterone also appears to have a permissive effect on the osmotic water flux response to vasopressin in the cortical collecting tubules *(46)*.

Aldosterone has multiple extrarenal actions, including actions on sweat glands, salivary glands, and gut *(44)*. In all these sites, the action favors the conservation of sodium and the secretion of potassium and hydrogen. In fact, an early screening test for hyperaldosteronism involved measurement of the Na:K ratio in saliva *(47)*.

PRIMARY VS SECONDARY ALDOSTERONISM

Conditions where there is increased secretion of aldosterone can be divided into two categories, primary aldosteronism and secondary aldosteronism. In primary aldosteronism, the stimulus to excessive production resides within the adrenal gland, and results either from an aldosterone-producing tumor or bilateral, usually nodular, hyperplasia. Because of the resultant sodium retention and extracellular volume expansion, plasma renin and angiotensin I and II levels are suppressed. When kidney function is normal, extracellular fluid volume expansion results in an increase in glomerular filtration rate combined with an inability of the proximal tubule to increase sodium reabsorption further (the latter probably related to increased atrial natriuretic peptide levels). With increased delivery of sodium to the distal tubule, there is increased renal excretion of sodium in spite of the action of aldosterone, and the "aldosterone escape" phenomenon occurs *(44,48)*. Because of the continuing action of aldosterone on the distal tubule, however, potassium and hydrogen secretion continue, and hypokalemic alkalosis can develop. In secondary aldosteronism, the stimulus is extra-adrenal, and usually begins with a decrease in effective blood volume or blood pressure causing stimulation of renin release. The aldosterone response to critical illness represents secondary aldosteronism. "Aldosterone escape" does not occur either because effective blood volume or blood pressure is restored and the stimulus to renin release is removed, or because of the underlying condition, effective blood volume or blood pressure cannot be restored in spite of significant and continuing sodium retention. In secondary aldosteronism, as in primary aldosteronism, the continuing action of aldosterone on the distal tubule can result in hypokalemic alkalosis.

Table 3
Secondary Aldosteronism in Critical Illness

Owing to extrarenal sodium and volume loss
    Acute blood loss
    Vomiting
    Diarrhea
    Burns
    Heavy perspiration
Owing to renal sodium and volume loss
    Sodium losing nephropathies
    Pseudohypoaldosteronism
    Severe hyperglycemia
    Diuretics
    Bartter's syndrome
    Gitelman's syndrome
Owing to sodium and volume redistribution
    Nephrotic syndrome
    Cirrhosis with ascites
    Congestive heart failure
Associated with hypertension
    Accelerated/malignant hypertension
    Polyarteritis nodosa
    Renal artery stenosis

One situation that does not appear to depend on volume and blood pressure changes should be addressed. That is acute stress *(33)*. Central nervous system activation with stimulation of renin release via neural pathways appears to be primary. Direct stimulation of aldosterone release by ACTH also is involved. This situation usually is short-lived and, therefore, may not have long-lasting effects on volume homeostasis.

Table 3 provides a classification of types of secondary aldosteronism seen in critical illness. The major categories are those involving true volume loss (either extrarenal or renal), those involving a redistribution of volume that is perceived by the volume and pressure receptors as volume loss, and those specifically involving decreased blood flow to one or both kidneys *(2)*. As discussed below, this classification is probably an oversimplification, but it does serve a useful purpose.

SECONDARY ALDOSTERONISM OWING TO EXTRARENAL SODIUM AND VOLUME LOSS

Numerous studies have demonstrated the stimulation of the RAA axis that results from volume loss owing to extrarenal causes. Acute blood loss owing to external trauma or to internal problems, such as a bleeding duodenal ulcer, is a good example. In fact, animal studies demonstrate a linear relationship between the amount of hemorrhage and the renin–angiotensin response *(49)*. Gastrointestinal fluid and electrolyte loss either by vomiting or diarrhea are also stimuli. It should be pointed out, however, that the potassium loss that usually accompanies gastrointestinal causes of volume depletion may blunt the angiotensin II-stimulated aldosterone production. Extensive burns are accompanied by significant loss of extracellular fluid directly through the burned surface area

(50,51). Perspiring heavily because of strenuous exertion and/or thermal exposure also can result in significant extracellular fluid volume loss *(52,53)*. In all these situations, activation of the RAA axis is appropriate and desirable, and provided the individual involved has access to salt and water, will serve to repair the defect.

SECONDARY ALDOSTERONISM OWING TO RENAL SODIUM AND VOLUME LOSS

Renal sodium loss also activates the RAA axis. The underlying cause for the sodium loss usually is such, however, that increasing levels of aldosterone, even when there is access to salt and water, may not be sufficient to repair the deficiency. The most clear-cut examples in this category are the sodium-losing nephropathies. In these forms of chronic renal failure, there is unusually pronounced loss of sodium in the urine. The usual pathologic finding in these conditions is a greater destruction of medullary and interstitial than of cortical and glomerular portions of the renal parenchyma. It appears that the damaged tubules in these areas are not able appropriately to reabsorb sodium, even when aldosterone levels are elevated *(54–56)*.

There is also a genetic disease in which the renal tubules do not respond to mineralocorticoids, but renal function is otherwise normal. Manifested clinically as salt wasting, hyperkalemia, and metabolic acidosis, this is seen mainly in infants. Plasma renin activity and aldosterone levels are greatly increased *(57,58)* in this disorder, referred to as pseudohypoaldosteronism (*see below* for a discussion of hypoaldosteronism).

The osmotic diuresis that occurs with severe hyperglycemia leads to sodium and volume depletion, and to stimulation of the RAA axis. This can be seen both in diabetic ketoacidosis and also in hyperosmolar nonketotic diabetic coma *(59,60)*. In ketoacidosis, vomiting also can contribute to volume loss. In these conditions, both insulin and iv saline are critical early steps in treatment. When the osmotic diuresis owing to glucose begins to abate secondary to appropriate treatment, then aldosterone can help to repair the volume deficit. As discussed subsequently, however, some diabetics may not be able to stimulate aldosterone secretion because of an impairment in renin synthesis and release.

Thiazide-type and loop diuretics, either when taken as directed as part of the treatment regimen for essential hypertension or edematous states, or when taken surreptitiously, can stimulate the RAA axis *(61–63)*. In these situations, the increased aldosterone secretion cannot overcome the pharmacologic effect of the diuretics to prevent sodium loss, but it will accentuate potassium and hydrogen loss. This will be particularly significant if the underlying condition already is accompanied by hyperaldosteronism (*see below*).

Though it represents a genetic disease with chronic manifestations, Bartter's syndrome should be listed here for completeness, since periodic paralysis may occur owing to potassium depletion. This is a syndrome characterized by hyperreninemia, hyperaldosteronism, hypokalemia, and alkalosis without hypertension or edema *(64)*. Several defects have been demonstrated, including decreased pressor responsiveness to angiotensin II, increased prostaglandin I_2 synthesis, and a chloride reabsorption defect in the thick ascending limb of the loop of Henle *(65)*. These all may be secondary, however *(66)*. Though it may not provide the complete explanation, certainly the hyperaldosteronism contributes to the hypokalemia and alkalosis seen in this syndrome.

Gitelman's syndrome, a recently described variant of Bartter's syndrome presenting in adult life, also deserves mention. In addition to the usual features of Bartter's syndrome, there is prominent hypomagnesemia, and there is hypocalciuria. Convulsions, presumably secondary to the hypomagnesium, can be a manifestation. The chloride resorptive defect in this syndrome has been localized to the distal convoluted tubule rather than the thick ascending limb of the loop of Henle as in Bartter's syndrome *(67,68)*.

SECONDARY ALDOSTERONISM OWING TO SODIUM AND VOLUME REDISTRIBUTION

The most clear-cut example of redistribution of extracellular fluid volume resulting in activation of the RAA axis would appear to be the nephrotic syndrome. This entity is the common end point of a variety of disease processes that increase the permeability of the glomerular capillary wall and result in leakage of plasma proteins into the urine. This sustained proteinuria leads to hypoalbuminemia and a decrease in plasma oncotic pressure. Fluid then migrates out of the vasculature and into the interstitial space. Edema will be evident on physical examination, but more important to this discussion, there will be a decrease in plasma volume, with a stimulation of renin release *(69)*. Aldosterone then will enhance renal sodium reabsorption, but this will not correct the plasma volume defect because of the continued low oncotic pressure. Instead, there will be further edema formation. This may well be the sequence in many patients; however, it does not provide a complete explanation in all, for not all have elevated angiotensin II and aldosterone levels. In those with elevated levels, the use of the ACE inhibitor captopril to block aldosterone production does not completely prevent sodium retention *(70)*. Furthermore, only a minority have low plasma volumes *(71)*. These observations have led to the alternate explanation that the primary defect is intrarenal, with a decreased fractional excretion of sodium as the earliest event *(69–72)*. Tubular insensitivity to atrial natriuretic peptide as part of the underlying renal disease has been offered as one possible intrarenal mechanism *(71)*.

Patients with cirrhosis and ascites also usually have secondary hyperaldosteronism. The sequence of events leading to the accumulation of ascites fluid is not clear. Three different hypotheses have been proposed *(73,74)*. The classic one begins with increased portal venous pressure leading to leakage of fluid into the abdominal cavity, and causing hypovolemia and stimulation of renal sodium and water retention. The second "overflow" hypothesis proposes that there is a hepato-renal interaction that results in primary renal sodium and water retention and then ascites formation. This could offer an explanation in those patients who do not have elevated aldosterone levels *(75)*. The more recent hypothesis begins with peripheral vasodilation leading to decreased filling of the arterial vascular tree, and then stimulation of renal sodium and water retention. Whatever the initiating event, several factors are known to be involved once fluid begins to accumulate. There is portal hypertension with increased hydrostatic pressure in the splanchnic bed. As in the case of nephrosis, there is hypoalbuminemia and decreased plasma oncotic pressure. As opposed to nephrosis, however, the hypoalbuminemia results from decreased production rather than from renal leakage. There is also weepage of hepatic lymph directly from the surface of the liver into the abdominal cavity. Though aldosterone levels are not always elevated, it is reasonable to conclude that aldosterone is a major factor responsible for sodium retention in most patients with advanced cirrhosis *(76)*. A correlation between sodium excretion and aldosterone levels can be demonstrated *(75,77–79)*. The aldosterone effect may be magnified by decreased hepatic removal *(41,75)*. Patients with cirrhosis and ascites who go on to develop the hepatorenal syndrome have an even more marked activation of the RAA axis, and this correlates with a further reduction in effective renal blood flow and with intense renal vasoconstriction. Here again, the exact sequence is not clear *(73,75,80)*. The hepatorenal syndrome is characterized by worsening azotemia, hyponatremia, progressive oliguria, and hypotension, and it is usually fatal.

The conflicting data regarding activation of the RAA axis in congestive heart failure appear to arise from the lack of a clear definition of the group of patients studied and the stage in disease progression. The best conclusion is that during acute decompensation or during severe chronic decompensation, angiotensin II and aldosterone levels are elevated *(81,82)*. The stimulus is low cardiac output, resulting both in activation of the sympathetic nervous system via carotid sinus baroreceptors and in activation of JG cells via decreased renal blood flow *(83)*. In fact, in patients with severe chronic heart failure, there is a correlation between unfavorable prognosis and marked elevation of angiotensin II levels *(84)*. With low cardiac output, there also can be decreased hepatic perfusion and decreased aldosterone clearance *(41)*. Evidence is accumulating to suggest that angiotensin II may be involved in the progression of heart disease in congestive failure by mechanisms beyond its effect on blood pressure and aldosterone secretion. Activation of both the systemic and local renin–angiotensin systems appears to play a part in promoting the hypertrophic myocardial response and interstitial fibrosis *(85–87)*.

SECONDARY ALDOSTERONISM IN HYPERTENSION

A discussion of the possible roles of the RAA axis in essential hypertension is beyond the scope of this chapter; however, the roles in accelerated/malignant hypertension and in hypertension owing to renal artery stenosis should be addressed.

The sequence of events in accelerated/malignant hypertension is not entirely clear. A sodium and water diuresis with volume contraction is an early event and may be precipitated by the severely elevated blood pressure itself. This volume contraction provides one possible explanation for the stimulation of the RAA axis that almost always occurs, but other factors must also contribute *(88)*. The persistent severely elevated blood pressure, probably in combination with markedly elevated angiotensin II levels, then leads to fibrinoid necrosis involving the walls of small renal arteries and arterioles. This results in further compromise to renal perfusion and further stimulation of renin release *(89)*.

A situation somewhat similar to accelerated/malignant hypertension is seen in some patients with polyarteritis nodosa. Renal vascular damage leads to renal ischemia and stimulation of the RAA axis, and these patients frequently have severe hypertension, high angiotensin II and aldosterone levels, and hypokalemia *(48,90)*.

Hypertension owing to renal artery stenosis often is severe and can lead to accelerated/malignant hypertension *(91)*. There is general agreement that activation of the RAA axis is responsible for the initial increase in blood pressure that results from critical narrowing of one renal artery. There are a number of subsequent adjustments that occur, however, such that the circulating levels of angiotensin II and aldosterone fall *(92)*. They still remain inappropriately high for the increased blood pressure and, furthermore, an increased level of plasma renin activity can consistently be measured from the vein of the involved kidney as compared to the uninvolved side *(93)*.

SECONDARY ALDOSTERONISM IN PREGNANCY

There is an early and sustained stimulation of the RAA axis in normal pregnancy *(94)*. It has been suggested that the estrogen-mediated increase in angiotensinogen offers an explanation for this observation; however, this seems unlikely *(95)*. Stimulation probably relates instead to the hemodynamic and fluid volume changes occurring during pregnancy and their effect on renal blood flow. Stimulation of the RAA axis may be a necessary contributor to maintenance of blood pressure in normal pregnancy *(95,96)*. When pre-eclampsia supervenes, with the appearance of hypertension, edema, and proteinuria, it might be anticipated that there would be further elevations in angiotensin II and aldosterone. Instead, these levels actually decrease *(96–98)*. There is, however, an increased vascular sensitivity to angiotensin II at this stage *(99)*.

RECOGNITION AND TREATMENT OF SECONDARY ALDOSTERONISM

What are the keys to the recognition of hyperaldosteronism in critical illness? Obviously, the first key is the recognition that the patient has a condition often associated with stimulation of the RAA axis, namely, one of those conditions just described and shown in Table 3. In patients with acute volume loss, either extrarenal or renal, there should be no problem in recognizing the relationship. In those patients with conditions involving redistribution of volume, hypokalemia (either spontaneous or easily induced by diuretic therapy) may be an indicator. In patients with severe hypertension, hypokalemia again may serve as the indicator. It should only rarely be necessary actually to measure plasma renin activity and aldosterone levels in these situations.

Treatment in those conditions owing to true volume loss is straightforward. The volume lost needs to be replaced either with blood, saline, or colloid solution, as appropriate. In those situations associated with volume redistribution, treatment should be addressed to the underlying disease when possible, for example, the use of steroids for certain forms of the nephrotic syndrome and measures to improve cardiac output in patients with congestive heart failure. The cautious use of standard diuretics may be necessary in patients with volume redistribution and edema, even in the face of secondary aldosteronism. Careful attention must be paid to the accentuated potassium and hydrogen loss that is likely to occur with diuretic administration. Adding the aldosterone antagonist spironolactone to the diuretic program may both enhance diuresis and aid in potassium conservation. Spironolactone alone has been shown to be very effective in reducing ascites in patients with cirrhosis *(100)*. ACE inhibitors have a special role in the treatment of congestive heart failure *(101–104)*; however, the role appears to be related more to reduction in peripheral vascular resistance and the consequent improvement in cardiac output than to the reduction in aldosterone level. A direct effect via blockade of the local cardiac renin-angiotensin system also may be important *(85–87)*. ACE inhibitors have been used effectively to lower blood pressure in patients with accelerated/malignant hypertension *(105)*. It is not evident that they are more effective than several other antihypertensive medications in reversing that process, however. There are insufficient data accumulated thus far to determine whether the new angiotensin II receptor-blocking agents offer significant advantages over the ACE inhibitors.

**Table 4
Causes of Clinical Hypoaldosteronism**

Hyporeninemic hypoaldosteronism
    Impaired extrinsic stimuli
        Primary autonomic insufficiency
        Diabetic neuropathy
        Central α_2-adrenergic receptor activators
        Renal β-adrenergic receptor blockers
    Impaired renin production
        Renal parenchymal disease
        Prostaglandin deficiency
        Diabetes mellitus
        AIDS
        Idiopathic
Hyperreninemic hypoaldosteronism
    Impaired conversion of angiotensin I
        Intrinsic converting enzyme inhibitors
        Extrinsic converting enzyme inhibitors
    Impaired aldosterone production
        Destruction of zona glomerulosa
        Hypokalemia
        ACTH deficiency
        Angiotensin II receptor defect
        Heparin
        Corticosterone methyl oxidase II deficiency

HYPOALDOSTERONISM

A number of cases have been described in which the anticipated response of the RAA axis does not occur, i.e., there is hypoaldosteronism *(106–108)*. Both endogenous and iatrogenic causes have been identified. In many of the conditions described above, this failure of response would be expected to have a compounding deleterious effect, especially in those with acute volume loss. Cases of hypoaldosteronism can be divided into two categories, those with low renin and low aldosterone levels and those with high renin, but low aldosterone levels. The causes are listed in Table 4 and discussed below.

HYPORENINEMIC HYPOALDOSTERONISM

The first category of hypoaldosteronism has been labeled hyporeninemic hypoaldosteronism, and includes both those cases where the extrinsic stimuli to renin release are inadequate and those where there is an intrinsic inability to produce renin. The former grouping includes patients with primary autonomic insufficiency syndromes and with diabetic neuropathy, as well as patients on antihypertensives, such as clonidine, which activates central α_2-adrenergic receptors and thus attenuates renal sympathetic nerve signals, and such as propranolol, which blocks renal β-receptors *(108–113)*. The latter grouping includes patients with renal parenchymal disease and some children who appear to have a genetic renal prostaglandin deficiency *(114–116)*. Prostaglandin deficiency owing to the effect of nonsteroidal anti-inflammatory drugs also has been reported *(117,118)*, and in fact, some of the patients with renal parenchymal disease also may have an acquired prostaglandin deficiency *(119,120)*. Recently, the acquired immunodeficiency syndrome (AIDS) has been reported to be associated with an inability to produce renin *(121)*.

In the majority of patients with hyporeninemic hypoaldosteronism, the exact cause is not apparent. These patients are usually elderly and have mild chronic renal failure, but with hyperkalemia out of proportion to the degree of renal failure. Half have diabetes mellitus *(122)*.

HYPERRENINEMIC HYPOALDOSTERONISM

The second category has been labeled hyperreninemic hypoaldosteronism. Impaired conversion of angiotensin I to angiotensin II represents one example. There is only one case report of an intrinsic defect in conversion of angiotensin I to angiotension II *(123)*; however, exogenous interference with the action of ACE is the expected consequence in patients who are treated with ACE inhibitors. Alternatively, aldosterone production can be deficient in spite of adequate angiotensin II levels. This can be the result of isolated destruction of the adrenal zona glomerulosa, for example, owing to an autoimmune process or to tumor invasion *(124–128)*. As noted previously, hypokalemia and ACTH deficiency can blunt the aldosterone response to angiotensin II *(29)*. Insensitivity of zona glomerulosa cells to the action of angiotensin II also has been reported in a patient with Sjögren's syndrome *(129)*. Heparin is the only medication that has been reported selectively to inhibit aldosterone secretion, and occasionally this can be clinically significant *(130–132)*.

Congenital adrenal hyperplasia can also be associated with high renin levels and hypoaldosteronism. A discussion of all the types of congenital adrenal hyperplasia that can result in hypoaldosteronism is beyond the scope of this chapter. It is, however, worth identifying corticosterone methyl oxidase type II (CMO II) deficiency, since this results in isolated hypoaldosteronism unaccompanied by cortisol deficiency or altered sexual development. The final conversion step of 18-hydroxycorticosterone to aldosterone is decreased when CMO II is deficient *(107)*. CMO deficiency typically presents as salt wasting in infancy *(133,134)*.

HYPOALDOSTERONISM IN CRITICAL ILLNESS

As noted above, a blunted response by the RAA axis would be expected to have a further deleterious effect in many of the conditions described previously. A listing here of these effects in each condition is not warranted, since they should be evident. There are, however, several situations that deserve special attention.

Since hyporeninemic hypoaldosteronism is common in patients with diabetes mellitus, one needs to be particularly alert to the possibility that the diabetic may not be able to generate angiotensin II and aldosterone in response to acute volume loss, either from hemorrhage or gastrointestinal problems, or from a glucose osmotic diuresis. The elderly diabetic should be particularly suspect *(122)*.

Because of the increasing impact of AIDS, one also needs to be alert to the possibility that patients with AIDS may have hyporenemic hypoaldosteronism *(121)*. These patients are prone to become volume depleted for a variety of reasons. Mild sustained hyperkalemia may be the clue to identifying the patient at risk.

Bilateral massive adrenal hemorrhage deserves special note. Both cortisol and aldosterone production will be affected, however; as emphasized in a recent review, the signs of mineralocorticoid deficiency, namely, volume contraction with hyponatremia, hyperkalemia, and mild acidosis, may be the early clues. Causes include fulminant meningococcemia, thromboembolic disease, and coagulopathies, the latter often induced by heparin or warfarin therapy *(135,136)*.

An interesting observation of uncertain significance is that many patients with critical illnesses in an intensive care unit, not necessarily associated with severe volume changes, do not respond appropriately to angiotensin II, (i.e., they appear to have hyperreninemic hypoaldosteronism). Aldosterone secretion is subnormal both in response to angiotensin II and ACTH *(137)*. Thus far, this appears to be an adaptive mechanism without adverse clinical consequences *(138)* as noted in Chapter 6.

RECOGNITION AND TREATMENT OF HYPOALDOSTERONISM

As implied above, the most common presentation of hypoaldosteronism is spontaneous hyperkalemia, usually mild, in the range of 5.5–6.5 mEq/L. If spontaneous hyperkalemia is not present, then the appearance of hyperkalemia, hyponatremia, and acidosis in response to volume contraction may provide evidence of hypoaldosteronism. In some instances, it may be warranted to make simultaneous measurements of plasma renin activity and plasma aldosterone, preferably when there is a stimulus present to increase both, such as volume contraction or upright posture. If hypoaldosteronism owing to CMO II deficiency is suspected, plasma 18-hydroxycorticosterone and plasma aldosterone can be measured, and the ratio can be calculated, preferably after a stimulus to secretion. The ratio of plasma 18-hydroxycorticosterone to plasma aldosterone will be high if the disorder is present.

When hypoaldosteronism is discovered, the first step is to discontinue any medications that are known to interfere with the RAA axis, such as clonidine, propranolol, ACE inhibitors, and heparin. If medications are not involved, the treatment for both hyporeninemic and hyperreninemic hypoaldosteronism is the administration of mineralocorticoid replacement orally, in the form of fludrocortisone, when possible. There is now no readily available mineralocorticoid for parenteral use; in an emergency situation, suprafysiologic doses of parenteral glucocorticoids may be used (particularly the agents with mineralocorticoid effect), but therapy should emphasize the restoration of volume and blood pressure with appropriate sodium-containing iv solutions, and correction of acidosis and hyperkalemia as needed.

ACKNOWLEDGMENT

The author thanks Jean Grigsby for her assistance in preparation of this chapter.

REFERENCES

1. Rolih CA, Ober KP. The endocrine response to critical illness. Med Clin North Am 1995;79:211–224.
2. Stockigt JR. Mineralocorticoid excess. In: James VHT, ed. The Adrenal Gland. Raven, New York, 1979, pp. 197–241.
3. Miller WL, Tyrrell JB. The adrenal cortex. In: Felig P, Baxter JD, Frohman LA, eds. Endocrinology and Metabolism. McGraw-Hill, New York, 1995, pp. 555–711.
4. Baxter JD, Perloff D, Hsueh W, Biglieri EG. The endocrinology of hypertension. In: Felig P, Baxter JD, Frohman LA, eds. Endocrinology and Metabolism. McGraw-Hill, New York, 1995, pp. 749–853.
5. Lindop GBM, Downie TT. New morphological evidence for the synthesis and storage of renin in the human kidney: an ultrastructural immunocytochemical study. J Hypertens 1984;2:7–16.

6. Weber PC, Siess W. Interactions of renal prostaglandins with the renin-angiotensin system. Pharm Ther 1981;15:321–337.
7. Hsueh WA, Goldstone R, Carlson EJ, Horton R. Evidence that the Beta-adrenergic system and prostaglandins stimulate renin release through different mechanisms. J Clin Endocrinol Metab 1985;61:399–403.
8. Margolius HS. Kallikreins and kinins. Molecular characteristics and cellular and tissue responses. Diabetes 1996;45(Suppl 1):S14–S19.
9. Hsueh WA, Baxter JD. Human prorenin. Hypertension 1991;17:469–479.
10. Campbell DJ, Kladis A, Skinner SL, Whitworth JA. Characterization of angiotensin peptides in plasma of anephric man. J Hypertens 1991;9:265–274.
11. Re RN. Cellular biology of the renin-angiotensin systems. Arch Intern Med 1984:144:2037–2041.
12. Ganong WF, Barbieri C. Neuroendocrine components in the regulation of renin secretion. In: Ganong WF, Martini L, eds. Frontiers in Neuroendocrinology. Raven, New York; 1982, pp. 231–262.
13. Davis JO, Freeman RH. Mechanisms regulating renin release. Physiol Rev 1976;56:1–56.
14. Taher MS, McLain LG, McDonald KM, Schrier RW. Effect of beta adrenergic blockade on renin response to renal nerve stimulation. J Clin Invest 1976;57:459–465.
15. Vander AJ. Inhibition of renin release in the dog by vasopressin and vasotocin. Circ Res 1968;23:605–609.
16. Cuneo RC, Espiner EA, Nicholls MG, Yandle TG, Joyce SL, Gilchrist NL. Renal, hemodynamic, and hormonal responses to atrial natriuretic peptide infusions in normal man, and effect of sodium intake. J Clin Endocrinol Metab 1986;63:946–953.
17. Martínez-Maldonado M, Gely R, Tapia E, Benabe JE. Role of macula densa in diuretics-induced renin release. Hypertension 1990;16:261–268.
18. Briggs JP, Lorenz JN, Weihprecht H, Schnermann J. Macula densa control of renin secretion. Renal Physiol Biochem 1991;14:164–174.
19. Lynch KR, Peach MJ. Molecular biology of angiotensinogen. Hypertension 1991;17:263–269.
20. Erdös EG, Skidgel RA. The unusual substrate specificity and the distribution of human angiotensin I converting enzyme. Special Lecture. Hypertension 1986;8(Suppl I):I34–I37.
21. Bernstein KE, Shai S-Y, Howard T, Balogh R, Frenzel K, Langford K. Structure and regulated expression of angiotensin-converting enzyme and the receptor for angiotensin II. Am J Kidney Dis 1993;21(Suppl 1):53–57.
22. Erdös EG. Angiotensin I converting enzyme. Circ Res 1975;36:247–255.
23. Guthrie GP. Angiotensin receptors: physiology and pharmacology. Clin Cardiol 1995;18(Suppl III): III29–III34.
24. Campbell DJ. Circulating and tissue angiotensin systems. J Clin Invest 1987;79:1–6.
25. Mulrow, PJ. The intrarenal renin-angiotensin system. Curr Opinion Neph Hypertens 1993;2:41–44.
26. Quinn SJ, Williams GH. Regulation of aldosterone secretion. Ann Rev Physiol 1988;50:409–426.
27. Dluhy RG, Axelrod L, Underwood RH, Williams GH. Studies of the control of plasma aldosterone concentration in normal man. II. Effect of dietary potassium and acute potassium infusion. J Clin Invest 1972;51:1950–1957.
28. Himathongkam T, Dluhy RG, Williams GH. Potassium-aldosterone-renin interrelationships. J Clin Endocrinol Metab 1975;41:153–159.
29. Fraser P, Mason PA, Buckingham JC, et al. The interaction of sodium and potassium status, of ACTH and of angiotensin II in the control of corticosteroid secretion. J Steroid Biochem 1979;11:1039–1042.
30. Schneider EG, Radke KJ, Ulderich DA, Taylor RE Jr. Effect of osmolality on aldosterone secretion. Endocrinology 1985;116:1621–1626.
31. Tucci JR, Espiner EA, Jagger PI, Pauk GL, Lauler DP. ACTH stimulation of aldosterone secretion in normal subjects and in patients with chronic adrenocortical insufficiency. J Clin Endocrinol Metab 1967;27:568–575.
32. Rayfield J, Rose LI, Dluhy RG, Williams GH. Aldosterone secretory and glucocorticoid excretory responses to alpha 1–24 ACTH (cortrosyn) in sodium depleted normal man. J Clin Endocrinol Metab 1973;36:30–35.
33. Aquilera G, Kiss A, Luo X, Akbasak B-S. The renin angiotensin system and the stress response. Ann NY Acad Science 1995;771:173–186.
34. Bethune JE, Nelson DH. Hyponatremia in hypopituitarism. N Engl J Med 1965;272:771–776.
35. Williams GH, Rose LI, Dluhy RG, Dingman JF, Lauler DP. Aldosterone response to sodium restriction and ACTH stimulation in panhypopituitarism. J Clin Endocrinol Metab 1971;32:27–35.

36. Guillon G, Trueba M, Joubert D, et al. Vasopressin stimulates steroid secretion in human adrenal glands: comparison with angiotensin II effect. Endocrinology 1995;136:1285–1295.
37. Atarashi K, Mulrow PJ, Franco-Saenz R. Effect of atrial peptides on aldosterone production. J Clin Invest 1985;76:1807–1811.
38. Cary RM. Physiologic and possible pathophysiologic relevance of dopamine mechanisms in the control of aldosterone secretion. In: Mantero F, Biglieri EG, Funder JW, Scoggins BA, eds. The Adrenal Gland and Hypertension. Raven, New York, Pr 1985, pp. 55–65.
39. Zipser RD, Meidar V, Horton R. Characteristics of aldosterone binding in human plasma. J Clin Endocrinol Metab 1980;50:158–162.
40. Chavarri M, Luetscher JA, Dowdy AJ, Ganguly A. The effects of temperature and plasma cortisol on distribution of aldosterone between plasma and red blood cells: influence on metabolic clearance rate and on hepatic and renal extraction of aldosterone. J Clin Endocrinol Metab 1977;44:752–759.
41. Vecsei P, Düsterdieck G, Jahnecke J, Lommer D, Wolff HP. Secretion and turnover of aldosterone in various pathological states. Clin Sci 1969;36:241–256.
42. Marver D, Kokko JP. Renal target sites and the mechanism of action of aldosterone. Min and Elect Metab 1983;9:1–18.
43. Morris DJ. The metabolism and mechanism of action of aldosterone. Endocr Rev 1981;2:234–247.
44. Gross F. 1974 Effects of aldosterone on blood pressure, water and electrolytes. In: Page IH, Bumpus FM, eds. Handbook of Experimental Pharmacology XXXVII. Angiotensin. Springer-Verlag, New York, 1974, pp. 369–399.
45. Sebastian A, Sutton JM, Hulter HN, Schambelan M, Poler SM. Effect of mineralocorticoid replacement therapy on renal acid-base homeostasis in adrenalectomized patients. Kidney Int 1980;18:762–773.
46. el Mernissi G, Bartlet-Bas C, Khadouri C, Cheval L, Marsy S, Doucet A. Short-term effect of aldosterone on vasopressin-sensitive adenylate cyclase in rat collecting tubule. Am J Physiol 1993;264(5 Pt 2):F821–F826.
47. Lauler DP, Hickler RB, Thorn GW. The salivary sodium-potassium ratio. A useful "screening" test for aldosteronism in hypertensive patients. N Engl J Med 1962;267:1136–1137.
48. Corry DB, Tuck ML. Secondary aldosteronism. Endocrinol Metab Clin North Am 1995;24:511–529.
49. Michailov ML, Schad H, Dahlheim H, Jacob ICM, Brechtelsbauer H. Renin-angiotensin system responses of acute graded hemorrhage in dogs. Circ Shock 1987;21:217–224.
50. Gore DC, Dalton JM, Gehr TWB. Colloid infusions reduce glomerular filtration in resuscitated burn victims. J Trauma Inj Infect Crit Care 1996;40:356–360.
51. Cioffi WG Jr, Vaughan GM, Heironimus JD, Jordon BS, Mason AD Jr, Pruett BA Jr. Dissociation of blood volume and flow in regulation of salt and water balance in burn patients. Ann Surg 1991;214:213–220.
52. Mitchell JB, Grandjean PW, Pizza FX, Starling RD, Holtz RW. The effect of volume ingested on rehydration and gastric emptying following exercise-induced dehydration. Med Sci Sports Exerc 1994;26:1135–1143.
53. Takamata A, Mack GW, Gillen CM, Nadel ER. Sodium appetite, thirst, and body fluid regulation in humans during rehydration without sodium replacement. Am J Physiol 1994;(5 Pt 2)266:R1493–R1502.
54. Fraser R, James VHT, Brown JJ, Davies DL, Lever AF, Robertson JIS. Changes in plasma aldosterone, cortisol, corticosterone, and renin concentration in a patient with sodium-losing renal disease. J Endocrinol 1966;35:311–320.
55. Popovtzer MM, Katz FH, Pinggera WF, Robinette J, Halgrimson CG, Butkus DE. Hyperkalemia in salt-wasting nephropathy. Study of the mechanism. Arch Int Med 1973;132:203–208.
56. Uribarri J, Oh MS, Carroll HJ. Salt-Losing Nephropathy. Clinical presentation and mechanism. Am J Neph 1983;3:193–198.
57. Dillon MJ, Leonard JV, Buckler JM, et al. Pseudohypoaldosteronism. Arch Dis Child 1980;55:427–434.
58. Throckmorton DC, Bia MJ. Pseudohypoaldosteronism: case report and discussion of the syndrome. Yale J Biol Med 1991;64:247–254.
59. Christlieb AR, Assal J-P, Katsilambros N, Williams GH, Kozak GP, Suzuki T. Plasma renin activity and blood volume in uncontrolled diabetes. Ketoacidosis, a state of secondary aldosteronism. Diabetes 1975;24:190–193.
60. Waldhäusl W, Kleinberger G, Korn A, Dudczak R, Bratusch-Marrain P, Nowatny P. Severe hyperglycemia: effects of rehydration on endocrine derangements and blood glucose concentration. Diabetes 1979;28:577–584.

61. Espiner EA, Tucci JR, Jagger PI, Paul GL, Lauler DP. The effect of acute diuretic-induced extracellular volume depletion on aldosterone secretion in normal man. Clin Sci 1967;33:125–134.
62. Dluhy RG, Cain JP, Williams GH. The influence of dietary potassium on the renin and aldosterone response to diuretic-induced volume depletion. J Lab Clin Med 1974;83:249–255.
63. Lijnen P, Fagard R, Staessen J, Amery A. Effect of chronic diuretic treatment on the plasma renin-angiotensin-aldosterone system in essential hypertension. Br J Clin Pharm 1981;12:387–392.
64. Bartter FC, Gill JR Jr, MacCardie RC. Hyperplasia of the juxtaglomerular complex with hyperaldosteronism and hypokalemic alkalosis. A new syndrome. Am J Med 1962;33:811–828.
65. Gill JR Jr. Bartter's syndrome. Ann Rev Med 1980;31:405–419.
66. Clive DM. Bartter's syndrome. The unsolved puzzle. Am J Kidney Dis 1995;25:813–823.
67. Zarraga Larrondo S, Vallo A, Gainza J, Muñiz R, Erauzkin GG, Lampreabe J. Familial hypokalemia-hypomagnesemia or Gitelman's syndrome: a further case. Nephron 1992;62:340–344.
68. Gibbs CJ, Millar JGB. Renin-angiotensin-aldosterone and kallekrein investigations in a patient with resistent hypomagnesaemia due to Gitelman's syndrome. Ann Clin Biochem 1995;32:426–430.
69. Usberti M, Gazzotti RM, Poiesi C, D'Avanzo L, Ghielmi S. Considerations on the sodium retention in nephrotic syndrome. Am J Neph 1995;15:38–47.
70. Brown EA, Markandu ND, Sagnella GA, Jones BE, MacGregor GA. Lack of effect of captopril on the sodium retention of the nephrotic syndrome. Nephron 1984;37:43–48.
71. Perico N, Remuzzi G. Renal handling of sodium in the nephrotic syndrome. Am J Neph 1993;13:413–421.
72. Bernard DB. Extrarenal complications of the nephrotic syndrome. Kidney Int 1988;33:1184–1202.
73. Schrier RW, Arroyo V, Bernardi M, Epstein M, Henriksen JH, Rodés J. Peripheral arterial vasodilation hypothesis: a proposal for the initiation of renal sodium and water retention in cirrhosis. Hepatology 1988;8:1151–1157.
74. Epstein M. The sodium retention of cirrhosis: a reappraisal. Hepatology 1986;6:312–315.
75. Gentilini P, LaVilla G, Romanelli RG, Foschi M, Laffi G. Pathogenesis and treatment of ascites in hepatic cirrhosis. Cardiology 1994;84(Suppl 2):68–79.
76. Arroyo V, Bosch J, Mauri M, et al. Renin, aldosterone and renal hemodynamics in cirrhosis with ascites. Eur J Clin Invest 1979;9:69–73.
77. Bernardi M, Trevisani F, Gasbarrini A, Gasbarrini G. Hepatorenal disorders: role of the renin-angiotensin-aldosterone system. Semin Liver Dis 1994;14:23–34.
78. Nicholls KM, Shapiro MD, Kluge R, Chung H-M, Bichet DG, Schrier RW. Sodium excretion in advanced cirrhosis: effect of expansion of central blood volume and suppression of plasma aldosterone. Hepatology 1986;6:235–238.
79. Jespersen B, Eiskjaer H, Jensen JD, Mogensen CE, Sorensen SS, Pedersen EB. Effects of high dose atrial natriuretic peptide on renal hemodynamics, sodium handling and hormones in cirrhotic patients with and without ascites. Scand J Clin Lab Invest 1995;55:273–288.
80. Laffi G, LaVilla G, Gentilini P. Pathogenesis and management of the hepatorenal syndrome. Semin Liver Dis 1994;14:71–81.
81. Dzau VJ, Colucci WS, Hollenberg NK, Williams GH. Relation of the renin-angiotensin-aldosterone system to clinical state of congestive heart failure. Circulation 1981;63:645–651.
82. Francis GS, Benedict C, Johnstone DE, et al. Comparison of neuroendocrine activation in patients with left ventricular dysfunction with and without congestive heart failure. A substudy of the studies of left ventricular dysfunction (SOLVD). Circulation 1990;82:1724–1729.
83. Cannon PJ. The kidney in heart failure. N Engl J Med 1977;296:26–32.
84. Lee WH, Packer M. Prognostic importance of serum sodium concentration and its modification by converting-enzyme inhibition in patients with severe chronic heart failure. Circulation 1986;73:257–267.
85. Packer ML. The neurohormonal hypothesis: a theory to explain the disease progression in heart failure. J Am Coll Cardiol 1992;20:248–254.
86. Dahlöf B. Effect of angiotensin II blockade on cardiac hypertrophy and remodelling: a review. J Hum Hypertens 9 1995;(Suppl 5):S37–S44.
87. Kawaguchi H, Kitabatake A. Renin-angiotensin system in failing heart. J Mol Cell Cardiol 1995;27:201–209.
88. Barraclough MA. Sodium and water depletion with acute malignant hypertension. Am J Med 1966;40:265–272.
89. Kindaid-Smith P. Understanding malignant hypertension. Aust NZ J Med 11 1981;(Suppl 1):64–68.

90. Thel MC, Mannon RB, Allen NB. Hyperrenin-hyperaldosterone-dependent malignant hypertension in polyarteritis nodosa. Southern Med J 1993;86:1400–1402.
91. Davis BA, Crook JE, Vestal RE, Oates JA. Prevalence of renovascular hypertension in patients with grade III or IV hypertensive retinopathy. N Engl J Med 1979;301:1273–1276.
92. Martinez-Maldonado M. Pathophysiology of renovascular hypertension. Hypertension 1991;17:709–719.
93. Michelakis AM, Foster JH, Liddle GW, Rhamy RK, Kuchel O, Gordon RD. Measurement of renin in both renal veins. Its use in diagnosis of renovascular hypertension. Arch Int Med 1967;120:444–448.
94. Wilson M, Morganti AA, Zervoudakis I, et al. Blood pressure, the renin-aldosterone system and sex steroids throughout normal pregnancy. Am J Med 1980;68:97–104.
95. August P, Mueller FB, Sealey JE, Edersheim TG. Role of renin-angiotensin system in blood pressure regulation in pregnancy. Lancet 1995;345:896–897.
96. Schrier RW, Briner VA. Peripheral vasodilation hypothesis of sodium and water retention in pregnancy: implications for pathogenesis of preeclampsia-eclampsia. Ob Gynecol 1991;77:632–639.
97. Brown JJ, Davies DL, Doak PB, Lever AF, Robertson JIS. Plasma renin concentration in the hypertensive diseases of pregnancy. J Ob Gynecol 1966;73:410–417.
98. August P, Lenz T, Ales KL, et al. Longitudinal study of the renin-angiotensin-aldosterone system in hypertensive pregnant women: deviations related to the development of superimposed preeclampsia. Am J Ob Gynecol 1990;163:1612–1621.
99. Gant NF, Daley GL, Chand S, Whalley PJ, MacDonald PC. A study of angiotensin II pressor response throughout primagravid pregnancy. J Clin Invest 1973;52:2682–2689.
100. Perez-Ayuso RM, Arroyo V, Planas R, et al. Randomized comparative study of efficiency of furosemide versus spironolactone in nonazotemic cirrhosis with ascites. Relationship between the diuretic response and the activity of the renin-aldosterone system. Gastroenterology 1983;84:961–968.
101. Chatterjee K, Parmley WW, Cohn JN, et al. A cooperative multicenter study of captopril in congestive heart failure: hemodynamic effects and long-term response. Am Heart J 1985;110:439–447.
102. Consensus Trial Study Group. Effects of enalapril on mortality in severe congestive heart failure. Results of the cooperative north Scandinavian enalopril survival study (CONSENSUS). N Engl J Med 1987;316:1429–1435.
103. SOLVD Investigators. Effect of enalapril on survival in patients with reduced left ventricular ejection fractions and congestive heart failure. N Engl J Med 1991;325:293–302.
104. Ramahi TM, Lee FA. Medical therapy and prognosis in chronic heart failure. Lessons from clinical trials. Cardiol Clin 1995;13:5–26.
105. Rutledge J, Ayers C, Davidson R, et al. Effect of intravenous enalaprilat in moderate and severe systemic hypertension. Am J Cardiol 1988;62:1062–1067.
106. Hudson JB, Chobanian AV, Relman AS. Hypoaldosteronism. A clinical study of a patient with an isolated adrenal mineralocorticoid deficiency, resulting in hyperkalemia and Stokes-Adams attacks. N Engl J Med 1957;257:529–536.
107. Veldhuis JD, Melby JC. Isolated aldosterone deficiency in man: acquired and inborn errors in the biosynthesis or action of aldosterone. Endocr Rev 1981;2:495–517.
108. Jagger PI. Hypoaldosteronism. Endocrinologist 1995;5:23–27.
109. Williams GH. Hyporeninemic hypoaldosteronism. N Engl J Med 1986;314:1041, 1042.
110. Polsky FI, Roque D, Hill PE. Hyporeninemic hypoaldosteronism complicating primary autonomic insufficiency. West J Med 1993;159:185–187.
111. Uribarri J, Oh MS, Carroll HJ. Hyperkalemia in diabetes mellitus. J Diabetes Complic 1990;4:3–7.
112. Farsang C, Varga K, Vajda L, Alföldi S, Kapocsi J. Effects of clonidine and guanfacine in essential hypertension. Clin Pharm Ther 1994;36:588–594.
113. Michelakis AM, McAllister RG. The effect of chronic adrenergic receptor blockade on plasma renin activity in man. J Clin Endocrinol Metab 1972;34:386–394.
114. Weidmann P, Reinhart R, Maxwell MH, Rowe P, Coburn JW, Massry SG. Syndrome of hyporeninemic hypoaldosteronism and hyperkalemia in renal disease. J Clin Endocrinol Metab 1973;36:965–977.
115. Schambelan M. Sebastian A, Biglieri EG. Prevalence, pathogenesis, and functional significance of aldosterone deficiency in hyperkalemic patients with chronic renal insufficiency. Kidney Int 1980;17:89–101.
116. Monnens L, Fiselier T, Bos B, van Munster P. Hyporeninemic hypoaldosteronism in infancy. Nephron 1983;35:140–142.

117. Tan SY, Shapiro R, Franco R, Stockard H, Mulrow PJ. Indomethacin-induced prostaglandin inhibition with hyperkalemia. A reversible cause of hyporeninemic hypoaldosteronism. Ann Intern Med 1979;90:783–785.
118. Tan SY, Burton M. Hyporeninemic hypoaldosteronism. An overlooked cause of hyperkalemia. Arch Intern Med 1981;141:30–33.
119. Kaufman JS, Peck M, Hamburger RJ, Flamenbaum W. Isolated hypoaldosteronism and abnormalities in renin, kallikrein, and prostaglandin. Nephron 1986;43:203–210.
120. Nadler JL, Lee FO, Hsueh W, Horton R. Evidence of prostacyclin deficiency in the syndrome of hyporeninemic hypoaldosteronism. N Engl J Med 1986;314:1015–1020.
121. Kalin MF, Poretsky L, Seres DS, Zumoff B. Hyporeninemic hypoaldosteronism associated with acquired immune deficiency syndrome. Am J Med 1987;82:1035–1038.
122. DeFronza RA. Hyperkalemia and hyporeninemic hypoaldosteronism. Kidney Int 1980;17:118–134.
123. Findling JW, Adams AH, Raff H. Selective hypoaldosteronism due to an endogenous impairment in angiotensin II production. N Engl J Med 1987;316:1632–1635.
124. Williams FA Jr, Schambelan M, Biglieri EG, Carey RM. Acquired primary hypoaldosteronism due to isolated zona glomerulosa defect. N Engl J Med 1983;309:1623–1627.
125. Carey RM, Schambelan M, Biglieri EG, Bright GM. Letter to the Editor. N Engl J Med 1984;310:1395.
126. Saenger P, Levine LS, Irvine WJ, et al. Progressive adrenal failure and polyglandular auto-immune disease. J Clin Endocrinol Metab 1982;54:863–868.
127. Otabe S, Muto S, Asano Y, et al. Hyperreninemic hypoaldosteronism due to hepatocellular carcinoma metastatic to the adrenal gland. Clin Nephrol 1991;35:66–71.
128. Thomas JP. Aldosterone deficiency in a patient with idiopathic haemochromatosis. Clin Endocrinol 1984;21:271–277.
129. Otabe S, Muto S, Asano Y, et al. Selective hypoaldosteronism in a patient with Sjögen's syndrome: insensitivity to angiotensin II. Nephron 1991;59:466–470.
130. O'Kelly R, Magee F, McKenna TJ. Routine heparin therapy inhibits adrenal aldosterone production. J Clin Endocrinol Metab 1983;56:108–112.
131. Aull L, Chao H, Coy K. Heparin-induced hyperkalemia. DICP Ann Pharmacother 1990;24:244–246.
132. Levesque H, Verdier S, Cailleux N, et al. Low molecular weight heparins and hypoaldosteronism. Br Med J 1990;300:1437–1438.
133. Hauffa BP, Sólyom J, Gláz E, et al. Severe hypoaldosteronism due to corticosterone methyloxidase type II deficiency in two boys: metabolic and gas chromatography-mass spectrometry studies. Eur J Pediatr 1991;150:149–153.
134. Picco P, Garibaldi L, Cotellessa M, DiRocco M, Borrone C. Corticosterone methyl oxidase type II deficiency: a cause of failure to thrive and recurrent dehydration in early infancy. Eur J Pediatr 1992;151:170–173.
135. Rao RH, Vagnucci AH, Amico JA. Bilateral Massive adrenal hemorrhage: early recognition and treatment. Ann Intern Med 1989;110:227–235.
136. Dahlberg PJ, Goellner MH, Pehling GB. Adrenal insufficiency secondary to adrenal hemorrhage. Two case reports and a review of cases confirmed by computerized tomography. Arch Intern Med 1990;150:905–909.
137. Zipser RD, Davenport MW, Martin KL, et al. Hyperreninemic hypoaldosteronism in the critically ill: a new entity. J Clin Endocrinol Metab 1981;53:867–873.
138. Parker LN, Levin ER, Lifrak ET. Evidence for adrenocortical adaptation to severe illness. J Clin Endocrinol Metab 1985;60:947–952.

8 Thyroid Response to Critical Illness

Jonathan S. LoPresti, MD, PhD and John T. Nicoloff, MD

CONTENTS

    INTRODUCTION
    MECHANISMS FOR PRODUCING THE LOW T_3 STATE
    LOW T_3–T_4 STATE
    GENESIS
    REGULATION OF SERUM TSH
    DIFFERENTIAL DIAGNOSIS
    THERAPEUTIC INTERVENTION
    VARIANTS OF NONTHYROID ILLNESS
    INTEGRATED ENDOCRINE RESPONSE
    SUMMARY
    ACKNOWLEDGMENT
    REFERENCES

INTRODUCTION

The imposition of a stress, such as systemic nonthyroidal illness (NTI) or caloric deprivation in euthyroid humans, produces characteristic alterations in serum thyroid hormone indices, which, in certain instances, may minimize the catabolic impact of these events *(1–3)*. The initial step in this process is characterized by the development of the so-called low T_3 state where serum total and free T_3 values are reduced, but serum T_4 levels remain normal. This represents the most common thyroid response observed in systemic illness. If the NTI progresses or is severe on presentation, then total serum T_4 concentrations may also become depressed producing a combined low T_3–T_4 state. Despite these reductions in circulating T_3 and T_4 levels, serum TSH values, for the most part, remain normal, justifying the use of the descriptive term euthyroid sick syndrome. Further, these patients typically do not display characteristic features suggestive of hypothyroidism. It is also of interest that these changes in thyroid hormone economy usually are paralleled by alterations in other anabolic endocrine systems, such as growth hormone/IGF-1 and the reproductive hormones *(4,5)*. Thus, systemic illnesses and nutritional deprivation induce an apparent integrated response involving multiple endocrine systems.

A wide variety of systemic illnesses are capable of producing the low T_3 and low T_3–T_4 states. These include trauma, burns, infectious disease, sepsis, myocardial infarction, surgery, and chronic diseases, as well as metabolic disorders, such as caloric restriction, poorly controlled diabetes mellitus, and fasting *(6–14)*. Indeed, the array of diseases capable of altering thyroid function is so vast that it is estimated that over 70% of hospitalized patients display changes in thyroid hormone indices without having any demonstrable underlying thyroid disease *(15,16)*. Since this condition is so common, it is imperative that the physician be aware that these alterations in thyroid function frequently occur and be able to differentiate them from changes resulting from true thyroid gland dysfunction. This diagnostic challenge will be discussed in detail later in this chapter. We will also speculate on the pathogenesis and metabolic impact of these alterations, discuss the diseases that may produce an aberrant thyroid hormone response, and summarize current experience relating to possible therapeutic interventions.

MECHANISMS FOR PRODUCING THE LOW T_3 STATE

Present evidence indicates that circulating T_3 levels are highly regulated in well-fed, healthy humans *(17)*. This regulation dominantly occurs in peripheral tissues rather than at the level of thyroid gland, since it is estimated that 80% of circulating T_3 normally originates from 5′-deiodination of T_4 in nonthyroidal tissues. Although it is generally believed that the liver is the likely site for the majority of T_4 to T_3 conversion, the actual location of this process has yet to be established in humans. The observation that serum T_3 concentrations are maintained within narrow limits with either T_4 excess or deficiency underscores the notion that circulating T_3 levels are highly regulated *(18)*. This phenomenon is referred to as autoregulation and is mediated by adjustments in the net T_4 to T_3 conversion rate, which maintain serum T_3 concentrations constant. It is also important to note that T_3 disposal is a complex metabolic process that includes inner-ring deiodination, sulfoconjugation, and side chain oxidative-decarboxylation and deamination *(19)*. The former two reactions, which are estimated to account for more than one-half of T_3's disposal under normal conditions, lead to T_3 inactivation *(20)*. However, side chain decarboxylation and deamination are responsible for the formation of triiodothyroacetic acid (T_3AC), which may act as a potent intercrine-paracrine form of thyroid hormone *(21)*. Thus, T_3 conversion to T_3AC may constitute a local activation as well as a disposal pathway for T_3. In any case, it is the combination of these processes associated with T_3 production and disposal that establishes circulating T_3 concentrations, which, in turn, serve as a clinical indicator of the patient's general state of health and nutrition.

With the advent of NTI, serum T_3 values progressively decline, as shown in Fig. 1. When critical illness intervenes, serum total and free T_3 values may actually fall below detection limits of many clinical T_3 assays, indicating a profound reduction in the availability of T_3 to peripheral tissues. Indeed, postmortem studies in humans have verified that tissue T_3 levels parallel the decline observed in serum T_3 values *(22)*. Further, since T_3 tracer studies in humans demonstrate that T_3 clearance is minimally affected in NTI, it is presumed that the decreases in circulating serum T_3 result from a decline in net T_4 to T_3 conversion *(23)*. Paradoxically, however, there is no indication that T_4 deiodination rate, which accounts for the majority of T_4 disposal, is altered to any significant degree in NTI *(24)*.

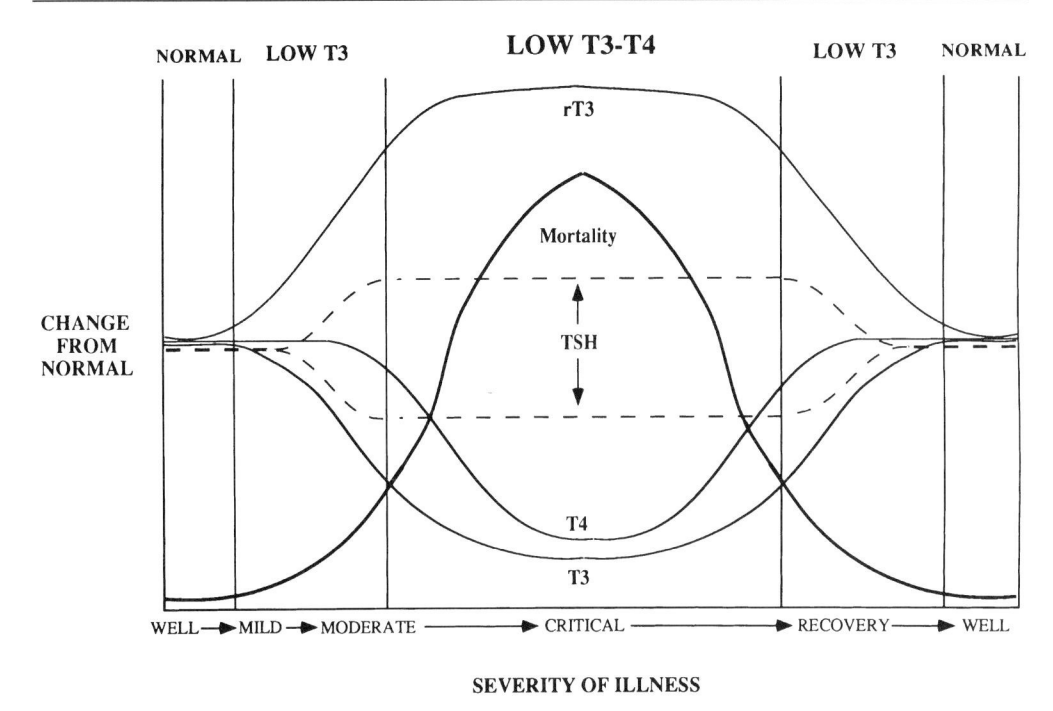

Fig. 1. This figure summarizes the temporal changes in serum thyroid hormone indices seen in illness and fasting. Note that an orderly progression from the low T_3 to the low T_3–T_4 state occurs as the severity of illness increases in these sick patients.

The most facile explanation for the lack of change in overall T_4 deiodination rate in NTI is that a greater inner-ring deiodination of T_4 to form reverse T_3(rT_3) occurs, which, in turn, is responsible for the reciprocal elevations in serum rT_3 commonly seen in NTI, as shown in Fig. 1. In other words, the decrease in T_3 formation (outer-ring deiodination of T_4) may occur at the expense of increased rT_3 production (inner-ring deiodination of T_4). However, this explanation has proven to be false, since rT_3 production rates measured in vivo are generally unaltered in NTI *(23)*. Thus, the increase in serum rT_3 concentrations in NTI results from diminished rT_3 clearance rather than increased production *(23)*. The reduction in T_4 to T_3 conversion combined with the maintenance of normal T_4 and rT_3 production rates leads to the inescapable conclusion that other routes of T_4 metabolism must be increased to compensate for the decreased conversion of T_4 to T_3, as shown in Fig. 2 *(25)*. Indeed, it is this diversion of T_4 metabolism away from T_3 production toward alternate pathways of metabolism that is currently considered to be the most likely explanation for the low T_3 state in humans.

Current evidence indicates that increased formation of T_3 sulfate (T_3S) and T_3AC at the expense of T_3 production most likely is responsible for the low T_3 state of NTI. T_3S, a biologically inactive product of T_3 metabolism, is formed by the addition of a sulfate moiety to the outer-ring hydroxyl group of the T_3 molecule *(26)*. This reaction is catalyzed by a specific thyronine arylsulfotransferase *(27)*. As expected, serum T_3S concentrations are elevated in NTI, supporting the view that there is increased diversion of T_3 to T_3S in NTI *(28)*. If T_3S generation from T_3 occurred in those tissues that convert T_4 to T_3, then T_3 would be shunted away from the circulation, thereby lowering serum T_3 concentrations

HEALTHY/FED   **NTI/FAST**

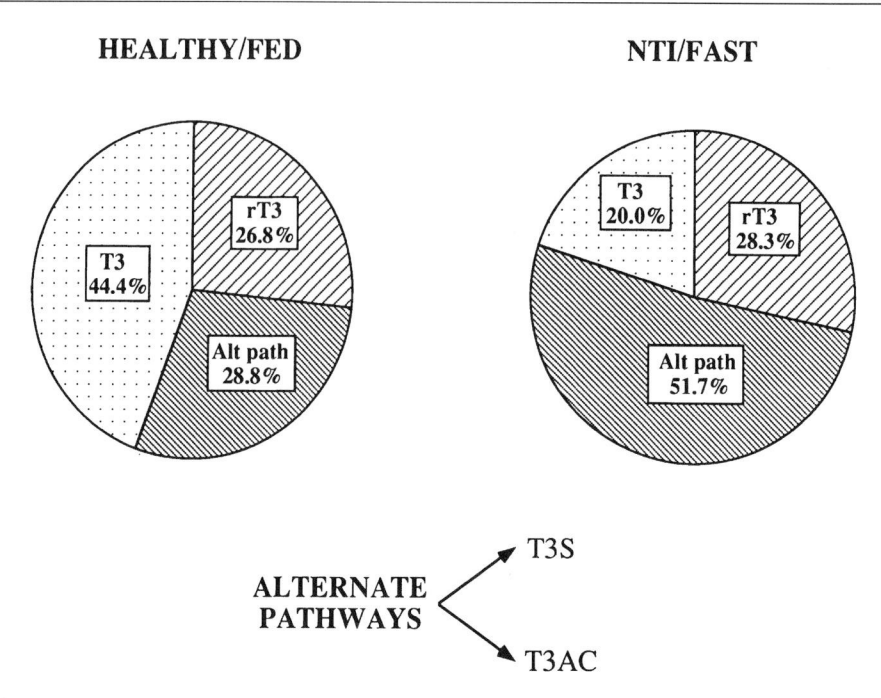

rT3 26.8%
T3 44.4%
Alt path 28.8%

T3 20.0%
rT3 28.3%
Alt path 51.7%

$$\text{ALTERNATE PATHWAYS} \diagup^{\text{T3S}}_{\text{T3AC}}$$

Fig. 2. The patterns of T_4 metabolism in healthy/fed and sick/fasting individuals are depicted. Hypertrophy of the alternate pathways of T_3 disposal to T_3 sulfate (inactive) and T_3AC (active) occur in illness and fasting.

and blood T_3 production rates. In addition to enhanced T_3S formation, increased generation of T_3AC may also contribute to the production of low T_3 states. In contrast to T_3S, T_3AC is a thyroid hormone that exceeds the potency of T_3 in vitro. However, because T_3AC is more rapidly cleared from the circulation than is T_3, it is a relatively weak systemic thyroid hormone in vivo *(29)*. This ineffectiveness as a systemic hormone would not, however, alter its ability to exert local thyroid hormone action at those tissue sites where it is generated. Indeed, such local T_3AC formation and action might explain the paradoxical euthyroid appearance and normal TSH levels seen in the low T_3 state. **A note of caution**: the local generation and action of T_3AC have not yet been firmly established from in vivo studies.

A central question that needs to be addressed in any discussion concerning the low T_3 state of NTI is the potential metabolic impact of the reduced serum T_3 levels. In other words, are some peripheral tissues hypothyroid? Studies conducted in fasting human subjects perhaps offer the best insight into this question. Clearly, successful adaptation to a fast requires maintenance of a minimum serum glucose level to satisfy central nervous system fuel requirements until the brain adapts to metabolizing ketone bodies formed from fat breakdown. For the first 12–24 h of a fast, hepatic glycolysis provides most of the endogenous glucose requirement. Subsequently, however, an increasing proportion of glucose originates from amino acids that are released from skeletal muscle breakdown and made available for gluconeogenesis. By 72 h into a fast, there is a reduction in the glucose required by the brain, since it has switched to a ketone-based source of energy *(30)*. The decline in serum T_3 values parallels these events in that the initial fall in serum T_3 occurs between 18 and 24 h after starting a fast and stabilizes after 4–5 d when ketone bodies now provide the major energy source *(14)*. Similar changes in urinary nitrogen losses reflecting protein turnover for gluconeogenesis are also seen. Initially, urinary nitrogen losses rapidly increase with the onset of gluconeogenesis, but then progressively fall with the switch to a fatty acid-based metabolism. This decrease in protein turnover would appear to be mediated through the fall in serum T_3 concentrations, since normalization of serum T_3 levels with exogenous T_3 administration rapidly restores urinary nitrogen losses to the levels seen in the early phases of fasting *(31)*. Also, the excretion of 3-methyl-histidine in the urine, a specific marker for skeletal muscle breakdown, is increased in T_3-supplemented fasting subjects *(32)*. Parenthetically, it is interesting to note that the amount of exogenous T_3 required to normalize serum T_3 concentrations in fasting is greater than would have been predicted from the reduction in T_3 levels, lending credence to the concept of augmented diversion of T_3 to alternate routes of disposal *(31)*. Further supporting the importance of the decline in circulating T_3 in orchestrating protein conservation is the observation that those patients having the greatest initial fall in serum T_3 in response to caloric restriction are also the same individuals who eventually develop the most efficient nitrogen conservation with prolonged caloric deprivation *(33)*. Taken together, these observations are consistent with the view that the low T_3 state likely produces some degree of peripheral tissue thyroid hormone deficiency, which may be adaptive by limiting protein breakdown for gluconeogenesis during a fast. Indeed, patients with prolonged caloric deprivation secondary to anorexia nervosa may actually display delayed deep tendon reflexes, supporting the view of a functional hypothyroidism of the skeletal muscle *(34)*.

Very recent studies have also suggested that the low T_3 state associated with caloric restriction may be necessary for the initiation of fasting-induced gluconeogenesis, since maintenance of normal T_3 levels during fasting prevents the expected increases in gluconeogenesis *(35)*. This finding suggests that the low T_3 levels, in addition to producing a form of adaptive peripheral tissue hypothyroidism to promote protein conservation, may also help initiate gluconeogenesis. Although the relevance of these studies may be limited because they were carried out in obese volunteers, further investigation of this phenomenon seems to be warranted to verify and extend these intriguing observations.

Whether these apparent adaptive metabolic responses to the low T_3 state also occur in systemic illness in a manner similar to that seen with reduced nutritional intake is unknown. However, it seems logical to assume that the decline in serum T_3 levels with NTI would be expected to mitigate the catabolic effects of illness as it does in fasting.

LOW T_3–T_4 STATE

Patients with more severe critical illnesses may transition from the low T_3 to a low T_3–T_4 state, as shown in Fig. 1. The time required for this change is variable, ranging from hours to days depending on the type and severity of the illness. The reduction in serum T_4 values seen in the low T_3–T_4 state primarily results from an increase in serum T_4 clearance rather than a decrease in T_4 secretion *(36)*. This has been verified by T_4 tracer kinetic studies carried out in severely ill patients in an ICU setting, which show a normal or near-normal T_4 production rate, but an increased T_4 clearance rate (reduced half-life) *(36)*. These T_4 kinetic changes result from an acquired defect in the ability of T_4 to bind to thyroxine binding globulin (TBG). Two different, but possibly complementary explanations, have been advanced to account for this acquired T_4-TBG binding defect. The first relates to the action of a circulating inhibitor with the chemical properties suggestive of a fatty acid that interferes with the binding of T_4 to TBG (37). This inhibitor appears to originate from injured tissues and is then released into the circulation. In addition, it may also impair hepatic intracellular T_4 binding as revealed by compartmental analysis of tracer T_4 kinetics (36). In addition to reducing T_4 binding to TBG and cytosolic proteins, this inhibitor has been proposed to suppress hepatic deiodinase activity, which would account for the decreased rT_3 clearance as well as impairing phagocytic activity of circulating leukocytes (38,39). However, questions still remain regarding the importance of this inhibitor, since some investigators have been unable to confirm these observations (40). A second explanation for this acquired protein binding defect is that illness induces a structural alteration in TBG, reducing its ability to bind T_4 (41). This defective TBG has been termed "slow TBG" because of its retarded electrophoretic migration. In either case, the finding that immunoassayable TBG concentrations are normal in the initial phases of critical illness lends credence to the concept that a T_4 binding inhibitor, a structurally defective TBG, or a combination of the two must be present in the low T_3–T_4 state of NTI.

An unanticipated facet of the low T_3–T_4 state is the finding of an inverse relationship between serum T_4 levels and mortality, as shown in Fig. 1. Several studies performed in surgical and medical intensive care units have clearly documented the value of serum T_4 measurement in predicting mortality (42–44). Despite the heterogeneity of the populations studied, a remarkably close inverse relationship between total T_4 and mortality exists. In fact, comparisons with more widely used prognostic methods have actually shown serum T_4 levels to be an equal or better predictor of mortality than the more conventional Apache II scoring system (45). Why total serum T_4 levels should serve as such an accurate prognostic indicator is unclear. Perhaps the proposed impairment of leukocytic phagocytosis by a circulating T_4 binding inhibitor provides the best explanation.

GENESIS

The cause of the low T_3 and low T_3–T_4 states of NTI likely have multiple origins. In most cases, the general pattern of alterations in thyroid hormone indices are remarkably predictable regardless of the inciting factors. Although the conditions producing the low T_3 and low T_3–T_4 states may range widely from undernutrition, poorly controlled diabetes, infection, trauma, and glucocorticoid administration, three general categories of promoters, namely cytokines, endocrine, and nutritional status, as shown in Fig. 3, seem to serve as primary initiators.

The actions of cytokines, the endocrine portion of the immune system, are undoubtedly responsible for inducing the low T_3 and low T_3–T_4 states seen with infection and trauma. The three classes of cytokines, interleukins (IL-1, IL-2, and so forth), interferons (α and β), and tumor necrosis factor (TNF), are polypeptide hormones secreted by the mononuclear cells, which produce the characteristic features of illness, including fever, inflammation, and the initiation of tissue repair (46). In addition, they also play an important role in regulating the changes in thyroid indices of NTI since parenteral administration of IL-1, IL-2, IL-6, and TNF to normal human volunteers results in the classic pattern of the low T_3 and low T_3–T_4 states (47–49). How these cytokines actually bring about these changes is not entirely known. In addition, in vitro studies have shown that some of these cytokines

```
         Cytokines  ⟷  Endocrine  ⟷  Nutrition
              \           |           /
               \          |          /
                \         ↓         /
                 ( Peripheral
                   Thyroid Hormone
                   Metabolism )
                 /         |         \
                /          |          \
               ↓           ↓           ↓
         HIGH rT3      LOW T3        LOW T4
         ↓ rT3 to T2   ↓ T4 to T3    Inhibitor
                       ↑ T3 to T3S   Slow TBG
                       ↑ T3 to T3AC
```

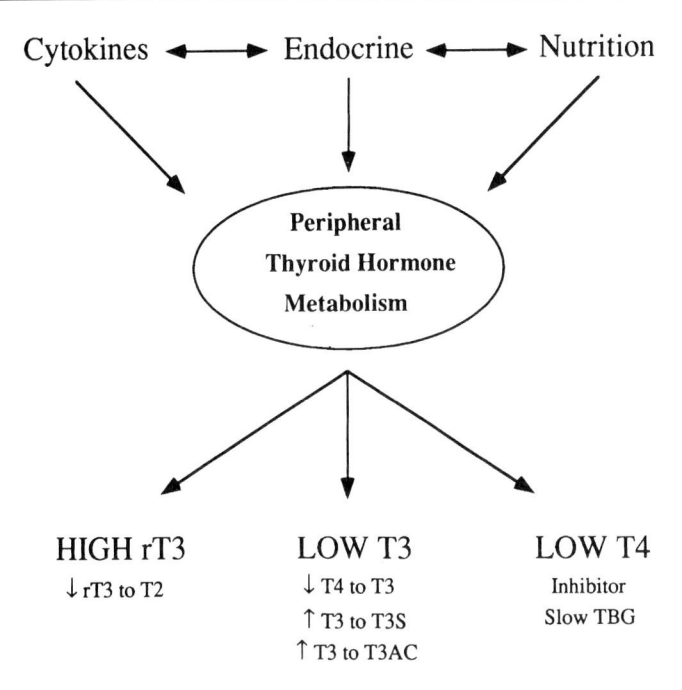

Fig. 3. The potential mediators of the low T_3 and low T_3–T_4 states are shown. Cytokine, endocrine, and nutritional signals initiate the changes in peripheral thyroid hormone metabolism responsible for the alterations in serum thyroid hormone indices present in illness and fasting.

may directly impair TRH biosynthesis and thyroid gland function (50,51). On the other hand, there is substantial support for the notion that these changes are also mediated through cytokine-induced activation of the CRH–ACTH–adrenal axis.

Increases in serum cortisol concentrations, either from endogenous or exogenous sources, are capable of producing the characteristic changes in thyroid hormone indices seen in NTI (52). This endocrinologic mechanism, whether initiated through cytokines, trauma, anesthesia, or glucocorticoid administration, produces alterations in serum thyroid hormone indices similar to those seen in the low T_3 state of NTI. The rapidity of this response is apparent in previously healthy individuals who have undergone elective surgery or sustained major burns (7,11). It seems particularly appropriate that cortisol excess should produce low serum T_3 levels, since it would counterregulate the gluconeogenic actions of glucocorticoids. It should also be emphasized, however, that cortisol elevations are not likely to be the sole cause of these changes in thyroid hormone indices observed in NTI. Even though the administration of glucocorticoids to healthy volunteers produces what appears to be a classic low T_3 state, subtle differences have been observed. Namely, the elevations in serum rT_3 concentrations produced with glucocorticoid administration result from an increase in T_4 to rT_3 conversion rather than from a decrease in rT_3 clearance as seen in spontaneous NTI and fasting (53). Therefore, increases in cortisol levels are not solely responsible for these changes, but probably play an important complementary role in the genesis of the low T_3 state of NTI.

Nutritional status is the third major factor capable of inducing changes in serum thyroid hormone indices in humans. Characteristically, fasting will initiate a fall in serum T_3 levels within 18–24 h after starting caloric deprivation and persists until refeeding takes place *(14)*. A marked decline in serum T_3 values is also seen in uncontrolled diabetes mellitus *(13)*, in essence a fasting response secondary to a lack of insulin action, which does not normalize until the premorbid nutritional status is achieved. As previously discussed, these changes in thyroid hormone values in fasting likely promote protein conservation and regulate gluconeogenesis. Less well-recognized is the fact that the nutrient content of the diet consumed can also influence serum T_3 levels. For example, ingestion of a minimum of at least 400 calories of either carbohydrate or protein/d is required to sustain normal serum T_3 levels, whereas a ketogenic diet, even with a normal caloric content, will result in the low T_3 state *(54,55)*. The specific endocrine signals that regulate T_3 levels in response to the diet are currently unknown, but one would have to speculate that one or a combination of the endocrine mediators of gluconeogenesis (glucagon, GH, IGF-1, insulin, cortisol) likely play an important role. Finally, the impact that caloric intake has on producing the low T_3 state in patients with a systemic illness is unknown, but it likely makes an important contribution.

REGULATION OF SERUM TSH

Circulating TSH normally displays a circadian variation with peak levels occurring near midnight and the trough values near noon. This pattern is lost early in the course of an illness or fasting when TSH concentrations usually become transiently suppressed as serum T_3 levels fall *(56)*. Recovery from illness or restoration of adequate nutritional intake will often reciprocally produce a "rebound" in serum TSH concentrations, as well. For the most part, these transient changes in the TSH concentrations occur within the normal range of TSH values and can last for a period of 3–7 d before a normal circadian pattern resumes. However, up to 15% of euthyroid patients admitted to a hospital with a nonthyroidal illness may demonstrate frankly abnormal TSH levels (2/3 low and 1/3 high) *(57)*. The majority of these changes, however, only deviate slightly from the normal range. Two to 3% patients will also display TSH values consistent with either thyrotoxicosis (<0.1 mU/L) or with hypothyroidism (>20 mU/L). It is this latter subset of patients that presents the major diagnostic dilemma to the clinician.

The mechanism(s) responsible for these transient changes in serum TSH values in illness is not well understood. Indeed, based on the known negative feedback actions of thyroid hormone on TSH release, it seems paradoxical that serum TSH would fall simultaneously with the declining circulating T_3 levels. Such a response suggests that an increased sensitivity to the negative feedback actions of T_3 must occur. Indeed, some animal models of NTI support this concept of enhanced negative feedback action of T_3 *(58)*. Interestingly, glucocorticoid administration, in addition to lowering T_3 levels, also rapidly depresses serum TSH levels, and on withdrawal will produce a rebound in TSH similar to that seen with NTI *(52)*. These glucocorticoid effects are probably mediated at the hypothalamus by inhibiting TRH secretion *(59)*. Certainly, as endogenous cortisol rises in response to systemic illness, it is reasonable to speculate that it may play a role in the pathogenesis of these TSH alterations in NTI. However, as previously pointed out, glucocorticoids cannot be the sole mediator of the changes in thyroid hormone indices, since their effects on peripheral thyroid hormone metabolism differ in some aspects to those described in fasting and illness. Cytokines, which can produce the low T_3 state, are also capable of altering TRH synthesis and decreasing TRH production, which could account for the typical initial transient decline in TSH concentrations *(47)*. Evidence for a potential role of TRH in altering the set point for TSH secretion in illness was recently gained when it was shown that the repetitive iv TRH administration to critically ill patients may restore TSH levels and thyroid gland responsiveness toward normal *(60)*. This response pattern is similar to that seen in patients with hypothalamic hypothyroidism where the repetitive administration of TRH restored thyroid function to normal *(61)*. Taken in sum, these studies suggest that the reset for TSH feedback response to circulating thyroid hormone may be mediated at the level of the hypothalamus, though the precise mediator(s) has not been identified. It is interesting to note that the reset of gonadal axis in fasting and illness also occurs at the level of the hypothalamus, leading to a functional hypogonadotropic hypogonadism *(14)*. Thus, the combination of the central and peripheral inhibition of the thyroid axis in fasting and illness appears to play an integral role in the development and maintenance of the low T_3 state.

DIFFERENTIAL DIAGNOSIS

A common problem confronting the physician is the interpretation of thyroid function tests obtained in the hospitalized patient; does the patient have true thyroid disease, or do the changes in thyroid indices reflect the low T_3 or T_3–T_4 state of NTI? It appears that the principal dilemma for the physician is to identify those few patients with underlying thyroid disease (<5%) from those who display changes in TSH secondary to NTI. Perhaps the simplest way to avoid this conflict is not to order thyroid tests in sick patients unless substantial clinical suspicion of underlying thyroid disease is present. Reasonable clinical indications of coexistent thyroid dysfunction that would warrant thyroid function testing in NTI include unexplained atrial fibrillation or congestive heart failure, history of thyroid disease, and current or past evidence of thyroid dysfunction, such as goiter or surgical scar in the neck. Other conditions that may occasionally sanction screening for thyroid disease include severe constipation, unexplained hyponatremia, or delayed return of DTRs on physical examination. Employing these simple clinical guidelines substantially enhances the ability of the physician to focus on those sick patient populations most likely to manifest underlying thyroid disease.

The spectrum of changes in serum TSH levels produced by illness can affect up to 15% of hospitalized patients with 2–3% having TSH concentrations consistent with true thyroid diseases (Fig. 4) *(57)*. Indeed, serious concern for true thyroid dysfunction should only be considered at the extremes of TSH aberrancy (<0.1 mU/L and >20 mU/L). Because of these limitations, the combination of a serum TSH and free T_4 estimate (FT_4E) seems to be the most cost-effective and rewarding approach to evaluate the thyroid status in a sick population suspected of harboring thyroid disease. If the serum TSH and FT_4E concentrations are normal, then the patient is likely euthyroid, and no further workup is needed as shown in Figs. 5 and 6. A normal FT_4E in conjunction with a TSH that is either modestly elevated (5–20 mU/L) or depressed (0.1–0.5 mU/L) is also suggestive that the changes in thyroid function are owing to illness *per se*. However, appropriate inverse relationships between FT_4E and TSH make the diagnosis of thyroid dysfunction more likely (low FT_4E, high TSH for hypothyroidism and high FT_4E, suppressed TSH for hyperthyroidism), and potentially justify therapeutic intervention. It cannot be emphasized enough that repeat thyroid function tests be obtained when the patient recovers from illness to verify the diagnosis.

The routine use of "third-generation" TSH assays has substantially helped with making the diagnosis of hyperthyroidism in patients with a concurrent nonthyroidal illness. In

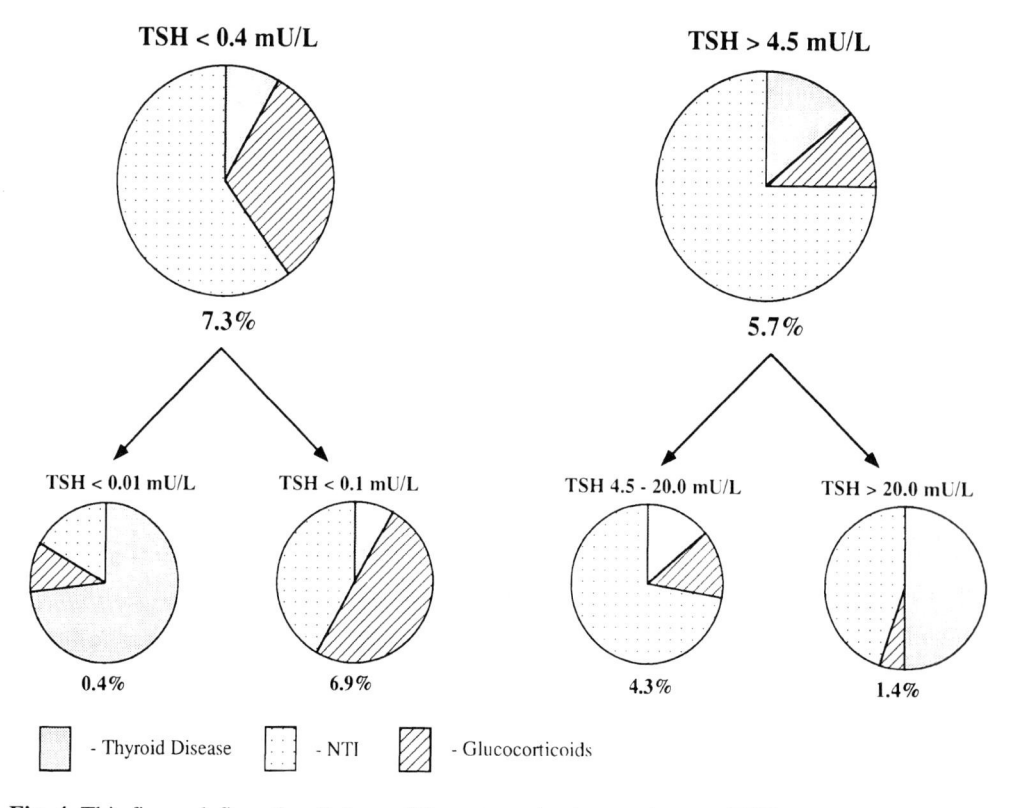

Fig. 4. This figure defines the etiology of the extremely abnormal serum TSH concentrations present in sick patients.

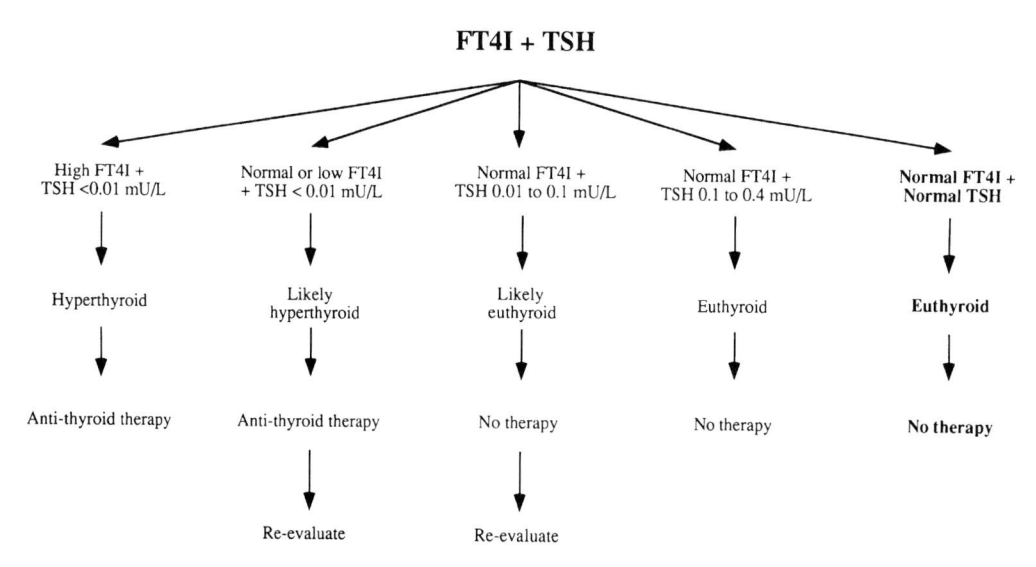

Fig. 5. Diagnosis of thyroid disease in NTI with low serum TSH values. An algorithm for diagnosing and treating potential thyroid disease in sick patients with low serum TSH values is outlined. Note that the algorithm is based on the physician obtaining a free T_4 estimate and TSH concentration, and that the patients are not taking drugs known to alter thyroid function.

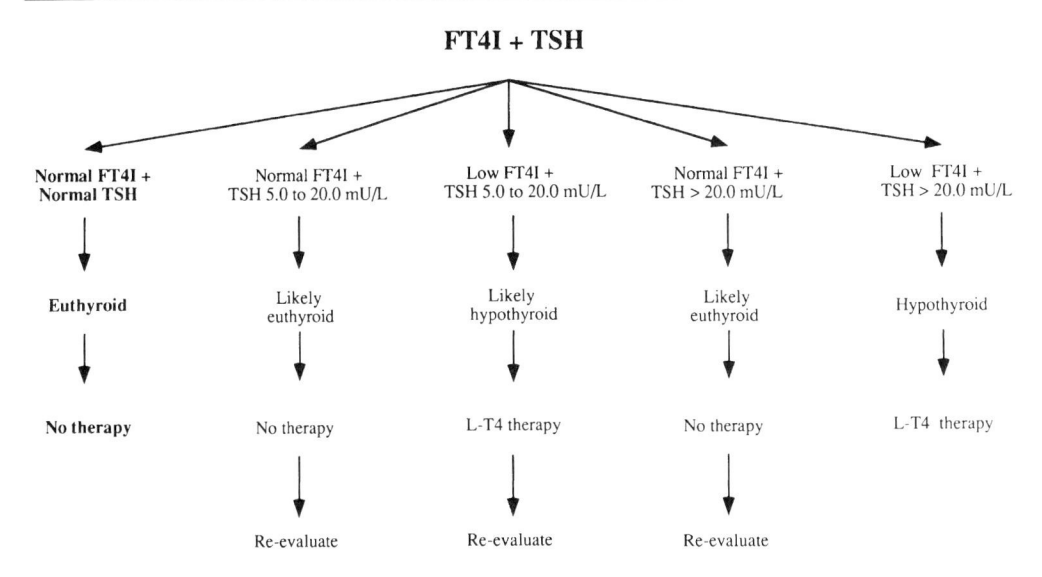

```
                        FT4I + TSH
         ┌─────────┬─────────┼─────────┬─────────┐
         ▼         ▼         ▼         ▼         ▼
  Normal FT4I +  Normal FT4I +  Low FT4I +   Normal FT4I +  Low FT4I +
  Normal TSH    TSH 5.0 to 20.0 mU/L  TSH 5.0 to 20.0 mU/L  TSH > 20.0 mU/L  TSH > 20.0 mU/L
         │         │         │         │         │
         ▼         ▼         ▼         ▼         ▼
    Euthyroid    Likely    Likely    Likely    Hypothyroid
                euthyroid  hypothyroid euthyroid
         │         │         │         │         │
         ▼         ▼         ▼         ▼         ▼
    No therapy  No therapy  L-T4 therapy  No therapy  L-T4 therapy
                   │         │         │
                   ▼         ▼         ▼
                Re-evaluate Re-evaluate Re-evaluate
```

Fig. 6. Diagnosis of thyroid disease in NTI with high serum TSH values. An algorithm for diagnosing and treating potential thyroid disease in sick patients with high serum TSH values is outlined. Note that the algorithm is based on the physician obtaining a free T_4 estimate and TSH concentration, and that the patients are not taking drugs known to alter thyroid function.

general, NTI produces considerably less suppression of serum TSH values than does hyperthyroidism. This reduction in TSH is also transient in nature. Thus, those individuals with a TSH level <0.01 mU/L should be considered thyrotoxic, whereas those with concentrations >0.01 mU/L should most likely be considered euthyroid (Fig. 5) *(57)*. If a third-generation TSH assay is not available and a TSH level is <0.1 mU/L in a second-generation assay, then TRH testing may be helpful in diagnosing the presence of hyperthyroidism. If TRH is administered and the serum TSH remains <0.1 mU/L, then a diagnosis of hyperthyroidism must seriously be weighed and appropriate antithyroid drug treatment initiated *(57)*. On the other hand, the patient should be considered euthyroid if a detectable TSH response (>0.1 mU/L) is observed. Other laboratory indicators of coexistent hyperthyroidism in a sick patient are the presence of an inappropriately normal serum T_3 and/or normal or a high FT_4E value. Regardless of the immediate decision reached, re-evaluation of the individual's thyroid status after recovery from NTI is mandatory to verify the diagnosis.

Elevated serum TSH values may also commonly accompany NTI. About one-third of sick patients with aberrant serum TSH values secondary to NTI display transient increases in TSH, which must be distinguished from true hypothyroidism. As with TSH depressions in NTI, it is reasonable to assume that a patient demonstrating a normal FT_4E and a modest rise in TSH is most likely euthyroid. However, a combination of a low FT_4E and an increased TSH level strongly supports a presumptive diagnosis of hypothyroidism in the hospital setting (Fig. 6). Again, the re-evaluation of the patient's thyroid status following recovery from the NTI is indicated.

The administration of pharmacologic doses of either glucocorticoids or dopamine alters serum thyroid hormone indices and may make the diagnosis of coexistent thyroid disease in a critically ill patient troublesome *(52,62)*. As previously discussed, exogenous glucocorticoids will produce the low T_3 state, including suppressed TSH values, whereas their withdrawal will lead to a rebound elevation (Fig. 4). In addition, dopamine infusions will also transiently suppress serum TSH concentrations by inhibiting TSH release from the thyrotrophs in the pituitary. The cessation of dopamine therapy will produce an abrupt rise in serum TSH levels *(62)*. Thus, the interpretation of thyroid function tests in a sick patient receiving these medications is quite difficult. It is highly recommended that if thyroid disease is suspected, serum thyroid hormone indices should be obtained prior to the initiation of either glucocorticoid or dopamine therapy.

Another diagnostic dilemma may occur when a low FT_4E and normal or low serum TSH values are observed in an ill patient. This combination most commonly presents in patients with serious critical illnesses where the question arises: do these changes in thyroid indices result from nonthyroidal illness alone (low T_3-T_4 state), or are they the result of central hypothyroidism? In such cases, advantage can be taken of the typical endocrine response to illness in differentiating between the two alternatives by assessing the endogenous cortisol response to the illness. Typically, serum cortisol values rise to >20 µg/dL in the severely sick patient *(63)*. If the cortisol concentrations are >20 µg/dL, then it is most likely that the hypothalamic–pituitary axis is intact, and the alterations in the thyroid hormone indices are owing to the underlying systemic illness and no therapeutic intervention is indicated required. On the other hand, if the cortisol values are <20 µg/dL, then the changes in thyroid function are more likely the result of diminished hypothalamic/pituitary function rather than the stress of the NTI. In such cases, appropriate hydrocortisone and L-T_4 therapy should be initiated. Although these criteria may be used as a guideline for the initiation of thyroid-glucocorticoid therapy, re-evaluation of the patient's status on recovery is necessary.

THERAPEUTIC INTERVENTION

An enticing question that needs to be addressed in any discussion involving euthyroid sick patients who display either the low T_3 or low T_3-T_4 state is: will they benefit from the administration of exogenous thyroid hormone? Recent studies have shown that giving small doses of iv T_3 (5 µg) to correct the low serum T_3 levels in patients undergoing open-heart surgery rapidly enhances cardiac performance by improving the inotropic performance of the heart. In addition, claims of better overall survival and reduced postoperative morbidity have also been made *(64,65)*. The rapidity of this response to T_3 administration also suggests that the effects may occur via nonnuclear-mediated thyroid hormone action. However, a very recently published study investigating the utility of the random administration of iv T_3 in patients undergoing cardiac bypass was unable to observe any discernible clinical benefit and only minimal differences in cardiac function *(66)*. These latter results are more consistent with earlier work showing that giving iv thyroxine to critically ill patients displaying the low T_3-T_4 state did not appear to influence the clinical course of the underlying illness *(67)*. Thus, thyroid hormone therapy cannot be recommended at this time in euthyroid patients with changes in serum thyroid hormone indices owing to nonthyroidal illness.

VARIANTS OF NONTHYROIDAL ILLNESS

The majority of metabolic derangements and systemic nonthyroidal illnesses in humans produce a predictable pattern of change in serum thyroid hormone indices (Fig. 1). Certain common diseases, however, may give what would be considered an atypical thyroid response pattern. The physician needs to be aware of these situations to avoid misinterpretation of thyroid function tests in such patients. The conditions most commonly associated with these variant patterns in thyroid function are summarized below.

Human Immunodeficiency Virus (HIV) Infection

Modest increases in serum T_3, T_3/T_4 ratios and TBG concentrations are observed in asymptomatic patients with HIV infection *(68)*. Although these changes are significant, they are modest in magnitude with many values remaining within the normal range. However, this is an unexpected finding given that these patients have an underlying chronic illness where a decline in T_3 levels would be expected *(69)*. In addition to the inappropriate normal to high T_3 values, decreased circulating rT_3 and rT_3/T_4 values are also seen. Further, these paradoxical changes in T_3 and rT_3 concentrations may also be observed in HIV patients who have experienced substantial wasting when very low T_3 and high rT_3 values would be expected. Whether this maintenance of the inappropriately normal serum T_3 concentrations contributes to this weight loss in some HIV-positive patients is the subject of current debate. The occurrence of opportunistic infections (i.e., *Pneumocystic carinii* pneumonia) in patients with HIV usually produces the anticipated decline in serum T_3 values, with undetectable levels being highly predictive of a poor outcome, that is, the lower the serum T_3 value at the onset of the opportunistic infection, the greater the likelihood of a fatal event *(70)*. Despite these changes in T_3 levels, TSH values typically remain normal in HIV infection, although they tend to be in the high normal range *(71)*. Additionally, serum TBG concentrations continue to rise with advancing HIV infection as reflected by falling CD4 counts *(72)*. This suggests that a progressive dysregulation in peripheral thyroid hormone metabolism parallels the downward course of HIV infection. The genesis of this aberrant response pattern is presently unknown, but it is interesting to speculate that derangements in cytokine responses in HIV infection may play a prominent role.

Liver Disease

Marked elevations in serum T_4 and T_3 concentrations are commonly observed in patients with both acute and chronic viral hepatitis *(73)*. Like those changes observed in HIV infection, serum rT_3 values tend to be lower in this group of patients. The rise in T_4 and T_3 levels appear, not to result from enhanced thyroidal secretion, but rather is secondarily an increase in TBG levels resulting from augmented synthesis by the hepatocyte *(74)*. When the disease progresses to liver failure, however, the classic low T_3 and low T_3-T_4 states will be seen. Similar to that seen in HIV-positive patients with a concurrent illness, a precipitous drop in serum T_3 levels in patients with end-stage alcoholic cirrhosis is also associated with a poor prognosis *(75)*. Earlier studies suggested that TSH levels may be elevated in liver disease, but confirmation of these findings with newer TSH assays has not been completed *(73)*.

Renal Disease

Patients with renal disease display the expected low serum T_3 levels as their disease advances, but in contrast to the classic low T_3 state, these individuals have paradoxically normal rather than elevated rT_3 values *(76)*. The normal rT_3 concentrations result from an unexpected maintenance of a normal rT_3 clearance rate. The mechanism(s) responsible for the unaltered rT_3 clearance is not completely understood. These observations clearly display the independence of the regulation of rT_3 from that of T_3 metabolism in nonthyroidal illness. As with liver disease, previous studies have shown that patients with renal failure may occasionally show high TSH values, but more recent studies have not confirmed these findings (77).

Psychiatric Illness

Patients with acute psychosis also commonly demonstrate aberrant patterns of serum thyroid hormone indices (78,79). These changes are transient in nature and tend to normalize in a few days as the underlying psychiatric disorder stabilizes. Typically, isolated elevations in total and free T_4 with normal T_3 levels are seen. Serum TSH levels are usually suppressed, but on occasion, they may be transiently elevated as well. Though no mechanism has been elucidated to explain these acute alterations, a temporary TRH-mediated TSH release, which subsequently causes a rise in T_4 release and secondarily decreases serum TSH levels, offers the most plausible explanation. Because these transient changes in serum thyroid hormone indices are commonly seen during the acute phase of illness, it is generally prudent to defer evaluation of the thyroid status of acutely psychotic patients.

Pregnancy

Although pregnancy is not classified as an illness, dramatic alterations in serum thyroid hormone indices are commonly observed. The most well-documented change is a rise in serum TBG levels producing an increase in total T_4 concentrations (80). The elevated TBG results from a change in the sialyation of the TBG molecule, which prolongs its biologic half-life (80). Free T_4 values, however, remain normal even though total T_4 levels are elevated. Although serum TSH concentrations generally remain within the normal range, a modest suppression in serum TSH levels is routinely seen in the first trimester of pregnancy (81). The TSH values typically decline to the low normal range, but up to 20% of women will show frankly low, but detectable values. The reduction in serum TSH most likely results from hCG stimulation of the TSH receptor, and an increase in T_4 secretion by the thyroid gland and secondary thyrotroph suppression. One aberrant pattern of the expected thyroid indices in pregnancy is with the superimposition of hyperemesis gravidarum, which is often associated with very high hCG levels. Serum thyroid hormone indices obtained in these patients are suggestive of hyperthyroidism with an elevation in total and free T_4 levels, normal to high serum T_3 values, but in distinction from true thyrotoxicosis, serum TSH concentrations, though suppressed, remain detectable (82). This syndrome, in both its clinical and chemical manifestations, is believed to be secondary to marked elevations in hCG levels measured in these women. Serum thyroid hormone indices normalize with resolution of the hyperemesis.

INTEGRATED ENDOCRINE RESPONSE

The chapter has primarily focused on the response of the thyroid axis to illness and caloric deprivation. However, this is a rather narrow view of the overall endocrine response to these catabolic stresses. Rather, a more global and complex endocrine adaptation occurs, which we have termed the integrated endocrine response to catabolic stress. This involves both anabolic and catabolic responses. In states of health and adequate nutrition, these systems act in concert to promote growth and reproduction, i.e., anabolism. In contrast, with the advent of catabolic stress, these systems interact in a cohesive manner to promote local tissue healing and, at the same time, limit growth and reproduction, i.e., conservation.

The onset of either illness or fasting with the resultant release of cytokines and, as of yet, undetermined nutritional signals, appear to be the prime factors in orchestrating this integrated endocrine response. A hypothalamically mediated inhibition of gonadotropin release leads to a drop in LH and FSH, which, in turn, decreases sex steroid levels. The hypogonadotropic hypogonadism reduces anabolism and probably facilitates protein breakdown while lessening the ability of the organism to reproduce. Simultaneously, serum IGF-1 levels drop, which also helps to minimize the stimulus for growth. Despite the fall in serum IGF-1 concentrations, circulating GH values rise to counterregulate this effect and minimize glucose utilization by fostering fatty acid breakdown. In conjunction with the low T_3 state and its metabolic impact, the combined effect is to reduce growth and reproduction (anabolism), decrease overall metabolic demands, and regulate gluconeogenesis as well as promote healing at sites of injury. On resolution of the catabolic insult, normalization of the anabolic endocrine system then occurs as the endocrine network responds to improved nutrition and/or a reduced cytokine influence.

SUMMARY

Nonthyroidal illnesses and caloric deprivation produce characteristic alterations in serum thyroid hormone indices that are a part of a more global integrated endocrine response. The most consistent feature of this thyroid hormone response is a drop in serum T_3 levels. Clearly, this low T_3 state appears to be adaptive in nature in that it likely serves to conserve protein and regulate gluconeogenesis during fasting or modest caloric deprivation. Enhanced protein losses in fasting patients with normalized serum T_3 values via exogenous T_3 administration is consistent with this view. Whether the same protein-sparing effects occur with the low serum T_3 concentrations associated with NTI is currently unknown, but it seems likely. Thus, it is plausible to assume that the low T_3 state of illness and caloric deprivation constitutes an adaptive form of hypothyroidism that mitigates the catabolic stress of these conditions.

The notion that hypothyroidism is present in all tissues in the low T_3 state may be naive. For example, the maintenance of normal or even slightly suppressed serum TSH values in illness when one would have expected elevated levels is the strongest argument against universal hypothyroidism. Corroborating this finding is the lack of clinical evidence of hypothyroidism in patients who are either ill or fasting. This suggests that variable tissue thyroid hormone action occurs in these conditions. Though the mechanism(s) responsible for this local regulation of thyroid hormone action has not been elucidated, it appears that the answer lies in the study of alternate routes of T_3 metabolism. The local generation of the inactive T_3S or active T_3AC from T_3 at the end organ may modify the autocrine and paracrine actions, and produce variable tissue action of thyroid hormone. Indeed, evidence already exists that these alternate T_3 pathways are hypertrophied in illness and fasting, but definitive proof of this hypothesis is still lacking. If this concept is true, then each tissue possesses the inherent ability to determine its own thyroid hormone needs dependent on its health and nutritional status, which makes the thyroid hormone adaption to NTI and caloric deprivation more complex than envisioned. Therefore, it must be concluded the low T_3 and low T_3-T_4 states of illness are an adaptive response for which only a embryonic understanding currently exists.

ACKNOWLEDGMENT

This work was supported in part by NCRR General Clinical Research Center Grant MO1-RR-43.

REFERENCES

1. Wartofsky L, Burman KD. Alterations in thyroid function in patients with systemic illnesses: the "euthyroid sick syndrome". Endocrinol Rev 1982;3:164–217.
2. Tibaldi JM, Surks MI. Effect of nonthyroidal illness on thyroid function. Med Clin North Am 1985;69:899–911.
3. Docter E, Krenning EP, deJong M, Hennemann G. The sick euthyroid syndrome: changes in thyroid hormone serum parameters and hormone metabolism. Clin Endocrinol 1993;39:499–518.
4. Moller S, Juul A, Becker U, Flyvbyers A, Skakkeback NE, Henriksen JH. Concentrations, release, and disposal of insulin-like growth factor (IGF)-binding proteins (IGFBP), IGF-1, and growth hormone in different vascular beds in patients with cirrhosis. J Clin Endocrinol Metab 1995;80:1148–1157.
5. Spratt DI, Gigas ST, Beitins I, Cox P, Longcope C, Orav J. Both hyper and hypogonadotropic hypogonadism occur transiently in acute illness: bio and immunoactive gonadotropins. J Clin Endocrinol Metab 1992;75:1562–1570.
6. Vitek V, Shatney CH. Thyroid hormone alterations in patients with shock and injury. Injury 1987;18:336–341.
7. Becker RA, Wilmore DW, Goodwin CW, et al. Free T_4, free T_3 and reverse T_3 in critically ill, thermally injured patients. J Trauma 1980;20:713–721.
8. Talwar KK, Sawhney RC, Rastogi RK. Serum levels of thyrotropin, thyroid hormones and their response to thyrotropin releasing hormone in infective febrile illness. J Clin Endocrinol Metab 1977;44:398–403.
9. Lutz JH, Gregerman RF, Spaulding SW, Hornick RB, Dawkins AT, Jr. Thyroxine binding proteins, free thyroxine and thyroxine turnover interrelationships during acute infectious illness in man. J Clin Endocrinol Metab 1972;35:230–249.
10. Smith SJ, Bas G, Gerbrandy J, Docter R, Visser TJ, Hennemann G. Lowering of serum 3,3'5-triiodothyronine thyroxine ratio in patients with myocardial infarction; relationship with extent of tissue injury. Eur J Clin Invest 1978;8:99–102.
11. Brandt MR, Skovsted L, Kehlet H, Hansen JM. Rapid decrease in plasma triiodothyronine during surgery and epidural anesthesia independent of afferent neurogenic stimuli and cortisol. Lancet 1976;2:1333–1335.
12. Chopra IJ, Solomon DH, Chopra U, Young RT, Chua Teco GN. Alterations in circulating thyroid hormones and thyrotropin in hepatic cirrhosis: evidence for euthyroidism despite subnormal serum triiodothyronine. J Clin Endocrinol Metab 1974;39:501–511.
13. Alexander CM, Kaptein EM, Lum SMC, Spencer CA, Kumar D, Nicoloff JT. Pattern of recovery of thyroid hormone indices associated with treatment of diabetes mellitus. J Clin Endocrinol Metab 1982;54:362–366.
14. Spencer CA, Lum SMC, Wilber JF, Kaptein EM, Nicoloff JT. Dynamics of the thyrotropin and thyroid hormone changes in fasting. J Clin Endocrinol Metab 1983;56:887–888.
15. Bermudez F, Surks MI, Oppenheimer JI. High incidence of decreased serum triiodothyronine concentration in patients with nonthyroidal disease. J Clin Endocrinol Metab 1975;41:27–40.
16. Rothwell PM, Udwadia ZF, Lawlser PG. Thyrotropin concentration predicts outcome in critical illness. Anesthesia 1993 1993;48:373–376.
17. Refetoff S and Nicoloff JT. Thyroid hormone transport and metabolism. In: DeGroot LJ, ed. Endocrinology, vol. 1. Saunders, Philadelphia, 1995, pp. 560–582.
18. Lum SMC, Nicoloff JT, Spencer, CA, Kaptein EM. Peripheral tissue mechanism for maintenance of serum T3 values in a T4-deficient state in man. J Clin Invest 1984;73:571–575.
19. Engler D, Merkelbach U, Steiger G, Burger AG. The monodeiodination of triiodothyronine and reverse triiodothyronine in man: a quantitative evaluation of the pathway by the use of turnover rate techniques. J Clin Endocrinol Metab 1984;58:49–61.
20. LoPresti JS, Nicoloff JT. 3,5,3'-triiodothyronine sulfate: a major metabolite in 3,5,3'-triiodothyronine metabolism in man. J Clin Endocrinol Metab 1993;78:688–692.

21. Dlott RS, Nicoloff JT, LoPresti JS. Does triiodothyroacetic accid (T_3AC) formation mediate the low T_3 state (LT_3S) in man? Program of 74th Annual Meeting of the Endocrine Society, San Antonio, TX 1992, 136 (338).
22. Arem R, Wiener GJ, Kaplan SG, Kim H-S, Reichlin S, Kaplan MM. Reduced tissue thyroid hormone levels in fatal illness. Metabolism 1993;42:1102–1108.
23. Faber J, Francis-Thomsen H, Lumholtz IB, Kirkegaard C, Sierbach-Nielsen K, Friis T. Kinetic studies of thyroxine, 3,5,3'-triiodothyronine, 3,3',5'-triiodothyronine, 3' diiodothyronine, 3,3'-diiodothyronine and 3'-monoiodothyronine in patients with liver cirrhosis. J Clin Endocrinol Metab 1981;53: 978–984.
24. LoPresti JS, Spencer CA, Nicoloff JT. Search for a missing deiodinative metabolite of T4 in fasting man. Program of the 72nd Endocrine Society, Atlanta, GA 1990, 211 (245).
25. Kaptein EM, Robinson WJ, Grieb DA, Nicoloff JT. Peripheral serum thyroxine, triiodothyronine, and reverse triiodothyronine kinetics in the low thyroxine state of acute nonthyroidal illness. J Clin Invest 1982;69:526–535.
26. Spaulding SW, Smith TJ, Hinkle PM, Davis FB, Kung M-P, Roth JA. Studies on the biological activity of triiodothyronine sulfate. J Clin Endocrinol Metab 1992;74:1062–1067.
27. Young WF, Gorman CA, Weinshilboum RM. Triiodothyronine: a substrate for thermostabile and thermolabile forms of human phenol sulfotransferase. Endocrinology 1988;122:1816–1824.
28. Chopra IS, Wu SY, Teio GNC, Santini F. A radioimmunoassay for measurement of 3,5,3'-triiodothyronine sulfate: studies in thyroidal and nonthyroidal diseases, pregnancy and neonatal life. J Clin Endocrinol Metab 1992;75:189–194.
29. Menegay C, Juge C, Burger AG. Pharmacokinetics of 3,5,3'-triiodothyroacetic acid and its effects on serum TSH levels. Acta Endocrinologica 1989;121:651–658.
30. DeFranzo RA, Ferrannini E. Regulation of intermediary metabolism during fasting and refeeding. In: DeGroot LJ, ed. Endocrinology, vol. 2. Saunders, Philadelphia, 1995;pp. 1389–1410.
31. Gardner DR, Kaplan MM, Stanley CA, Utiger RD. Effect of triiodothyronine replacement on the metabolic and pituitary responses to starvation. N Engl J Med 1979;300:579–584.
32. Burman KD, Wartofsky L, Dinterman RE, Kesler P, Wannemacher RW, Jr. The effect of T_3 and reverse T_3 administration on muscle protein catabolism during fasting as measured by 3-methylhistidine excretion. Metabolism 1979;28:805–813.
33. Fisler JS, Kaptein EM, Drinick EJ, Nicoloff JT, Yoshimura NN, Swendseid ME. Metabolic and hormonal factors as predictors of nitrogen retention in obese men consuming very low calorie diets. Metabolism 1985;34:101–105.
34. Croxson MS, Ibbertson HK. Low serum triiodothyronine (T_3) and hypothyroidism in anorexia nervosa. J Clin Endocrinol Metab 1977;44:167–174.
35. Byerley LO, Helier D. Metabolic effects of triiodothyronine replacement during fasting in obese subjects. J Clin Endocrinol Metab 1996;81:968–976.
36. Kaptein EM, Grieb DA, Spencer CA, Wheeler WS, Nicoloff JT. Thyroxine metabolism in the low thyroxine state of critical nonthyroidal illness. J Clin Endocrinol Metab 1981;53:764–771.
37. Chopra IJ, Huang TS, Hurd RE, Beredo A, Solomon DH. A competitive ligand binding assay for measurement of thyroid hormone-binding inhibitor in serum and tissues. J Clin Endocrinol Metab 1984;58:619–628.
38. Chopra IJ, Huang TS, Beredo A, Solomon DH, Chua-Teco GN, Mead JF. Evidence for an inhibitor of extrathyroidal conversion of thyroxine to 3,5,3'-triiodothyronine in serum of patients with nonthyroidal illnesses. J Clin Endocrinol Metab 1985;60:666–672.
39. Huang TS, Hurd RE, Chopra IJ, Stevens P, Solomon DH, Young LS. Inhibition of phagocytosis and chemiluminescence in human leukocytes by a lipid soluble factor in normal tissues. Infect Immun 1984;46:544–550.
40. Haynes IG, Lockett SJ, Farmer MJ, et al. Is oleic acid the thyroxine binding inhibitor in the serum of ill patients? Clin Endocrinol 1989;31:25–30.
41. Reilly CP, Welley ML. Slow thyroxine binding globulin in the pathogenesis of increased dialyzable fraction of thyroxine in nonthyroidal illness. J Clin Endocrinol Metab 1983;57:15–18.
42. Slag MF, Morley JE, Elson MK, Croxson TW, Nuttall FQ, Shafer RB. Hypothyroxinemia in critically ill patients as a predictor of high mortality. JAMA 1981;245:43–45.
43. Kaptein EM, Weiner JM, Robinson WJ, Wheeler WS, Nicoloff JT. Relationship of altered thyroid hormone indices to survival in nonthyroidal illness. Clin Endocrinol 1982;16:565–579.
44. Phillips RH, Valente WA, Caplan ES, Connor TB, Wisweil JG. Circulating thyroid hormone changes in acute trauma: prognostic implications for clinical outcome. J Trauma 1984;24:116–119.

45. Kaufman DA, Dlott R, Townsend R, Mizuno L, Weiner J, Nicoloff J. Indices of thyroid function as predictors of outcome in critically ill patients. Clin Res 1988;36:101A.
46. Whicher JT, Evans SW. Cytokines in disease. Clin Chem 1990;26:1269–1281.
47. Kakuscka I, Romero LI, Clark BD, et al. Suppression of thyrotropin-releasing hormone gene expression by interleukin-1-beta in the rat: implications for nonthyroidal illness. Neuroendocrinology 1994;59:129–134.
48. Stouthard JML, Van der Poll T, Endert E, et al. Effects of acute and chronic interleukin-6 administration on thyroid hormone metabolism in humans. J Clin Endocrinol Metab 1994;79:1342–1346.
49. vanderPall T, Romijn JA, Wiersinga WM, Sauerwein HP. Tumor necrosis factor: a putative mediator of the sick euthyroid syndrome in man. J Clin Endocrinol Metab 1990;71:1567–1572.
50. Dubuis JM, Dayer JM, Siegrist-Kaiser CA, Burger AG. Human recombinant interleukin I-β decreases plasma thyroid hormone and thyroid stimulating hormone levels in rats. Endocrinology 1988;123:2175–2181.
51. Pang X-P, Hershman JM, Mirell CJ, Pekary EA. Impairment of hypothalamic-pituitary-thyroid function in rats treated with human recombinant tumor necrosis factor-α (cachetin). Endocrinology 1989;125:76–84.
52. Brabant G, Brabant A, Ranft U, et al. Circadian and pulsatile thyrotropin secretion in euthyroid man under the influence of thyroid hormone and glucocorticoid administration. J Clin Endocrinol Metab 1987;65:83–88.
53. LoPresti JS, Eigen A, Kaptein E, Anderson KP, Spencer CA, Nicoloff JT. Alterations in 3,3′,5′-triiodothyronine metabolism in response to propylthiouracil, dexamethasone, and thyroxine administration in man. J Clin Invest 1989;84:1650–1656.
54. Davidson MB, Chopra IJ. Effect of carbohydrate and noncarbohydrate series of calories on plasma 3,5,3′-tiiodothyronine concentrations in man. J Clin Endocrinol Metab 1979;48:577–581.
55. Otten MH, Hennemann G, Docter R, Visser TJ. The role of dietary fat in peripheral thyroid hormone metabolism. Metabolism 1980;29:930–935.
56. Hamblin PS, Dyer SA, Mohn VS, et al. Relationship between thyrotropin and thyroxine changes during recovery from severe hypothyroxinemia of critical illness. J Clin Endocrinol Metab 1986;62:717–722.
57. Spencer CA, Eigen A, Shen D, et al. Sensitive TSH tests—specificity limitations for screening for thyroid disease in hospitalized patients. Clin Chem 1987;33:1391–1396.
58. Hughes J-N, Enjalbert A, Burger AG, Voiral M-J, Sebaoun J, Epelbaum J. Sensitivity of thyrotropin (TSH) secretion to 3,5,3′-triiodothyronine and TSH-released hormone in rat during starvation. Endocrinology 1986;119:253–269.
59. Samuels MH, Luther M, Ridgway EC. Effect of hydrocortisone on pulsatile pituitary glycoprotein secretion. J Clin Endocrinol Metab 1994;78:211–215.
60. vanderBergh G, deZeghe F, Vlasselaers D, Scheta M, Verwaest C, Ferdinande P, Lauer's P. Thyrotropin-releasing hormone in critical illness: from a dopamine-dependent test to a strategy for increasing low serum triiodothyronine, prolactin, and growth hormone concentrations. Crit Care Med 1996;24:590–595.
61. Beck-Peccoz P, Amr S, Menezes-Ferreira MM, Faglia G, Weintraub BD. Decreased receptor binding of biologically inactive thyrotropin in central hypothyroidism. Effect of treatment with thyrotropin-releasing hormone. N Engl J. Med 1985;312:1085–1090.
62. Kaptein EM, Spencer CA, Kamiel MB, Nicoloff JT. Prolonged dopamine administration and thyroid hormone economy in normal and critically ill patients. J Clin Endocrinol Metab 1980;51:387–393.
63. Zipser RD, Davenport MW, Martin KL, Swinney RR, Davis CL, Horton R. Hyperreninemic hypoaldosteronism in the critically ill: a new entity. J Clin Endocrinol Metab 1981;53:867–873.
64. Novitsky D, Cooper DKC, Swanepoel A. Inotropic effect of triiodothyronine (T_3) in low cardiac output following cardioplegic arrest and cardiopulmonary bypass: an initial experience in patients undergoing open heart surgery. Eur J Cardiothoracic Surg 1989;3:140–143.
65. Novitsky D, Cooper DKC, Barton CI, et al. Triiodothyronine as an inotropic agent after open heart surgery. J Thoracic Cardiovasc Surg 1989;98:972–976.
66. Klemperer JD, Klein I, Gomez M, Helm RE, Ojamaa K, Thomas SJ, Isom OW, Kreiger K. Thyroid hormone treatment after coronary-artery bypass surgery. N Engl J Med 1995;333:1522–1527.
67. Brent GA, Hershman JM. Thyroxine therapy in patients with severe nonthyroidal illness and low serum thyroxine concentration. Ann Intern Med 1986;103:1–7.
68. LoPresti JS, Fried JC, Spencer CA, Nicoloff JT. Unique alterations of thyroid hormone indices in the acquired immunodeficiency syndrome (AIDS). Ann Intern Med 1989;110:970–975.

69. Coodley GO, Loveless MO, Nelson HD, Coodley MK. Endocrine function in the HIV wasting syndrome. J Acquired Immune Defic Syndrome 1994;7:46–53.
70. Fried JC, LoPresti JS, Micon M, Bauer M, Tuchschmidt J, Nicoloff JT. Serum triiodothyronine values. Prognostic indicators of acute mortality due to pneumocystis carinii pneumonia associated with acquired immunodeficiency syndrome. Arch Int Med 1990;150:406–409.
71. Hommes MJT, Romijn JA, Endert E, et al. Hypothyroid-like regulation of the pituitary thyroid axis in stable human immunodeficiency virus infection. Metabolism 1993;42:556–561.
72. O'Connor CB, Sanvito M, DeCherney GS. Falling CD4 counts in HIV infection: relationship to thyroid hormone and thyroid hormone binding globulin (TBG). A review and new findings. Endocrinology 1995;5:371–376.
73. Yamanaka T, Ido K, Kumura K, Saito T. Serum levels of thyroid hormones in liver disease. Clin Chim Acta 1980;101:45–55.
74. Schussler GC, Schaffner F, Karn F. Increased serum thyroid hormone binding and decreased free hormone in chronic active liver disease. N Engl J Med 1978;299:510–515.
75. Walfish PG, Orrego H, Israel Y, Blake J, Kalant H. Serum triiodothyronine and other clinical and laboratory indices of alcoholic liver disease. Ann Intern Med 1979;91:13–16.
76. Kaptein EM, Feinstein EI, Nicoloff JT, Massry SG. Serum reverse triiodothyronine and thyroxine kinetics in patients with chronic renal failure. J Clin Endocrinol Metab. 1983;57:181–189.
77. Soffer E, Pelet D, Segal S, Bar-Khayim Y. Thyroid function in hemodialysis. Israel J Med Sci 1979;15:836–839.
78. Spratt DI, Pont A, Miller MB, et al. Hyperthyroxinemia in patients with acute psychiatric disorders. Am J Med 1982;73:41–48.
79. Hein MD, Jackson IM. Review: thyroid function in psychiatric illness. Gen Hosp Psychiatry 1990;12:232–244.
80. Ain KB, Mau Y, Refetoff S. Reduced clearance rate of thyroxine binding globulin (TBG) with increased sialylation: a mechanism for estrogen-induced elevations of serum TBG concentration. J Clin Endocrinol Metab 1987;65:689–692.
81. Glinoer D, DeNayer P, Bourdoux P. Regulation of maternal thyroid function during pregnancy. J Clin Endocinol Metab 1990;71:276–287.
82. Goodwin TM, Montoro M, Mestman JH, Pekary EA, Hershman JM. The role of chorionic gonadotropin in transient hyperthyroidism of hyperemesis gravidarum. J Clin Endocrinol Metab 1992;75:1333–1337.

9 Pathophysiology of Water Metabolism During Critical Illness

Mary H. Parks, MD
and Joseph G. Verbalis, MD

CONTENTS
    INTRODUCTION
    NORMAL PHYSIOLOGY OF WATER METABOLISM
    EFFECTS OF DRUG AND AGE ON WATER AND SOLUTE
       HOMEOSTASIS
    DISORDERS OF WATER METABOLISM
    WATER METABOLISM IN CRITICAL ILLNESSES
    CONCLUSION

INTRODUCTION

Maintenance of blood volume and pressure that is adequate for perfusion of vital body tissues and organs is crucial for the survival of organisms during periods of acute stress, such as critical illnesses. As might be expected of such important functions, many complex and overlapping physiological defense mechanisms have evolved to defend body fluid homeostasis during such periods. The efficacy of these mechanisms is attested to by the fact that derangements of body water and electrolytes do not occur even more frequently during disease states. Nonetheless, hypo- and hypernatremia represent the most common electrolyte disorders encountered in clinical practice today, and in order to understand both the pathogenesis and the appropriate therapy of these disorders in critically ill patients, it is crucial to understand body water metabolism and its disorders, since this accounts for the major part of regulation of the concentration in the extracellular fluid and blood. This chapter briefly summarizes the normal regulation of body water and then reviews in greater detail specific disorders associated with disruption of this normally finely tuned system for maintaining body fluids at physiologically appropriate volumes and solute concentrations.

NORMAL PHYSIOLOGY OF WATER METABOLISM

Water homeostasis in humans involves a balance of fluid intake and renal water excretion. Total fluid intake is comprised of a regulated amount determined by thirst and

From: *Contemporary Endocrinology: Endocrinology of Critical Disease*
Edited by K. P. Ober   Humana Press Inc., Totowa, NJ

an unregulated amount that is consumed with meals and social beverages. The renal excretion of water is regulated by the hypothalamus through release of arginine vasopressin (AVP), which binds to AVP V_2 receptors located on the distal collecting tubules causing insertion of water channels (aquaporins) along the luminal surface with subsequent reabsorption of water through these channels *(1)*. This system is tightly regulated to maintain the serum osmolality within a narrow range (275–290 mOsm/kg H_2O), with minor fluctuations of the serum osmolality resulting in a rapid hormonal response and more pronounced alterations of the serum osmolality affecting the thirst center with changes in fluid intake to maintain total fluid balance.

The primary regulator of pituitary AVP secretion is the effective osmotic pressure of plasma, with sodium being the most significant effective solute. Changes in plasma osmolality are detected by osmoreceptors located in the anterolateral hypothalamus and bear a directly proportional relation to AVP secretion (Fig. 1). The slope of this relationship is relatively steep, with a 1% change in serum osmolality leading to a change in plasma AVP levels of approx 1 pg/mL. There is also a positive linear relationship between plasma AVP levels and urine osmolality, with increasing AVP levels resulting in increasing urine osmolality. However, once plasma AVP levels reach approx 5 pg/mL, urinary concentration is maximal, and no further antidiuresis can occur despite further increases in AVP secretion *(2)*.

Higher levels of AVP produce vasoconstriction by acting at AVP V_1 receptors located on arterial blood vessels. This function of AVP is the basis for its response to hypotension and hypovolemia as a result of stimulation of baroreceptors located in the great vessels of the aorta and in the heart. These sensors detect changes in blood pressure and volume with decreases in these hemodynamic parameters leading to stimulation of AVP release through activation of the vagal and glossopharyngeal nerves. In contrast to the extremely sensitive osmotic regulation of AVP secretion, a fall in blood pressure of at least 20–30% is required before a significant AVP response is noted *(3)*. However, the amount of AVP released to hypovolemic stimuli is markedly greater than that required for antidiuresis in order to cause vasoconstriction and thereby stabilize perfusion pressure (Fig. 1). Although this function and response of AVP is critical for the maintenance of perfusion to vital organs, it can also contribute to disturbances of water metabolism seen during critical illness.

Other stimuli known to activate AVP release include hypoxia, hypercapnia, and hypoglycemia. These conditions most likely mediate their effects through baroreceptor stimulation as opposed to direct stimulation of the neurohypophysis. Nausea is the most potent stimulus to AVP secretion, which is mediated by activation of afferent vagal pathways from the gastrointestinal tract to the area postrema and nucleus tractus solitarius of the medulla (emetic center), though usually this is a short-lived stimulus. Recent studies have demonstrated stimulation of AVP secretion by hormones, such as cholecystokinin and angiotensin II, but the significance of these factors as potential contributors to disorders of water metabolism have yet to be elucidated *(4)*.

EFFECTS OF DRUGS AND AGE ON WATER AND SOLUTE HOMEOSTASIS

Drugs

The effects of drugs on water balance have been recognized since 1966 when the oral sulfonylurea, chlorpropamide, was found to have an antidiuretic effect in patients with diabetes insipidus *(5)*. Since that time the number of drugs shown to potentiate antidiuresis

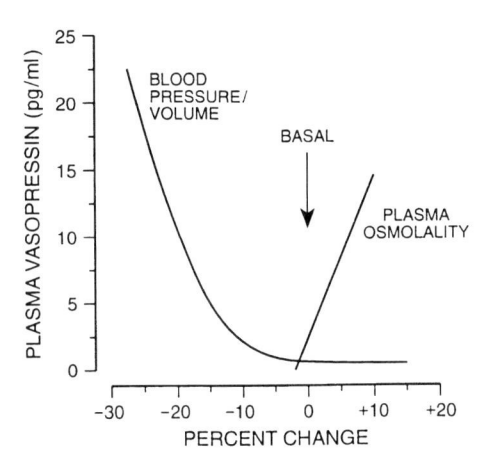

Fig. 1. Comparative sensitivity of AVP secretion in response to increases in plasma osmolality decreases in blood volume or blood pressure in human subjects. The arrow indicates the low plasma AVP concentrations found at basal plasma osmolality (modified with permission from ref. *3*).

and potentially induce hyponatremia has increased dramatically, acting through various mechanisms including enhanced AVP secretion, direct activation of renal AVP receptors, potentiation of the antidiuretic effects of AVP, or some combination of these. Other pharmacologic agents cause hyponatremia via non-AVP-mediated actions, such as diuretics or agents that impair renal sodium conservation. However, even in these cases, plasma AVP levels may still be inappropriately elevated if there is accompanying volume contraction with secondary baroreceptor-mediated AVP secretion *(6)*.

Drug-induced hyponatremia usually arises in conjunction with ingestion or administration of hypotonic fluids, or in the elderly. As an example, severe hyponatremia has recently been reported in conjunction with administration of a variety of psychotropic agents with resolution of the hypoosmolar symptoms following discontinuation of the drug and institution of fluid restriction *(7,8)*. The hyponatremia seen with this class of drugs is often associated with a tendency for compulsive water drinking in these patients, or when they are prescribed to older patients who have impaired free water excretion *(see below)*. As more medications are reported to cause the syndrome of inappropriate antidiuretic hormone secretion (SIADH) and dilutional hyponatremia, clinicians must therefore be cognizant of this potential complication of many different types of medications, take a detailed drug history in all cases, and recognize factors, such as excessive fluid intake and age that predispose patients to develop hypoosmolality while on these medications.

In contrast to the many different drugs that induce hyponatremia, there are only a few pharmacologic agents that interfere with AVP action; some of these agents have been employed as treatment for chronic SIADH. Their mechanisms of action include impairment of cyclic 3′,5′-adenosine monophosphate action in the distal nephron (e.g., demeclocycline, lithium), induction of an osmotic diuresis (e.g., urea), and inhibition of AVP release (e.g., phenytoin, ethanol) *(9)*. Unfortunately, therapeutic use of these agents for SIADH is limited by their many side effects, including renal toxicity, idiosyncratic drug toxicity, and tolerability. However, the recent development of selective nonpeptide AVP V_2 receptor antagonists provides a potential new treatment option for SIADH and other hyponatremic states associated with elevated plasma AVP levels *(10)*.

Increasing Age

The physiologic mechanisms that regulate water and sodium balance are commonly affected by the normal aging process. Electrolyte disorders, particularly sodium derangements, are frequently seen in the elderly, with various studies reporting incidences as high as 18 and 4% for hyponatremia and hypernatremia, respectively (11,12). These patients often have medical or neurologic illnesses that can affect AVP secretion, alter renal concentrating mechanisms, and/or alter thirst perception. Furthermore, these patients are often on medications that can disrupt the finely tuned mechanisms that regulate water and solute homeostasis.

Most studies have not shown an age-related decrease in neurosecretory functions of the supraoptic or paraventricular nuclei (13) of the hypothalamus. Instead, there appears to be an increased osmoreceptor hypersensitivity with elevated plasma AVP levels in older vs younger patients with similar serum osmolalities (14). In contrast, AVP release appears to be blunted in response to decreased blood volume and pressure stimuli, suggesting a decreased baroreceptor sensitivity for AVP secretion (15). Based on these findings, it has been hypothesized that impaired baroreceptor function accompanying normal aging leads to decreased inhibitory input to AVP neurons and that this loss of inhibition results in heightened osmoreceptor sensitivity for AVP secretion (16). Renal water and sodium concentrating ability also diminishes with age, as has been demonstrated in both healthy and hospitalized elderly patients (17). A reduced glomerular filtration rate (GFR) and impaired free water clearance contribute to the impaired renal concentrating and diluting capacities associated with aging (18). The role of chronic plasma AVP elevations contributing to age-related impairments of renal diluting ability has been studied in rats, with evidence that chronic exposure to AVP may result in diminished renal responsiveness to this hormone (19), although this finding has not yet been demonstrated in humans.

Along with renal water conservation and excretion, the intake of fluids is an integral part of maintaining water homeostasis. In this regard, it is significant that the thirst mechanism in the elderly is altered, especially in those patients who have had cerebral vascular accidents or are demented. In these extreme settings, the perception of thirst can be blunted or absent, and such patients are at increased risk of developing dehydration and hyperosmolality during conditions of increased fluid losses (e.g., diarrhea, fever, exposure). Interestingly, studies of healthy, elderly individuals also demonstrate a significantly blunted thirst perception. When subjected to water deprivation then allowed free access to water, older subjects reported less sensation of thirst and drank less than younger subjects despite identical weight losses and changes in plasma volume (14). Mechanisms for the diminished thirst perception in healthy, older patients are unclear, but possibilities include cerebral cortical dysfunction or selectively altered osmoreceptor sensitivity to thirst, since some studies have suggested the presence of separate osmoreceptors for thirst and AVP secretion (20).

Despite these perturbations in the regulation of water and solute homeostasis in the elderly, plasma sodium concentrations ([Na^+]) are usually normal in healthy individuals, which likely reflects maintenance of homeostasis from adequate intake of palatable liquids and food in conjunction with renal water and sodium conservation. Nonetheless, it is important to be aware of the increased susceptibility of this population to the development of hyponatremia and hypernatremia during critical illness, physical incapacity, and in association with certain medications. For example, administration of hypotonic IV fluids to the older patient who has an elevated baseline plasma AVP level coupled with a defective renal-sodium conservation capacity, or who is on diuretic drugs, may easily lead to hyponatremia. Conversely, the use of hypertonic nutritional supplements in the older patient with increased isotonic fluid losses and a diminished renal water conservation capacity can just as easily result in hypernatremia. Both of these types of patients can present with a decreased sensorium, which may erroneously be attributed to age-related cortical dysfunction, but following appropriate correction of the water and electrolyte derangements, a marked improvement of cognitive mental function often results.

DISORDERS OF WATER METABOLISM

Disturbances in the regulation of water homeostasis associated with critical illnesses may result in a clinical picture that is clinically indistinguishable from primary disorders of AVP action. The purpose of this section is to familiarize the clinician with those disorders of insufficient or excess AVP effect. A complete review of the pathophysiology of these disorders is beyond the scope of this chapter, and the reader is referred to several recent review articles that address this topic *(21–23)*.

Disorders of Insufficient AVP Secretion or AVP Effect

Diabetes insipidus (DI) refers to the insufficient release or action of AVP and is characterized by excretion of large volumes of hypotonic urine (typically >2.5 L/d) in the absence of significant glucosuria. The inability to secrete an adequate amount of AVP in response to an osmotic stimulus is commonly referred to as central or neurogenic DI, and may result from acquired (e.g., pituitary-hypothalamic surgery, head trauma), genetic (e.g., autosomal-dominant AVP gene defect), or idiopathic diseases that destroy the AVP-producing neurons or posterior pituitary. Renal resistance to AVP effect with normal or elevated plasma levels of AVP is referred to as nephrogenic DI. Nephrogenic DI can also result from acquired (e.g., drugs, hypercalcemia), genetic (e.g., X-linked recessive defect in the vasopressin V_2 receptor), or idiopathic causes. An excessive daily intake of fluid can also result in diminished AVP secretion in the setting of polyuria. This condition is called primary polydipsia and may be secondary to an abnormal thirst mechanism (dipsogenic polydipsia) or from psychiatric disorders with compulsive drinking behavior (psychogenic polydipsia).

Patients with neurogenic or nephrogenic DI are typically able to maintain a normal serum osmolality from adequate oral intake of fluids. However, hypernatremia, hyperosmolality, and dehydration can occur if the patient is unable to drink fluids as a result of incapacitation or a defective thirst mechanism. Similarly, primary polydipsic patients rarely develop significant hypoosmolality unless they have a renal diluting defect or an antidiuretic agent is inadvertently or inappropriately administered. In this setting, the primary polydipsic patient can continue to consume large amounts of fluids leading to water intoxication with hyponatremia, central nervous system impairment, and death. Accurate diagnosis of the different causes of polyuria is therefore critical, since proper treatment will relieve the symptoms of true central DI, whereas inappropriate use of an antidiuretic agent can lead to significant morbidity and mortality in patients with primary polydipsia. The correct diagnosis can generally be made based on the clinical history and results of urine volumes, osmolality, and response to exogenous AVP plus measurement of plasma AVP levels during a water-deprivation test. This test can still occasionally yield equivocal results, especially if the patient has a partial defect of AVP secretion or action. In this setting, the patient may be given a short trial of exogenous AVP or the long-acting vasopressin V_2 receptor agonist dDAVP (desmopressin) with careful monitoring of urine volumes and plasma [Na^+] or osmolality.

Disorders of Excess AVP Secretion or AVP Effect

Disorders of excess AVP secretion or action commonly result in hyponatremia and hypoosmolality. However, the presence of hypoosmolality does not always indicate inappropriate secretion of AVP, since diverse disorders can lead to imbalances of water metabolism. A detailed discussion of the many causes of hypoosmolality is beyond the scope of this chapter, and this section will briefly focus on the syndrome of inappropriate antidiuretic hormone release (SIADH), the most common cause of euvolemic hyponatremia.

The diagnostic criteria for SIADH requires that the patient have true hypoosmolality with a urinary osmolality that is greater than maximally dilute (<100 mOsm/kg H_2O) and an elevated urinary Na^+ excretion. Clinical euvolemia must also be demonstrated since hypo- or hypervolemic hyponatremia may not be due to inappropriate AVP secretion. Finally, the clinician must be aware that SIADH is a diagnosis of exclusion and that other causes of hyponatremia must be excluded, including hypothyroidism, hypocortisolism, renal insufficiency, and diuretic use. Despite these defining criteria, SIADH may at times be difficult to distinguish between renal salt-wasting syndromes, and the patient may require a therapeutic trial of volume replacement via isotonic saline solution, which generally will not correct the hyponatremia of SIADH. Patients with SIADH can also develop secondary disorders of hypovolemia or hypervolemia, and under these conditions, they must be rendered euvolemic prior to applying the above diagnostic criteria.

With the development of sensitive radioimmunoassays for plasma AVP levels, it had been thought that measurement of the hormone would allow more definitive diagnosis of SIADH. However, plasma levels have been found to be within the normal range as well as undetectable in patients with all the classical features of SIADH. For this reason, some investigators have proposed using the term syndrome of inappropriate antidiuresis (SIAD) as opposed to the older term used in the original description of this disorder. Finally, measurements of plasma AVP have demonstrated elevated levels in certain hypoosmolar states in which the AVP secretion is inappropriate for the degree of plasma hypoosmolality, but appropriately secreted in response to other nonosmotic stimuli, such as volume depletion. This important physiologic response of AVP secretion is often the cause of impaired free water excretion in many critical illnesses, as will be discussed in many of the subsequent sections.

WATER METABOLISM IN CRITICAL ILLNESSES

Acquired Immune Deficiency Syndrome (AIDS)

Hyponatremia is a fairly common finding in patients with AIDS and the AIDS-related complex (ARC; Fig. 2). Retrospective and prospective studies report incidences of 28–57% (24) with significantly higher mortality rates and prolonged hospitalization compared to normonatremic patients (25). The etiologies for this electrolyte abnormality are varied, reflecting the multiple organ systems affected by this disease.

Approximately one-third of these cases are due to volume depletion, usually from vomiting, diarrhea, and unreplaced insensible fluid losses. These patients frequently

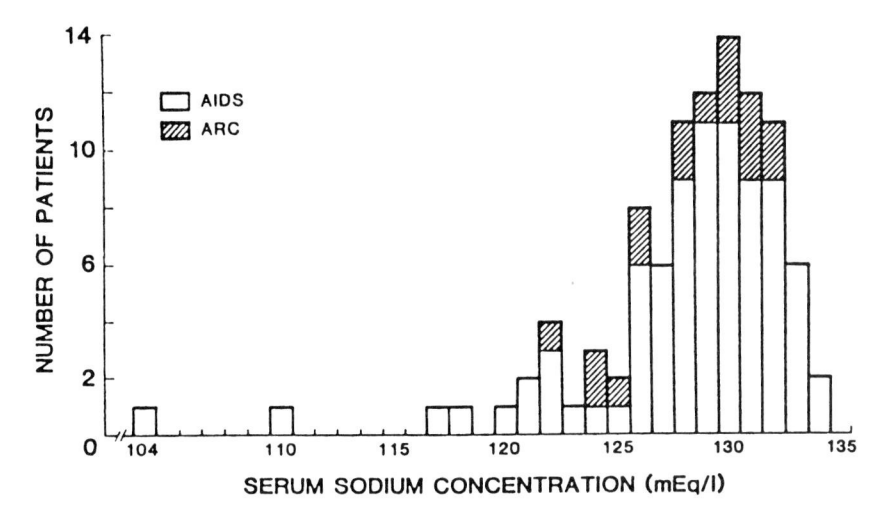

Fig. 2. Distribution of serum sodium concentrations in 83 hospitalized hyponatremic patients with AIDS (open bars) or ARC (shaded bars) (reproduced with permission from ref. 25).

have a urinary Na$^+$ concentration ≤20 mEq/L and clinical findings of hypovolemia. The hyponatremia in this setting is usually easily corrected with rehydration using isotonic saline. Most of the hyponatremic patients, however, are euvolemic with a high urinary Na$^+$ concentration (typically ≥70 mEq/L) and an inappropriately elevated urine osmolality in relation to the plasma osmolality. If assayed, measurable AVP levels are detectable despite hypoosmolality (Fig. 3). After assessing thyroid and adrenal function, one-half to two-thirds of these cases have been shown to be due to SIADH (25,26).

The etiology of the SIADH in AIDS and ARC patients is not easily defined. Prospective analysis of this subgroup revealed a high incidence of pulmonary and central nervous system infections. *Pneumocystis carinii* pneumonia accounted for the majority of the pulmonary infections, although the studies did not evaluate the degree of hypoxemia present or the need for ventilatory support in these patients, both of which could contribute to the SIADH (25,26). As expected, treatment in this group consisted of strict fluid restriction and only on rare occasions the use of demeclocycline.

An infrequent, but important potential cause of hyponatremia in AIDS is adrenal insufficiency. Autopsy studies have revealed a >50% incidence of adrenal pathology in patients with AIDS, with the most common being infection with cytomegalovirus (27,28). Symptoms of hypocortisolism, such as weakness, nausea, vomiting, and orthostatic hypotension, are relatively nonspecific and commonly seen in AIDS patients. However, the true incidence of adrenal insufficiency based on an inadequate cortisol response to rapid ACTH stimulation is estimated to be <10% (29). Interestingly, several reports have indicated a supranormal baseline cortisol level compared with controls, but a blunted response in the 17-deoxysteroid pathway after both rapid and prolonged ACTH stimulation, consistent with a decreased adrenal reserve (30). This suggests that such patients may be at increased risk of becoming adrenally insufficient when challenged with stressors or placed on drugs that either interfere with adrenal function or enhance glucorticoid clearance. Because of the above considerations, the possibility of

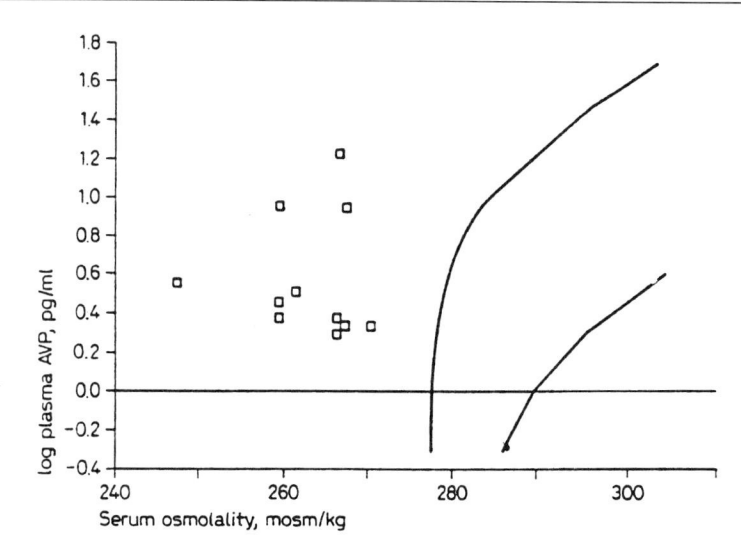

Fig. 3. Plasma AVP levels in relation to plasma osmolality in 11 hyponatremic euvolemic patients with AIDS. Normal levels of AVP in relation to plasma osmolaity should be within the area bounded by the two solid lines; below these ranges, AVP should be suppressed to levels beneath the detection limits for this hormone (reproduced with permission from ref. 26 et al.,1989).

adrenal insufficiency should always be entertained and evaluated in a patient with AIDS and hyponatremia, especially since in this case, the electrolyte abnormality as well as the patient's symptoms can be easily corrected with glucocorticoid replacement.

A less common cause of hyponatremia in patients with AIDS is hyporeninemic hypoaldosteronism (31,32). These patients often present with hyperkalemia and a mild metabolic acidosis, although there have been reported cases with plasma [Na$^+$] <130 mEq/L. After rapid ACTH stimulation testing, glucocorticoid secretion appears intact, but baseline renin and aldosterone levels are low as is their response to furosemide and upright posture. Distinguishing this entity from primary adrenal insufficiency is important, because the former requires only replacement with mineralocorticoids, thereby avoiding unnecessary use of glucocorticoids, which could further compromise immune function in these already immunosuppressed patients.

In view of the multiple organs affected by HIV, it is not surprising that patients with ARC and AIDS can develop cardiomyopathy, HIV nephropathy, and/or cirrhosis. Hyponatremia in this setting is frequently due to hypervolemia, and treatment should be directed at correcting or controlling the edema-forming state. This may require the judicious use of diuretics, and fluid restriction or afterload reduction to improve cardiac function.

AIDS patients are also at risk for developing hypernatremia, although this occurs much less often than does hyponatremia. This disorder is most commonly seen in patients with an impaired sensorium and an abnormal thirst mechanism in the setting of large free water losses from decreased renal concentrating ability (33). DI is seldom seen in AIDS despite the extensive CNS pathology that can occur in these patients. Recently, a 30-yr-old male was reported who presented with DI and negative neuroimaging studies. Two months later, he developed panhypopituitarism, and repeat imaging studies revealed lesions consistent with cerebral toxoplasmosis (34). Consequently, symptoms suggestive of DI should be evaluated with magnetic resonance imaging of the brain and cerebrospinal fluid analysis for CNS infection, since underlying infections can respond to antimicrobials with possible alleviation of the polyuria and polydipsia.

In summary, sodium and water disturbances are frequent findings in patients with AIDS and ARC, with hyponatremia being the most common disorder. The potential causes of the electrolyte imbalance are numerous, but an approach focusing on the history, physical exam, and pertinent laboratory data with particular emphasis on the volume status, body fluid losses, and urinary Na$^+$ concentration will generally be successful in diagnosing and directing appropriate therapy in most such patients.

Hypothyroidism

Defects of free water clearance are well recognized in hypothyroid patients. However, hyponatremia rarely develops in mild hypothyroidism, but is limited to patients with more severe degrees of myxedema. Even in myxedematous patients, hyponatremia generally occurs in more elderly patients with concurrent medical problems, such as heart failure, infection, and renal failure *(35,36)*. In this setting, the pathophysiology of the hyponatremia may not be due to hypothyroidism alone, but rather to the complications of these accompanying medical problems. Despite the frequent occurrence of these other factors, which may contribute to the hypoosmolality, studies of hypothyroid patients without concomitant glucocorticoid deficiency have consistently revealed an inability to excrete an acutely administered water load *(37–39)*. This impairment appears to be neither dependent on AVP action nor is it due to impaired renal sodium transport, but rather appears to be a result of thyroid hormone deficiency and can be corrected by thyroid hormone replacement.

When hypothyroid patients are given a standard oral water load of 20 mL/kg of their body weight, they demonstrate a delay in the excretion of free water and a decreased peak urine flow compared to euthyroid patients *(37,40)*. Hypothyroid patients, however, are usually able to dilute their urine to <100 mOsm/kg H$_2$O (although values often still remain somewhat above those found in the euthyroid state), thus arguing against a significant contribution from inappropriate AVP secretion *(40;* Fig. 4). These findings are also supported by experimental animal studies involving normal controls, hypothyroid rats, and hypothyroid rats with congenital DI. Both strains of hypothyroid rats had a similar decreased fraction of water excretion compared to control animals, but urine osmolalities were similar in all groups regardless of their thyroid state or the presence or absence of AVP *(41)*.

Studies that have measured plasma AVP levels during hypothyroidism have produced conflicting data, with some investigators demonstrating appropriately suppressed AVP levels, whereas others detected normal to elevated AVP levels despite the presence of plasma hypoosmolality *(38,42–44)*. In one study of 20 myxedematous patients, plasma AVP levels were elevated in 15 patients and did not completely suppress after water loading despite the development of plasma hypoosmolality (267 ± 2 mOsm/kg H$_2$O) *(38)*. However, the functional effects of AVP in these subjects were quite variable, since 20% of the patients with elevated plasma AVP levels were capable of excreting >80% of the administered water load and 60% of the patients with suppressed AVP levels were incapable of excreting a maximally dilute urine. These inconsistencies may reflect different degrees of hypothyroidism, such that the patients with more extreme thyroid-deficient states stimulated AVP release via nonosmotic mechanisms (e.g., baroreceptors), whereas the patients with milder hypothyroidism had AVP-independent causes of impaired water excretion.

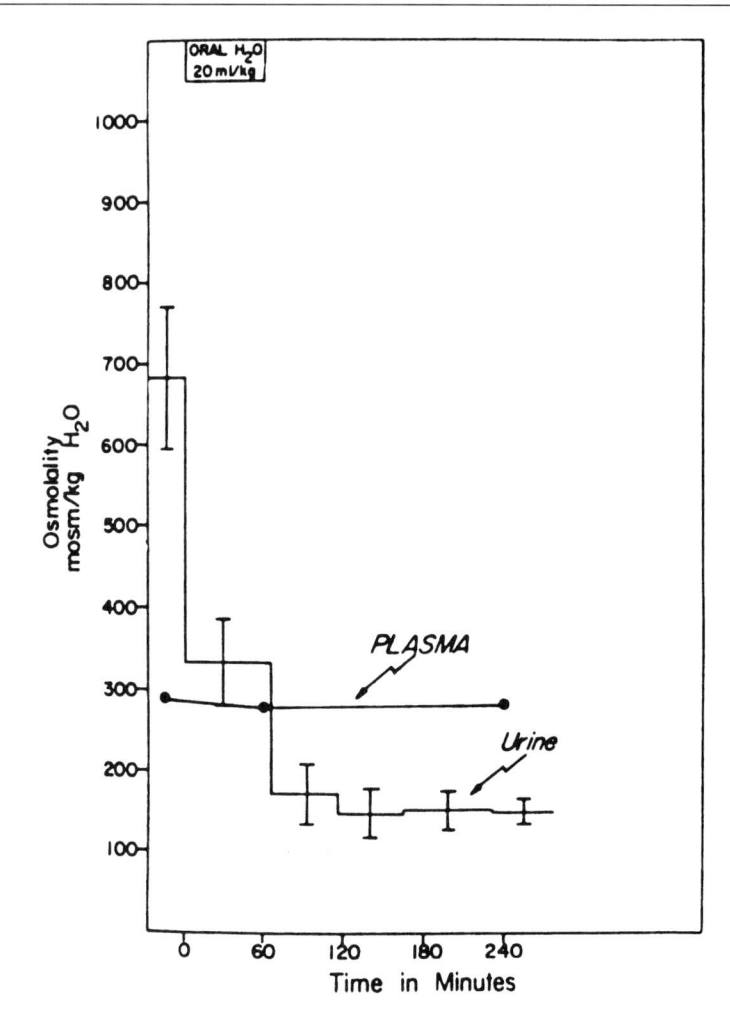

Fig. 4. Mean plasma and urine osmolalities in 16 patients with untreated myxedema for 6 h following an oral water load (20 mL/kg body wt). Urine osmolalities decreased significantly to <200 mosM/kg H2O by 4 h after the water load, indicating fairly normal renal diluting mechanisms in these patients (reproduced with permission from ref. *37*).

Although the pathological role of AVP remains unsettled, the sodium reabsorptive ability of the distal diluting segment of the nephron is clearly intact in patients with hypothyroidism. In both human and rat studies, urinary Na^+ concentrations were similar in both euthyroid and hypothyroid states *(37,41)*. Furthermore, tissue osmolality measured in different segments of rat kidneys during maximal water diuresis revealed similar fractional distal sodium reabsorption in both control and hypothyroid animals *(41)*. Therefore, the hyponatremia observed in hypothyroidism is clearly not due to excess natriuresis from defective renal sodium transport.

As mentioned previously, the defects of water metabolism in hypothyroidism can be completely corrected with thyroid hormone replacement. Interestingly, these defects can also be reversed with isotonic saline volume expansion or with administration of carbonic anhydrase inhibitors that block proximal Na^+ reabsorption, thereby increasing volume delivery to the distal tubule *(37)*. Based on all of these findings, the most likely mechanism accounting for the impaired water clearance of hypothyroidism is a reduced glomerular filtration rate, resulting in increased proximal sodium reabsorption and reduced volume delivery to the distal diluting segments of the kidney. This in turn appears to be secondary to a reduced renal blood flow from poor cardiac output and increased peripheral vascular resistance, which are commonly seen in severe hypothyroidism *(45,46)*. According to this perspective, hyponatremia can result either when fluid intake exceeds the impaired free water excretion capacity of the hypothyroid kidney, or alternatively when nonosmotic stimuli to AVP secretion cause even further decrements in free water excreting capacity of hypothyroid patients.

Adrenal Insufficiency

Similar to hypothyroidism, impaired water excretion is also a common manifestation of adrenal insufficiency *(47,48)*. As a result of this defect, hypoosmolality and hyponatremia are frequent laboratory findings in adrenally insufficient patients. The mechanism of impaired water clearance in this setting is multifactorial, reflective of the different functions of the adrenal cortex. The zona glomerulosa produces the mineralocorticoid aldosterone, which is primarily regulated by the renin–angiotensin system. The zona fasciculata is the site of glucocorticoid production and is regulated mainly by adrenocorticotropic hormone (ACTH) produced in the anterior pituitary, which in turn is under control of the hypothalamus via corticotropin-releasing hormone (CRH). Several studies in which either glucocorticoids or mineralocorticoids were given to adrenalectomized animals to produce isolated hormone deficiencies clearly demonstrated that each of these hormones is independently capable of causing a defect in water metabolism *(49–51)*. With the subsequent development of sensitive radioimmunoassays for plasma AVP, several studies have demonstrated elevated AVP levels during hypoosmolality in adrenally insufficient animals *(49,51,52)*. Therefore, multiple factors are involved in defective free water clearance of adrenal insufficiency, both AVP-independent (i.e., directly as a result of glucocorticoid or mineralocorticoid deficiency) and AVP-dependent.

Glucocorticoid deficiency is well recognized as a cause of impaired water excretion in both animals and humans. Mechanisms responsible for this defect have long been studied and debated, with a focus on impaired systemic and renal hemodynamics and/or elevated plasma AVP levels from nonosmotic stimuli. In support of AVP-independent factors is the observation that patients with damage to the neurohypophysis and absent or inadequate AVP secretion do not manifest symptoms of DI if there is concomitant glucocorticoid deficiency *(53)*. Green et al. *(54)* evaluated this phenomenon in adrenalectomized Brattleboro rats with congenital hypothalamic DI. When given a standard water load, adrenalectomized DI rats who were only given mineralocorticoid replacement had a significantly lower urine flow compared to control DI rats, suggesting an important role for glucocorticoids even in the absence of AVP as a cause for the impaired water excretion in hypocortisolism. Other investigators have evaluated the role of acute and chronic isolated glucocorticoid deficiency in rats with either an intact neurohypophysis or congenital DI, and found evidence supporting both AVP-dependent and AVP-independent factors in impaired renal excretion *(49)*. In this study, plasma AVP levels measured following an acute water load were significantly elevated in the 24-h (2.5 ± 0.2 pg/mL) and 14-d (2.4 ± 0.3 pg/mL) glucocorticoid-deficient animal compared to controls (1.1 ± 0.1 pg/mL). Defects in amount of urine excreted and urinary dilution were noted in the glucocorticoid-deficient animals at both 24 h and 14 d, whereas in the adrenalectomized DI rats, a defect in water excretion was not noted until after 14 d of glucocorticoid deficiency. Measurement of hemodynamic parameters revealed a significant decrease in systemic arterial pressure and glomerular filtration rate (GFR) at 24 h, and a decrease in the cardiac index and renal blood flow accompanied by an increase in systemic and renal vascular resistance compared to controls after 14 d of glucocorticoid deficiency. Therefore, glucocorticoid deficiency in rats causes impaired free water excretion that appears to be mediated acutely by AVP-dependent mechanisms as a result of decreased systemic pressure and GFR with stimulated AVP secretion, and chronically by AVP-independent mechanisms as a result of cardiovascular and renovascular compromise with decreased renal perfusion, resulting in decreased volume delivery to the distal diluting segment of the kidney leading to defective water clearance.

Mineralocorticoid deficiency contributes to impaired water metabolism only in primary adrenal insufficiency, since the renin–angiotensin system remains intact in pituitary or hypothalamic causes of adrenal insufficiency. Aldosterone acts at the distal collecting tubule to enhance sodium reabsorption, potassium, and hydrogen ion excretion. In primary adrenal insufficiency, the deficiency of aldosterone leads to excessive urine Na^+ losses *(55)*, in response to which most animals and some patients manifest a craving for salt. This behavior has clinical significance, since studies on adrenalectomized dogs have shown an ability to overcome impaired urinary dilution when the animals were allowed to drink isotonic saline rather than tap water *(56)*. Boykin et al. *(57)* documented elevated plasma AVP levels in adrenalectomized, glucocorticoid-replaced dogs despite hypoosmolality; these animals manifested weight loss, decreased glomerular filtration rate, and an increased serum creatinine, implicating volume depletion as a likely nonosmotic stimulus to AVP release. Analogous studies have shown correction of plasma AVP levels to near-normal levels following sodium chloride replacement *(58)*. Therefore, an adequate intake of sodium is able to overcome the excess natriuresis associated with mineralocorticoid depletion and can maintain a normal volume status, thereby preventing stimulation of AVP secretion secondary to volume depletion.

In summary, adrenal insufficiency can produce derangements of free water clearance via multiple etiologies. The primary defect associated with mineralocorticoid deficiency is the inability to reabsorb sodium in the distal collecting tubules; prolonged salt wasting leads to volume depletion, which in turn stimulates AVP secretion with subsequent antidiuresis. The urinary diluting defect can be corrected with either mineralocorticoid replacement or volume repletion. In contrast, acute glucocorticoid deficiency appears to cause defective free water clearance primarily via baroreceptor-mediated stimulation of AVP secretion secondary to cardiovascular dysfunction. However, with more chronic glucocorticoid deficiency, the cardiac stroke volume decreases further, causing decreased renal blood flow and leading to impaired water excretion as a result of decreased volume delivery to the distal tubule. Clinical improvement in water metabolism, cardiac, and renal function generally occurs promptly following adequate glucocorticoid replacement.

Edema-Forming States

Edema-forming states commonly encountered in medical patients include congestive heart failure (CHF), nephrotic syndrome, and cirrhosis. Although each disease has its own unique pathogenesis, they share a common finding of avid renal sodium and water retention, despite a generalized hypervolemic edematous state. This disorder of body fluid volume has long been of interest to numerous investigators, and many studies have attempted to define the underlying disturbance of the volume regulatory system in these disorders. Many hypotheses have been postulated, but the primary focus has centered around extrarenal mechanisms that regulate sodium and water excretion. The term "effective blood volume" was proposed in 1948 *(59)* to explain how a single component of the total body fluid volume can be diminished, thereby enhancing renal sodium and water reabsorption. Although used frequently, the exact nature of the effective blood volume has remained elusive. In an attempt to unify the multiple derangements described in edema-forming states, Schrier recently proposed that it is the arterial circulation that primarily serves to regulate body fluid volume. "Underfilling" of the arterial circulation in various disease states activates a cascade of events leading to stimulation of the sympathetic nervous system, the renin–angiotensin system, and AVP secretion, thereby resulting in renal sodium and water retention in an attempt to maintain the "effective arterial blood volume" (EABV) *(60–62;* Fig. 5). Decreases in EABV (underfilling) can occur either with states of low cardiac output or high cardiac output in association with peripheral arterial vasodilatation. The primary focus of this section will be on the contribution of AVP to the pathogenesis of edema-forming states.

Induced states of high- and low-output cardiac failure in animal models clearly demonstrated elevated plasma levels of AVP in association with abnormal water excretion *(63,64)*, and this impairment of free water clearance could be reversed with AVP-receptor antagonists *(64)*. Furthermore, Brattleboro rats with central DI with induced heart failure were able to excrete an acute water load normally, presumably from a lack of AVP effect *(65)*. The association between stimulated AVP secretion and water retention in CHF is also supported by the demonstration of increased hypothalamic AVP messenger RNA (mRNA) transcription in rats with chronic CHF compared to control animals *(66)*. The stimulus for AVP synthesis and secretion in this setting is clearly nonosmotic due to the fall in arterial pressure that activates the baroreceptors located in the heart and great vessels *(67)*. Although the action of AVP on the renal collecting tubules further exacerbates the hypoosmolar state of CHF, it is the vasoconstrictive properties of this hormone that constitute the basis for baroreceptor-mediated stimulation of AVP secretion during states of diminished EABV.

As expected, many patients with CHF have been demonstrated to have elevated plasma AVP levels *(68,69)*. However, this is not a consistent finding and is clearly related to the degree of cardiac decompensation. Bichet et al. studied the clinical characteristics of CHF patients with elevated vs suppressed plasma AVP concentrations *(69)*. Those patients with higher plasma AVP levels had lower plasma [Na^+] and serum osmolalities than patients with lower AVP levels. The former group of patients also had a lower cardiac index and higher pulmonary capillary wedge pressure indicative of a more severe state of heart failure, and this group excreted a smaller percentage of an administered water load. Interestingly, treatment of the CHF with afterload reducers, such as angiotensin-converting enzyme (ACE) inhibitors or α_1-adrenergic blockers, improved cardiac output, enhanced water excretion, and lowered plasma AVP levels. These findings will likely provide new treatment options for heart failure patients in the near future, since it has been unequivocally shown that improvement of left ventricular function with afterload reducers improves survival *(70–72)*; in conjunction with this proven treatment modality, the addition of an AVP receptor antagonist can be expected to improve water excretion further and any additional morbidity associated with plasma hypoosmolality in such patients.

The role of AVP in the abnormal water excretion of cirrhosis has also been evaluated. Water loading of cirrhotic patients revealed two types of response: patients who excreted

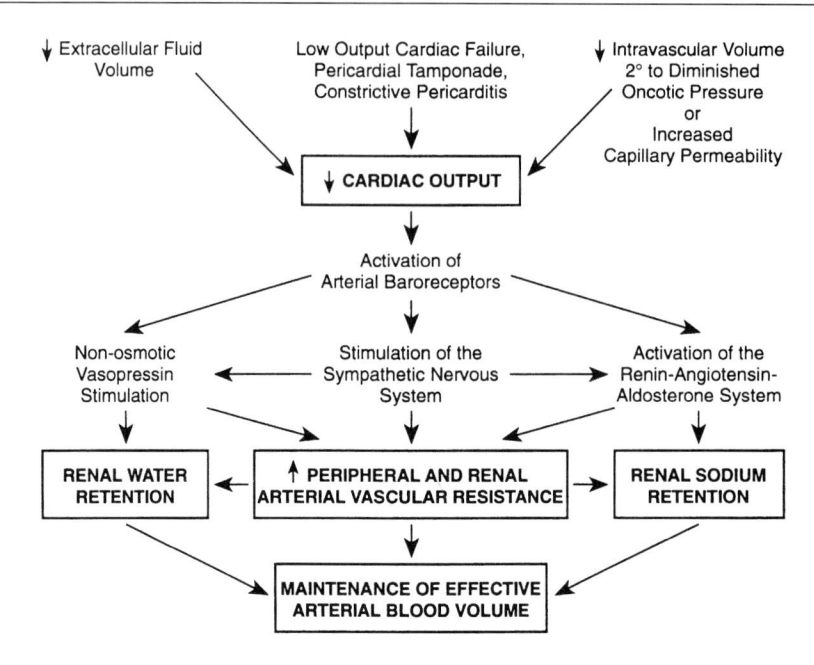

Fig. 5. Schematic summary of the secondary effects of decreased CO on neural and humoral systems that act to maintain effective arterial blood volume by promoting renal Na⁺ and water retention, and stimulating arterial vasoconstriction (reproduced with permission from ref. 62).

<80% of the water load at 5 h (nonexcretors) and those who had a normal excretion pattern (excretors) (73). Clinically, the nonexcretors had moderate to tense ascites with a more significant amount of peripheral edema. Serum osmolality and plasma [Na⁺] were also lower in this group. Despite the hypoosmolality, the nonexcretors had significantly higher plasma AVP levels compared to the excretors, indicating the presence of a nonosmotic stimulus for AVP release. Although the mean arterial blood pressure and hematocrit were similar in the two groups of patients, the nonexcretors had a significantly lower plasma albumin concentration, a higher pulse rate, and more elevated plasma renin activities and aldosterone levels. These findings are consistent with a decreased EABV secondary to the splanchnic and peripheral vasodilatation known to occur in cirrhotic patients (74). Therefore, similar to CHF patients, a diminished effective arterial circulation appears to provide a nonosmotic stimulus for AVP release in cirrhotic patients with subsequent water retention and induced hypoosmolality.

Treatment for cirrhosis has produced fewer successful outcomes compared with vasodilator therapy in heart failure. Placement of surgical or transjugular intrahepatic portal shunts along with treatment using aldosterone antagonists and β-blockers has provided temporary relief of symptoms, but has not resulted in significant decreases in mortality. Future use of AVP receptor antagonists may nonetheless prove to be beneficial in these patients as an adjunctive treatment to improve ascites and edema, and in addition, correction of hypoosmolality may have further beneficial effects on the quality of life and life expectancy in such patients.

Both intrarenal and extrarenal mechanisms, causing abnormal sodium and water retention appear to contribute to the edema associated with the nephrotic syndrome.

However, attempts at studying the role of AVP in this syndrome have been complicated by an inability to measure blood volume status accurately. Usberti et al. *(75)* evaluated the role of AVP in the impaired water excretion of patients with nephrotic syndrome and found that plasma AVP levels were elevated in patients despite hypoosmolality induced via a water load. However, isoosmotic volume expansion with a 20% albumin infusion led to decreased plasma AVP levels and produced an increased water diuresis only in those patients with low baseline blood volumes. A significant inverse correlation was found between plasma AVP levels and blood volume, supporting a volume-mediated stimulation of AVP release in nephrotic patients. However, in patients with normal to increased blood volumes, an AVP-independent intrarenal mechanism likely contributes more to the sodium and water retention *(76)*.

In summary, the pathogenesis of edema in CHF, cirrhosis, and nephrotic syndrome is complex and remains incompletely understood despite many years of study. It is clearly multifactorial, with the sympathetic nervous system, the renin–angiotensin system, and AVP all acting in concert in order to attempt to maintain an effective arterial circulation. Many such patients are often hyponatremic and hypoosmolar, indicating a greater reabsorption of water than sodium, and in this setting, AVP secretion appears to be stimulated by nonosmotic activation of the arterial baroreceptors. Although the vasoconstrictive properties of AVP at high plasma levels are important for maintaining arterial perfusion, its antidiuretic activity further exacerbates the interstitial fluid accumulation associated with these disorders. With the likely availability of selective V_2-specific AVP receptor antagonists on the horizon, the potential exists for new treatment options in these patients to correct their defect in free water clearance, while maintaining EABV by virtue of intact AVP effects at V_1 vascular AVP receptors.

Respiratory Failure

Patients with respiratory failure are known to have impairments of water and solute excretion. The mechanisms responsible for these disturbances involve both hormonal and hemodynamic factors that result from hypoxemia, hypercapnia, positive-pressure ventilation, or a combination of all these variables in the setting of an acutely ill patient with multiple organ system failure. This section discuss the role of AVP in the impaired water excretion that occurs in the setting of respiratory failure.

Several investigators have studied the role of hypoxemia and hypercapnia as stimuli for AVP secretion and their contribution to impaired free water clearance in respiratory failure. Early studies in animal models demonstrated an increase in plasma AVP levels in association with hypoxemia and hypercapnia *(77,78)*. However, these studies relied on less sensitive bioassays for AVP measurement and did not adequately control for other variables, such as the use of positive-pressure ventilation or hemodynamic changes, which may have affected AVP release. Conversely, other studies that failed to demonstrate an effect of hypoxemia on AVP release may not have induced a sufficient lowering of blood arterial oxygen content to stimulate AVP release *(79)*. Anderson et al. *(80)* studied the effect of isolated hypoxemia on renal water excretion in dogs in which the arterial oxygen content was lowered to <50 mmHg with maintenance of a normal arterial pH and pCO_2. Under these conditions, there was a significant antidiuresis and increased urine osmolality with induced hypoxemia in association with a significant increase in plasma AVP levels. Cardiac output (CO), mean arterial pressure (MAP), GFR, solute excretion rate, and filtration fraction did not change with the development of hypoxemia. The authors also attempted to determine the stimulus for AVP release by inducing hypoxemia under different conditions. Hypoxemia was induced in one group of hypophysectomized rats, a group with one denervated kidney, another group with chemoreceptor denervation, and a group with baroreceptor denervation. The effect of hypoxemia on the renal response to exogenous AVP was also evaluated in hypophysectomized animals. The results revealed that hypoxemia did not induce a significant antidiuresis in hypophysectomized animals, supporting the role of AVP in defective water clearance with severe hypoxemia. Animals with one denervated kidney or chemoreceptor denervation still demonstrated a marked antidiuresis, but the baroreceptor denervated group demonstrated a normal excretion of urine with no significant increase in urine osmolality. The renal response to exogenous AVP was unaltered by the hypoxemia. These results clearly supported a role for endogenous AVP secretion in the impaired water excretion of severe hypoxemia that was independent of CO, MAP, GFR, renal nerve activity, and chemoreceptors, since this impairment was abolished in the absence of AVP. The stimulus for AVP release appeared to be baroreceptor-mediated, although the exact nature of this baroreceptor activation has yet to be determined.

The role of hypercapnia as a stimulus to AVP stimulation in respiratory failure is more controversial. Most studies to date have been performed in patients with chronic obstructive pulmonary disease (COPD). Farber et al. evaluated COPD patients at different stages of their illness, and found that patients with hypoxemia, but no hypercapnia or edema exhibited similar clinical and hormonal responses to water loading and hypertonic saline infusion as did control patients *(81)*. In contrast, COPD patients with hypoxemia, hypercapnia, and edema had inappropriately elevated AVP levels and hyponatremia, and demonstrated a delayed excretion of an acute water load *(81,82)*. However, it is well recognized that hypercapnia is a potent vasodilator that decreases systemic vascular resistance *(83)*, and this can stimulate AVP release via activation of nonosmotic receptors. To investigate this variable further, Chabot, et al. *(84)* studied the independent effect of hypercapnia on hormonal systems involved in sodium and water homeostasis. When hypercapnia was induced in patients while maintaining constant cardiac filling pressures and normal arterial O_2 content, they did not demonstrate any significant increases in plasma AVP levels. Therefore, hypercapnia appears to impair water excretion mostly through its ability to alter systemic hemodynamics and only secondarily due to stimulation of AVP secretion.

Progressive respiratory failure often culminates in intubation and mechanical ventilation. Positive end expiratory pressure (PEEP) ventilation has been associated with antidiuresis and a decrease in fractional excretion of sodium, which contributes to the fluid retention often seen in critically ill patients *(85)*. PEEP causes an increase in intrathoracic pressure with a resultant decrease in CO, blood pressure, and GFR *(86)*, thus potentially activating baroreceptors and stimulating AVP release *(87,88)*. However, in a recent study, patients undergoing PEEP ventilation did not show an elevation of plasma AVP levels, and the authors concluded that intrarenal mechanisms causing activation of the renin–angiotensin–aldosterone system were responsible for the sodium and water retention in mechanically ventilated patients *(89)*. The discrepancies between these studies are likely due to the presence of multiple factors found in critically ill and intubated patients, many of which can alter the neurohormonal systems that control water balance.

Intrinsic pulmonary disease is often cited as a cause of SIADH. This has been best described in patients with lung cancer where AVP production has been demonstrated in tumor cell lines *(90,91)*. Pulmonary infections have also been associated with hyponatremia, with several cases of advanced tuberculosis demonstrating antidiuretic properties of infected lung tissue *(92–96)*. Significant hypoosmolality does not appear to occur in this setting unless there is severe hypoxemia and may be exacerbated by positive-pressure ventilation. Typically, these patients respond rapidly to fluid restriction and correction of the underlying pulmonary disturbance. These findings demonstrate the need for clinicians to be aware of impaired free water excretion in patients with any cause of respiratory failure, including acute pneumonias, and to monitor closely the volume and electrolyte status of such patients.

Other Causes of Impaired Water Metabolism in Critical Illness

Impaired water excretion and hyponatremia have been described in other critical disease states, such as sepsis, the postoperative setting, and acute hemorrhage. Plasma AVP levels are often elevated in these states secondary to nonosmotic activation of baroreceptors, signifying the importance of maintaining perfusion pressure via the vasoconstrictive properties of AVP regardless of its antidiuretic effects with subsequent exacerbation of plasma hypoosmolality. Hyponatremia in the postoperative setting is typically related to inappropriate replacement of body fluid losses with hypotonic solutions, but there is one unique situation, sexual dimorphism, which warrants additional discussion. In a study by Ayus et al. *(97)*, the likelihood of developing postoperative hyponatremia appears to be similar between men and women. However, they also evaluated the factors associated with postoperative hyponatremic encephalopathy and found an increased incidence and severity of this neurologic event in menstruating females. Of the cases with significant neurologic deficit or death, 97% of the patients were female, and among this group, 76% were premenopausal. Although these figures are quite significant and suggest a potential role for estrogen in exacerbating hyponatremic encephalopathy, several unanswered questions persist about this theory. First, some of the male patients in this study underwent a transurethral prostatectomy involving transurethral irrigation with large volumes of hypotonic glycine-containing solutions. This practice is well recognized as causing hyponatremia, so the physicians may have been more alert to this potential complication with early recognition of the signs and symptoms of hyponatremia and sooner treatment of the patients' hypoosmolality. Second, the theory of an estrogen milieu affecting brain volume regulation has been studied in several animal models, but with sometimes inconsistent results *(98,99)*. Therefore, the clinician should certainly be aware of the potentially deleterious effects of developing hyponatremia in the postoperative setting and the possibility that encephalopathy may be worse in menstruating women, but the exact incidence and severity of gender-associated differences in neurologic complications will need to be further evaluated via future prospectively controlled studies.

Malignancies have long been associated with SIADH, since the initial description of this syndrome by Bartter and Schwartz *(100)* in a patient with bronchogenic carcinoma. Since then, SIADH has become a well-recognized paraneoplastic syndrome associated with a variety of malignancies *(101,102)*. Hypoosmolality associated with cancer may also occur secondary to chemotherapeutic regimens, and this may result from direct stimulation of the neurohypophysis, nausea, or renal salt wasting. Significant hyponatremia has been described in patients receiving cyclophosphamide or cis-platinum *(103–106)*. Cyclophosphamide in high doses, such as employed in conditioning regimens for bone marrow transplantation, can cause hyponatremia with elevated urine osmolality consistent with SIADH. This event typically occurs early in the course of chemotherapy and generally responds to fluid restriction. Cyclophosphamide and cis-platinum are also nephrotoxic agents and can induce acute tubular necrosis with subsequent electrolyte disturbances. The electrolyte disturbances usually associated with cis-platinum toxicity are hypocalcemia and hypomagnesemia, but prolonged severe hyponatremia has also been reported, especially in patients who have received multiple-dosing chemotherapeutic regimens. Correction of the hyponatremia in this setting requires volume replacement with isotonic saline and only rarely hypertonic saline infusion.

The role of chronic stress on AVP secretion has been evaluated, but still remains controversial. Some investigators have studied the hypothalamic–pituitary–adrenal axis as a modulator of AVP secretion in stressed states. In a recent study, ovine CRH was given to healthy volunteers, and a significant increase in inferior petrosal AVP concentrations was demonstrated *(107)*. Although there was no significant hyponatremia noted with this study, the authors concluded that certain stressed states that are associated with chronic CRH elevation can potentially lead to impaired free water excretion. Interleukin-6 (IL-6), a cytokine often elevated in certain disease states, has also been shown to activate the hypothalamic–pituitary–adrenal axis *(108)* and AVP secretion. These findings suggest another mechanism for hyponatremia in critically ill patients whose acute or chronic stress may induce CRH hypersecretion or IL-6 secretion with subsequent impairment of water diuresis. Although these findings are provocative, the role of cytokines and CRH as significant contributors to the hypoosmolality of critical illnesses in humans will require further evaluation.

CONCLUSION

This chapter has attempted to provide the reader with an overview of water homeostasis during a variety of critical illnesses in humans. Although it is apparent that a great deal is known about how the body maintains constancy of cellular, extracellular, and intravascular fluids during times of stress, much more still needs to be learned about the basic pathophysiologic mechanisms responsible for disorders of body fluid homeostasis. Hopefully, continued basic and clinical research in both humans and experimental animal models will provide the answers to some of the many unanswered questions that we have posed in our discussion of this important group of disorders.

REFERENCES

1. Robertson GL. Physiology of vasopressin, oxytocin, and thirst. In: Becker KL, ed. Principles and Practice of Endocrinology and Metabolism. Lippincott, Philadelphia, 1995, pp. 248–256.
2. Robertson GL. Thirst and vasopressin function in normal and disordered states of water balance. J Lab Clin Med 1983;101:351–371.
3. Robertson GL. Diseases of the posterior pituitary. In: Felig P, Baxter J, Brodus A, Frohman L, eds. Endocrinology and Metabolism. McGraw-Hill, New York, 1986, pp. 338–385.
4. Verbalis JG, Hoffman GE, Sherman TG. Use of immediate early genes as markers of oxytocin and vasopressin neuronal activation. Curr Opinion Endocrinol Diabetes 1995;2:157–168.
5. Arduino F, Ferraz FPJ, Rodrigues J. Antidiuretic action of chlorpropamide in idiopathic diabetes insipidus. J Clin Endocrinol Metab 1966;26:1325–1328.

6. Fichman MP, Vorherr H, Kleeman CR, Telfer N. Diuretic-induced hyponatremia. Ann Intern Med 1971;75:853–863.
7. Spigset O and Hedenmalm K. Hyponatremia and the syndrome of inappropriate antidiuretic hormone secretion (SIADH) induced by psychotropic drugs. Drug Safety 1995; 12(3):209–225.
8. Taylor IC and McConnell JG. Severe hyponatremia associated with selective serotonin reuptake inhibitors. Scott Med J 1995;40:147–148.
9. Miyagawa CI. The pharmacologic management of the syndrome of inappropriate secretion of antidiuretic hormone. Drug Intel Clin Pharmacol 1986;20:527–531.
10. Shimizu K. Aquaretic effects of the nonpeptide V_2 antagonist OPC-31260 in hydropenic humans. Kidney Int 1995;48:220–226.
11. Miller M, Morley JE, Rubenstein LZ. Hyponatremia in a nursing home population. J Am Geriatr Soc 1995;43:1410–1413.
12. Borra SI, Beredo R, Kleinfeld M. Hypernatremia in the aging: causes, manifestations, and outcomes. J Nat Med Assoc 1995;87(3):220–224.
13. Fliers E, Swaab DF, Pool CW, Verwer RW. The vasopressin and oxytocin neurons in the human supraoptic and paraventricular nucleur: change with aging and in senile dementia. Brain Res 1985;342:45–53.
14. Phillips PA, Rolls BJ, Ledinghan JGG, Ledingham DM, Forsling ML, Morton JJ, Crowe MJ, Wollner L. Reduced thirst after water deprivationin healthy elderly man. N Engl J Med 1984;311:753–759.
15. Bevilacqua M, Norbiato G, Chebat E, Raggi U, Cavaiani P, Guzzetti R, Bertora P. Osmotic and nonosmotic control of vasopressin release in the elderly: effect of metoclopramide. J Clin Endocrinol Metab. 1987;65:1243–1247.
16. Robertson GL, Rowe JW. The effect of aging on neurohypophysial function. Peptides 1 1980; (Suppl 1):159.
17. Anderson S, Brenner BM. Effects of aging on the renal glomerulus. Am J Med 1986;80:435–442.
18. Crowe MJ, Forsling ML, Rolls BJ, Phillips PA, Ledingham JG, Smith RF. Altered water excretion in healthy elderly men. Age Ageing 1987;16:285–293.
19. Bengele HH, Mathias RS, Perkins JH, Alexander EA. Urinary concentrating defect in the aged rat. Am J Physiol 1981;240:F147–F150.
20. Baylis PH, Gaskill MR, Robertson GL. Vasopressin secretion in primary polydipsia and cranial diabetes insipidus. Q J Med 1981;50:345–358.
21. Robertson GL. Diabetes insipidus. In: Dluhy RG, ed. Endocrinology and Metabolism Clinics and North America. Saunders, Philadelphia, Co 1995;pp. 549–572.
22. Verbalis JG. Hyponatremia: epidemiology, pathophysiology, and therapy. Curr Opin Nephrol Hyperten 1993; 2:636–652.
23. Verbalis JG. Clinical aspects of body fluid homeostasis in humans. In: Handbook of Behavioral Neurobiology, Vol. 10. Plenum, New York, 1990, pp. 421–462.
24. Bevilacqua, M. Hyponatraemia in AIDS. Bailliere's Clin Endocrinol Metab 1994; 8(4):837–848.
25. Tang WW, Kaptein EM, Feinstein EI, Massry SG. Hyponatremia in hospitalized patients with the acquired immunodeficiency syndrome (AIDS) and the AIDS-related complex. Am J Med 1993;94:169–174.
26. Agarwal A, Soni A, Ciechanowsky M, Chander P, Treser G. Hyponatremia in patients with the acquired immunodeficiency syndrome. Nephron 1989;53:317–321.
27. Tapper ML, Rotterdam HZ, Lerner CW, Al'Khafaji K, Seitzman PA. Adrenal necrosis in the acquired immunodeficiency syndrome. Ann Intern Med 1984;100:239–241.
28. Glasgow BJ, Steinsapir BS, Anders K, Layfield LJ. Adrenal pathology in the acquired immune deficiency syndrome. Am J Clin Pathol 1985;84:594–597.
29. Dobbs AS, Dempsey MA, Ladenson PW, Polk BF. Endocrine disorders in men infected with human immunodeficiency virus. Am J Med 1988;84:611–616.
30. Membreno L, Irony I, Dere W, Klein R, Biglieri EG, Cobb E. Adrenocortical function in acquired immunodeficiency syndrome. J Clin Endocrinol Metab 1987;65:482–487.
31. Kalin MF, Poretsky L, Seres DS, Zumoff B. Hyporeninemic hypoaldosteronism associated with acquired immune deficiency syndrome. Am J Med 1987;82:1035–1038.
32. Cobbs R, Pepper GM, Torres JG, Gruenspan HL. Adrenocortical insufficiency with normal serum cortisol levels and hyporeninaemia in a patient with acquired immunodeficiency syndrome (AIDS). J Intern Med 1991;230:179–181.
33. Seney FD, Burns DK, Silva FG. Acquired immunodeficiency syndrome and the kidney. Am J Kidney Dis 1990;16:1–13.

34. Brandle M, Vernazza PL, Oesterle M, Galeazzi RL. Cerebral toxoplasmosis with central diabetes insipidus and panhypopituitarism in a patient with AIDS. Schweiz Med Wochenschr 1995;125(14): 684–687.
35. Catz B, Russell S. Myxedema, shock and coma. Arch Intern Med 1961;108:407–417.
36. Curtis RH. Hyponatremia in primary myxedema. Ann Intern Med 1956;44:376–385.
37. Derubertis FR, Michelis MF, Bloom ME, Mintz DH, Field JB, Davis BB. Impaired water excretion in myxedema. Am J Med 1971;51:41–53.
38. Skowsky WR, Kikuchi TA. The role of vasopressin in the impaired water excretion of myxedema. Am J Med 1978;64:613–621.
39. Crispell KR, Parson W, Sprinkle P. A cortisone-resistant abnormality in the diuretic response to ingested water in primary myxedema. J Clin Endocrinol Metab 1954;14:640–644.
40. Discala VA, Kinney MJ. Effects of myxedema on the renal diluting and concentrating mechanism. Am J Med 1971;50:325–335.
41. Emmanouel DS, Lindheimer MD, Katz AI. Mechanisms of impaired water excretion in the hypothyroid rat. J Clin Invest 1974;54:926–934.
42. Pettinger WA, Talner L, Ferris TF. Inappropriate secretion on antidiuretic hormone due to myxedema. N Engl J Med 1965;272:362–364.
43. Iwasaki Y, Oiso Y, Yamauchi K, Takatsuki Kensuke, Kunikazu K, Haruhiko H, Tomita A. Osmoregulation of plasma vasopressin in myxedema. J Clin Endocrinol Metab 1990;70(2): 534–539.
44. Macaron C, Famuyiwa O. Hyponatremia of hypothyroidism. Appropriate suppression of antidiuretic hormone levels. Arch Intern Med 1978;138:820–822.
45. Amidi M, Leon DF, DeGroot WJ, Kroetz FW, Leonard JJ. Effect of the thyroid state on myocardial contractility and ventricular ejection rate in man. Circulation 1968;38:229–239.
46. Graettinger JS, Muenster JJ, Checchia CS, Grissom RL, Campbell JA. A correlation of clinical and hemodynamic studies in patients with hypothyroidism. J Clin Invest 1958;37:502–510.
47. Gaunt R, Birnie JH, Eversole WJ. Adrenal cortex and water metabolism. Physiol Rev 1949;29: 281–310.
48. Kleeman CR, Czaczkes JW, Cutler R. Mechanisms of impaired water excretion in adrenal and pituitary insufficiency: IV. Antidiuretic hormone in primary and secondary adrenal insufficiency. J Clin Invest 1964;43:1641–1648.
49. Linas SL, Berl T, Robertson GL, Aisenbrey GA, Schrier RW, Anderson RJ. Role of vasopressin in the impaired water excretion of glucocorticoid deficiency. Kidney Int 1980;18:58–67.
50. Ishikawa S, Schrier RW. Effect of arginine vasopressin antagonist on renal water excretion in glucocorticoid and mineralocorticoid deficient rats. Kidney Int 1982;22:587–593.
51. Boykin J, DeTorrente A, Erickson A, Robertson G, Schrier RW. Role of plasma vasopressin in impaired water excretion of glucocorticoid deficiency. J Clin Invest 1978;62:738–744.
52. Mandell IN, DeFronzo RA, Robertson GL, Forrest JN. Role of plasma arginine vasopressin in the impaired water diuresis of isolated glucocorticoid deficiency in the rat. Kidney Int 1980;17:186–195.
53. Martin MM. Coexisting anterior and neurohypophyseal insufficiency: A syndrome with diagnostic implication. Arch Intern Med 1969;123:409–416.
54. Green HH, Harrington AR, Valtin H. On the role of antidiuretic hormone in the inhibition of acute water diuresis in adrenal insufficiency and the effects of gluco- and mineralocorticoids in reversing the inhibition. J Clin Invest 1970;49:1724–1736.
55. Harrop GA, Soffer LJ, Ellsworth R, Trescher JH. Studies on the suprarenal cortex. III. Plasma electrolytes and electrolyte excretion during suprarenal insufficiency in the dog. J Exp Med 1933;58:17–38.
56. Ufferman RC, Schrier RW. Importance of sodium intake and mineralocorticoid hormone in the impaired water excretion in adrenal insufficiency. J Clin Invest 1972;51:1639–1646.
57. Boykin J, Detorrente A, Robertson GL, Erickson A, Schrier RW. Mechanism of impaired water excretion in mineralocorticoid deficient dogs. Miner Electrolyte Metab 1979;2:310–315.
58. Share L, Travis RH. Plasma vasopressin concentration in the adrenally insufficient dog. Endocrinology 1970;86:196–201.
59. Peters JP. The role of sodium in the production of edema. N Engl J Med 1948;239:353–362.
60. Schrier RW. Pathogenesis of sodium and water retention in high-output and low-output cardiac failure, nephrotic syndrome, cirrhosis, and pregnancy (1). N Engl J Med 1988;319(16):1065–1072.

61. Schrier RW. Pathogenesis of sodium and water retention in high-output and low-output cardiac failure, nephrotic syndrome, cirrhosis, and pregnancy (2). N Engl J Med 1988;319(17):1127–1134.
62. Schrier RW. Body fluid volume regulation in health and disease: a unifying hypothesis. Ann Intern Med 1990;113:155–159.
63. Riegger AJG, Liebau G. The renin-angiotensin-aldosterone system, antidiuretic hormone and sympathetic nerve activity in an experimental model of congestive heart failure in the dog. Clin Sci 1982;62:465–469.
64. Ishikawa S, Saito T, Okada K, Tsutsui K, Kuzuya T. Effect of vasopressin antagonist on water excretion in inferior vena cava constriction. Kidney Int 1986;30:49–55.
65. Handelman WA, Lum GM, Schrier RW. Impaired water excretion in high output cardiac failure in the rat (abstract). Clin Res 1979;27:173A.
66. Kim JK, Michel JB, Soubrier F, Durr J, Corvol P, Schrier RW. Arginine vasopressin gene expression in congestive heart failure (abstract). Kidney Int 1988;33:270.
67. Robertson GL. The regulation of vasopressin function in health and disease. Recent Prog Horm Res 1977;33:333–375.
68. Riegger AJG, Liebau G, Kochsiek K. Antidiuretic hormone in congestive heart failure. Am J Med 1982;72:49–57.
69. Bichet DG, Kortas C, Mettauer B, Manzini C, Marc-Aurele J, Rouleau JL, Schrier RW. Modulation of plasma and platelet vasopressin by cardiac function in patients with heart failure. Kidney Int 1986;29:1188–1196.
70. The Consensus Trial Study Group. Effects of enalapril on mortality in severe congestive heart failure: results of the cooperative North Scandinavian Enalapril Survival Study (CONSENSUS). N Engl J Med 1987;316:1429–1435.
71. Konstam MA, Kronenberg MW, Rousseau MF, Udelson JE, Melin J, Stewart D, Dolan N, Edens TR, Ahn S, Kinan D. Effects of the angiotensin converting enzyme inhibitor enalapril on the long-term progression of left ventricular dilatation in patients with asymptomatic systolic dysfunction. SOLVD (Studies of Left Ventricular Dysfunction) Investigators. Circulation 1993;88:2277–2283.
72. Ziesche S, Cobb FR, Cohn JN, Johnson G, Tristani F. Hydralazine and isosorbide dinitrate combination improves exercise tolerance in heart failure. Results from V-HeFT I and V-HeFT II. The V-HeFT VA Cooperative Studies Group. Circulation 1993;87(6 Suppl):SV 156–164.
73. Bichet DG, Szatalowicz V, Chaimovitz C, Schrier RW. Role of vasopressin in abnormal water excretion in cirrhotic patients. Ann Intern Med 1982;96:413–417.
74. Schrier RW, Arroyo V, Bernardi M, Epstein M, Henriksen JH, Rodes J. Peripheral arterial vasodilation hypothesis: a proposal for the initiation of renal sodium and water retention. J Hepatol 1987;6:239–257.
75. Usberti M, Federico S, Meccariello S, Cianciaruso B, Balletta M, Pecoraro C, Sacca L, Ungaro B, Pisanti N, Andreucci VE. Role of plasma vasopressin in the impairment of water excretion in nephrotic syndrome. Kidney Int 1984;25:422–429.
76. Ichikawa I, Rennke HG, Hoyer JR, Badr KF, Schor N, Troy JL, Lechene CP, Brenner BM. Role for intrarenal mechanisms in the impaired salt excretion of experimental nephrotic syndrome. J Clin Invest 1983;71:91–103.
77. Forsling ML, Rees M. Effects of hypoxia and hypercapnia on plasma vasopressin concentration. J Endocrinol 1975;67:62p.
78. Forsling ML, Ullman EA. Release of vasopressin during hypoxia. J Physiol 1974;241:35P.
79. Farber MO, Kiblawi SSO, Strawbridge RA, Robertson GL, Weinberger MH, Manfredi F. Studies on plasma vasopressin and the renin-angiotensin-aldosterone system in chronic obstructive lung disease. J Lab Clin Med 1977;90(2):373–380.
80. Anderson RJ, Pluss RG, Berns AS, Jackson JT, Arnold PE, Schrier RW, McDonald KE. Mechanism of effect of hypoxia on renal water excretion. J Clin Invest 1978;62:769–777.
81. Farber MO, Roberts LR, Weinberger MH, Robertson GL, Fineberg NS, Manfredi F. Abnormalities of sodium and water handling in chronic obstructive lung disease. Arch Intern Med 1982;142:1326–1330.
82. Farber MO, Weinberger MH, Robertson GL, Fineberg NS, Manfredi F. Hormonal abnormalities affecting sodium and water balance in acute respiratory failure due to chronic obstructive lung disease. Chest 1984;85:49–54.
83. Weinberger SE, Schwartzstein RM, Weiss JW. Hypercapnia. N Engl J Med 1989;321:1223–1231.
84. Chabot F, Mertes PM, Delorme N, Schrijen FV, Saunier CG, Polu JM. Effect of acute hypercapnia on alpha atrial natriuretic peptide, renin, angiotensin II, aldosterone, and vasopressin plasma levels in patients with COPD. Chest 1995;107:780–786.

85. Sladen A, Laver MB. Pulmonary complications and water retention in prolonged mechanical ventilation. N Engl J Med 1968;279:448–453.
86. Robotham JL, Sharf SM. Effects of positive and negative pressure ventilation on cardiac performance. Clin Chest Med 1983;4:161–187.
87. Bark H, Le Roith D, Myska M, Glick SM. Elevations in plasma ADH levels during PEEP ventilation in the dog: mechanisms involved. Am J Physiol 1980;239:E474–E48.
88. Khambatta HJ, Baratz RA. IPPB plasma ADH and urine flow in conscious man. J Appl Physiol 1972;33:362–364.
89. Farge D, De La Coussaye JE, Beloucif S, Fratacci MD, Payen DM. Interactions between hemodynamic and hormonal modifications during PEEP-induced antidiuresis and antidiuresis. Chest 1995;107:1095–1100.
90. Sorensen JB, Andersen MK, Hansen HH. Syndrome of inappropriate secretion of antidiuretic hormone (SIADH) in malignant disease. J Intern Med 1995;238:97–110.
91. Gross AJ, Steinberg SM, Reilly JG, Bliss DP, Brennan J, Le PT, Simmons A, Phelps R, Mulshine JL, Ihde DC, Johnson BE. Atrial natriuretic factor and arginine vasopressin production in tumor cell lines from patients with lung cancer and their relationship to serum sodium. Cancer Res 1993;53:67–74.
92. Weiss H, Katz S. Hyponatremia resulting from apparently inappropriate secretion of antidiuretic hormone in patients with pulmonary tuberculosis. Am Rev Respir Dis 1965;92:609–616.
93. Vorherr H, Massry SG, Fallet R, Kaplan L, Kleeman CR. Antidiuretic principle in tuberculous lung tissue of a patient with pulmonary tuberculosis and hyponatremia. Ann Intern Med 1970;72:383–387.
94. Rosenow EC, Segar WE, Zehr JE. Inappropriate antidiuretic hormone secretion in pneumonia. Mayo Clin Proc 1972;47:169–174.
95. Pollard RB. Inappropriate secretion of antidiuretic hormone associated with adenovirus pneumonia. Chest 1975;68(4):589–591.
96. Breuer R, Rubinow A. Inappropriate secretion of antidiuretic hormone and mycoplasma pneumonia infection. Respiration 1981;42:217–219.
97. Ayus JC, Wheeler JM, Arieff AI. Postoperative hyponatremic encephalopathy in menstruant women. Ann Intern Med 1992;117:891–897.
98. Verbalis JG. Hyponatremia induced by vasopressin or desmopressin in female and male rats. J Am Soc Nephrol 1993;3:1600–1606.
99. Fraser CL, Kucharczyk J, Arieff AI, Rollin C, Sarnacki P, Norman D. Sex differences result in increased morbidity from hyponatremia in female rats. Am J Physiol 1989;256:R880–R885.
100. Bartter FC, Schwartz WB. The syndrome of inappropriate secretion of antidiuretic hormone. Am J Med 1967;42:790–806.
101. Campling BG, Sarda IR, Baer KA, Pang SC, Baker HM, Lofters WS, Flynn TG. Secretion of atrial natriuretic peptide and vasopressin by small cell lung cancer. Cancer 1995;75:2442–2451.
102. Sorensen JB, Andersen MK, Hansen HH. Syndrome of inappropriate secretion of antidiuretic hormone (SIADH) in malignant disease. J Intern Med 1995;238:97–110.
103. Weshl AE, Thieblemont C, Cottin V, Barbet N, Catimel G. Cisplatin-induced hyponatremia and renal sodium wasting. Acta Oncologica 1995;34:264–265.
104. Lammers PJ, White L, Ettinger LJ. Cis-platinum-induced renal sodium wasting. Med Pediatr Oncol 1984;12:343–346.
105. Abe T, Takaue Y, Okamoto Y, Yamaue T, Nakagawa R, Makimoto A, Sato J, Kawano Y, Kuroda Y. Syndrome of inappropriate antidiuretic hormone secretion (SIADH) in children undergoing high-dose chemotherapy and autologous peripheral blood stem cell transplantation. Pediatr Hematol Oncol 1995;12(4):363–369.
106. Bissett D, Cornford EJ, Sokal M. Hyponatraemia following cisplatin chemotherapy. Acta Oncol 1989;28(6):823.
107. Mastorakos G, Weber JS, Magiakou M, Gunn H, Chrousos GP. Hypothalamic-pituitary-adrenal axis activation and stimulation of systemic vasopressin secretion by recombinant interleukin-6 in humans: potential implications for the syndrome of inappropriate vasopressin secretion. J Clin Endocrinol Metab 1994;79:934–939.
108. Kalogeras KT, Nieman LK, Friedman TC, Doppman JL, Cutler GB, Chrousos GP, Wilder RL, Gold PW, Yanovski JA. Inferior petrosal sinus sampling in healthy human subjects reveals a unilateral corticotropin-releasing hormone-induced arginine vasopressin release associated with ipsilateral adrenocorticotropin secretion. J Clin Invest 1996;97:2045–2050.

10 Alterations in Fuel Metabolism in Critical Illness
Hyperglycemia

Barry A. Mizock, MD, FACP

CONTENTS

THE STRESS RESPONSE TO CRITICAL ILLNESS
STRESS-INDUCED ALTERATIONS
 IN CARBOHYDRATE METABOLISM
OTHER CAUSES OF HYPERGLYCEMIA DURING STRESS
CLINICAL MANAGEMENT OF HYPERGLYCEMIA DURING STRESS
REFERENCES

THE STRESS RESPONSE TO CRITICAL ILLNESS

Claude Bernard *(1)*, in the late 19th century, was one of the first to recognize that acute injury was associated with the development of hyperglycemia. His observation was subsequently confirmed by others who applied the terms "traumatic diabetes," "diabetes of injury," or "stress diabetes" to this state. It has been suggested that the evolutionary value of a hyperglycemic response to injury is to compensate for volume loss by promoting movement of cellular fluid into the intravascular compartment or liberating water bound to glycogen *(2)*. It has also been proposed that hyperglycemia is beneficial by satisfying an increased requirement for glucose by cells active in the immune response to severe injury or infection (e.g., neutrophils, macrophages); the wound may be viewed from this perspective as an "organ of repair," which generates a hyperglycemic milieu through the release of neuroendocrine and cytokine mediators *(3)*. In 1942, Sir David Cutherbertson *(4)* introduced the terms "ebb" and "flow" to describe the phases of hypo- and hypermetabolism, which follow traumatic injury. The ebb phase begins immediately following injury; it is characterized by tissue hypoperfusion and peripheral vasoconstriction, which are accompanied by a decrease in metabolic activity. Hyperglycemia during the ebb phase roughly parallels the severity of injury; it is promoted by hepatic glycogenolysis secondary to catecholamine release, as well as by direct sympathetic stimulation of glycogen breakdown *(5,6)*. The ebb phase typically lasts 12–24 h, but may last longer depending on the severity of injury and adequacy of resuscitation. Restoration of oxygen delivery and metabolic substrate appear to signal

From *Contemporary Endocrinology: Endocrinology of Critical Disease*
Edited by K. P. Ober   Humana Press Inc., Totowa, NJ

the onset of the flow phase (also known as the catabolic phase). The duration of the flow phase varies depending on the severity of injury and complications, but typically peaks around 3–5 d after injury; it gradually subsides by 7–10 d and merges into an "anabolic" phase over the next few weeks. Hyperglycemia is a prominent feature of the flow phase in patients who sustain more severe injury or in whom septic complications develop; it results from augmented glucose production in the presence of insulin resistance in peripheral tissues *(7)*. The flow phase is clinically expressed as a syndrome consisting of: hypermetabolism (as manifest by hyperglycemia, hyperlactatemia, and protein catabolism), a hyperdynamic cardiovascular state, and clinical manifestations of fever or hypothermia, tachycardia, tachypnea, and leukocytosis *(8)*. The term "stress response to critical illness" has been used to describe this syndrome, since it can also be elicited by nontraumatic insults (e.g., sepsis, pancreatitis, hemorrhage) *(8)*. The hypermetabolic response to stress may be prolonged when there is a stimulus for continuing formation of mediators (e.g., a persistant focus of injury or infection). A prolonged stress response in associated with a progressive decrease in the ability of normal mechanisms to modulate substrate flow and utilization (as manifest by peripheral and hepatic insulin resistance, hypertriglyceridemia, protein catabolism); this is typically accompanied by clinical evidence of organ dysfunction (e.g., jaundice, encephalopathy, renal failure) *(8)*.

Three systems are responsible for translating the initial insult into the stress response: nervous, endocrine, and humoral (cytokine). These systems are interrelated; a maximal metabolic response to stress requires participation of all three. The neuroendocrine system can be triggered by a variety of factors including: hypoglycemia, alterations in intravascular volume, acidosis, hypoxia, and pain. Afferent inputs from the focus of injury or infection and efferent signals are integrated in the brain by areas within the hypothalamus (and medulla). Hypoglycemia causes increased firing of nuclei in the lateral hypothalamus and tractus solitarius *(9)*. This in turn increases sympathetic outflow, which elevates blood glucose by promoting glycogenolysis and inhibiting insulin secretion. In contrast, hyperglycemia stimulates receptors in the ventromedial hypothalamus, which in turn promote insulin release by decreasing sympathetic inhibition on β-cells of the pancreas *(9)*. Several cytokines, such as tumor necrosis factor (TNF) and interleukin-1 (IL-1), have also been shown to be capable of directly activating the neuroendocrine response *(10–12)*. The term "immune–hypothalamic–pituitary–adrenal axis" has been proposed to emphasize the important role of cytokines in initiating and modulating this response *(see below) (13)*. As mentioned, hyperglycemia during the ebb phase is primarily owing to catecholamine and adrenergically mediated hepatic glycogenolysis; the magnitude of increase in blood glucose within 3 h of injury has been shown to be proportional to the plasma epinephrine concentration *(6)*. Peak plasma catecholamine concentrations are typically achieved 24–48 h after injury; however, interpretation of isolated values of catecholamines may be difficult, because norepinephrine metabolism does not occur in a single-compartment system *(14,15)*. Serum glucagon is usually normal acutely post trauma and may require 12 h to rise above baseline (portal venous glucagon may show a greater and more rapid response) *(16,17)*. It is unlikely that glucagon plays a significant role in the genesis of hyperglycemia immediately following injury, since the initial increase in blood sugar has been shown to be independent of glucagon secretion *(18)*. Glucagon release is largely the consequence of adrenergic stimulation and catecholamine activation of α-receptors in the pancreas. It is also possible that glucagon release may be mediated by cytokines; studies have indicated that both IL-1 and TNF stimulate glucagon secretion *(19,20)*. Patients with prolonged septic stress exhibit the most prominent elevation in plasma glucagon; this in turn serves to promote hyperglycemia by stimulating hepatic glucose production *(see below) (7)*. A number of investigators have measured plasma insulin postinjury with widely variable results owing in part to differences in type and severity of disease *(6,21–23)*. Barton summarized these studies by stating that insulin levels during the ebb phase demonstrate "an increase in variability, with little change in the mean value" *(5)*. It can be argued, however, that a "normal" value of insulin is actually low relative to the degree of hyperglycemia. It has also been noted that the metabolic clearance rate of insulin is increased nearly twofold following trauma; this could diminish the value of plasma insulin as an index of pancreatic secretion in this setting *(24)*. During the flow phase, insulin levels usually show a modest rise; this could be owing in part to the pancreatic and/or central effects of cytokines (e.g., IL-1) on insulin secretion *(7,25,26)*. Plasma cortisol is generally elevated during stress as the result of pituitary release of ACTH. However, the increase is not great; cortisol appears to play more of a "permissive" role in the maintenance of hepatic glucose production by potentiating the actions of glucagon and epinephrine on the liver *(27)*. Growth hormone (GH) may also play a role in the pathogenesis of hyperglycemia during critical illness. The hypothalamus promotes pituitary secretion of GH during stress; the effects of GH are mediated by secondary release of insulin-like growth factor (IGF-1), formerly called somatomedin *(14)*. Several studies have suggested that critical illness is associated with a switch from anabolic effects of GH (normally mediated by an increase in IGF-1) to catabolic, counterregulatory effects, which are associated with decreased levels of IGF-1 *(28,29)*.

Although hormones are responsible for many of the metabolic alterations of the ebb phase, they do not completely explain the changes observed during the flow phase. Bessey et al. demonstrated that infusion of counterregulatory hormones into normal volunteers resulted in metabolic alterations similar to those seen in septic or injured patients *(30)*; however, these hormones did not promote skeletal muscle catabolism, which is characteristic of the flow phase *(31)*. As mentioned, it is likely that cytokines play a significant role in mediating the metabolic response to acute injury or infection. Several investigators have shown that short-term TNF infusion produces alterations in glucose metabolism that are similar to what is observed during stress. Meszaros et al. *(32)* noted that TNF increased glucose utilization in macrophage-rich tissues. Lang et al. *(33)* demonstrated that TNF infusion resulted in hyperglycemia, increased glucose production, and hepatic and peripheral insulin resistance. In a subsequent study, ip zymosan was used to induce a hypermetabolic response in rats. Arterial TNF levels were found to be increased, and pretreatment with a neutralizing anti-TNF antibody prevented increased glucose flux and lessened the severity of insulin resistance *(34)*. Cytokines have also been shown to influence glucose metabolism by their direct actions on the central nervous system; Lang et al. were able to produce hyperglycemia by an intraventricular injection of IL-1 α, which augmented glucose production by increasing insulin, glucagon, and corticosterone secretion *(35)*. Petit et al. found that intraventricular administration of IL-1 α produced hyperglycemia accompanied by elevations in plasma glucagon, insulin, epinephrine, and norepinephrine; preadministration of α- and β-antagonists blocked this response, which suggested adrenergic mediation *(19)*. Despite these impressive findings, several objections to cytokines as the sole mediator of stress metabolism have been raised: *(31)*.

1. The inability to demonstrate consistently blood levels of cytokines following injury;
2. The failure of infused cytokines to produce a sustained effect; and
3. The inability of cytokines to cause skeletal muscle catabolism directly, one of the key features of the metabolic response to injury or infection.

STRESS-INDUCED ALTERATIONS IN CARBOHYDRATE METABOLISM

Increased Glucose Production

Although glycogenolysis increases hepatic glucose output during the ebb phase, this effect is transient because glycogen stores are rapidly depleted *(5,6)*. In contrast, the flow phase is characterized by a sustained increase in gluconeogenesis (GNG), which in turn promotes hyperglycemia *(36,37)*. Glucagon is the primary hormonal stimulator of GNG during critical illness *(7)*; Jahoor et al. *(38)* in a study of burn patients, noted that hepatic glucose production was reduced when glucagon secretion was inhibited by somatostatin. The adrenergic nervous system appears to have a smaller role, since combined α- and β-blockade does not reduce GNG *(39)*. Similarly, increased peripheral production of gluconeogenic precursors is not of major importance, since infusion of alanine does not stimulate GNG *(40)*. Both TNF and IL-1 have been shown to promote hepatic glucose production; they may also act synergistically as well as interacting with hormones to augment GNG *(31,34,41)*. Granulocyte macrophage colony-stimulating factor has also been shown to increase glucose production *(42)*. Enhanced GNG during stress is resistant to the inhibitory effects of insulin and glucose infusion; this is likely to be owing to persistant stimulation by glucagon or cytokines *(36,37)*. A progressive decrease in the ability of normal inhibitors to modulate GNG (metabolic dysregulation) is characteristic of a prolonged hypermetabolic stress state, which in turn may progress to the multiple-system organ failure syndrome *(7,8)*.

Lactate, alanine, pyruvate, glutamine, and glycerol are the major gluconeogenic substrates; of these, lactate and alanine are the most important during stress *(43,44)*. Skeletal muscle, because of its large mass, makes the greatest contribution to lactate production *(45)*. Acute injury results in glycogen breakdown in muscle with a concomitant increase in glucose-6-phosphate; this in turn is channeled into the glycolytic pathway, where it results in hyperlactatemia by virtue of a mass effect on glycolytic flux *(46,47)*. Wound is also a significant source of lactate, since its energy demands are met largely via glycolysis *(3)*. Alanine release during stress exceeds its constitution in muscle (only 30% of alanine in blood is derived from catabolism of skeletal muscle); the majority of alanine originates from *de novo* synthesis. Its carbon skeleton is derived from pyruvate, whereas the ammonia moiety originates from deamination of branched-chain amino acids *(48)*. Lactate and alanine are reconstituted to glucose in the lactic acid (Cori) and glucose-alanine cycles, respectively (Fig. 1) *(43,44)*. Glutamine and glycerol are also substrates for GNG. Glycerol is a major source of new carbons, since unlike lactate or alanine, it is not recycled *(49,50)*. Although the contribution of glycerol to glucose production is minimal during normal conditions, fat mobilization induced by stress can increase its contribution to glucose production by as much as 20% *(51)*.

Although GNG is typically increased following injury, septic stress may be associated with a biphasic response in which an initial phase of hyperglycemia is followed by decreased glucose production and hypoglycemia *(52,53)*. The mechanism has been postulated to involve an inhibition (possibly cytokine-mediated) of phosphoenolpyruvate carboxykinase (PEPCK) gene expression *(54)*. In support of this theory, Deutschman et al.

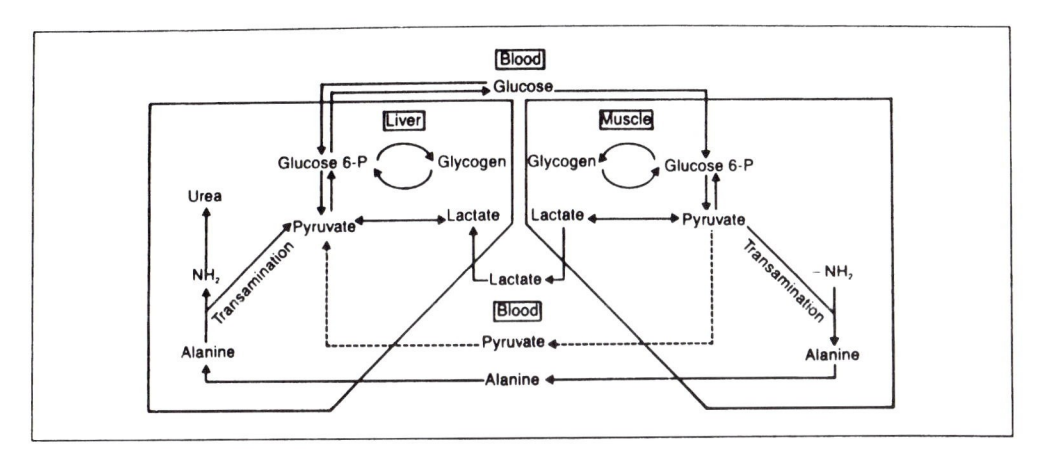

Fig. 1. Lactic acid (Cori) and glucose-alanine cycles. Glucose 6-P, glucose 6-phosphate; –NH$_2$, ammonia. (From ref *80* with permission.)

found that the induction of sepsis in rats was associated with a 66% reduction in levels of PEPCK mRNA and an attenuated response of PEPCK expression to stimulation by glucagon *(55)*.

In summary, hyperglycemia during the catabolic phase of stress is intimately linked with augmented hepatic glucose production. This occurs as the result of hormonal and cytokine stimulation of GNG in which lactate and alanine are the most important substrates. Prolonged stress is characterized by progressive metabolic dysregulation in which GNG exhibits resistance to inhibition by insulin and glucose. Severe sepsis may be associated with a biphasic response in glucose production, which terminates in hypoglycemia.

Increased Glucose Uptake and Utilization

Severe injury or infection is associated with enhanced cellular uptake of glucose *(56,57)*. Although the precise mechanism is not entirely clear, current evidence supports a central role for cytokines in mediating this process *(42)*. Under basal conditions, 80% of whole-body glucose utilization is by noninsulin-mediated uptake (NIMGU), mainly by the central nervous system *(58)*. Twenty percent of glucose uptake is by skeletal muscle of which 1/2 is NIMGU and 1/2 insulin-mediated (IMGU) *(59)*. Glucose transport in most cells occurs by a process of facilitated diffusion in which carrier proteins facilitate the movement of glucose across the cell membrane down its concentration gradient. Five transporter isoforms have been described; three of the isoforms (GLUT1, GLUT2, and GLUT4) are thought to play important roles in glucose uptake *(60)*. The GLUT1 isoform is responsible for basal glucose uptake and can be found in many tissues. Augmented cellular glucose uptake during stress occurs predominately via NIMGU by the GLUT1 receptor; this process is most prominent in organs involved in the immune response to severe injury or infection (e.g., spleen, lung, liver, wound) *(56,61)*. Glucose uptake by the GLUT1 receptor is maintained during stress even in the presence of hypoglycemia *(62)*. Current evidence suggests that cytokines can promote glucose uptake by increasing the synthesis, plasma membrane concentration, or activity of the GLUT1 transporter *(63–66)*. TNF appears to play a important role in this process; a recent study demonstrated that pretreatment with anti-TNF antibodies blocked a zymosan-induced augmentation of glucose uptake *(34)*. The GLUT2 transporter is involved in bidirectional glucose transport in hepatocytes and in the regulation of glucose-stimulated insulin secretion in pancreas. It is possible that downregulation of the GLUT2 transporter (resulting in decreased hepatic export of glucose) could play a role in hypoglycemia, which is occasionally observed in patients with prolonged sepsis *(67)*. The GLUT4 isoform is present only in tissues where glucose uptake is mediated by insulin (e.g., muscle, fat, heart). Certain tissues may contain more than one isoform; skeletal muscle, for example, contains both GLUT1 and GLUT4 isoforms (GLUT4 is more numerous, however). Under basal conditions, GLUT4 is localized to intracellular vesicles with little in the plasma membrane, whereas GLUT1 is distributed equally between the plasma membrane and vesicles. Insulin appears to promote glucose uptake by inducing a postbinding signal (mediated by tyrosine kinase) for migration of GLUT4 transporters from an intracellular location to the plasma membrane; it may also increase intrinsic activity *(V_{max})* of carrier proteins *(68–70)*. Alterations in the synthesis, activity, degradation, or translocation of the GLUT4 receptor may play a role in insulin resistance by decreasing insulin-mediated glucose transport *(see below) (71–74)*. Once taken up by the cell, glucose is directed into either glycogen formation or glycolysis. Glycogen formation in liver and muscle is inhibited during stress; this may be the result of persistant hormonal stimulation of glycogen breakdown or by decreased glycogen synthase activity *(46,72,75,76)*. Inhibition of glycogen storage may have evolved as a mechanism that directs glucose into the glycolytic pathway, thereby providing energy for injured, infected, or immune tissues *(75)*. Decreased glycogenesis may also play a role in stress-induced insulin resistance *(see below) (72)*. Stress stimulates glycolytic activity by virtue of a mass effect resulting from increased cellular glucose uptake *(46,47)*. This process has been termed "aerobic glycolysis," since most studies have failed to provide evidence of a hypoxic stimulus for glycolysis in the setting of resuscitated stress *(77)*. Although it is not known why certain cells chose to meet their energy needs in this fashion, it is possible that an accelerated rate of aerobic glycolysis may be necessary to sustain processes that require high rates of cytoplasmic ATP turnover *(78,79)*. In addition to producing ATP, glycolysis also generates pyruvate, which is directed into:

1. Conversion to lactate;
2. Oxidation to carbon dioxide;
3. Transamination to alanine; and
4. Recycling to glucose via oxaloacetate.

Increased blood lactate resulting from augmented aerobic glycolysis has been termed stress hyperlactatemia *(80)*. It differs from hypoxic hyperlactatemia in part because buffering capacity is preserved; that is, there is no metabolic acidosis since oxygenation is intact *(80)*. In addition, a normal lactate/pyruvate ratio of 10–15:1 is maintained, because it results from a equilibrium effect (tissue hypoxia manifests an increased lactate/pyruvate ratio) *(7)*. The degree of hyperlactatemia is a useful indicator of the severity of stress, since it increases in parallel with the systemic oxygen consumption and the level of insulin resistance *(see below) (7,81)*. Oxidative utilization of pyruvate during stress was previously thought to be decreased, which in turn promoted hyperglycemia; this position was supported by studies that indicated downregulation of pyruvate dehydrogenase (PDH) during stress *(7,82)*. Long et al. *(44)* were the first to demonstrate that hyperglycemia is not owing to an inability to oxidize glucose by infected or injured tissue. Recent data obtained using a stable isotope technique in burn patients also casts doubt on downregulated PDH, since pyruvate oxidation was shown to be markedly (300%) increased *(46)*.

In summary, stress is associated with increased cellular uptake of glucose. This is largely the result of a cytokine-mediated increase in NIMGU by cells involved in the immune response to injury or infection; this in turn stimulates glycolytic flux by a mass action effect. The reason why these cells satisfy their energy requirements glycolytically despite adequate oxygenation is unknown. Current evidence fails to support earlier theories that hyperglycemia during stress occurs secondary to inhibited oxidative utilization of glucose.

Insulin Resistance

One of the earliest descriptions of insulin resistance during stress was by Howard in 1955, who noted that military casualties demonstrated a response to oral glucose loading that was similar to diabetics *(83)*. Although the concept of the "diabetes of injury" is well recognized, this terminology is misleading in that it implies a lack of insulin. Stress is more appropriately viewed as an insulin-resistant state, since hyperglycemia typically occurs in the setting of a normal or increased plasma insulin concentration. Insulin resistance is usually defined in terms of the action of insulin on glucose homeostasis; however, stress is also associated with resistance to other effects of insulin, such as the failure to suppress lipolysis *(84)*. As mentioned, the degree of insulin resistance is directly proportional to the severity of the stress response; for reasons that are not clear, septic stress is particularly prone to induce insulin resistance *(7,8,76)*. Skeletal muscle is the primary site of peripheral insulin resistance during stress owing in part to its large mass; IMGU in fat, liver, and heart may also be reduced *(85–89)*.

Insulin resistance may result from a receptor and/or postreceptor defect in insulin action. Receptor defects are manifest as decreased sensitivity to insulin in which the dose–response relationship between no effect and maximal effect is shifted to the right; decreased sensitivity can usually be overcome by increasing the insulin concentration. A postreceptor defect is expressed as decreased responsiveness to insulin in which the maximal response to insulin is reduced (e.g., increasing insulin will not further increase glucose uptake). Although experimental evidence exists that supports impaired insulin binding in critical illness *(90,91)*, the majority of the data favor a postreceptor defect *(24,72,74,76)*. The mechanism for insulin resistance has not been precisely identified. However, as previously mentioned, it is likely that a combined effect of the neuroendocrine and cytokine systems plays a major role in this process; for example, insulin resistance induced by TNF appears to be mediated by β-adrenergic stimulation *(92)*. It is also likely that the mechanism for insulin resistance involves the rate-limiting step for glucose disposal (i.e., the process or metabolic step that ultimately determines the amount of glucose metabolized in tissue). Although data are stress is lacking, Fink et al. observed that under normal conditions, glucose transport is rate-limiting for glucose up-take *(93)*. Glucose transport was also shown to be rate limiting in type I and II diabetes *(94,95)*. Counterregulatory hormones and cytokines may antagonize insulin-mediated glucose transport in muscle or fat by causing translocation of transporters from the plasma membrane to an internal location or by decreasing the intrinsic activity or synthesis of the GLUT4 transporter isoform *(73,96–99)*. Glucose transport could also be inhibited by a cytokine-mediated defect in the postbinding signaling process *(74)*. TNF has been shown to mediate insulin resistance in animal models of obesity-diabetes by inhibiting insulin receptor tyrosine kinase in muscle and fat *(100)*; however, no data currently exist that have explored this mechanism during stress. Alternately, it has been proposed that in the setting of hyperinsulinemia, the rate-limiting step in IMGU in muscle shifts from glucose transport to some step beyond transport *(101)*. Inhibition of glycogenesis in skeletal muscle has been proposed as a posttransport mechanism for insulin resistance; the resulting decrease in glucose utilization could inhibit glucose diffusion by promoting a rise in intracellular glucose concentration (which is normally close to zero) *(72,75,76,81)*. Manchester et al. *(102)* also provided evidence supporting a posttransport mechanism for insulin resistance. Using a single cultured myocyte preparation, they observed that hexokinase was saturated with glucose in the presence of insulin and physiological concentrations of glucose; in this setting, glucose phosphorylation rather than glucose transport was the rate-limiting step for insulin-stimulated glucose utilization. Finally, it has been suggested that insulin resistance may occur secondary to downregulation of pyruvate dehydrogenase in skeletal muscle *(7,47)*. Shangraw et al. recently explored this hypothesis by observing the effect of dichloroacetate on glucose kinetics during insulin stimulation in septic humans and rats; dichloroacetate did not influence whole-body insulin-stimulated glucose utilization in either group *(103)*. It therefore appears that decreased pyruvate dehydrogenase activity does not mediate sepsis-induced insulin resistance.

In summary, hyperglycemia is common following injury or infection, despite the fact that many tissues exhibit increased cellular uptake and utilization of glucose. Peripheral insulin resistance is central to this process by limiting IMGU in skeletal muscle. In addition, hepatic insulin resistance also plays a role in the genesis of hyperglycemia during stress *(72,104)*. Teleologically, insulin resistance is an effective means to maintain a hyperglycemic milieu; this aids in meeting substrate demands of tissues that have an increased obligatory requirement for glucose as an energy substrate. Although the precise mechanism for insulin resistance is unknown, it is likely that the defect occurs at a site proximal to mitochondrial glucose oxidation *(76,103)*.

Hyperglycemia, Insulin Resistance, and Stress Stratification

In general, the degree of hyperglycemia and insulin resistance is directly proportional to the severity of the stress response; hyperlactatemia and oxygen consumption also increase concurrently with the severity of stress *(8,81)*. These parameters can be used to stratify the level of stress (i.e., low, mid, or high) (Table 1). This is valuable not only as an indicator of response to treatment (a persistently high level of stress may indicate the presence of a complication, such as an occult abscess), but also as a way to assess nutritional requirements *(105)*.

OTHER CAUSES OF HYPERGLYCEMIA DURING STRESS

Administration of glucose-based parenteral nutrition is a common cause of hyperglycemia in the stressed patient. Although glucose is the preferred fuel for tissues involved in the immune response to injury, once glucose uptake is maximized, administration of additional glucose calories may result in significant hyperglycemia (e.g., glucose > 250 mg/dL) *(3,106)*. Blood glucose must therefore be frequently monitored (at least twice daily) in stressed patients receiving parenteral nutrition. Patients with underlying cirrhosis also may exhibit glucose intolerance ("hepatogenous diabetes") owing to a limited ability to store glycogen *(107)*. Pancreatitis is also a well-described cause of hyperglycemia, owing in part to associated hyperglucagonemia *(108)*. A vari-

Table 1
Stress Stratification by Metabolic Criteria[a]

Stress level	Urine nitrogen, g/d	Plasma[b] lactate, mM/L	Plasma[c] glucose, mg/dL	Insulin resistance	Oxygen consumption, mL/min/m²
Low	<10	<1.5	<150	No	<140
Mid	10–20	1.5–3.0	150–250	Some	140–180
High	>20	>3	>250	Yes	>180

[a]Adapted from ref 8 with permission.
[b]With a lactate/pyruvate ratio <20 mM/L.
[c]In the absence of diabetes mellitus, pancreatitis, and steroid therapy.

ety of drugs may worsen glucose tolerance and result in hyperglycemia. Although corticosteroids are probably the major cause, hyperglycemia may also be promoted by thiazide diuretics, pentamidine, phenytoin, or phenothiazines (109). Hypokalemia promotes hyperglycemia on the basis of impaired insulin secretion (110). Glucose intolerance has been described in association of chromium deficiency (111). Chromium is required for the synthesis of the glucose tolerance factor, which facilitates insulin binding to its receptor site. The requirements for chromium during critical illness have not been precisely determined, however. Finally, previously undiagnosed diabetes mellitus may present with hyperglycemia during stress (112).

CLINICAL MANAGEMENT OF HYPERGLYCEMIA DURING STRESS

There is no good evidence that maintaining normoglycemia (e.g., blood glucose of 90–120 mg/dL) during stress is beneficial. In fact, modest hyperglycemia (e.g., blood glucose > 160 < 220 mg/dL) may be of potential benefit by promoting cellular glucose uptake (113). However, severe hyperglycemia may be associated with complications, such as hypertonicity, osmotic diuresis, volume depletion, hypotension, and electrolyte imbalance; this in turn could result in end-organ dysfunction (e.g., renal failure, myocardial infarction, altered mental status).

The initial approach to the management of severe hyperglycemia during stress involves correcting hypokalemia and eliminating any drugs that worsen glucose tolerance. However in many cases, hyperglycemia occurs secondary to the administration of parenteral nutrition, particularly when glucose calories are dosed in excess of requirements. Infusing excess glucose calories may also stimulate catecholamine release, causing diaphoresis and tachycardia (114,115), as well as promoting hepatic lipogenesis and fatty liver (116). It is therefore important to assess energy requirements accurately in the critically ill; indirect calorimetry may be of value in some instances (113). Supplying the predicted caloric requirements of morbidly obese patients without inducing hyperglycemia may be particularly difficult; some authorities have recommended caloric restriction in this setting (117). Insulin can be used to control plasma glucose, with the understanding that it does not alter the metabolism of glucose through oxidative pathways (118). Only modest doses of insulin should be used; the requirement for more than 5 U regular insulin/hour to maintain a blood glucose <250 mg/dL in a nondiabetic, nonpancreatic patient implies that significant insulin resistance is present and that further increases in insulin dosing are not likely to be of benefit (119). In this instance, glucose calories should be reduced; any caloric deficit resulting from glucose restriction can be satisfied by increasing the fractional proportion of lipid calories. However, iv fat is not without problems in the critically ill; administration of excess lipids is potentially associated with a fat overload syndrome and iatrogenic immunosuppression *(120,121)*. Lipids should therefore be limited to 0.5–1.0 g/kg/d, and serum triglyceride levels should not be allowed to exceed 350 mg/dL during continuous infusion of parenteral nutrition *(122)*. There may be also be a role for alternate caloric sources; data exist that support the use of glycerol or xylitol during stress *(123,124)*.

REFERENCES

1. Bernard C. Leçons sur le diabete et la Glycogenase Animale. Bailliere, Paris, 1877.
2. Jarhult J. Osmotic fluid transfer from tissue to blood during hemorrhagic hypotension. Acta Physiol Scand 1973;89:213–226.
3. Wilmore DW. The wound as an organ. In: Little RA, Frayn KN, eds. The Scientific Basis for the Care of the Critically Ill. Manchester University Press, Manchester, UK, 1986, pp. 45–59.
4. Cuthbertson DP. Post-shock metabolic response. Lancet 1942;1:433–437.
5. Barton RN. Neuroendocrine mobilization of body fuels after injury. Br Med Bul 1985;41:218–225.
6. Frayn KN, Little RA, Maycock PF, Stoner HB. The relationship of plasma catecholamines to acute metabolic and hormonal responses to injury in man. Circ Shock 1985;16:229–240.
7. Siegel JH, Cerra FB, Coleman B, Giovannini I, Shetye M, Border JR, McMenamy RH. Physiological and metabolic correlations in human sepsis. Surgery 1979;86:163–193.
8. Cerra FB. Multiple organ failure syndrome. In: Bihari DJ, Cerra FB, eds, Multiple Organ Failure. Society of Critical Care Medicine, Fullerton, CA, 1989, pp. 1–24.
9. Abumrad NN, Molina PE. The role of the nervous system in modulating the catabolic state. In: Revhaug A, ed. Acute Catabolic State: Update in Intensive Care and Emergency Medicine, vol. 21. Springer, Berlin, 1996, pp. 23–33.
10. Dunn AJ. The role of interleukin-1 and tumor necrosis factor alpha in the neurochemical and neuroendocrine responses to endotoxin. Brain Res Bull 1992;29:807–812.
11. Ovadia H, Abramsky O, Barak V, Confortini N, Saphier D, Weidenfeld J. Effect of interleukin-1 on adreno-cortical activity in intact and hypothalamic deafferentated male rats. Exp Brain Res 1989;76:246–249.
12. Rivier C, Chizzonite R, Vale W. In the mouse, the activation of the hypothalamic–pituitary–adrenal axis by a lipopolysaccharide (endotoxin) is mediated through interleukin-1. Endocrinology 1989;125:2800–2805.
13. Bateman A, Singh A, Kral T, Solomon S. The immune-hypothalamic–pituitary–adrenal axis. Endocr Rev 1989;10:92–112.
14. Foster AH. The early endocrine response to injury. In: Revhaug A, ed. Acute Catabolic State: Update in Intensive Care and Emergency Medicine, vol. 21. Springer, Berlin, 1996, pp. 35–77.
15. Linares O, Jacquez J, Zech L, Smith MS, Sanfield JA, Morrow LA, Rosen SG, Halter JB. Norepinephrine metabolism in humans: kinetic analysis and model. J Clin Invest 1987;80:1332–1341.
16. Frayn KN. Hormonal control of metabolism in trauma and sepsis. Clin Endocrinol 1986;24:577–599.
17. Blackard WG, Nelson NC, Andrews SS. Portal and peripheral vein immunoreactive glucagon concentrations after arginine or glucose infusions. Diabetes 1974;23:199–202.
18. McLeod MK, Carlson DE, Gann DS. Hormonal responses associated with early hyperglycemia after graded hemorrhage in dogs. Am J Physiol 1986;251:E597–E606.
19. Petit F, Jarrous A, Dickinson RD, Molina PE, Abumrad NN, Lang CH. Contribution of central and peripheral adrenergic stimulation to IL-1 alpha-mediated gluco-regulation. Am J Physiol 1994;267:E49–E56.
20. Michie HR, Spriggs DR, Manogue KR, Sherman ML, Revhaug A, O'Dwyer ST, Arthur K, Dinarello CA, Cerami A, Wolff SM, Kufe DW, Wilmore DW. Tumor necrosis factor and endotoxin induce similar metabolic responses in human beings. Surgery 1988;104:280–286.
21. Meguid MM, Brennan MF, Aoki TT, Muller WA, Ball MR, Moore FD. Hormone-substrate interrelationships following trauma. Arch Surg 1974;109:776–783.
22. Vitek V Lang DJ, Cowley RA. Admission serum insulin and glucose levels in 247 accident victims. Clinica Chimica Acta 1979;95:93–104.

23. Stoner HB, Frayn KN, Barton RN, Threlfall CJ, Little RA. The relationships between plasma substrates and hormones and the severity of injury in 277 recently injured patients. Clin Sci 1979;56:563–573.
24. Black PR, Brooks DC, Bessey PQ, Wolfe RR, Wilmore DW. Mechanisms of insulin resistance following injury. Ann Surg 1982;196:420–435.
25. Zawalich WS, Zawalich KC. Interleukin 1 is a potent stimulator of islet insulin secretion and phosphoinositide hydrolysis. Am J Physiol 1989;256:E19–E24.
26. Cornell RP, Schwartz DB. Central administration of interleukin 1 elicits hyperinsulinemia in rats. Am J Physiol 1989;256:R772–R777.
27. Felig P, Sherwin RS, Soman V, Warren J, Hendler R, Sacca L, Eigler N, Goldberg D, Walesky M. Hormonal interactions in the regulation of blood glucose. Recent Prog Horm Res 1979;35:501–532.
28. Ross R, Miell J, Freeman E, Jones J, Matthews D, Preece MA, Buchanan C. Critically ill patients have high basal growth hormone levels with attenuated oscillatory activity associated with low levels of insulin-like growth factor-1. Clin Endocrinol (Oxford) 1991;35:47–54.
29. Ross RJM, Miell JP, Holly JMP, Maheshwari H, Norman M, Abdulla AF, Buchanan CR. Levels of GH, IGF BP-1, insulin, blood glucose and cortisol in intensive care patients. Clin Endocrinol (Oxford) 1991;35:361–367.
30. Bessey PQ, Watters JM, Aoki TT, Wilmore DW. Combined hormonal infusion simulates the metabolic response to sepsis. Ann Surg 1984;200:264–281.
31. Hill AG, Wilmore DW. The history of the metabolic response to injury. In: Revhaug A, ed. Acute Catabolic State: Update in Intensive Care and Emergency Medicine, vol. 21. Springer, Berlin, 1996, pp. 5–14.
32. Meszaros K, Lang CH, Bagby GJ, Spitzer JJ. Tumor necrosis factor increases in vivo glucose utilization of macrophage-rich tissues. Biochem Biophys Res Commun 1987;149:1–6.
33. Lang CH, Dobrescu C, Bagby GJ. Tumor necrosis factor impairs insulin action on peripheral glucose disposal and hepatic glucose output. Endocrinology 1992;130:43–52.
34. Petit F, Bagby GJ, Lang CH. Tumor necrosis factor mediates zymosan-induced increase in glucose flux and insulin resistance. Am J Physiol 1995;268:E219–E228.
35. Lang CH, Molina PE, Yousef KA, Tepper PG, Abumrad NN. Role of IL-1 alpha in central nervous system immunomodulation of glucoregulation. Brain Res 1993;624:53–60.
36. Wolfe RR, Burke JF. Effect of glucose infusion on glucose and lactate metabolism in normal and burned guinea pigs. J Trauma 1978;18:800–805.
37. Gump FE, Long CL, Geiger JW, Kinney JM. The significance of altered gluconeogenesis in surgical catabolism. J Trauma 1975;15:704–713.
38. Jahoor F, Herndon DN, Wolfe RR. Role of insulin and glucagon in the response of glucose and alanine kinetics in burn-injured patients. J Clin Invest 1986;78:807–814.
39. Durkot MJ, Wolfe RR. Effects of adrenergic blockade on glucose kinetics in septic and burned guinea pigs. Am J Physiol 1984;241:R222–R227.
40. Wolfe RR, Jahoor F, Herndon DN, Wolfe MH. The glucose-alanine cycle: origin of control. J Parenter Enteral Nutr 1985;8:107 (Abstract).
41. Roh MS, Moldawer LL, Ekman LG, et al. Stimulatory effect of interleukin-1 upon hepatic metabolism. Metabolism 1986;35:419–424.
42. Bagby GJ, Lang CH, Spitzer JJ. Cytokine modulation of glucose metabolism. In: Schlag G, Redl H, eds. Pathophysiology of Shock, Sepsis and Organ Failure. Springer Verlag, Berlin, 1993, pp. 593–608.
43. Wolfe RR, Burke JF. Effect of glucose infusion on glucose and lactate metabolism in normal and burned guinea pigs. J Trauma 1978;18:800–805.
44. Long CL, Spencer JL, Kinney JM, Geiger JW. Carbohydrate metabolism in man: effect of elective operations and major injury. J Appl Physiol 1971;31:110–116.
45. Daniel AM, Shizgal HM, MacLean LD. The anatomic and metabolic source of lactate in shock. Surg Gynecol Obstet 1978;147:697–700.
46. Wolfe RR, Jahoor F, Herndon D, Miyoshi H. Isotopic evaluation of the metabolism of pyruvate and related substrates in normal adult volunteers and severely burned children: effect of dichloroacetate and glucose infusion. Surgery 1991;110:54–67.
47. Vary TC, Siegel JH, Tall BD, Morris JG. Metabolic effects of partial reversal of pyruvate dehyrogenase activity by dichloroacetate in sepsis. Circ Shock 1988;24:3–18.
48. Haymond MW, Miles JM. Branched chain amino acids as a major source of alanine nitrogen in man. Diabetes 1982;31:86–89.

49. Bortz WM, Paum P, Haff AC, Holmes WL. Glycerol turn-over and oxidation in man. J Clin Invest 1972;51:1537–1546.
50. Boija PO, Nulander G, Ware J. The effect of hemorrhagic stress on liver gluconeogenesis. Acta Chir Scand 1987;153:273–278.
51. Wolfe RR. Carbohydrate metabolism in the critically ill patient. Crit Care Clin 1987;3:11–24.
52. Wolfe RR, Burke JF. Glucose and lactate metabolism in experimental septic shock. Am J Physiol 1978;235:R219–R227.
53. Yelich MR, Witek-Janusek L, Filkins JP. Glucose dyshomeostasis in endotoxicosis: direct versus monokine-mediated mechanisms of endotoxin action. In: Szentivanyi A, Friedman H, Nowotny A, eds. Immunobiology and Immunopharmacology of Bacterial Endotoxins. Plenum, New York, 1986, 111–132.
54. Hill M, McCallum R. Altered transcriptional regulation of phosphoenolpyruvate carboxykinase in rats following endotoxin treatment. J Clin Invest 1991;88:811–816.
55. Deutschman CS, DeMaio A, Buchman TG, Clemens MG. Sepsis-induced alterations in phosphoendolpyruvate carboxykinase expression: the role of insulin and glucagon. Circ Shock 1993;40:295–302.
56. Meszaros K, Lang CH, Bagby GJ, Spitzer JJ. Contribution of different organs to increased glucose consumption after endotoxin administration. J Biol Chem 1987;262:10,965–10,970.
57. Lang CH, Dobrescu C. Gram-negative infection increases noninsulin-mediated glucose disposal. Endocrinology 1991;128:645–653.
58. Huang SC, Phelps ME, Hoffman EJ, Sideris K, Selin CJ, Kuhl DE. Noninvasive determination of local cerebral metabolic rate of glucose in man. Am J Physiol 1980:238:E69–E82.
59. Baron AD, Brechtel G, Edelman SV. Rates and tissue sites of non-insulin- and insulin-mediated glucose uptake in humans. Am J Physiol 1988;255:E769–E774.
60. Pessin JE, Bell G. Mammalian facilitative glucose transporter family: structure and molecular regulation. Ann Rev Physiol 1992;54:911–930.
61. Stephens JM, Bagby GJ, Pekala PH, Shepherd RE, Spitzer JJ, Lang CH. Differential regulation of glucose transporter gene expression in adipose tissue of septic rats. Biochem Biophys Res Commun Res Commun 1992;183:417–422.
62. Lang CH, Dobrescu C. Sepsis-induced increases in glucose uptake by macrophage-rich tissues persist during hypoglycemia. Metabolism 1991;40:585–593.
63. Lee MD, Zentella A, Pekala PH, Cerami A. Effect of endotoxin-induced monokines on glucose metabolism in the muscle cell line L6. Proc Natl Acad Sci USA 1987;84:2590–2594.
64. Meszaros K, Lang CH, Bagby GJ, Spitzer JJ. Tumor necrosis factor increases in vivo glucose utilization of macrophage-rich tissues. Biochem Biophys Res Commun 1987;149:1–6.
65. Bird TA, Davies A, Baldwin SA, Saklatvala J. Interleukin-1 stimulates hexose transport in fibroblasts by increasing the expression of glucose transporters. J Biol Chem 1990;265:13578–13583.
66. Cornelius P, Lee MD, Marlow M, Pekala PH. Monokine regulation of glucose transporter mRNA in L6 myotubes. Biochem Biophys Res Commun 1989;165:429–436.
67. Zeller WP, Sian WT, Sweet M, Goto M, Gottschalk ME, Hurley RM, Filkins JP, Hofman C. Altered glucose transporter mRNA abundance in a rat model of endotoxic shock. Biochem Biophy Res Commun 1991;176:535–540.
68. Baly DL, Horuk R. The biology and biochemistry of the glucose transporter. Biochem Biophys Acta 1988;947:571–590.
69. Cushman SV, Wardzala JL. Potential mechanism of insulin action on glucose transport in the isolated rat adipose cell. J Biol Chem 1980;255:4758–4762.
70. Cheatham B, Kahn CR. Insulin action and the insulin signaling network. Endocr Rev 1995;16:117–142.
71. Moller DE, Flier JS. Insulin resistance-mechanisms, syndromes, and implications. N Engl J Med 1991;325:938–948.
72. Virkamaki A, Puhakainen I, Koivisto VA, Vuorinen-Markkola H, Yki-Jarvinen H. Mechanisms of hepatic and peripheral insulin resistance during acute infections in humans. J Clin Endo Met 1992;74:673–679.
73. Sato N, Irie M, Kajinuma H, Suzuki K. Glucagon inhibits insulin activation of glucose transport in rat adipocytes mainly through a postbinding process. Endocrinology 1990;127:1072–1077.
74. Lang CH. Mechanism of insulin resistance in infection. In: Schlag G, Radl H, eds. Pathophysiology of Shock, Sepsis and Organ Failure. Springer Verlag, Berlin 1993, pp. 609–625.
75. Lang CH, Bagby GJ, Buday AZ, Spitzer JJ. The contribution of gluconeogenesis to glycogen repletion during glucose infusion in endotoxemia. Metabolism 1987;36:180–187.

76. Shangraw RE, Jahoor F, Miyoshi H, Neff WA, Stuart CA, Herndon DN, Wolfe RR. Differentiation between septic and postburn insulin resistance. Metabolism 1989;38:983–989.
77. Hotchkiss RS, Karl IE. Reevaluation of the role of cellular hypoxia and bioenergetic failure in sepsis. JAMA 1992;267:1503–1519.
78. Brooks GA. Lactate production under fully aerobic conditions: the lactate shuttle during rest and exercise. Fed Proc 1986;45:2924–2929.
79. Cohen SR. Why does brain make lactate? J Theor Biol 1985;112:429–432.
80. Mizock BA. Lactic acidosis. Disease-a-Month 1989;35:233–300.
81. Mizock BA. Alterations in carbohydrate metabolism during stress: a review of the literature. Am J Med 1995;98:75–84.
82. Vary TC, Siegel JH, Nakatani T, Sato T, Aoyam H. Regulation of glucose metabolism by altered pyruvate dehydrogenase activity. I. Potential site of insulin resistance in sepsis. J Parenter Enteral Nutr 1986;10:351–355.
83. Howard JM. Studies of the absorption and metabolism of glucose following injury. The systemic response to injury. Ann Surg 1955;141:321–326.
84. Little RA, Carlson GL. Insulin resistance and tissue fuels. In: Kinney JM, Tucker HN, eds. Organ Metabolism and Nutrition: Ideas for Future Critical Care. Raven, New York, 1994, pp. 49–68.
85. Lang CH, Dobrescu C, Meszaros K. Insulin-mediated glucose uptake by individual tissues during sepsis. Metabolism 1990;39:1096–1107.
86. Clemems MG, Chaudry IH, Daigneau N, Baue AE. Insulin resistance and depressed gluconeogenic capability during early hyperdynamic sepsis. J Trauma 1984;24:701–708.
87. Holley DC, Spitzer JA. Insulin action and binding in adipocytes exposed to endotoxin in vitro and vivo. Circ Shock. 1980;7:3–12.
88. Raymond RM, McLane MP, Law WR, King NF, Leutz DW. Myocardial insulin resistance during acute endotoxin shock in dogs. Diabetes 1988;37:1684–1688.
89. Igarashi M, Yamatani K, Fukase N, Daimon M, Ohnuma H, Takahashi H, Manaka H, Tominaga M, Sasaki H. Sepsis inhibits insulin-stimulated glucose transport in isolated rat adipocytes. Diabetes Res Clin Pract 1992;15:213–218.
90. Chaudry IH, Sayeed MM, Baue AE. The effect of insulin on glucose uptake in soleus muscle during hemorrhagic shock. Can J Physiol Pharmacol 1975;53:67–73.
91. Raymond RM, Klein DM, Gibbons DA, Jacobs MK, Emerson TE. Skeletal muscle insulin unresponsiveness during chronic hypermetabolic sepsis in the dog. J Trauma 1985;25:845–855.
92. Lang CH. Beta-adrenergic blockade attenuates insulin resistance induced by tumor necrosis factor. Am J Physiol 1993;264:R984–R991.
93. Fink RI, Wallace P, Brechtel G, Olefsky JM. Evidence that glucose transport is rate-limiting for in vivo glucose uptake. Metabolism 1992;41:897–902.
94. Yki-Jarvinen H, Sahlin K, Ren JM, Koivisto VA. Localization of rate-limiting defect for glucose disposal in skeletal muscle of insulin-resistant type I diabetic patients. Diabetes 1990;39:157–167.
95. Kashiwagi A, Verso MA, Andrews J, Vasquez B, Reaven G, Foley JE. In vitro insulin resistance of human adipocytes isolated from subjects with noninsulin-dependent diabetes mellitus. J Clin Invest 1983;72:1246–1252.
96. Kuroda M, Honnor RC, Cushman SW, Londos C, Simpson IA. Regulation of insulin-stimulated glucose transport in the isolated rat adipocyte. J Biol Chem 1987;262:245–253.
97. Horner HC, Munck A, Lienhard GE. Dexamethasone causes translocation of glucose transporters from the plasma membrane to an intracellular site in human fibroblasts. J Biol Chem 1987;262:17696–17702.
98. Smith U, Kuroda M, Simpson IA. Counter-regulation of insulin-stimulated glucose transport by catecholamines in the isolated rat adipose cell. J Biol Chem 1984;259:8758–8763.
99. Stephens JM Pekeala PH. Transcriptional repression of the GLUT4 and C/EBP genes in 3T3-L1 adipocytes by tumor necrosis factor-alpha. J Biol Chem 1991;266:21,839–21,845.
100. Hatamisligil GS, Budaavari A, Murray D, Spiegelman BM. Reduced tyrosine kinase activity of the insulin receptor in obesity-diabetes: central role of tumor necrosis factor alpha. J Clin Invest 1994;94:1543–1594.
101. Kubo K, Foley JE. Rate-limiting steps for insulin-mediated glucose uptake into perfused rat hindlimb. Am J Physiol 1986;250:E100–E102.
102. Manchester J, Kong Z, Nerbonne J, Lowry OH, Lawrence JC Jr. Glucose transport and phosphorylation in single cardiac myocytes: rate-limiting steps in glucose metabolism. Am J Physiol 1994;266:E326–E333.

103. Shangraw RE, Jahoor F, Wolfe RR, Lang CH. Pyruvate dehydrogenase inactivity is not responsible for sepsis-induced insulin resistance. Crit Care Med 1996;24:566–574.
104. McLane MP, Tomasik TW, Law WR, Raymond RM. Hepatic insulin resistance during canine sepsis. Circ Shock 1991;33:207–215.
105. Mizock BA. Branched-chain amino acids in sepsis and hepatic failure. Arch Int Med 1985;145:1284–1288.
106. Wolfe RR. Metabolic response to burn injury: nutritional implications. Semin Nephrol 1993;13:382–390.
107. Megyesi C, Samols E, Marks V. Glucose intolerance and diabetes in chronic liver disease. Lancet 1967;2:1051–1055.
108. Donowitz M, Hendler R, Spiro HM, Binder HJ, Felig P. Glucagon secretion in acute and chronic pancreatitis. Ann Int Med 1975;83:778–781.
109. Kahn CR, Shechter Y. Insulin, oral hypoglycemic agents, and the pharmacology of the endocrine pancreas. In: Goodman Gilman A, Rall TW, Nies AS, Taylor P, eds. Goodman and Gilman's The Pharmacological Basis of Therapeutics, 8th ed. Pergamon, New York, 1990, p. 1483.
110. Rowe JW, Tobin JD, Rosa RM, Andres R. Effect of experimental potassium deficiency on glucose and insulin metabolism. Metabolism 1980;29:498–502.
111. Baumgartner TG. Trace elements in clinical nutrition. Nutr Clin Pract 1993;8:251–263.
112. Husband DJ, Alberti KG, Julian DG. Stress hyperglycemia during acute myocardial infarction: an indicator of pre-existing diabetes? Lancet 1983;2:179–181.
113. Bursztein S, Elwyn DH, Askanazi J, Kinney JM. Energy Metabolism, Indirect Calorimetry, and Nutrition. Saunders, Baltimore, 1989.
114. Askanazi J, Carpentier YA, Elwyn DH, Nordenstrom J, Jeevanandan M, Rosenbaum SH, Gump FE, Kinney JM. Influence of total parenteral nutrition on fuel utilization in injury and sepsis. Ann Surg 1980;191:40–46.
115. Nordenstrom J, Jeevanandam M, Elwyn DH, Carpentier YA, Askanazi J, Robin A, Kinney JM. Increasing glucose intake during total parenteral nutrition increases norepinephrine excretion in trauma and sepsis. Clin Physiol 1981;1:525–534.
116. Nussbaum MS, Li S, Bower RH, McFadden SW, Dayal R, Fischer JE. Addition of lipid to total parenteral nutrition prevents hepatic steatosis in rats by lowering the portal venous insulin/glucagon ratio. J Parent Ent Nutr 1992;16:106–109.
117. Pasulka PS, Kohl D. Nutrition support of the stressed obese patient. Nutr Clin Pract 1989;4:130–132.
118. Cerra F. The syndrome of hypermetabolism and multiple system organ failure. In: Hall JB, Schmidt GA, Wood LDH, eds. Principles of Critical Care. McGraw Hill, New York, 1992, pp. 656–666.
119. Pruett TL, Cerra FB. The physiologic and metabolic response to stress and sepsis. Med Times 1985;113:98–107.
120. Fischer GW, Hunter KW, Wilson SR, Mease AD. Diminished bacterial defences with Intralipid. Lancet 1980;2:819–820.
121. Sobrado J, Moldawer LL, Pomposelli JJ, Mascioli EA, Babayan VK, Bistrian BR, Blackburn GL. Lipid emulsions and reticuloendothelial system function in healthy and burned guinea pigs. Am J Clin Nutr 1985;42:855–863.
122. Negro F, Cerra FB. Nutritional monitoring in the ICU: rational and practical application. Crit Care Clin 1988;4:559–572.
123. Karlstad MD, DeMichele SJ, Bistrian BR, Blackburn GL. Effect of total parenteral nutrition with xylitol on protein and energy metabolism in thermally injured rats. J Parent Ent Nutr 1991;15:445–449.
124. Waxman K, Day AT, Stellin GP, Tominaga GT, Gazzaniga AB, Bradford RR. Safety and efficacy of glycerol and amino acids in combination with lipid emulsion for peripheral parenteral nutition support. J Parent Ent Nutr 1992;16:374–378.

11 Alterations in Fuel Metabolism in Critical Illness
Hypoglycemia

K. Patrick Ober, MD

CONTENTS
> INTRODUCTION
> METABOLIC NEED FOR GLUCOSE
> CLINICAL MANIFESTATIONS
> PHYSIOLOGY OF GLUCOSE MAINTENANCE
> COUNTERREGULATION
> DIAGNOSIS OF HYPOGLYCEMIA
> CAUSES OF HYPOGLYCEMIA
> THERAPY OF HYPOGLYCEMIA
> REFERENCES

INTRODUCTION

Glucose has an essential function as the fundamental energy source for the brain. This critical fuel requirement creates a need for a consistently available and uninterrupted supply of glucose. Because of the crucial need for glucose, an intricate homeostatic system has evolved to assure adequate availability of glucose at all times: Postabsorptive (fasting) levels of plasma glucose are generally kept within the fairly narrow range of 60–100 mg/dL or 3.3–5.6 m*M*/L *(1)*. This stability is maintained even under the disruptive circumstances of caloric deprivation and increased energy requirements, which occur with severe trauma, febrile illnesses, and other catabolic states. The maintenance of adequate serum glucose levels is, in fact, a paramount goal of the stress response, and the increased secretion of "stress hormones," such as cortisol, catecholamines, and growth hormone, contributes to the provision of consistent glucose availability; if the system for glucoregulation is going to be off-target, it will err by promoting an elevation of glucose levels, rather than risking the potential catastrophe of an inadequate glucose supply. Thus, an elevation of the serum glucose level is the most common clinical disorder of glucose metabolism in critical illness, as discussed in detail in Chapter 10. However, some patients with critical illness will have a failure in the life-sustaining system for maintaining serum glucose levels; this inability to provide an adequate energy supply can lead to severe dysfunction of many organs, and it ultimately may cause the demise of the affected individual.

From *Contemporary Endocrinology: Endocrinology of Critical Disease*
Edited by K. P. Ober   Humana Press Inc., Totowa, NJ

METABOLIC NEED FOR GLUCOSE

The central nervous system (CNS) is the major site of glucose utilization *(2)*. In the infant, the brain uses 85–90% of the glucose that is produced *(3)*. In the adult, about 50% of the glucose produced by the body is metabolized by the brain *(4)*. A higher ratio of brain to body weight and high rates of insulin-independent use of glucose by the brain put infants and children at greater risk than adults for developing hypoglycemia *(5)*. Glucose moves down a concentration gradient across the blood–brain barrier; this movement is facilitated by glucose transport proteins *(3,6)*. There are five glucose-transporter proteins in the human. The importance of these transport proteins is demonstrated by an "experiment of nature" in which two children were found to have a decreased number of the type of glucose transporters found in brain tissue (type 1, or GLUT1, transporters); in spite of normal serum glucose levels, the ratio of serum:cerebrospinal fluid glucose concentration was reduced to the range of 0.19–0.35 (compared to the normal of 0.65), and the patients experienced typical symptoms of hypoglycemia (including seizures and impaired psychomotor development) *(7)*. With deficient GLUT1, the defect in glucose transporters functionally creates the same consequences as those that occur in the more typical hypoglycemic individuals who lack sufficient amounts of glucose for presentation to the transporters (Fig. 1). The situation with the GLUT-deficient individuals is a contrast to normal physiology, in which glucose transport across the blood–brain barrier is not the rate-limiting step in cerebral glucose metabolism—typically, about half of the transported glucose actually diffuses back into the bloodstream, and under normal conditions, the metabolism of glucose in the brain is limited by the intracellular phosphorylation of glucose to glucose-6-phosphate, not by the transport process (in a rat model, the rate of glucose uptake by the whole brain is maintained even with a sustained reduction of plasma glucose concentration to approx 2.3 mM/L, although more severe hypoglycemia (<2 mM/L) does result in decreased cerebral glucose utilization *[8]*).

The system of glucose transport into the CNS is an adaptable one, and the effectiveness of the transport system can be increased to compensate for the challenges of hypoglycemia. In vitro, capillary endothelial cells in the brain will increase the transcription and translation of GLUT1 if they are deprived of glucose *(9,10)*. Prolonged hypoglycemia in rodents will lead to an increased number of glucose transporters in the brain (Fig. 1), which augments the extraction of glucose *(11,12)*. In a study of patients with insulin-dependent diabetes mellitus *(13)*, brain glucose transport was evaluated in the context of lowering the plasma glucose from 105 mg/dL (5.8 mM/L) to 54 mg/dL (3.0 mM/L). The patients with the lowest glycosylated hemoglobin levels (7.2 ± 0.5%), who also have the greatest frequency of hypoglycemia *(14)*, were able to maintain normal brain glucose transport at the lower glucose level, whereas brain glucose transport was less effective in diabetic subjects with chronically higher mean glucose levels (glycosylated hemoglobin 8.5 ± 0.4 and 10.2 ± 1.3%) when glucose levels were lowered. Nondiabetic subjects also showed less effective glucose transport at the lower glucose range. As would be anticipated, the group that maintained more effective glucose transport also had the lowest responses of plasma epinephrine and pancreatic polypeptide to lower blood sugars, and also had the lowest frequency of hypoglycemic symptoms. This seemingly beneficial adaptive response to hypoglycemia can be a mixed blessing, however. On the positive side, enhanced glucose uptake in the setting of hypoglycemia allows the individual at the greatest risk of low blood sugar level (such as the tightly controlled insulin-dependent

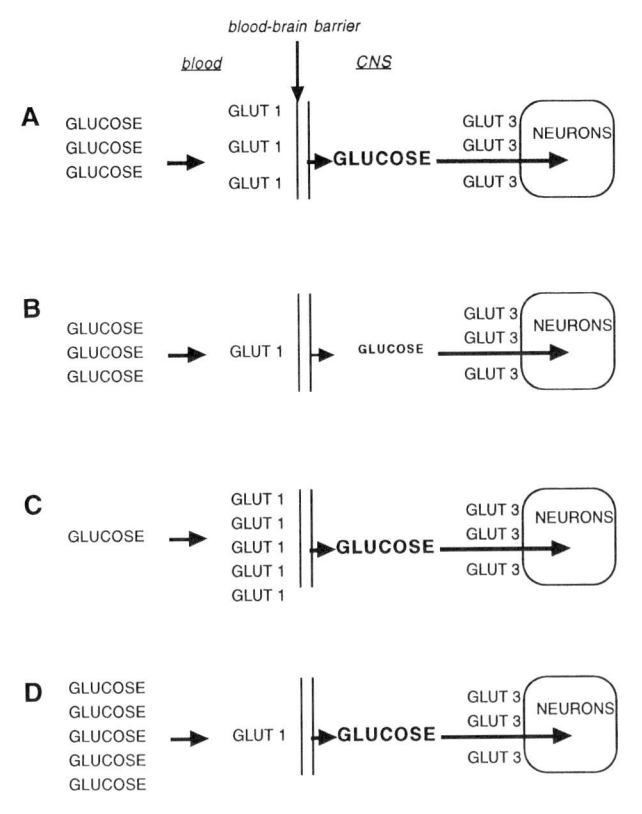

Fig. 1. Relationships of glucose transporters. The blood–brain barrier is depicted in the middle. Glucose transfer from the bloodstream to the CNS is mediated by GLUT1 transporters on the vascular cells of the CNS, and GLUT3 transporters move glucose into the neurons. (**A**) Normal physiology. (**B**) GLUT1-deficient individuals have decreased glucose transport into the CNS, in spite of normal blood glucose concentrations. (**C**) Upregulation of GLUT1 in the setting of chronic hypoglycemia, resulting in enhanced availability of glucose to the CNS, but preventing CNS awareness of low blood glucose levels. (**D**) Downregulation of GLUT1 in the context of chronic hyperglycemia, potentially explaining symptoms of neuroglycopenia at "normal" blood glucose levels in patients with poorly controlled diabetes mellitus. (Modified from ref. 87.)

diabetic) to maintain better an adequate glucose supply to the brain in the face of hypoglycemia; on the negative side, the enhanced uptake prevents the brain from recognizing that the plasma glucose is lower than normal, thereby creating a considerable risk for continuing (but unrecognized and thus undefended) declines in glucose levels to a point where hypoglycemia is so profound that even the augmented uptake cannot provide the brain with sufficient glucose. As a result, the role of the brain as the consumer of plasma glucose usurps its role as the protector of the plasma glucose level because of this adaptation; the enhanced glucose transport allows the brain to receive an adequate amount of glucose for a longer duration, which simultaneously denies the CNS the chance to recognize hypoglycemia, and thus removes the opportunity to promote the processes of counterregulation and caloric ingestion needed to protect the plasma glucose level. By the time the plasma glucose is low enough to impair cerebral metabolism, the resultant neuroglycopenia may be severe enough to render the patient incapable of correcting the defect, and the seemingly protective ability to increase glucose uptake in the brain has become a maladaptive response *(13)*.

Since the increased brain uptake of glucose that follows hypoglycemia tends to preserve cerebral metabolism in the setting of low blood sugar levels, the blunting of the expected autonomic and counterregulatory responses creates an unawareness of hypoglycemia that creates an environment for recurrent hypoglycemic episodes *(13)*. The phenomenon is not unique to patients with insulin-treated diabetes mellitus *(15)*: When nondiabetic subjects are made hypoglycemic for <2 h, they have less vigorous autonomic and symptomatic responses to hypoglycemia the following day *(16)*. Similarly, at any given level of hypoglycemia, patients with insulinomas demonstrate a reduction in the autonomic and symptomatic responses to a low blood sugar, with less impairment of their cognitive function; removal of the insulinoma reverses these changes *(17)*. The reversibility of this effect has also been show in intensively treated diabetic patients with hypoglycemia unawareness; efforts to avoid hypoglycemia (reflected in an increase in glycosylated hemoglobin from 5.8 to 6.9%) have resulted in normalization of responses to hypoglycemia, including symptomatic, cognitive, and biochemical (pancreatic polypeptide, growth hormone, and cortisol) responses *(18)*.

The adverse effects of hypoglycemia are owing to a depression of central synaptic transmission, which is caused by energy deprivation. In rat hippocampal slices, the hypoglycemia-mediated defect is caused by the release of adenosine, which acts at a presynaptic site and suppresses the release of transmitters *(19)*. (Endogenous adenosine release is also the mediator of hypoxia-induced suppression of synaptic transmission.) Although an activation of ATP-sensitive K^+ channels (resulting from falling cellular ATP) could theoretically be another possible mechanism by which hypoglycemia might cause synaptic failure, this does not seem to be the case *(19)*.

There are regional differences in glucose metabolism throughout the brain, and as a result, the susceptibility to adverse effects of the hypoglycemia varies on a regional basis *(2)*. The explanation for the varying regional effects of hypoglycemia is not clearcut. Even though the oxygen consumption of the brain is closely linked to glucose metabolism *(2)* (cerebral oxygen consumption decreases proportionately to decreases in blood sugar), hypoglycemia and hypoxia provoke different responses in terms of physiologic, biochemical, and cellular changes *(6)*. For example, even though the functional changes resulting from hypoglycemia and hypoxia appear to be similar, the effect of hypoglycemia is more likely to affect cortical areas, especially the temporal lobes, whereas hypoxia's effects are more localized to the posterior brain *(2)*. Hypoglycemia tends to spare the brainstem and spinal cord, but causes damage to the middle layers of the cerebral cortex and hippocampus *(20)*. Hypoglycemia is associated with an increase in tissue pH, contrasted to the tissue acidosis, which occurs with hypoxia *(2)*.

Neurophysiologic consequences of hypoglycemia include nonspecific abnormalities in the electroencephalogram and impairment of event-related brain potentials, with conflicting reports regarding visual, auditory, and somatosensory evoked potentials *(21)*.

CLINICAL MANIFESTATIONS

The clinical consequences of hypoglycemia are variable, and undoubtedly are related to duration and severity of the hypoglycemic insult. Although most symptomatology is short-lived, with reversal occurring promptly after restoration of blood glucose levels, some neurologic deficits can persist for days or even weeks if the hypoglycemia has been particularly severe or prolonged; in some cases, the neurological damage may be irreversible, but such an outcome is very rare *(2)*. The neurologic effects of hypoglycemia as seen clinically are protean, with confusion, disorientation, and combativeness being relatively common. Seizures are also frequently seen, and other described problems include ataxia, hemiparesis, coma, decortication, decerebration, choreoathetosis, and "locked-in" syndrome *(20)*. A case of bilateral cortical blindness, with full recovery after 5 mo, has been described *(22)*. There has been concern about possible long-term intellectual impairment following hypoglycemia, although the Diabetes Control and Complications Trial did not find any difference in neuropsychologic function in the intensive insulin treatment group (followed for an average of 6.5 yr) in spite of a threefold increase in severe hypoglycemia *(14)*. However, in another study, the frequency of severe hypoglycemia has been correlated with the magnitude of intellectual decline in 100 patients with insulin-dependent diabetes *(23)*.

In a Danish survey of patients with diabetes mellitus diagnosed before the age of 31 yr, 5% of the deaths can be attributed to hypoglycemia *(24)*. A United Kingdom study suggests that 4% of deaths in diabetic patients <50 yr old are caused by hypoglycemia *(25)*.

In addition to its CNS effects, hypoglycemia can cause a peripheral neuropathy (which is predominantly motor-sensorimotor) *(26)*.

The maintenance of normal glucose levels is also critical for the function of nonneuronal tissues. Euglycemia is essential for the normal function of phagocytic cells; the ability of the reticuloendothelial system to remove bacteria or endotoxin from the circulation is depressed by hypoglycemia *(27)*.

Hypothermia is a well-recognized accompaniment of hypoglycemia *(28)*; the degree of hypothermia is related to the severity of the hypoglycemia *(29)*. In healthy human subjects, hypoglycemia causes an early increase in metabolic heat production owing to increased sympathoadrenal activity (which can be abolished by β-blockade). Even with the increase in metabolic heat production, heat dissipation at the skin surface causes a subsequent fall in core temperature as a consequence of a prompt and sustained sympathetically mediated sweating response, with evaporative heat loss and conduction of heat to the periphery *(29)*. There is evidence that the hypothermia of hypoglycemia may be a protective response: mortality in hypoglycemic rats is increased if hypothermia is prevented *(30)*, and lower brain temperature during hypoglycemia has been shown to limit hypoglycemic neuronal loss *(31)*.

PHYSIOLOGY OF GLUCOSE MAINTENANCE

In view of the primacy of glucose as fuel for the CNS and the fact that it takes the CNS several days to convert to the use of alternative fuels, such as ketones *(32)*, it is not surprising that numerous and complex control mechanisms have evolved for the maintenance of euglycemia. These mechanisms are directed toward achieving a balance between the systemic utilization of glucose and the entry of glucose into the bloodstream by means of the gastrointestinal tract, glycogenolysis, and gluconeogenesis.

The diet is the most obvious source of glucose for the meeting of energy requirements. After a meal, insulin secretion in response to carbohydrate ingestion promotes hepatic glucose storage in the form of glycogen, and stimulates glucose uptake by muscle and fat

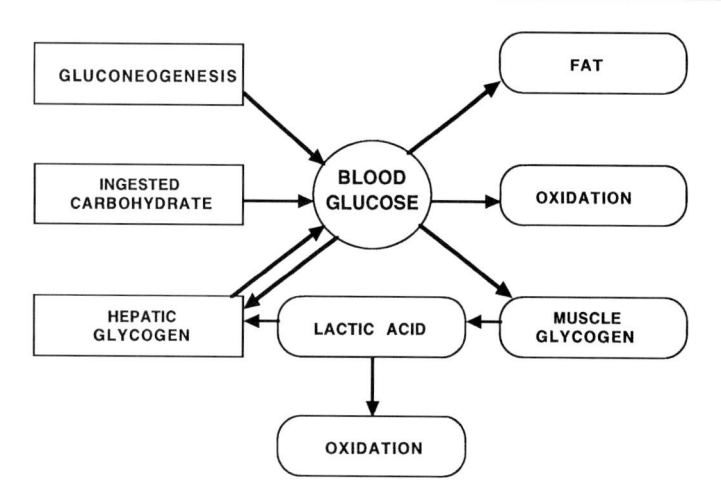

Fig. 2. Sources of glucose and products of glucose metabolism. (From ref. *34*.)

tissue. In the absence of caloric intake, the liver becomes responsible for maintenance of the serum glucose level. Insulin plays a critical role in suppressing hepatic glucose output, and a decline in serum insulin concentration is the single most important hormonal response to decreasing glucose levels; plasma insulin levels approach zero as the blood glucose approaches 40 mg/dL *(33)*. For the first 8–12 h of a fast, a decrease in insulin levels permits the liver to liberate glucose from the breakdown of glycogen stores (glycogenolysis) in order to maintain the serum glucose (Fig. 2). When glycogen stores are depleted, the liver switches to production of glucose from noncarbohydrate precursors (gluconeogenesis). The precursors for gluconeogenesis become more readily available owing to the declining insulin effect in peripheral tissues; the substrates of gluconeo-genesis include products of protein breakdown (especially alanine), end products of glucose metabolism (lactate and pyruvate), and a product of triglyceride breakdown (glycerol). Because of the low insulin levels of fasting, there is little glucose uptake in insulin-sensitive tissues, and glucose utilization is predominantly directed to the CNS. After glycogen stores are depleted, the glucose concentration represents the balance between gluconeogenesis and the body's relatively constant noninsulin-mediated glucose consumption (primarily by the brain); thus, most conditions that cause altered glucose balance reflect abnormalities in gluconeogenesis *(34)*.

With prolonged fasting (on the order of weeks), fat breakdown becomes the dominant source of energy supply as the brain adapts to the use of ketone bodies for an energy source and body proteins are spared.

Even though the physiological need to maintain adequate glucose levels is well established, the definition of the "normal" serum glucose concentration has been enigmatic. There are several variables, including gender, which appear to influence this measurement. Two obvious stresses on the glucose-maintenance system are the cessation of caloric intake (fasting) and the acceleration of energy utilization (exercise); studies of fasting and exercising humans have given some insights into the physiological set points which appear to be relevant to glucose homeostasis. These studies also provide intriguing information that runs counter to many popular concepts of glucose balance, including a demonstration that surprisingly low blood sugar measurements can occur in very healthy people who fast or exercise intensely, and that these low glucose concentrations do not result in any of the defined functional impairments that are classically associated with hypoglycemia in other contexts.

With fasting, the plasma glucose measurements gradually drift downward and eventually level off at a fairly consistent steady-state value. When normal subjects were fasted for 72 h, the lowest glucose levels in men were found to be 61.9 mg/dL *(35)* and 66.4 ± 2.9 mg/dL *(36)*, compared to values of 52.0 mg/dL *(35)* and 47.8 ± 2.9 mg/dL in premenopausal women *(36)*. Based on these results, plasma glucose measurements within the first 24 h of fasting would have to be <55 mg/dL in men and <35 mg/dL in women before they can be considered abnormal (i.e., more than 2 SD below the mean nadir); at 72 h of fasting, the glucose measurements that would define the lower limits of normal are 50 mg/dL for men and 14.5 mg/dL for premenopausal women *(36)*! In studies of 72-h fasts in healthy subjects, the lowest measurement found in men is consistent at 55 mg/dL *(35,36)*; this is in contrast to the lowest levels found in asymptomatic women of 22 *(36)*, 36 *(35)*, and 47 mg/dL *(37)*. Thus, it appears that there is no clinically meaningful lower limit for glucose levels in premenopausal women who are fasting for prolonged intervals—as a result, there is not any way to differentiate a physiologically low from a pathologically low glucose level on the basis of glucose measurements alone (Fig. 3). The reason for this sex difference is unclear. Theorized considerations include an effect of sex hormones, a decrease in gluconeogenesis in women (owing to reduced muscle mass, with decreased availability of the amino acids needed for gluconeogenesis), or impairment of gluconeogenesis precursors owing to the ketosis of fasting (which is greater in women than in men).

Prolonged and intensive physical activity is also a severe challenge to glucose balance. With exercise for more than 90 min, liver glycogen stores are depleted; glucose production does not keep up with glucose utilization, and serum glucose levels fall. Approximately one-third (37%) of men who exercised to exhaustion at 60–65% maximal aerobic power following a 10–14 h fast developed blood glucose levels under 45 mg/dL (2.5 mM/L) (Fig. 4). The hypoglycemic range was reached after 60–150 min of exercise; however, in spite of blood glucose levels of 25–48 mg/dL (1.4–2.7 mM/L), the hypoglycemic subjects exercised at the same intensity for another 15–70 min, and their exhaustion time was not significantly different from that of the euglycemic group *(38)*. The hypoglycemia was not a physiologically silent event; plasma epinephrine was inversely related to blood glucose, and in the hypoglycemic subjects, reached levels that were three times higher than in the normoglycemic individuals. Glucose ingestion prevented the hypoglycemia (and attenuated the rise in epinephrine), but did not affect the perception of exertion or delay exhaustion.

COUNTERREGULATION

The importance of maintaining a fairly constant level of serum glucose is reflected in the elaborate system for defending against falling glucose concentrations. Four major counterregulatory hormones are of varying importance and effectiveness in counteracting a hypoglycemic threat, and there is a hierarchy of responses of the factors that counterbalance the threat of hypoglycemia. Each factor has a somewhat different threshold for activation *(39,40)*, and the physiological importance of each component in the system of defense against hypoglycemia tends to be reflected by its position in the hierarchy. Small

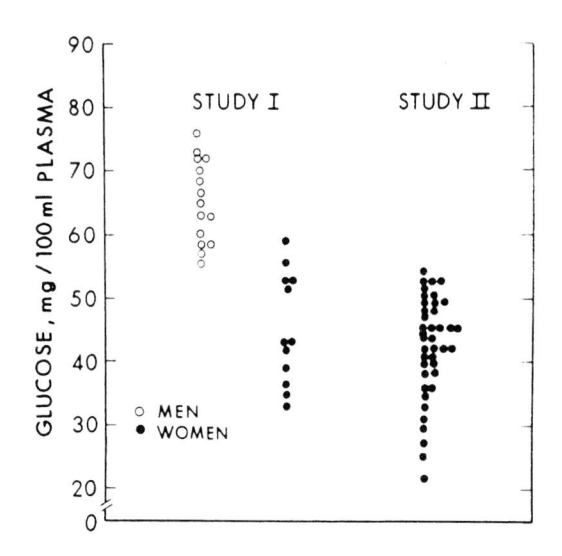

Fig. 3. Effect of fasting on blood glucose levels in men and in premenopausal women. Each circle represents the lowest plasma glucose concentration recorded for an individual during a 72-h fast. (From ref. *36*.)

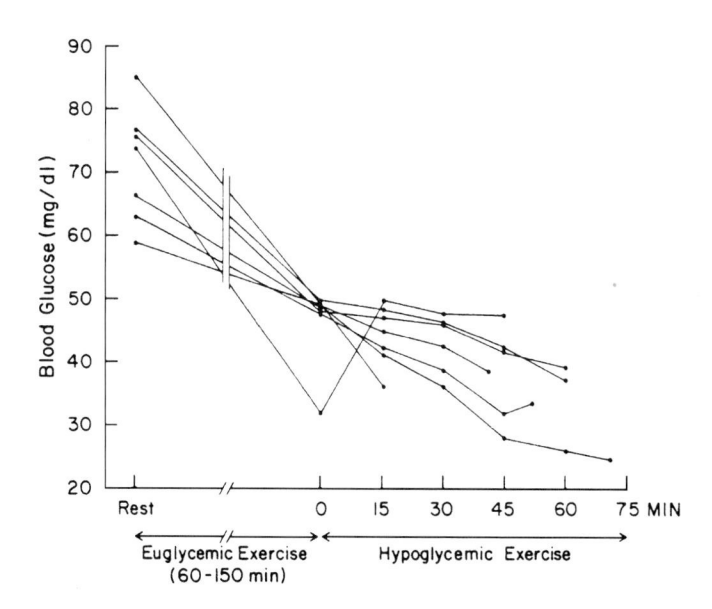

Fig. 4. Effect of vigorous exercise on blood glucose levels. Of 19 healthy men who exercised to exhaustion on a cycle ergometer, the seven shown in this figure became hypoglycemic (blood glucose <45 mg/dL [<2.5 mM/L]). "Euglycemic Exercise" denotes the interval of exercise in which the blood glucose remained >50 mg/dL (>2.8 mM/L), and "Hypoglycemic Exercise" indicates the period of exercise after the blood glucose concentration fell below 50 mg/dL (2.8 mM/L). (From ref. *38*.)

decreases in the plasma glucose concentration to the threshold of 65 mg/dL (3.6 m*M*/L) are usually sufficient to trigger the secretion of glucagon and epinephrine *(40,41)*, the hormones that are of greater counterregulatory importance. Cortisol levels do not increase until the blood glucose falls below 55 mg/dL.

The single most important counterregulatory hormone is glucagon, which enhances hepatic glycogenolysis and gluconeogenesis; without glucagon, full recovery from hypoglycemia does not occur *(1)*. Epinephrine, which has an additional action of inhibiting insulin secretion, is not necessary for counterregulation of hypoglycemia when glucagon is present, but it becomes essential in the absence of glucagon (a common occurrence in the patient with insulin-dependent diabetes). Growth hormone and cortisol are slower to act as counterregulatory agents, and these hormones do not make any substantial contribution to glucose counterregulation during acute insulin-induced hypoglycemia *(42)*; since growth hormone and cortisol cannot compensate effectively for hypoglycemia in the absence of glucagon and epinephrine, they are of secondary importance in the counterregulatory scheme *(34)*. Although cortisol production is increased with severe hypoglycemia, its effect as an insulin antagonist develops over a somewhat longer time frame *(40)*. Deficiencies of growth hormone and cortisol do not impair the recovery from prolonged insulin-induced hypoglycemia, but will result in lower plasma glucose concentrations in such a setting *(43)*.

As the major user of glucose, it is not surprising that the brain is a primary organ for recognizing and directing the counterregulatory response to hypoglycemia. However, the previously described counterregulatory factors have a higher glycemic threshold than that of the CNS, and thus the counterregulatory hormones are activated before CNS symptoms develop or cognitive function becomes impaired *(40)*. As plasma glucose levels reach the 60–66 mg/dL range, the triggering of catecholamine release causes the adrenergic symptoms of tachycardia, palpitation, tremor, and pallor, and these symptoms become even more severe with further decline in glucose concentrations *(40)*. If the plasma glucose falls lower than 65 mg/dL (3.6 m*M*/L), the level where glucagon and epinephrine release are provoked, to the range of 55 mg/dL (3.1 m*M*/L), the increasing production of counterregulatory hormones is joined by the onset of autonomic symptoms (including anxiety, hunger, irritability, trembling, and sweating), which are mediated by specific glucose-sensing centers in the ventromedian hypothalamic nuclei of the brain *(44)*. With further lowering of glucose, neuroglycopenic symptoms appear (weakness, confusion, faintness, headache, impaired concentration, cognitive impairment, behavioral abnormalities, and even coma and seizures) *(41,45,46)*.

In a measurement of the latency of a brain potential related to decision time, a threshold for neuroglycopenia was identified between 50 and 60 mg/dL *(47)*; most studies suggest that the threshold for neuroglycopenia is near 50 mg/dL *(32,40)*. The symptomatic responses to hypoglycemia promote actions that compensate for the falling glucose, such as the increased caloric intake which is stimulated by the autonomic symptoms. Although the suggestion has been made that the rate of fall of glucose (independent of the absolute glucose levels) might be a trigger for the release of catecholamines (and thus the development of adrenergic symptoms), the bulk of available information indicates that the development of symptoms and signs of hypoglycemia is not influenced by the rate of decrease of the plasma glucose level, but is related to the glycemic threshold level *per se (48–50)*. The precise threshold level reported for the triggering of these responses varies somewhat from investigator to investigator. With arterialized venous blood, plasma glucose concentrations near 60 mg/dL will result in symptoms in healthy persons during acute insulin-induced hypoglycemia; impaired brain function is noted around 50 mg/dL (2.8 m*M*/L) *(15,39,40)* (these values should be lowered by 3 mg/dL [0.17 m*M*/L] in venous blood *[51]*).

In spite of the sophistication and intricacy of this elaborate counterregulatory system, it can fail under several circumstances. One such situation occurs in the insulin-treated patient who is unaware of hypoglycemia because of the compensatory enhancement of glucose transport efficiency in response to previous hypoglycemia, as noted above *(13)*. Such an individual becomes aware of hypoglycemia only when the fall in glucose is so profound as to induce severe brain dysfunction, by which time the patient may not be capable of reacting to the problem *(41)*.

The specific sites in the CNS that detect glucopenia and initiate the counterregulatory response have not been clearly identified. When hypoglycemia is selectively induced in only the carotid or in only the vertebrobasilar circulation of dogs, the humoral response to hypoglycemia (and the subsequent increase in hepatic glucose production) is only mildly attenuated in comparison to the effect of whole brain hypoglycemia *(52)*. The response to selective hypoglycemia in the vertebrobasilar circulation suggests that glucose-sensitive neurons are found in the brainstem and/or posterior hypothalamus, whereas the response to carotid system hypoglycemia indicates that other sites are also important. Since significant counterregulation occurs when hypoglycemia develops in either of these circulations, it is not likely that there is a single center for hypoglycemic counterregulation; instead, it appears that redundant glucose-sensing neurons are located in widespread brain regions.

Factors other than hypoglycemia may play a role in the counterregulatory response. In insulin-dependent diabetes, there is evidence that insulin itself may modulate neuroendocrine counterregulation, the perception of hypoglycemia, and cerebral function *(53)*. When blood glucose levels are maintained at comparable levels, higher levels of hyperinsulinemia within the physiological range enhance neuroendocrine response and symptom awareness, and are associated with deterioration of electrophysiological activity and neuropsychological skills. Although the brain has traditionally been considered to be insensitive to insulin, it is possible for insulin to enter the CNS directly, without passing through the blood–brain barrier, by way of the circumventricular organs (median eminence and arcuate nucleus), or indirectly (through insulin receptor-mediated active transport across the blood–brain barrier *[54]*). The facilitated receptor-mediated transport of insulin across the blood–brain barrier *(55)* leads to a suppressive effect of insulin on glucose utilization in the CNS *(56,57)*. In view of the fact that hyperinsulinemia is linked with hyperglycemia under normal physiological circumstances, the role of insulin as a suppressor of CNS glucose use has been suggested as a teleologic mechanism to avoid "inundation of the brain with glycolytic products" *(53)*. Thus, in the insulin-treated patient, the impairment of glucose utilization which is mediated by insulin (resulting in subsequent neuroglycopenia of the glucoregulatory centers) could be a trigger of autonomic activation by insulin.

DIAGNOSIS OF HYPOGLYCEMIA

From a clinical perspective, the measurement of a low blood glucose level is certainly an essential component of the diagnosis. However, as discussed previously, remarkable nadirs of blood sugar can occur in perfectly healthy people under varying physiological conditions (such as intense exercise by athletes and fasting in healthy premenopausal women). As a result, the isolated finding of a low blood sugar (defined by criteria that are intrinsically arbitrary) is not in its own right sufficient for diagnosing hypoglycemia, a term that connotes a pathological state. Instead, "Whipple's triad" must be employed to define the criteria for establishing the diagnosis of hypoglycemia:

1. CNS manifestations of low glucose ("neuroglycopenic symptoms"), which can include confusion, disorientation, unusual behavior, seizures, and coma;
2. A simultaneous blood glucose level <40 mg/dL (2.2 mmol/L); and
3. Recovery from the symptoms following glucose administration *(32)*.

Thus, although the finding of a low plasma glucose level is required for the diagnosis of hypoglycemia, it is not sufficient by itself.

The diagnosis of hypoglycemia can be excluded if hypoglycemic signs or symptoms fail to occur during a 72-h fast *(1)*. It should be emphasized that even though the "β-adrenergic" manifestations of tachycardia, tremor, palpitation, and diaphoresis can be seen with hypoglycemia, these symptoms are quite nonspecific (they are commonly associated with anxiety, fear, and a multitude of other stresses), and they should not be considered indicative of a hypoglycemic disorder unless they are associated with neuroglycopenic symptoms and the measurement of a low serum glucose level. In fact, the diagnosis of "reactive hypoglycemia" (which traditionally has been used as an explanation or rationalization for isolated autonomic symptoms) is now defunct, and its associated "diagnostic test," the 5-h oral glucose tolerance test, has been discredited: "there are no bona fide hypoglycemic disorders characterized solely by autonomic symptoms" *(1)*.

CAUSES OF HYPOGLYCEMIA

Even after the presence of hypoglycemia has been firmly established by the criteria contained in Whipple's triad, the differential diagnosis can be a tricky clinical challenge. There are many potential causes of hypoglycemia, iatrogenic and organic, and many patients may have several coexisting problems that could contribute to hypoglycemia.

Insulin excess is probably the most obvious cause of hypoglycemia. In an insulin-treated patient, the source of hypoglycemia is usually quite evident (especially in the patient who has had decreased or delayed caloric intake or increased activity prior to the hypoglycemic episode). This is a particularly commonplace problem in hospitalized patients with diabetes who have decreased caloric intake because of illness and hospital routine *(58)*. Following treatment of insulin-induced hypoglycemia by either glucose or glucagon administration, most patients will recover without sequelae. However, seizures are common, and a small percentage of deaths in diabetic patients can be attributed to hypoglycemia *(2)*. The possibility that patients with recurring episodes of hypoglycemia may experience long-term impairment of intellectual or cognitive function has been a topic of concern; there is some evidence to suggest that this may occur, although the data are not consistent or clear-cut *(2)*.

There may be additional confounding factors in the patient with insulin-induced hypoglycemia: the kidneys play a role in insulin metabolism, and the patient with frequent hypoglycemia or decreasing insulin requirements should be assessed for possible renal insufficiency. In addition, insulin-dependent diabetes (as an autoimmune disorder) can also be associated with other immunologically mediated diseases, and thus, the possibility of Addison's disease should be considered as a possible contributor to hypoglycemia in such patients.

The differential diagnosis becomes more complicated when hypoglycemia occurs in an individual who is not insulin-treated. The possibility of insulin-mediated hypoglycemia should be strongly considered in the healthy-appearing patient. This is in contrast to many patients who are hypoglycemic because of noninsulin-related problems (such as end-stage renal disease, hepatic failure, malignancy, and so forth, as discussed below) in whom the underlying disease is usually severe and apparent, and thus the cause of the hypoglycemia is evident (1).

The classic evaluation of the hypoglycemic patient with no obvious cause for the low glucose includes a prolonged fast (up to 72 h), and requires demonstration of nonsuppressed insulin levels in combination with documented and symptomatic hypoglycemia. The differential diagnosis of a patient with hypoglycemia and nonsuppressed insulin levels includes insulinoma and surreptitious insulin administration (insulin has been used as a means of suicide and homicide [59]), and the simultaneous measurement of C-peptide becomes a critical component of the evaluation. C-peptide and insulin, the two breakdown products of proinsulin, are produced in equimolar amounts; therefore, elevated measurements of both insulin and C-peptide are seen with an insulinoma, in contrast to the findings in a patient who surreptitiously uses exogenous insulin (where the insulin level will be high, but the C-peptide will be low owing to the hypoglycemia-induced suppression of endogenous insulin production).

In the hypoglycemic patient, the finding of a lowered level of β-hydroxybutyrate also strongly suggests that the hypoglycemia is mediated by insulin or an insulin-like factor, and a brisk increase in plasma glucose following the iv administration of glucagon is further support of the same conclusion.

In the patient with factitious hypoglycemia owing to the surreptitious use of exogenous insulin, the symptoms usually involve neuroglycopenic symptoms, which are erratic in their occurrence; this disorder is seen mostly in women, especially if they are employed in a health-related job (60). With confrontation, about half of them will admit to the activity, and most will discontinue the practice (59). Insulin autoimmune hypoglycemia is a biochemically similar disorder (with elevated free insulin and suppressed C-peptide levels at the time of hypoglycemia), and may be difficult to differentiate from factitious hypoglycemia. In this disorder, some of the insulin secreted in response to a meal is presumably bound to antibodies; later, as the insulin dissociates from the antibodies (in the postabsorptive phase when less insulin is needed), the free insulin level becomes higher than the physiological need, and the hyperinsulinemia promotes hypoglycemia. Autoimmune hypoglycemia appears to be a self-limiting disorder, and many of the patients with this process can be identified because of the presence of other coexisting autoimmune diseases (1,61,62). In other patients, autoantibodies to the insulin receptor may exert an agonist action instead of the expected antagonist effect, with resultant hypoglycemia; coexisting autoimmune disorders may be a clue to the diagnosis (63).

The finding of simultaneously increased insulin and C-peptide does not absolutely confirm the presence of insulinoma: ingestion of sulfonylureas, which stimulate β-cell insulin secretion, will also result in elevation of both insulin and C-peptide levels.

Hypoglycemia also occurs in the setting of nonislet cell tumors. These are typically large tumors of mesenchymal, hepatocellular, hematological, or neuroendocrine origin. The mechanisms proposed for the hypoglycemia have included increased glucose utilization by the large tumors, suppression of hepatic glucose production, or enhanced peripheral glucose utilization. There is now convincing evidence that insulin-like growth factor 2 (IGF-2) is the hormonal mediator of the hypoglycemia *(64–66)*. Total IGF-2 levels may be normal, but are inappropriate for the associated low growth hormone (GH) state, and increased amounts of free IGF-2 and "big IGF-2" (a prohormone of IGF-2) are found. Elevated free IGF-2 inhibits insulin and pituitary GH secretion, which subsequently suppresses production of IGF-1; there is a decrease in levels of the major IGF binding protein IGFBP-3 (its levels are related to GH levels), but increased production of IGFBP-2 (its levels are inversely related to GH). These changes in IGFBPs appear to make IGF more available to tissues (because of the greater capillary permeability of IGFBP-2's smaller molecular weight and its more rapid turnover *[67]*); the hypoglycemia occurs as the result of IGF interaction with receptors for both insulin and IGF *(66)*. The major cause of hypoglycemia is a substantial increase in glucose disposal, primarily into muscle tissue, where large numbers of both insulin and IGF-1 receptors are found *(65)*. Although suppression of hepatic glucose output contributes to the hypoglycemia of nonislet cell tumors, this is a relatively minor effect; the liver has few IGF-1 receptors, and thus the hepatic effects of IGF-2 and big IGF-2 are probably mediated through the insulin receptor (with resultant attenuation of signal transduction *(65)*, as IGF-2 binds to the insulin receptor with about 1/100 the affinity of insulin *[32]*).

If the underlying tumor is not surgically resectable, it appears that euglycemia can be maintained (at least for some tumors) with GH therapy, which reverses some of the metabolic disturbances: the increase in GH increases insulin resistance, and the associated elevation of IGF-1 levels stimulates IGFBP-3 and suppresses IGFBP-2, thereby offsetting the derangements induced by the increase in IGF-2 and big IGF-2 *(66)*. However, GH has not been successful for all tumors *(68)*. Somatostatin infusion has also been shown to reduce the elevated levels of IGF-2 and decrease whole-body glucose disposal, but hepatic glucose output was also reduced simultaneously (probably because of somatostatin-induced suppression of pancreatic glucagon). As a result, somatostatin alone could not control hypoglycemia, but required the concurrent use of exogenous glucose or glucagon to be effective *(65)*.

End-stage renal disease is frequently cited as a cause of hypoglycemia. The typical patient is severely ill, and the hypoglycemia is frequently a component of the terminal illness. The mechanism for the hypoglycemia is uncertain; renal failure has been associated with impairment of glycogenolysis *(69)* and limitations of gluconeogenesis *(70,71)*, and both of these factors may contribute, particularly in the patient with impaired caloric intake. In addition to impaired hepatic glycogenolysis and gluconeogenesis, a reduction of renal gluconeogenesis is another potential contributor to hypoglycemia (renal gluconeogenesis may provide 45% of new glucose during prolonged starvation *[58]*). Enhanced glucose utilization may also be responsible for the hypoglycemia of renal failure in some patients, although the mechanism for this phenomenon is unknown *(72)*. Ultimately, however, renal failure-associated hypoglycemia is probably multifactorial, and may not be an immediate or direct consequence of the renal failure alone *(73)*. In most cases, one or two factors in addition to the renal disease can be identified; these include chronic malnutrition or an acute reduction of caloric intake; possible limitation of alanine as substrate for gluconeogenesis; a prolonged half-life of insulin; concomitant failure of other organs (hepatic disease or cardiac failure); drug effect (particularly β-adrenergic blockers); infection; use of glucose-free dialysate; and impaired counterregulation *(58,73)*.

Not surprisingly, a variety of liver diseases can be associated with hypoglycemia, reflecting the central role of hepatic function in glucose homeostasis through the crucial processes of glycogenolysis and gluconeogenesis. Passive venous congestion of the liver from congestive heart failure can cause sufficient liver dysfunction to interfere with hepatic glucose output, perhaps because of a defect in release of stored glucose, which is reversible with improvement of cardiac function *(74)*.

Endocrine deficiencies, such as GH deficiency and cortisol deficiency, are also associated with hypoglycemia, with impairment of gluconeogenesis being the presumed mechanism for the hypoglycemia *(32)*. GH deficiency has been associated with an impairment of gluconeogenic substrate from the decreased alanine delivery from muscle stores, which results in hypoglycemia in children (GH-deficient adults appear to be spared from hypoglycemia, although the reasons for this protection are not clear).

In children with hypoglycemia, other liver-related causes should also be considered. Compared to adults, children have impaired abilities of sustaining serum glucose levels with a lengthy fast, and limitations in maintaining sufficient alanine availability to the liver for support of hepatic gluconeogenesis may be an important factor (although the relatively higher proportion of brain mass to body mass in children may also play a role). Ketotic hypoglycemia accounts for 90% of the hypoglycemia in children past infancy. The cause is uncertain, but a popular suggestion is that it is related to an inadequate amount of substrate for gluconeogenesis (particularly alanine); this would be consistent with the fact that it typically occurs in small-sized children with limited muscle mass, and is "outgrown" as the child gains size (and muscle mass). Ketotic hypoglycemia may be no more than an exaggeration of the normal childhood predilection for hypoglycemia with fasting *(75)*. In hypoglycemic children, other considerations include disorders of hepatic gluconeogenesis, which are caused by enzyme deficiencies, such as glucose-6-phosphatase or fructose-1,6-diphosphatase deficiency, and abnormalities in fatty acid metabolism caused by carnitine deficiency. Acquired hepatic dysfunction, as in Reye's syndrome, can cause the same consequences as diffuse liver disease in adults.

Infectious diseases have also been associated with hypoglycemia. Because of the number of coexisting medical problems that can occur in patients with serious infections, the relationship between any particular infectious process and hypoglycemia is not always clear. In recent years, hypoglycemia has become recognized as a serious complication of falciparum malaria *(76)*. The prognosis of these patients is poor; in part, this may be because of a tendency to attribute all neurological signs in infected patients to cerebral malaria, with failure to recognize the coexisting hypoglycemia. The pathophysiology of the hypoglycemia is not clear; increased insulin production triggered by quinine therapy and increased glucose consumption by the parasite appear to be major contributors to the problem, and poor nutritional status of afflicted patients may also play a role. The level of parasitemia may be the most significant correlation, and clearing of parasitemia is a good predictor of resolution of hypoglycemia *(77)*.

Hypoglycemia may also be a manifestation of overwhelming sepsis. In one series, nine patients were identified with mean serum glucose of 22 mg/dL in the setting of severe bacterial sepsis *(78)*. Hypotension, altered mental status, and metabolic acidosis were common findings in these patients. *Streptococcus pneumoniae* was found in three cases and *Hemophilus influenzae*, type b, in two cases. Possible causes for the hypoglycemia may include depletion of glycogen stores, impaired gluconeogenesis, and increased peripheral glucose utilization. Five of the nine patients had other possible contributors to the hypoglycemia, with alcoholism in four and chronic renal insufficiency in one. The mortality was 67%. Hypoglycemia has been noted to be a particularly common finding in cirrhotic patients with septicemia (found in 15 of 30 patients), and is indicative of an extremely poor prognosis (with death in 11 of the 15 affected patients within 48 h *[79]*). In an animal model in which sepsis was induced by injection of *Escherichia coli* into rats, whole-body glucose disposal increased by 53%; this was because of an increased rate of glucose removal by macrophage-rich tissues (liver, spleen, and lung) as well as by barrier tissues that have an immunologic function (ileum and skin) *(8)*. This increased glucose uptake was observed even in the setting of hypoglycemia and insulinopenia; sepsis-related decreases in serum glucose are mediated by noninsulin-mediated glucose transport through the GLUT1 and GLUT3 isoforms of the glucose transporters (which are present in most insulin-insensitive tissues and which are responsible for basal glucose uptake). A number of macrophage secretory products (including tumor necrosis factor and interleukin-1) may be capable of promoting insulin-independent glucose uptake.

Infectious diarrhea is the major cause of death in children 1–5 yr of age in developing countries, and hypoglycemia appears to be a contributor to these deaths, occurring in 4.5% of children who require hospitalization and in 43% of those who die *(80)*. In these patients, counterregulatory hormones are appropriately elevated, and inappropriately low levels of gluconeogenetic substrates appear to be the cause of the hypoglycemia. In the most malnourished patients, concentrations of alanine were as low as in patients with ketotic hypoglycemia (where insufficient mobilization of alanine for gluconeogenesis is believed to be the cause of hypoglycemia); in the better-nourished patients, alanine concentrations were normal, but lactate concentrations were higher than in normal children, suggesting impairment of the hepatic enzymes involved in gluconeogenesis *(80)*.

Of the many potential causes of hypoglycemia, medications and toxins are the most common causes of acute hypoglycemia *(32)*. Prescribed drugs and other substances with pharmacological effects can cause or contribute to hypoglycemia. All sulfonylureas (acetohexamide, chlorpropamide, tolazamide, tolbutamide, glipizide, glyburide, glimepiride) work through the mechanism of stimulating insulin production by pancreatic β-cells. Thus, it is not surprising that all sulfonylureas have been associated with hypoglycemia *(81)*, with the frequency of reported hypoglycemia being related to the half-life of each drug and its metabolites. Chlorpropamide, with the longest half-life of 35 h, is responsible for the largest number of reported hypoglycemic episodes and associated deaths. Since this drug is primarily excreted by the kidneys, its half-life (and thus its toxicity) increases considerably in patients with renal impairment. Some physicians preferentially choose chlorpropamide because of the availability of low-cost generic forms, but this practice can be particularly problematic in some elderly patients in whom inconsistent caloric intake combined with renal disease and the long drug half-life are very substantial risk factors for hypoglycemia. Currently, the "second generation" sulfonylureas (glyburide, glipizide, and glimepiride) account for the vast majority of sulfonylurea usage; of these, glyburide is second only to chlorpropamide in the number of reported cases of severe hypoglycemia and death, reflecting the drug's relatively long half-life and the frequency with which it is prescribed. The presence of a toxin, such as ethanol, can contribute to prolonged episodes of hypoglycemia with the use of chlorpropamide or glyburide *(82)*. Because of the duration of drug effect with the longer-acting agents (especially chlorpropamide), the normalization of blood sugar by glucose administration should not be considered to be the end point of therapy; a recurrent episode of hypoglycemia at home, before the drug has been completely metabolized, could prove fatal. Thus, it may be prudent to admit some patients for further observation (and continued glucose infusion) even after the glucose level has been restored by glucose administration, especially if the patient is an elderly individual who has experienced hypoglycemia from one of the longer-acting agents.

As in other situations involving drug toxicity, the issue of sulfonylurea-induced hypoglycemia is particularly difficult if the drug ingestion is surreptitious. Sulfonylurea levels should be measured in any patient with hypoglycemia of uncertain cause, especially if that person might have access to the drugs (either through prior prescription or from a treated family member). As with factitious insulin administration, a particularly high index of suspicion is warranted for patients with a medical background who have access to these agents, especially if there is any reason to suspect emotional instability.

In some cases, the patient may be the innocent victim of a prescription or dispensing error, receiving a sulfonylurea instead of a drug with a similar name: patients have received Diabenese (chlorpropamide) instead of Diamox (acetazolamide) or Tolinase (tolazamide) instead of Tolectin (tolmetin) *(59)*. A particularly treacherous situation occurs with Diamox (acetazolamide) and Dymelor (acetohexamide) because of the similarities in both trade and generic names *(81)*. Deaths have also occurred in newborns of women who have been treated with sulfonylureas during the third trimester of pregnancy (which is a contraindication to sulfonylurea use), patients who have been administered iv tolbutamide during diagnostic testing for insulinoma, and in individuals who have been treated with chlorpropamide for therapy of diabetes insipidus *(81)*.

Many other agents are capable of causing hypoglycemia. Ethanol is by far the most common cause of severe and life-threatening hypoglycemia in the United States *(81)*. Frequently seen in binge drinkers, the development of ethanol-related hypoglycemia requires an interval of inadequate calorie ingestion during the drinking spree with eventual depletion of liver glycogen stores; in these circumstances, the hepatic conversion of nicotine adenine dinucleotide (NAD) to NADH, which occurs as alcohol is metabolized, renders the liver incapable of providing new glucose formation (because of the dependency of gluconeogenesis on NAD), and hypoglycemia follows *(32)*. In the absence of hepatic glycogen stores, these patients cannot respond to administration of glucagon, and therefore the hypoglycemia must be treated by glucose administration; possible vitamin deficiencies and other nutritional deficiencies, which may be associated with chronic alcoholism, need to be considered and treated—thiamine administration is a particularly crucial intervention in order to avoid the Wernicke-Korsakoff syndrome, which is associated with the glucose therapy.

Salicylate poisoning has also been associated with hypoglycemia (with most reports in children) *(81)*. In addition, β-blocking drugs (particularly the nonselective agents propranolol, pindolol, and nadolol) have been implicated as causes of hypoglycemia, probably because of inhibition of hepatic glucose production *(81)*. This may be of particular concern in dialysis patients in whom the drugs or their metabolites can accumulate. Other drugs that have been associated with hypoglycemia include pentamidine, disopyramide (Norpace), ritodrine (a β-sympathomimetic drug used to inhibit premature labor, with hypoglycemia reported in either mother or baby), and quinine; most of these agents seem to stimulate insulin release from the islet cells to variable degrees. Haloperidol is also associated with hypoglycemia, and in the setting of renal failure, both trimethoprim-sulfamethoxazole and propoxyphene have been implicated *(1)*. The rodenticide Vacor is particularly toxic to pancreatic β-cells, inducing a massive release of stored insulin, which may may result in profound hypoglycemia; eventually, β-cell destruction occurs with resultant diabetes (similar to the result of streptozotocin).

Hypoglycemia can also result from the ingestion of naturally occurring substances, such as unripened Caribbean akee fruit. The mature fruit is a safely ingested dietary staple in Jamaica, but the unripened form contains a substance known as "hypoglycin." This inhibitor of hepatic fatty acid oxidation leads to impaired hepatic gluconeogenesis and resultant hypoglycemia, a disorder referred to "Jamaican vomiting illness" *(32)*.

Approximately 1.2% of adults who are hospitalized in a tertiary care hospital develop hypoglycemia. In an analysis of patients who developed hypoglycemia (serum glucose of 49 mg/dL or less) in a tertiary care hospital, 45% had diabetes mellitus, and the hypoglycemia was attributable to insulin administration in 90% of these, with decreased caloric intake owing to effects of illness or hospital procedures being an important cofactor *(58)*. Chronic renal failure was found in 49% of the hypoglycemic patients; although 43% of the renal failure patients had coexisting diabetes, renal failure in the nondiabetic patient represented the second most common cause of hypoglycemia. Chronic malnutrition was found in 30% of the patients with kidney disease, and 57% had acute caloric deprivation. Liver disease (including passive hepatic congestion, hepatitis, fulminant hepatic failure, and metastatic infiltration) was found in 19% of hypoglycemic patients. Of the 9% who had malignancy, additional factors included liver metastases, malnutrition, and diabetes. Other cases of hypoglycemia were associated with infections, shock, pregnancy, and burns. The overall hospital mortality in this group of hypoglycemic patients was 27%, and was related to the number of risk factors for hypoglycemia and the degree of hypoglycemia, even though hypoglycemia was not the apparent cause of death in any patient.

Inaccuracy of measurement is a potential problem in assessing the patient with possible hypoglycemia. This appears to be a particularly common occurrence with the use of fingerstick glucose measurements in hypotensive patients; 32% of severely hypotensive patients (with systolic blood pressure <81 mmHg) were incorrectly diagnosed as hypoglycemic (glucose <3.89 mM/L [70 mg/dL]) when glucose was measured on fingerstick samples using typical glucose oxidase reagent strips and meters *(83)*. The fingerstick values were significantly lower than simultaneous measurements of venous blood by reagent strips or by laboratory measurements (the fingerstick values were 67.5% of the laboratory-measured levels), even though the measurement of glucose in venous blood by reagent strips correlated well with the laboratory results. This discrepancy cannot be explained by recognized differences in results related to the source of the sample (capillary glucose levels are 7–8% higher than venous glucose values, and plasma glucose values are 15% higher than whole blood measurements *[84]*). It has been suggested that peripheral vasoconstriction with continuous tissue glucose consumption may lead to the decreased peripheral glucose values in this setting *(83)*.

THERAPY OF HYPOGLYCEMIA

The immediate therapy of hypoglycemia is fairly straightforward, requiring simply the administration of glucose to the affected patient *(2)*, and the specific cause of the hypoglycemia is a secondary issue at the time (although simultaneous measurement of insulin and C-peptide levels at the time of hypoglycemia will eventually provide critical diagnostic information in the patient for whom the cause of the low blood sugar is unknown). In the patient who is awake and alert and aware of hypoglycemic symptoms (as in the individual with insulin-dependent diabetes mellitus and insulin-induced hypoglycemia), 20 g of oral glucose or 40 g of carbohydrate as orange juice are sufficient to correct hypoglycemia; a smaller amount of orange juice (20 g of carbohydrate) and milk (20 g of carbohydrate) provides partial correction *(85)*. For patients who are confused, combative, or comatose, glucose should be administered intravenously, with a dose of 25 g being effective in most cases; attempts to administer glucose solutions orally in such patients are strongly discouraged because of a very real risk of aspiration. Another option with comparable efficacy in most patients is the use of 1 mg of iv glucagon *(86)*. Glucagon should be considered only in patients in whom there is a good likelihood that glycogen stores are available in the liver, or else the agent will have no effect; practically speaking, this will be the known insulin-treated patient (in whom the interference of insulin with metabolism of hepatic glycogen stores is a major contributing factor to hypoglycemia). In the patient who is hypoglycemic from causes such as a prolonged alcoholic binge, the absence of hepatic glycogen stores will render the use of glucagon a futile activity. In such patients, glucose should be administered in amounts sufficient to keep the serum glucose within normal limits.

REFERENCES

1. Service FJ. Hypoglycemic disorders. N Engl J Med 1995;332:1144–1152.
2. Service FJ. Hypoglycemia. Med Clin North Am 1995;79:1–8.
3. Zeller J, Bougneres P. Hypoglycemia in infants. Trends Endocrinol Metab 1992;3:366–370.
4. Huang S, Phelps E, Hoffman E, et al. Noninvasive determination of local cerebral metabolic rate of glucose in man. Am J Physiol 1981;238:E69–E82.
5. Haymond MW. Diarrhea, malnutrition, euglycemia, and fuel for thought. N Engl J Med 1990;322:1390–1391.
6. McCall AL. Effects of glucose deprivation on glucose metabolism in the central nervous system. In Frier BM, Fisher BM, eds. Hypoglycemia and Diabetes: Clinical and Physiological Aspects. Edward Arnold, London, 1993, pp. 56–71.
7. De Vivo DC, Trifiletti RR, Jacobson RI, et al. Defective glucose transport across the blood-brain barrier as a cause of persistent hypoglycorrhachia, seizures, and developmental delay. N Engl J Med 1991;325:703–709.
8. Lang CH, Dobrescu C. Sepsis-induced increased in glucose uptake by macrophage-rich tissues persist during hypoglycemia. Metabolism. 1991;40:585–593.
9. Takakura Y, Kuentzel SL, Raub TJ, et al. Hexose uptake in primary cultures of bovine brain microvessel endothelial cells. I. Basic characteristics and effects of D-glucose and insulin. Biochim Biophys Acta 1991;1071:1–10.
10. Boado RJ, Pardridge WM. Glucose deprivation causes posttranscriptional enhancement of brain capillary endothelial glucose transporter gene expression via GLUT1 mRNA stabilization. J Neurochem 1993;60:2290–2296.
11. Koranyi L, Bourrey RE, James D, et al. Glucose transporter gene expression in rat brain: pretranslational changes associated with chronic insulin-induced hypoglycemia, fasting and diabetes. Mol Cell Neurosci 1991;2:244–252.
12. McCall AL, Fixman LB, Fleming N, et al. Chronic hypoglycemia increases brain glucose transport. Am J Physiol 1986;251:E442–E447.
13. Boyle PJ, Kempers SF, O'Connor AM, Nagy RJ. Brain glucose uptake and unawareness of hypoglycemia in patients with insulin-dependent diabetes mellitus. N Engl J Med 1995;333:1726–1731.
14. The Diabetes Control and Complications Trial Research Group. The effect of intensive treatment of diabetes on the development and progression of long-term complications in insulin-dependent diabetes mellitus. N Engl J Med. 1993;329:977–986.

15. Cryer PE. Hypoglycemia begets hypoglycemia in IDDM. Diabetes 1993;42:1691–1693.
16. Heller SR, Cryer PE. Reduced neuroendocrine and symptomatic responses to subsequent hypoglycemia after one episode of hypoglycemia in nondiabetic humans. Diabetes 1991;40:223–226.
17. Mitrakou A, Fanelli C, Veneman T, et al. Reversibility of unawareness of hypoglycemia in patients with insulinomas. N Engl J Med 1993;329:834–839.
18. Fanelli CG, Epifano L, Rambotti AM, et al. Meticulous prevention of hypoglycemia normalizes the glycemic threshold and magnitude of most neuroendocrine responses to, symptoms of, and cognitive function during hypoglycemia in intensively treated patients with short-term IDDM. Diabetes 1993;42:1683–1689.
19. Zhu PJ, Krnjevic K. Adenosine release is a major cause of failure of synaptic transmission during hypoglycemia in rat hippocampal slices. Neuroscience Letters. 1993;155:128–131.
20. Lins PE, Adamson H. Neurologic manifestations of hypoglycemia. In Frier BM, Fisher BM, eds. Hypoglycaemia and Diabetes: Clinical and Physiological Aspects. Edward Arnold, London, 1993, pp. 347–354.
21. Bendtson I. Neurophysiological changes of hypoglyceamia. In Frier BM, Fisher BM, eds. Hypoglycemia and Diabetes: Clinical and Physiological Aspects. Edward Arnold, London, 1993, pp. 72–79.
22. Odeh M, Oliven A. Hypoglycemia and bilateral cortical blindness. Diabetes Care. 1996;19:272–273.
23. Langan SJ, Deary IJ, Hepburn DA, et al. Cumulative cognitive impairment following recurrent severe hypoglyceamia in adult patients with insulin-treated diabetes mellitus. Diabetologia 1991;34:337–344.
24. Deckert T, Poulsen JE, Larsen M. Prognosis of diabetics with diabetes onset before the age of thirty-one: I. Survival, causes of death, and complications. Diabetologia 1978;14:363–370.
25. Tunbridge WM. On behalf of the Medical Services Study Group and British Diabetic Association: Factors contributing to deaths of diabetics under fifty years of age. Lancet 1981;2:569–572.
26. Jaspan JB, Wollman RL, Bernstein L, et al. Hypoglycemic peripheral neuropathy in association with insulinoma: Implication of glucopenia rather than hyperinsulinism. Medicine 1982;61:33–44.
27. Buchanan BJ, Filkins JP. Hypoglycemic depression of RES function. Am J Physiol 1976;231:265–269.
28. Strauch B, Felig P, Baxter J, Schimpff S. Hypothermia in hypoglycemia. JAMA 1969;210:345–346.
29. Maggs DG, Scott AR, MacDonald IA. Thermoregulatory responses to hyperinsulinemic hypoglycemia and euglycemia in humans. Am J Physiol 1994;267:R1266–R1272.
30. Buchanan T, Cane P, Eng C, Sipos G, Lee C. Hypothermia is critical for survival during prolonged insulin-induced hypoglycemia in rats. Metabolism 1991;40:330–334.
31. Agardh C, Smith M, Siesjo B. The influence of hypothermia on hypoglycemia-induced brain damage in the rat. Acta Neuropathol 1992;83:379–385.
32. Comi RJ. Approach to acute hypoglycemia. Endocrinol Metab Clin North Am 1993;22:247–262.
33. Comi RJ, Gorden P, Doppman JL, et al. Insulinoma. In Go VLW, ed. The Exocrine Pancreas. Raven, New York, 1986, pp. 745–761.
34. Kitabchi AE, Goodman RC. Hypoglycemia. Pathophysiology and diagnosis. Hosp Pract 1987; 22:45–56, 59–60.
35. Fajans SS, Floyd JC Jr. Fasting hypoglycemia in adults. N Engl J Med. 1976;294:766–772.
36. Merimee TJ, Tyson JE. Stabilization of plasma glucose during fasting: normal variations in two separate studies. N Engl J Med. 291:1275–1278.
37. Felig P, Lynch V. Starvation in human pregnancy: hypoglycemia, hypoinsulinemia and hyerketonemia. Science 1970;170:990–992.
38. Felig P, Cherif A, Minagawa A, et al. Hypoglycemia during prolonged exercise in normal men. N Engl J Med 1982;306:895–900.
39. Schwartz NS, Clutter WE, Shah SD, Cryer PE. Glycemic threshold for activation of glucose counterregulatory systems are higher than the threshold for symptoms. J Clin Invest 1987;79:777–781.
40. Mitrakou A, Ryan C, Veneman T, et al. Hierarchy of glycemic thresholds for counterregulatory hormone secretion, symptoms, and cerebral dysfunction. Am J Physiol 1991;260:E67–E74.
41. Bolli GB, Fanelli CG. Unawareness of hypoglycemia. N Engl J Med 1995;333:1771–1772.
42. Cryer PE. Glucose counterregulation: the physiological mechanisms that prevent or correct hypoglycaemia. In: Frier BM, Fisher MB, eds. Hypoglycaemia and Diabetes: Clinical and Physiological Aspects. Edward Arnold, London, 1993, pp. 34–55.
43. Boyle PJ, Cryer PE. Growth hormone, cortisol, or both are involved in defense against, but are not critical to recovery from, prolonged hypoglycemia. Am J Physiol 1991;260:E395–E402.
44. Borg WP, During MJ, Sherwin RS, Borg MA, Brines ML, Shulman GI. Ventromedial hypothalamic lesions in rats suppress counterregulatory responses to hypoglycemia. J Clin Invest 1994;93:1677–1682.

45. Hepburn DA, Deary IJ, Frier BM, Patrick AW, Quinn JD, Fisher BM. Symptoms of acute insulin-induced hypoglycemia in humans with and without IDDM: factor-analysis approach. Diabetes Care 1991;14:949–957.
46. Service FJ, Dale AJD, Elveback LR, Jiang NS. Insulinoma: clinical and diagnostic features of 60 consecutive cases. Mayo Clin Proc 1976;51:417–429.
47. Blackman JD, Towle VL, Lewis GF, et al. Hypoglycemia thresholds for cognitive dysfunction in humans. Diabetes 1990;39:828–835.
48. DeFronzo RA, Andres R, Bedsoe TA, Boden G, Faloona GA, Tobin JD. A test of the hypothesis that the rate of fall in glucose concentration triggers counterregulatory hormonal responses in man. Diabetes. 1972;26:445–452.
49. Santiago JV, Clarke WL, Shah SD, Cryer PE. Epinephrine, norepinephrine, glucagon, and growth hormone release in association with physiological decrements in plasma glucose concentration in normal and diabetic man. J Clin Endocrinol Metab. 1980;51:877–883.
50. Field JB. Hypoglycemia. Endocrinol Clin North Am. 1989;18:27–43.
51. Liu D, Moberg E, Kollind M, Lin PE, Adamson U, Macdonald IA. Arterial, arterialized venous, venous and capillary blood glucose measurements in normal man during hyperinsulinemic euglycemia and hypoglycemia. Diabetologia 1992;35:287–290.
52. Frizzell RT, Jones EM, Davis SN, et al. Counterregulation during hypoglycemia is directed by widespread brain regions. Diabetes 1993;42:1253–1261.
53. Lingenfelser T, Overkamp D, Renn W, Buettner U, Kimmerle K, Schmalfuss A, Jakober B. Insulin-associated modulation of neuroendocrine counterregulation, hypoglycemia perception, and cerebral function in insulin-dependent diabetes mellitus: evidence for an intrinsic effect of insulin on the central nervous system. J Clin Endocrinol Metab 1996;81:1197–1205.
54. Pardridge WM, Eisenberg J, Yang J. Human blood-brain barrier insulin receptor. J Neurochem 1985;44:1771–1778.
55. Baura GD, Foster DM, Porte D, et al. Saturable transport of insulin from plasma into the central nervous system of dogs *in vivo*. J Clin Invest 1993;92:1824–1830.
56. Grundstein JS, James DE, Storlien LH, Smythe GA, Kraegen EW. Hyperinsulinemia suppresses glucose utilization in specific brain regions: *in vivo* studies using the euglycaemic clamp in the rat. Endocrinology 1985;116:604–610.
57. Marfaing P, Penicaud L, Broer Y, Mraovitch S, Calando Y, Picon L. Effects of hyperinsulinemia on local cerebral insulin binding and glucose utilization in normoglycemic awake rats. Neurosci Lett 1985;115:1675–1679.
58. Fischer KF, Lees JA, Newman JH. Hypoglycemia in hospitalized patients. Causes and outcomes. N Engl J Med 1986;315:1245–1250.
59. Service FJ. Factitial hypoglycemia. The Endocrinologist 1992;2:173–176.
60. Grunberger G, Weiner JL, Silverman R, et al. Factitious hypoglycemia due to surreptitious administration of insulin. Ann Intern Med 1988;108:252–257.
61. Goldman J, Baldwin D, Rubenstein AH, et al. Characterization of circulating insulin and proinsulin-binding antibodies in autoimmune hypoglycemia. J Clin Invest 1979;63:1050–1059.
62. Hirata Y. Methimazole and insulin autoimmune syndrome with hypoglycaemia. Lancet 1983;2:1037–1038.
63. Moller DE, Ratner RE, Borenstein DH, Taylor SI. Autoantibodies to the insulin receptor as a cause of autoimmune hypoglycemia in systemic lupus erythematosus. Am J Med 1988;84:334–338.
64. Phillips LS, Robertson DG. Insulin-like growth factors and non-islet cell tumor hypoglycemia. Metabolism 1993;42:1093–1101.
65. Chung J, Henry RR. Mechanisms of tumor-induced hypoglycemia with intraabdominal hemangiopericytoma. J Clin Endocrinol Metab 1996;81:919–925.
66. Katz LEL, Liu F, Baker B, Agus MSD, Nunn SE, Hintz RL, Cohen P. The effect of growth hormone treatment on the insulin-like growth factor axis in a child with nonislet cell tumor hypoglycemia. J Clin Endocrinol Metab 1996;81:1141–1146.
67. Daughaday WH, Kapadia M. Significance of abnormal serum binding of insulin-like growth factor II in the development of hypoglycemia in patients with non-islet cell tumors. Proc Natl Acad Sci USA 1989;86:6778–6782.
68. Wing JR, Panz VR, Joffe BI, et al. Hypoglycemia in hepatocellular carcinoma: failure of short-term growth hormone administration to reduce enhanced glucose requirements. Metabolism 1991;40:508–515.
69. Frizzell M, Larsen PR, Field JB. Spontaneous hypoglycemia associated with chronic renal failure. Diabetes 1973;22:493–498.

70. Gorden AJ, Bier DM, Cryer PE, et al. Hypoglycemia in compensated chronic renal insufficiency: substrate limitation of gluconeogenesis. Diabetes 1974;23:982–986.
71. Peitzman SJ, Agarwal BN. Spontaneous hypoglycemia in end-stage renal failure. Nephron 1977;19:131–139.
72. Bansal VK, Brooks MH, York JC, Hano JE. Intractable hypoglycemia in a patient with renal failure. Arch Intern Med 1979;139:100–102.
73. Toth EL, Lee DW. "Spontaneous"/uremic hypoglycemia is not a distinct entity: substantiation from a literature review. Nephron 1991;58:325–329.
74. Benzing G, Schubert W, Huq G, et al. Simultaneous hypoglycemia and acute congestive heart failure. Circulation 1969;40:209–216.
75. Haymond MW, Pagliara AS. Ketotic hypoglycaemia. Clin Endocrinol Metab 1983;12:447–462.
76. Phillips RE. Hypoglycemia is an important complication of falciparum malaria. Q J Med 1989;71:477–483.
77. Shalev O, Tsur A, Rahav G. Falciparum malaria-induced hypoglycaemia in a diabetic patient. Postgrad Med J 1992;68:281–282.
78. Miller AI, Wallace RJ, Musher DM, et al. Hypoglycemia as a manifestation of sepsis. Am J Med 1980;68:649–654.
79. Nouel O, Bernuau J, Rueff B, Benhamou J-P. Hypoglycemia. A common complication of septicemia in cirrhosis. Arch Intern Med 1981;141:1477–1478.
80. Bennish ML, Azad AK, Rahman O, Phillips RE. Hypoglycemia during diarrhea in childhood. Prevalence, pathophysiology, and outcome. N Engl J Med 1990;322:1357–1363.
81. Seltzer HS. Drug-induced hypoglycemia. Endocrinol Metab Clin North Am 1989;18:163–131.
82. Jennings AM, Wilson RM, Ward JD. Symptomatic hypoglycemia in NIDDM patients treated with oral hypoglycemic agents. Diabetes Care 1989;12:203–208.
83. Atkin SH, Dasmahapatra A, Jaker MA, Chorost MI, Reddy S. Fingerstick glucose determination in shock. Ann Intern Med 1991;114:1020–1024.
84. Rasaiah B. Self-monitoring of the blood glucose level: potential sources of inaccuracy. Can Med Assoc J 1985;132:1357–1361.
85. Brodows RG, Williams C, Amatruda JM. Treatment of insulin reactions in diabetics. JAMA 1984;252:3378–3381.
86. Collier A, Steedman DJ, Patrick AW, et al. Comparison of intravenous glucagon and dextrose in treatment of severe hypoglycemia in an accident and emergency department. Diabetes Care 1987;10:712–715.
87. Karam JH, Young CW. Hypoglycemic disorders. In: Greenspan FS, Baxter JD, eds. Basic and Clinical Endocrinology. Appleton & Lange, East Norwalk, CT, pp. 635–648.

12 Critical Illness and Calcium Metabolism

Jack F. Tohme, MD, and John P. Bilezikian, MD

CONTENTS

INTRODUCTION
CALCIUM HOMEOSTASIS
MEASUREMENT OF THE SERUM CALCIUM CONCENTRATION
PREVALENCE OF HYPOCALCEMIA AND HYPERCALCEMIA
CLINICAL MANIFESTATIONS OF HYPOCALCEMIA
 AND HYPERCALCEMIA
CAUSES OF HYPOCALCEMIA AND HYPERCALCEMIA
 IN CRITICALLY ILL PATIENTS
TREATMENT OF HYPOCALCEMIA AND HYPERCALCEMIA
REFERENCES

INTRODUCTION

Calcium is a vital ion serving a variety of extracellular and intracellular functions. Extracellular calcium is predominantly in the skeleton (over 99% of total body calcium) where it supports bodily movement and protects vital organs. Extracellular calcium also plays important roles in blood clotting, in maintenance of cell membrane integrity, and in mechanisms of intercellular adhesion. Basic intracellular functions include muscle contraction, intracellular signaling, cell movement, enzyme activation, and neurohumoral secretion *(1)*. Alterations in the concentration of serum ionized calcium can therefore be expected to have clinically significant consequences. An acute reduction in serum calcium concentration can lead to hyperexcitability of nerve and muscle tissues, presenting a constellation of symptoms and signs that are encompassed by the term, "tetany." Hypocalcemia can be a medical emergency when symptoms are manifest as laryngeal spasm or seizures. An acute increase in the serum calcium concentration can also be life-threatening when neurological functions are depressed, especially if the central nervous system is involved. A wide variety of acute illnesses can cause or be accompanied by hypocalcemia and hypercalcemia *(1–4)*. This chapter reviews the clinical

From: *Contemporary Endocrinology: Endocrinology of Critical Disease*
Edited by K. P. Ober   Humana Press Inc., Totowa, NJ

syndromes associated with acute alterations in calcium metabolism and summarizes current concepts in management.

CALCIUM HOMEOSTASIS

Because of its important role in maintaining normal physiologic processes, rapid homeostatic response systems have developed in mammalian life that regulate the extracellular calcium concentration within a narrow range *(5)*. In contrast, the intracellular calcium concentration varies more widely owing, in part, to a concentration of free calcium inside the cell that is 10,000-fold lower than the extracellular free calcium concentration. Tight control of the extracellular calcium concentration is exerted by a complex system of adaptive mechanisms that protect against hypocalcemia or hypercalcemia. The key sensor to a change in extracellular calcium concentration is the parathyroid cell. An increase in extracellular calcium will signal the cell to reduce secretion and synthesis of PTH. A decrease in extracellular calcium will trigger an increase in PTH secretion and synthesis. Because PTH is a major regulator of 1,25-dihydroxyvitamin D formation, an increase or decrease in PTH will lead directly to an increase or decrease in 1,25-dihydroxyvitamin D levels. In response to a hypocalcemic signal, these hormones increase movement of calcium into the intravascular space by way of reduced renal excretion, increased calcium release from the skeleton, and enhanced intestinal calcium absorption. A slight reduction in the ionized calcium concentration, even on the order of 1–2%, leads to a prompt increase, within seconds, in PTH secretion from small stores of preformed hormone. This is followed within hours by enhanced PTH synthesis; a prolonged hypocalcemic stimulus over days will cause parathyroid cell hypertrophy and proliferation.

The target organs of PTH are the kidneys and the skeleton. In bone, PTH leads to calcium release by osteoclast-activated bone resorption. PTH is believed to activate bone resorption indirectly through its direct effect of stimulating osteoblasts, bone-forming cells. The osteoblasts then communicate with and activate osteoclasts via intercellular signaling events that are unknown. In the kidney, PTH enhances distal tubular reabsorption of calcium, decreases proximal tubular reabsorption of phosphate, and stimulates the conversion of 25-hydroxyvitamin D to 1,25-dihydroxyvitamin D. 1,25-dihydroxyvitamin D, the most active vitamin D metabolite, in turn acts on small intestinal cells to facilitate calcium absorption and on bone cells to activate the bone resorption process much like PTH. The excess phosphate mobilized from bone and intestine along with calcium is excreted in the urine through the phosphaturic action of PTH. Interestingly, 1,25-dihydroxyvitamin D also acts to inhibit PTH secretion, directly limiting the glands' response to hypocalcemia. Production of 1,25-dihydroxyvitamin D is virtually absent in advanced renal failure, helping to explain, in part, parathyroid gland enlargement in chronic renal disease *(6,7)*. The role of PTH-related protein (PTHrP) in normal physiology is unclear. This hormone was originally described as a tumor-derived hypercalcemic factor *(8–10)*. It does have physiologic properties, unrelated to cancer, but insofar as regulation of calcium metabolism is concerned, PTHrP is believed to function only in fetal and very early neonatal life, and with respect to mammary gland and placental calcium metabolism *(11)*.

MEASUREMENT OF THE SERUM CALCIUM CONCENTRATION

Routinely, calcium is measured as the sum total of three intravascular calcium components: ionized, physiologically active calcium (45%); albumin-bound calcium (45%);

and calcium complexed with serum anions (10%). In the patient with a normal concentration of albumin and with normal acid-base balance, the total serum calcium concentration accurately reflects the ionized or free concentration *(12)*. With reductions in serum albumin, the total calcium concentration will be low, but the ionized fraction is usually normal. Hypoalbuminemia is common in critically ill patients, especially when the illness is prolonged. Because reliable methods to measure the ionized calcium concentration may not be generally available, one can utilize a formula to estimate its concentration: the total serum calcium concentration is reduced by approx 0.8 mg/dL for every 1 g/dL by which the serum albumin concentration is reduced below the normal mean of 4 g/dL. Further perturbations in the partition between free and bound calcium may be seen in the critically ill patient owing to changes in the pH, fatty acid concentration, and complexing ions. In acidosis, binding to albumin is decreased, making more calcium available in the free form. In alkalosis, binding to albumin is increased, and less calcium is available in the free form. Abrupt increases in the concentration of phosphate, citrate, or bicarbonate ions that complex with the calcium ion can lead to significant and sometimes marked reductions in ionized calcium levels. Examples include rapid blood transfusions with concomitant infusions of citrate and acute rhabdomyolysis with a rapid release of intracellular phosphate into the circulation. When the partition between free, bound, and complexed calcium is altered, the level of total calcium in the blood may be misleadingly normal, and in these circumstances, direct measurements of ionized calcium are not only helpful, but often necessary. The blood sample must be collected under strictly anaerobic conditions, and the ion-selective electrode must be properly calibrated for reliable determination.

PREVALENCE OF HYPOCALCEMIA AND HYPERCALCEMIA

Hypocalcemia is now very commonly seen in the setting of acute illness. The availability of automated blood chemistry panels has led to greater awareness of hypocalcemia, particularly in the asymptomatic hospitalized patient, in whom hypoalbuminemia or hypomagnesemia *(13)* is quite prevalent. In a survey of patients in the medical intensive care unit *(14)*, 70% of patients were found to have low serum calcium levels. Surprisingly, both total and ionized calcium levels were reduced. Known causes could be identified in only 45% of patients. They included hypomagnesemia, renal insufficiency, and acute pancreatitis. There was a strong association between sepsis and hypocalcemia. In another retrospective study of critically ill patients, 64% were hypocalcemic *(15)*. About half of these patients were also alkalotic. Patients with hypocalcemia had greater mortality than normocalcemic patients. Patients with gastrointestinal hemorrhage and intra-abdominal surgery were more likely to become hypocalcemic than patients with cardiac or neurosurgical illnesses. Predisposing factors were renal failure, blood transfusions, sepsis, hypoalbuminemia, and hypomagnesemia. In patients with malignancy, hypoproteinemia is common, but true reductions in the free calcium concentration have been reported in patients with prostate and breast cancer with osteoblastic metastases. The uptake of calcium into osteoblastic lesions can cause hypocalcemia if the kinetics of this flux into bone is sufficiently great. In the study of Derasmo et al. *(16)*, hypocalcemia was present in 13% of 82 patients hospitalized with cancer. Hypocalcemia is also being seen more frequently in pediatric and neonatal intensive care units. In a study of over 13,000 infants, hypocalcemia was very common in infants with low gestational age and in those with low Apgar scores *(17)*.

Hypercalcemia in the setting of acute illness is also common *(18,19)*. It is seen most often in patients who are in the terminal phase of malignant diseases associated with hypercalcemia. It is caused by excessive bone resorption owing to tumor cells or to humoral factors, such as PTHrP, released by tumor cells. Primary hyperparathyroidism may also be the cause of severe life-threatening hypercalcemia. The major pathophysiologic mechanism is accelerated calcium mobilization from bone owing to osteoclast activation. Another important mechanism of acute hypercalcemia is a decline in the ability of the kidneys to excrete the excessive calcium presented to them. When PTH or PTHrP is involved, tubular reabsorption of calcium is greater than normal, thus adding to the inability of the kidneys to dispose of the calcium load. Hypercalcemia interferes further with the renal mechanisms of salt and water handling, leading to polyuria. When anorexia and nausea ensue as a result of worsening hypercalcemia, fluid intake is decreased and further dehydration develops, leading to even higher calcium levels. This cycle can develop over a relatively short period of time with rapid clinical deterioration *(18)*.

CLINICAL MANIFESTATIONS OF HYPOCALCEMIA AND HYPERCALCEMIA

Clinical features of hypocalcemia and hypercalcemia are most pronounced in the neurologic, muscular, and cardiovascular systems *(1,2,18,19)*. They are both a function of the actual level of the serum calcium and the rate of its fall (or rise), such that the patient is more likely to be symptomatic if hypocalcemia or hypercalcemia develops quickly. In the critically ill patient, hypocalcemia or hypercalcemia is mostly either asymptomatic or the patient is too ill to manifest clearly the usual symptomatology, and therefore hypocalcemia (and hypercalcemia) may go unnoticed. The availability of routine blood chemistry testing has increased early awareness of this situation.

Clinical Manifestations of Hypocalcemia

Early signs of hypocalcemia can include circumoral numbness and distal paresthesias in the hands and feet. Neuromuscular irritability follows with muscle cramps and stiffness. Fasciculations, spasms, and frank tetany are extreme manifestations. The hands can contract involuntarily in a particular posture with flexed elbow and wrist, adducted thumb and flexed metacarpal-phalangeal joints, and extended interphalangeal joints: a similar posture can be seen in the feet. The disposition is referred to as carpopedal spasm. Neuromuscular irritability can often be elicited by certain bedside maneuvers: Chvostek's sign is demonstrated by tapping the facial nerve just anterior to the ear. A positive Chvostek's sign is involuntary spasm of the percussed facial muscle. However, the sign can be seen in about 10% of healthy individuals. It has more clinical value if it is known to have been absent beforehand, for example, prior to thyroid or parathyroid surgery. Trousseau's sign is elicited by inflating the blood pressure cuff for 3–5 min at the level of the systolic blood pressure. The ensuing mild ischemia unmasks latent muscular irritability, and carpal spasm is observed. Both Chvostek's and Trousseau's signs can be absent despite significant hypocalcemia. With more severe hypocalcemia, involuntary muscle contractions can become automatic, and tetany can occur in the bronchial or laryngeal muscles with life-threatening consequences. Hypocalcemia also affects the central nervous system with early symptoms, such as restlessness and difficulty sleeping, with nonspecific changes seen on electroencephalography, and with seizures in severe cases.

Cardiovascular manifestations of hypocalcemia are related to reduced muscle tone in the vascular smooth muscle and in the myocardium. Hypotension, impaired myocardial contractility, and arrhythmias can ensue *(2)*. There is often resistance to pressors, inotropic agents, and volume replacement. Classical signs of hypocalcemia on the electrocardiogram include a prolonged QT interval. Nonspecific ST and T wave changes are also seen. A prolonged QT interval, in the absence of other etiologies, can be an important clue to unsuspected hypocalcemia.

The physical exam can also be helpful if signs of chronic hypocalcemia are present. Long-standing hypocalcemia can be suspected when subcapsular cataracts, dry skin, brittle nails, and coarse hair are seen. A surgical scar in the anterior neck might provide a clue to surgical hypoparathyroidism. Mucocutaneous candidiasis and adrenal insufficiency are often seen in idiopathic autoimmune hypoparathyroidism *(20)*. Pseudohypoparathyroidism, a disorder of parathyroid hormone resistance *(21,22)*, is seen in its classic form (type 1a) with characteristic skeletal and physical abnormalities: a short, rotund appearance with short neck, shortened metacarpal and metatarsal bones (especially fourth and fifth digits), and diminished intelligence. Intracranial calcifications, particularly of the basal ganglia, can be seen on CAT scanning in many patients with pseudohypoparathyroidism or long-standing hypoparathyroidism. In type 1a pseudohypoparathyroidism, the guanine nucleotide binding protein, Gs, is reduced by 50%, consistent with a heterozygous genetic disorder *(21–23)*. A reduction of this protein, critically involved in coupling of PTH/PTHrP receptor to adenylyl cyclase, helps to explain a deficient response of target tissues to PTH. In type 1b pseudohypoparathyroidism, PTH resistance is present, but physical features are absent. The resistance in this form of pseudohypoparathyroidism, which is limited to PTH, is not associated with a G-protein deficiency, nor does it appear to be owing to an abnormality of the PTH/PTHrP receptor. The molecular abnormality in the type 1b variant remains obscure.

Clinical Manifestations of Hypercalcemia

Hypercalcemia can also have wide-ranging clinical manifestations or can be asymptomatic. It can affect the gastrointestinal tract, causing anorexia, nausea, vomiting, constipation, and rarely, acute pancreatitis. Hypercalcemia can also affect the cardiovascular system leading to hypertension, a shortened QT interval on the electrocardiogram, and enhanced sensitivity to digitalis. Symptoms of renal involvement include polyuria, polydipsia, and on occasion, nephrocalcinosis. Various symptoms related to central nervous system dysfunction include mild lethargy, cognitive impairment, and when severe, coma. The physical exam does not often give specific clues to the underlying diagnosis. A total body erythematous rash associated with generalized lymphadenopathy can be almost diagnostic of HTLV-1-associated lymphoma *(24,25)*.

CAUSES OF HYPOCALCEMIA AND HYPERCALCEMIA IN CRITICALLY ILL PATIENTS

Hypocalcemia

Table 1 summarizes the causes of hypocalcemia in critically ill patients. Certain illnesses are associated in particular with hypocalcemia. In acute pancreatitis, for example, pancreatic destruction leads to fatty acid release with precipitation, and deposition of large amounts of calcium salts in the hemorrhagic and damaged pancreas and surrounding

Table 1
Causes of Hypocalcemia[a]

Hypoparathyroidism (insufficient or absent PTH secretion)
  Postsurgical
  Transient suppression (neonatal, postparathyroidectomy)
  Autoimmune
    Isolated
    End-organ endocrine deficiency syndrome
  Genetic (DiGeorge's syndrome, Kearns-Sayre syndrome)
    Mutations in the PTH gene
    Mutations in the Ca sensing receptor
  Infiltrative
    Hemochromatosis, sarcoidosis, Wilson's disease, amyloidosis, metastatic cancer
  Irradiation
  Severe magnesium deficiency
Resistance to PTH action
  Pseudohypoparathyroidism
  Severe magnesium deficiency
Deficiency in or disorders of vitamin D metabolism
  Inadequate intake or absorption of vitamin D (primary deficiency or malabsorption)
  Inadequate formation of 25-hydroxyvitamin D (severe liver disease)
  Inadequate formation of 1,25-dihydroxyvitamin D
    Renal insufficiency
    1-α hydroxylase deficiency (vitamin D-dependent rickets, type 1)
  Resistance to 1,25-dihydroxyvitamin D (vitamin D-dependent rickets, type 2)
Acute complexing, sequestration, or altered partitioning of calcium
  Acute pancreatitis
  Rhabdomyolysis
  Massive tumor lysis
  Phosphate infusion
  Massive blood transfusion
  Toxic shock syndrome
  Acute, severe illness
  Alkalosis
Increased osteoblastic activity
  Osteoblastic metastases (prostate, breast cancer)
  Hungry bone syndrome (postparathyroidectomy)
Drugs
  Anticalcemic agents
    Bisphosphonates
    Plicamycin
    Calcitonin
    Gallium nitrate
    Phosphate
  Antineoplastic agents
    Asparaginase
    Doxorubicin
    Cytosine Arabinoside
    WR2721
    Cisplatinum
  Others
    Ketaconazole
    Pentamadine
    Foscarnet

[a]Adapted from ref. *(2)* with permission.

retroperitoneal fat *(26)*. There may also be an inadequate response of the parathyroid glands to the hypocalcemic stimulus, possibly related to magnesium deficiency commonly seen in patients with alcoholism, a predisposing toxin to the pancreas. The degree of hypocalcemia seems to correlate with the severity of the pancreatitis, and its presence in general is a poor prognostic sign.

Another common mechanism of hypocalcemia in the acute setting is a sudden influx of phosphate into the intravascular space. Patients with rhabdomyolysis are most vulnerable *(27)*. Rhabdomyolysis can alter renal function with oliguria followed by polyuria. Hypocalcemia is seen in the oliguric phase, whereas hypercalcemia can be seen in the polyuric phase of rhabdomyolysis. Another setting for acute hypocalcemia is chemotherapy for lymphomas and leukemias in which there is massive release of intracellular phosphate. The hypocalcemia can be severe. Calcium can also be complexed by excess citrate following multiple blood transfusions. Toxic shock syndrome, Gram-negative sepsis, and other catastrophic illnesses can be associated with hypocalcemia, but the mechanisms are unclear. As noted earlier, the exact cause of hypocalcemia is frequently not readily identified.

In situations of markedly increased osteoblastic activity, as is seen following successful surgical correction of severe hyperparathyroidism, calcium is rapidly deposited into bone-forming skeletal sites. The resulting "hungry bone syndrome" can lead to a hypocalcemic emergency. The hungry bone syndrome can be distinguished from hypoparathyroidism after parathyroid surgery by the PTH concentration. In hungry bone syndrome, the PTH level will be elevated, as would be expected when a major hypocalcemic stimulus is presented to the remaining parathyroid glands. In hypocalcemia owing to postsurgical hypoparathyroidism, PTH levels are undetectable *(28)*.

Renal disease, one of the most common causes of hypocalcemia, has a complex pathogenesis *(6,7)*. Decreased glomerular function leads to reduced clearance of phosphorus. The tendency for the serum phosphorus to be elevated has two consequences. The serum calcium is lowered by virtue of its physicochemical relationship with phosphorus and the renal 1-α-hydroxylase enzyme, responsible for producing 1,25-dihydroxyvitamin D, is inhibited. The reduction in 1,25-dihydroxyvitamin D has three consequences: the serum calcium is reduced further, because the gastrointestinal tract no longer absorbs calcium efficiently; the gene for parathyroid hormone controlled, in part, by 1,25-dihydroxyvitamin D is stimulated; and several protooncogenes that help to regulate parathyroid cell growth, also under the control of 1,25-dihydroxyvitamin D, are activated. Hypocalcemia in renal failure can be profound, but it is not usually symptomatic unless the renal failure is acute.

The body's defense against hypocalcemia involves mobilizing the key calciotropic hormones, PTH and 1,25-dihydroxyvitamin D. Thus, hypocalcemia is often the result of a deficiency of either (Table 1). In hypoparathyroidism, the lack of PTH leads to impaired mobilization of calcium from bone and loss of PTH's calcium-conserving renal actions. Phosphate is conserved owing to the loss of PTH's phosphaturic renal actions. PTH deficiency and hyperphosphatemia inhibits renal conversion of 25-hydroxyvitamin D to 1,25-dihydroxyvitamin D. Thus, hypocalcemia, hyperphosphatemia, and reduced PTH and 1,25-dihydroxyvitamin D levels are characteristic features of patients with hypoparathyroidism independent of its etiology.

Idiopathic hypoparathyroidism can be autoimmune either affecting the parathyroid glands alone or in association with the polyglandular autoimmune syndrome. Postsurgical hypoparathyroidism usually occurs after thyroid surgery, either a transient event related to ischemic injury to the parathyroids, or uncommonly as a result of injury or removal of all four parathyroids, as for example after extensive thyroid cancer surgery. It can also occur after surgery for primary hyperparathyroidism. Permanent hypoparathyroidism is more likely to occur after parathyroid surgery in patients with hyperparathyroidism owing to four-gland hyperplasia. Hypoparathyroidism can also be the result of an underlying genetic disorder of the calcium-sensing receptor or a disorder in intracellular trafficking mechanisms for the molecule *(29–34)*. Rarely, external or internal neck irradiation leads to permanent parathyroid damage. The parathyroid glands can be infiltrated in diseases, such as hemochromatosis, sarcoidosis, Wilson's disease, amyloidosis, and metastatic cancer. In infants and children, congenital absence of the parathyroids can be associated with DiGeorge's syndrome, where cell-mediated immunity is deficient (along with facial abnormalities and aortic arch defects, such as Tetralogy of Fallot).

Vitamin D deficiency can also lead to hypocalcemia. Reduced absorption of calcium from the gastrointestinal tract leads to secondary hyperparathyroidism and phosphaturia. The basic biochemical profile is therefore quite different from hypoparathyroidism. In hypocalcemia owing to vitamin D deficiency, hypocalcemia, hypophosphatemia, and elevated PTH levels are characteristic. In this setting, the most helpful vitamin D metabolite to measure is 25-hydroxyvitamin D. This measurement reflects body stores of vitamin D. Levels of 1,25-dihydroxyvitamin D are not always low. They may be low, but they may also be normal or even elevated. Worldwide, the most common cause of vitamin D deficiency is nutritional, believed to be rare in the US because of the widespread availability of fortified milk, cereals, and vitamin supplements. The latitude of the US also ensures adequate sunlight of sufficient wavelength (290–315 nm) to permit conversion of skin 7-dehydrocholesterol to vitamin D, at least in the summer months *(25)*. In the US, the leading causes of overt vitamin D deficiency with hypocalcemia are malabsorption syndromes, renal failure, and severe liver disease. In children, hypocalcemia can be related to rare vitamin D resistance syndromes secondary to defective renal 1-α-hydroxylase activity (vitamin D-dependent rickets type 1) or to defective vitamin D receptors (vitamin D-dependent rickets type 2). Vitamin D-resistant rickets is not usually associated with hypocalcemia.

A special category of hypocalcemia is that associated with magnesium deficiency. Magnesium deficiency is a relatively common problem because of its frequent association with a variety of disorders (Table 2). The associated hypocalcemia is multifactorial in origin. If there is a malabsorption syndrome, hypocalcemia and hypomagnesemia can coexist without being causally related. However, magnesium deficiency *per se* can cause hypocalcemia by three different mechanisms. First, severe hypomagnesemia impairs PTH secretion. Second, there is peripheral resistance to the actions of PTH that can persist for several days after magnesium administration and restitution of normal circulating levels of parathyroid hormone. Third, hypomagnesemia can be associated with a reduction in the formation of 1,25-dihydroxyvitamin D *(35)*.

In the differential diagnosis of hypocalcemia, early laboratory testing can be decisive in directing the investigation to the leading possibilities. Adjustment of the total calcium level to the ambient albumin level will sometimes obviate the need for further evaluation. In the acute care setting, hypomagnesemia should always be considered. An elevated serum creatinine and urea nitrogen accompanied by hyperphosphatemia points to renal failure as a likely cause. In the presence of normal renal function, hyperphosphatemia

Table 2
Causes of Hypomagnesemia[a]

Endocrine disorders	Renal magnesium wasting
Primary hyperparathyroidism	Diuretics
Hypoparathyroidism	Alcohol
Hyperthyroidism	Osmotic diuresis
Primary hyperaldosteronism	Gentamycin
Diabetic ketoacidosis	Cisplatin
Disorders of the gastrointestinal tract	Chronic renal tubular disorders
Malabsorption syndrome	Nutritional
Alcoholic cirrhosis	Protein-calorie malnutrition
Chronic diarrheal states	Excessive, chronic alcohol ingestion
Bowel or biliary fistulas	
Parenteral hyperalimentation	
Pancreatitis	
Short bowel syndrome	

From ref. *(2)* with permission.

usually indicates a form of hypoparathyroidism of pseudohypoparathyroidism. Hypophosphatemia, on the other hand, argues for syndromes of vitamin D deficiency or resistance. Distinction of the hypocalcemic states between those associated with hypophosphatemia and those associated with hyperphosphatemia is further sharpened by the measurement of the circulating parathyroid hormone level. The two-site immunoradiometric and immunochemiluminometric assays, highly specific for intact parathyroid hormone, are extremely useful *(36)*. PTH will be low in a hypoparathyroid state and high in vitamin D-deficiency states. PTH will be high in PTH resistance syndromes, but normal in vitamin D-resistance syndromes where the serum calcium is usually normal. The measurement of vitamin D metabolites focuses on 25-hydroxyvitamin D, when body stores are being assessed, and on 1,25-dihydroxyvitamin D when a defect in conversion from 25-hydroxyvitamin D to 1,25-dihydroxyvitamin D is being considered.

Hypercalcemia

Virtually any cause of hypercalcemia can present in the acute care setting. Because the differential diagnosis of hypercalcemia is overwhelmingly the result of primary hyperparathyroidism or malignancy, these two etiologies dominate the differential diagnosis of life-threatening hypercalcemia. Acute primary hyperparathyroidism should not be overlooked. Some of the highest serum calcium levels ever recorded have been owing to acute primary hyperparathyroidism. One-fourth of patients with acute primary hyperparathyroidism (also called parathyroid crisis or parathyroid poisoning) have a history of antecedent mild hypercalcemia *(37)*. What causes the parathyroid gland to release rather suddenly extraordinary amounts of parathyroid hormone in this syndrome, thus causing life-threatening hypercalcemia is not known. Typically, the parathyroid hormone level in acute primary hyperparathyroidism is 10–20 times above the upper limits of normal. This is to be contrasted in more typical asymptomatic primary hyperparathyroidism in which the parathyroid hormone level is about twice the normal range *(38)*. Although these patients are obviously ill, they typically do not present in a debilitated state as is more typical in patients whose hypercalcemia is the result of underlying malignancy.

Virtually any malignancy can be associated with life-threatening hypercalcemia. Lung cancer, breast cancer, lymphoma, and multiple myeloma are particularly notorious. As is true for acute primary hyperparathyroidism, these patients usually have become less ambulatory; sometimes they are bedridden. The negative calcium balance, worsened further by the immobilization, is a major stimulus to osteoclast-mediated bone resorption.

The patient becomes symptomatic of hypercalcemia by the same pathophysiologic mechanisms described earlier with the gastrointestinal tract and the kidney being critically important. The distinction between acute primary hyperparathyroidism and hypercalcemia of malignancy is made readily by measuring the parathyroid hormone level. Even when the hypercalcemia in malignant disease is caused by parathyroid hormone-related protein, the PTH level as measured by the immunoradiometric assay is suppressed.

The extent to which other causes of hypercalcemia will be sought in acute hypercalcemic states depends on the initial evaluation that considers either primary hyperparathyroidism or malignancy. Among the long list of other diagnostic possibilities for hypercalcemia, any of the granulomatous diseases, other forms of vitamin D toxicity, treatment regimens, including large amounts of vitamin D, vitamin A toxicity, milk alkali syndrome, and, rarely, adrenal insufficiency, can all be associated with marked hypercalcemia. Less likely causes of severe hypercalcemia are hyperthyroidism, use of lithium or thiazide diuretics, and familial hypocalciuric hypercalcemia *(39)* (Table 3).

TREATMENT OF HYPOCALCEMIA AND HYPERCALCEMIA

Hypocalcemia

The primary objective of therapy for hypocalcemia is to alleviate symptoms of hypocalcemia. The secondary objective is to restore the serum calcium concentration to within normal limits. Acute therapy attempts to meet the first objective; it is usually not necessary or indicated to return the serum calcium concentration to the normal range with iv therapy. Urgent therapy with iv calcium is clearly indicated for patients with tetany, laryngospasm, seizures, or arrhythmias. It is also indicated for those without frank tetany, but in whom the serum calcium concentration has fallen to a point that is usually associated with symptoms, or places the patient at substantial risk for complications. Most experts would set this level at or below a corrected serum calcium of 7.0 mg/dL. The agent of choice is calcium gluconate. A 10-mL vial of 10% calcium gluconate contains 93 mg of elemental calcium. When life-threatening symptoms are present, two vials can be infused over 10–20 min. The formula for children is 0.2 mL/kg of 10% calcium gluconate. If symptoms persist, two more vials can be administered. As is true for the iv administration of any electrolyte solution, caution is always advised. Rapid administration can have adverse consequences on cardiac function, precipitating acute elevation in blood pressure, ventricular arrhythmias, and even systolic arrest. Intravenous calcium can also cause local irritation. If there is an ongoing process that could lead to recurrent severe hypocalcemia (as in rhabdomyolysis, hungry bone syndrome, acute pancreatitis, and so forth), a continuous infusion of calcium gluconate over 4–8 h can be started. A popular formula is to use 15 mg/kg of elemental calcium. For a 65-kg patient, 10 ampules of 10% calcium gluconate are added to a liter of normal saline or 5% dextrose in water. Administration of this infusion over 4–8 h will elevate the serum calcium by approx 2–4 mg/dL. In patients with severe hypocalcemia, but without symptoms, the infusate can be started without initial bolus administration.

Table 3
Differential Diagnosis of Hypercalcemia[a]

Primary hyperparathyroidism
   Sporadic (adenoma, hyperplasia or carcinoma)
   Familial
      Isolated
      Cystic
      Multiple endocrine neoplasia type 1 or 2
Malignancy
   Parathyroid hormone-related protein
   Excess production of 1,25-dihydroxyvitamin D
   Other factors (cytokines, growth factors)
Disorders of vitamin D
   Exogenous vitamin D toxicity—parent D compound. 25(OH)-D, 1,25-(OH)2D
   Endogenous production of 25-hydroxyvitamin D—Williams syndrome
   Endogenous production of 1,25-dihydroxyvitamin D
      Granulomatous diseases
         Sarcoidosis
         Tuberculous
         Histoplasmosis
         Coccidiomycosis
         Leprosy
         Others
      Lymphoma
Nonparathyroid endocrine disorders
   Thyrotoxicosis
   Pheochromocytoma
   Acute adrenal insufficiency
   Vasointestinal polypeptide hormone-producing tumor (VIPoma)
Medications
   Thiazide diuretics
   Lithium
   Estrogens/antiestrogens, testosterone in breast cancer
   Milk-alkali syndrome
   Vitamin A toxicity
Familial hypocalciuric hypercalcemia
Immobilization
Parenteral nutrition
Aluminum excess
Acute and chronic renal disease

[a]Reproduced from ref. (39) with permission.

If magnesium deficiency is present in symptomatic patients, parental calcium is required to alleviate the signs of hypocalcemia. These patients also should receive magnesium. One to two grams of magnesium sulfate (8–16 mEq) can be administered intravenously every 6 h for several days. Magnesium sulfate can also be used intramuscularly, but injections can be painful. The purpose of parenteral therapy with magnesium is to begin the process of total body replenishment and to restore normal secretory dynamics and sensitivity to PTH. Following acute management, magnesium stores are replaced by oral supplements and dietary sources of magnesium, which include red meat, green vegetables, and dairy products.

With iv calcium therapy, close monitoring of serum calcium, phosphate, magnesium, and creatinine is indicated. Care should be taken to avoid extravasation of the calcium infusate in the skin. Severe soft tissue reactions have been seen with calcium chloride, which should not be used for this purpose. In order to avoid iv precipitation of calcium salts, bicarbonate and phosphate should not be used along with the calcium solution. Another cautionary note regarding the acute administration of calcium is in order when hyperphosphatemia is present. Damaging precipitation of calcium phosphate salts in soft tissues can result. Measures to reduce the serum phosphorous should be undertaken first, unless the hypocalcemia is severe and life-threatening.

Most critically ill patients with hypocalcemia will not require long-term therapy, because resolution of the acute illness usually restores serum calcium levels to normal. However, there are many situations discussed above in which underlying abnormalities in parathyroid hormone or vitamin D metabolism are associated with chronic hypocalcemia. After acute management, a plan for satisfactory chronic therapy should be implemented. Vitamin D therapy is the cornerstone of this strategy, because vitamin D deficiency is a feature of virtually all hypocalcemic states. Hypoparathyroid states are treated with 1,25-dihydroxyvitamin D, because formation of this metabolite is impaired. Malabsorption syndromes are characterized by lack of the parent vitamin D compound, chronic liver disease by inability to form 25-hydroxyvitamin D, and renal insufficiency by inability to form 1,25-dihydroxyvitamin D. In these individual cases, therapy can be tailored to the pathophysiology. Therefore, malabsorption syndrome can be treated with vitamin D, liver disease can be treated with 25-hydroxyvitamin D, and renal disease with 1,25-dihydroxyvitamin D. Alternatively, 1,25-dihydroxyvitamin D simplifies the options, because it can be used in all conditions. Moreover, it is much easier to reverse its toxicity, because 1,25-dihydroxyvitamin D has a very short half-life and is not stored appreciably in fat tissues. In contrast, hypercalcemia from overadministration of parent vitamin D can be protracted. Sufficient dietary calcium in the chronic care of the hypocalcemic patient is also important. Total calcium intake ranges between 1 and 2.5 g daily. It is most unusual to meet this requirement from dietary calcium alone even when foods fortified with calcium are used. Oral calcium salt preparations are virtually always needed. There are many calcium salts available for this purpose, such as calcium carbonate, citrate, phosphate, lactate, gluconate, and glubionate. The most convenient preparation to use is calcium carbonate, because it contains the most elemental calcium as a percentage of the compound (40%). In patients with hypochlorhydria or achlorhydria, it is said that calcium citrate is preferable because this form of calcium does not require gastric acid for absorption in the fasting state *(40–42)*. If the patient is to take calcium supplementation while fasting, this advice is sound. On the other hand, when calcium salts are taken with food, gastric acid is not required for absorption *(43–45)*. Moreover, there seems to be an added efficiency of calcium absorption when the supplement is taken with food. An attractive alternative therefore is to use calcium preparation with meals. In some patients with chronic hypocalcemia, especially those with hypercalciuria, thiazide diuretics have been used because they enhance renal tubular reabsorption of calcium.

Hypercalcemia (18,46)

In the patient with symptomatic hypercalcemia, volume replacement is key, because dehydration is virtually always present. The choice of fluid is saline, because saline will facilitate volume replacement and induce a calciuresis. The actual amount of fluid to be administered depends on the patient's state. If hypotension is present, vigorous fluid therapy is in order, sometimes with central monitoring. If the patient has a history of marginal cardiovascular tolerance or renal function is unknown, one has to be more cautious. An initial rate of 200 mL/h is reasonable, but it should be monitored closely. A loop diuretic like furosemide can help to facilitate renal tubular excretion of salt and obligatorily also induce a calciuresis. It is also helpful if the patient's tolerance to vigorous saline administration is in doubt or unknown. Furosemide should never be used before the patient has been rehydrated. Its use subsequently is a matter of clinical judgment. If furosemide is to be used, a dosage of 10–20 mg when needed, but not more often than 6–12 h is reasonable.

Specific therapy for hypercalcemia is critically important, because general measures of fluid, saline, and furosemide do not control ongoing osteoclast-mediated bone resorption, the major source of intravascular calcium. The bisphosphonates, potent osteoclast inhibitors, are ideally suited for specific management of hypercalcemia. Parenteral preparations are necessary, because they are poorly absorbed, especially in this setting when the patient is likely to be symptomatic with upper gastrointestinal symptoms. Intravenous preparations of etidronate and pamidronate are available in the US. They can be given as single-dose infusions. Etidronate (25 mg/kg) and pamidronate (60–90 mg, total amount) lead to a reduction in the serum calcium within 2–3 d. Depending on the initial calcium value and the ongoing stimulus to bone resorption, the serum calcium concentration can be lowered substantially, sometimes to normal.

Other specific approaches to hypercalcemia include plicamycin, calcitonin, and gallium nitrate. Although each of these osteoclast inhibitors has a potential role in the specific management of acute hypercalcemia, the uniform success with the bisphosphonates and rather uncertain record of calcitonin and gallium nitrate combined with the toxicities of plicamycin have relegated these three anticalcemic drugs to second-line agents.

In situations of life-threatening hypercalcemia, one would like to have access to an agent that is faster than the bisphosphonates. Intravenous phosphate is probably the fastest way to reduce the serum calcium, but it is fraught with potential for disastrous precipitation of calcium-phosphate salts in soft tissues and the vasculature. It cannot be recommended. An alternative approach to gaining a fast therapeutic response is to use calcitonin together with a bisphosphonate *(47)*. Calcitonin does not usually have a profound anticalcemic effect, but its time-course of action is extremely rapid. Thus, the combination of a bisphosphonate and calcitonin unites the features of speed and potency. If 200 IU of calcitonin are used with pamidronate, 60–90 mg, at the time specific therapy for life-threatening hypercalcemia is implemented, the patient will experience a rapid, but not profound reduction in the serum calcium (calcitonin effect) followed by a more substantial reduction (bisphosphonate effect).

Some disorders of hypercalcemia are best treated with glucocorticoids. In the vitamin D sensitivity or toxic conditions (vitamin D toxicity, granulomatous disease, some lymphomas), steroids can be very effective. Also, in patients with HTLV1-associated lymphoma, glucocorticoid therapy can be very effective in reducing the serum calcium. Glucocorticoids are typically ineffective in primary hyperparathyroidism.

In the patient with life-threatening hypercalcemia whose diagnosis is not known, treatment is obviously indicated. In patients whose underlying disease is known and treatment is ongoing, anticalcemic measures are clearly indicated. However, there are patients who present with life-threatening hypercalcemia whose underlying disorder is known to be in its terminal stages. In this setting, the wisest course is sometimes to make sure the patient is comfortable. Heroic measures to control the serum calcium under these desperate conditions are not always the best course of action.

REFERENCES

1. Tohme JF, Bilezikian JP. Diagnosis and treatment of hypocalcemic emergencies. The Endocrinologist 1996;6:10–18.
2. Tohme JF, Bilezikian JP. Hypocalcemic emergencies. Endocrinol Metab Clin North Am 1993;22:363–376.
3. Bilezikian JP. Hypercalcemia. In: Bardin CW, ed. Current Therapy in Endocrinology and Metabolism. Mosby-Year Book, St. Louis, 1994, pp. 511–514.
4. Bilezikian JP. The hypercalcemic states: Their differential diagnosis and acute management. In: Coe FL, Favus MJ, eds. Disorders of Bone and Mineral Metabolism. Raven, New York, 1992, pp. 493–522.
5. Brown EM. Homeostatic mechanisms regulating extracellular and intracellular calcium metabolism. In: Bilezikian JP, Marcus R, Levine MA, eds. The Parathyroids. Raven, New York, 1994, pp. 15–51.
6. Martin KJ, Slatopolsky E. Parathyroid gland function in renal disease. In: Bilezikian JP, Marcus R, Levine MA, eds. The Parathyroids. Raven, New York, 1994, pp. 711–719.
7. Feinfeld D, Sherwood LM. Parathyroid hormone and 1,25-dihydroxyvitamin D in chronic renal failure. Kidney Int 1988;33:1049–1058.
8. Broadus AE, Mangin M, Ikeda K, et al. Humoral hypercalcemia of cancer. Identification of a novel parathyroid hormone-like peptide. N Engl J Med 1988;319:556–563.
9. Moseley GM, Kubota M, Diefenbach-Jagger H, et al. Parathyroid hormone related protein purified from a lung cancer cell line. Proc Natl Acad Sci USA 1987;84:5048–5052.
10. Strewler GJ, Stern GH, Jacobs JW, et al. PTH-like protein from human renal carcinoma cells: structural and functional homology with PTH. J Clin Invest 1987;80:1803–1807.
11. Broadus AE, Stewart AF. Parathyroid hormone related protein, structure, processing and physiologic actions. In: Bilezikian JP, Marcus R, Levine MA, eds. The Parathyroids. Raven, New York, 1994, pp. 259–294.
12. Guise T, Mundy GR. Evaluation of hypocalcemia in children and adults. J Clin Endocrinol Metab 1995;80:1473–1478.
13. Rude RK. Magnesium metabolism and deficiency. Endocrinol Metab Clin North Am 1993;22:377–395.
14. Desai TK, Carlson RW, Geheb MA. Prevalence and clinical implications of hypocalcemia in acutely ill patients in the medical intensive care setting. Am J Med 1988;84:209–214.
15. Chernow B, Zaloga G, McFadden E, et al. Hypocalcemia in critically ill patients. Crit Care Med 1982;10:848–851.
16. Derasmo AU, Leli FS, Acc M, et al. Hypocalcemia and hypomagnesemia in cancer patients. Biomed Pharmacol 1991;45:315–317.
17. Mimouni CP, Loughead JL, Tsang RC. A case control study of hypocalcemia in high-risk neonates: Racial but no seasonal differences. J Am Coll Nutr 1991;10:196–199.
18. Bilezikian JP. Management of acute hypercalcemia. N Eng J Med 1992;326:1196–1203.
19. Burtis NJ, Yang KH, Stewart AF. Nonparathyroid hypercalcemia. In: Becker KL, ed. Principles and Practice of Endocrinology and Metabolism, 2nd ed. JB Lippincott Co., Philadelphia, 1995, pp. 521–532.
20. Whyte MP. Autoimmune aspects of hypoparathyroidism. In: Bilezikian JP, Marcus R, Levine MA, eds. The Parathyroids. Raven, New York, 1994, pp. 753–764.
21. Streeten EA, Levine MA. Hypoparathyroidism and other causes of hypocalcemia. In: Becker KL, ed. Principles and Practice of Endocrinology and Metabolism, 2nd ed. Lippincott, Philadelphia, 1995, pp. 532–546.

22. Levine MA, Schwindinger WF, Downs RW, Moses AM. Pseudohypoparathyroidism: Clinical, biochemical and molecular features. In: Bilezikian JP, Marcus R, Levine MA, eds. The Parathyroids. Raven, New York, 1994, pp. 781–800.
23. Levine MA. Pseudohypoparathyroidism. In: Bilezikian JP, Raisz LR, Rodan GA, eds. Principles of Bone Biology. Academic, San Diego, 1996, in press.
24. Fukumoto S, Matsumoto T, Ikeda K, et al. Clinical evaluation of calcium metabolism in adult T-cell leukemia/lymphoma. Arch Intern Med 1988;148:921–925.
25. Johnston SRD, Hammond PJ. Elevated serum parathyroid hormone related protein and 1,25-dihydroxycholecalciferol in hypercalcemia associated with adult T-cell leukaemia-lymphoma. Postgrad Med J 1992;68:753–755.
26. Stewart AF, Longo W, Kreutter D, Jacob R, Burtis WJ. Hypocalcemia due to calcium soap formation in a patient with a pancreatic fistula. N Eng J Med 1986;315:496–498.
27. Llach F, Felsenfeld D, Haussler M. The pathophysiology of altered calcium metabolism in rhabdomyolysis-induced acute renal failure. N Engl J Med 1981;305:117–123.
28. Brasier AR, Wang CA, Nussbaum SR. Recovery of parathyroid hormone secretion after parathyroid adenomectomy. J Clin Endocrinol Metab 1988;66:495–500.
29. Arnold A, Horst SA, Gardella TJ, et al. Mutations of the signal peptide encoding region of pre-proparathyroid hormone gene in isolated hypoparathyroidism. J Clin Invest 1990;86:1084–1087.
30. Karaplis AC, Lim SC, Baba H, et al. Inefficient membrane targeting, translocation, and proteolytic processing by signal peptidase of a mutant preproparathyroid hormone protein. J Biol Chem 1995;27:1629–1635.
31. Pollak MR, Brown EM, Estep HL, et al. Autosomal dominant hypocalcemia caused by a calcium-sensing receptor gene mutation. Nature Genet 1994;8:303–307.
32. Perry YM, Finegold DN, Armitage MM, et al. A missense mutation in the Ca-sensing receptor causes familial autosomal dominant hypoparathyroidism. Am J Hum Genet 1994;55:A17.
33. Pearce SHS, Williamson C, Kifor O, et al. A familial syndrome of hypocalcemia with hypocalciuria due to mutations in the calcium-sensing receptor gene. N Engl J Med 1996; 335:1115–1122.
34. Baron J, Winer KK, Yanovski JA, et al. Mutations in the Ca2+-sensing receptor gene cause autosomal dominant and sporadic hypoparathyroidism. Hum Mol Genet 1996;5:601–606.
35. Rude RK. Magnesium metabolism. In: Becker KL, ed. Principles and Practice of Endocrinology and Metabolism, 2nd ed. JB Lippincott, Co., Philadelphia, 1995, pp. 616–621.
36. Endres DB. Villanueva R, Sharp CR Jr, Singer FR. Immunochemiluminometric and immunoradiometric determinations of intact and total immunoreactive parathyrin: performance in the differential diagnosis of hypercalcemia and hypoparathyroidism. Clin Chem 1991;37:162–168.
37. Fitzpatrick LA, Bilezikian JP. Acute primary hyperparathyroidism. Am J Med 1987;82:275–282.
38. Silverberg SJ, Fitzpatrick LA, Bilezikian JP. Primary hyperparathyroidism. In: Becker KL, ed. Principles and Practice of Endocrinology and Metabolism, 2nd ed. Lippincott, Philadelphia, 1995, pp. 512–520.
39. Chan FKW, Koberle LMC, Thys-Jacobs S, Bilezikian JP. Differential diagnosis, etiologies and management of hypercalcemia. Curr Problems in Surg 1997, in press.
40. Harvey JA, Kenny P, Poindexter J, Pak CYC. Superior calcium absorption from calcium citrate than calcium carbonate using external forearm counting. J Am Coll Nutr 1990;9:6:583.
41. Nicar MJ, Pak CYC. Calcium bioavailability from calcium carbonate and calcium citrate. J Clin Endocrinol Metab 1985;61:391.
42. Bilezikian JP. Viewpoint: Osteoporosis: Why calcium is important. J Women's Health 1995;4:483–494.
43. Heaney RP. Calcium supplements: Practical considerations. Osteoporosis Int 1991;1:65.
44. Heaney RP, Smith KT, Recker RR, Hinders SM. Meal effects on calcium absorption. Am J Clin Nutr 1989;49:372.
45. Recker RR. Calcium absorption and achlorhydria. N Engl J Med 1985;313:70.
46. Bilezikian JP, Singer FR. Acute management of hypercalcemia due to parathyroid hormone and parathyroid hormone-related protein. In: Bilezikian JP, Marcus R, Levine MA, eds. The Parathyroids. Raven, New York, 1994, pp. 359–372.
47. Fatemi S, Singer FR, Rude RK. Effect of salmon calcitonin and etidronate on hypercalcemia of malignancy. Calcif Tissue Int 1992;50:107–109.

13 Skeletal Metabolism in Critical Illness

Steven R. Gambert, MD, and Stephen J. Peterson, MD

CONTENTS

INTRODUCTION
NORMAL BONE: STRUCTURE, FUNCTION, AND HOMEOSTASIS
MEASURES OF BONE RESORPTION AND TURNOVER
MEDICATION-INDUCED METABOLIC BONE DISEASE
GLUCOCORTICOIDS
MANAGING GLUCOCORTICOID BONE LOSS
HEPARIN
CAFFEINE/THEOPHYLLINE
CATECHOLAMINES
ANTICONVULSANTS
EFFECT OF DISEASE ON THE SKELETON
THYROID DISEASE
OSTEOMALACIA AND RICKETS
PAGET'S DISEASE OF BONE
HYPERCALCEMIA
PRIMARY HYPERPARATHYROIDISM
SECONDARY HYPERPARATHYROIDISM AND RENAL FAILURE
IMMOBILIZATION
METASTATIC BONE DISEASE
MULTIPLE MYELOMA
SUMMARY
REFERENCES

INTRODUCTION

Although a wealth of information has accumulated concerning physiological changes that may occur in the setting of critical illness, little has been written specifically regarding critical illness and its potential effects on the skeletal system. Not only may individual problems alter normal skeletal homeostasis, but treatment modalities used both short and long

From: *Contemporary Endocrinology: Endocrinology of Critical Disease*
Edited by K. P. Ober   Humana Press Inc., Totowa, NJ

term must be considered. The skeletal system is the largest "organ" in the body, and serves a structural function and as a reservoir for calcium and other nutrients necessary for normal homeostasis and cellular action. Bone is a complex tissue and has a developmental process; it is constantly being remodeled throughout life. Its mechanical properties provide strength for skeletal support as well as protection for other organs. Changes that occur may have significance for one's functional capacity and ability to conduct necessary activities of daily living, as well as may compromise function of internal organs. Although most changes in bone take months to years to become clinically significant, even small changes may alter the balance in individuals with pre-existing pathology or decreased reserve capacity.

We have become quite sophisticated in our ability to measure bone turnover, calcium balance, and bone density; small changes can now be noted, resulting from a variety of internal and external influences. Although the principal interest of those caring for individuals with critical illness will most certainly be to treat the "critical illness" under consideration, the effects that it has had on the skeleton may last for years to come. Changes may be additive to other life events. Although perhaps less life-threatening than other organs that may be affected, these changes are no less worthy of note and remedy if one is to continue to attempt to maximize one's functioning ability and quality of life.

NORMAL BONE: STRUCTURE, FUNCTION, AND HOMEOSTASIS

In order to understand how critical illness may affect bone homeostasis, it is important first to understand normal bone physiology. Bone is best described as a constantly evolving, dynamic tissue. The skeleton is in a constant state of formation and resorption, and under normal circumstances receives approx 10% of the body's cardiac output. It not only provides rigid support to the extremities and joints for mobility, but also protects neural structures and key organs. It is a reservoir of essential nutrients, including calcium, phosphorus, and magnesium, among others that allow normal cellular metabolism to take place. Structurally, bone consists of both dense compact bone and cancellous bone. Organized in a system of canals and supporting lamellae, bone is three times lighter than cast iron with similar tensile strength. Despite this, it remains flexible. An inorganic mineral component comprises approximately two-thirds of the weight of bone. A small amount of water, an organic portion consisting primarily of type I collagen, and a mineral component largely represented by calcium phosphate are also present. Recent research has focused on numerous proteins that are thought to play a major role in bone remodeling and maintenance. Most of the identified proteins are thought to be derived from osteoblasts. Osteocalcin, identified as a specific product, is often referred to as GLA protein or BGP and has a mol w of 6000. It is a product of both osteoblasts and odontoblasts; 1,25-dihydroxyvitamin D3 is capable of stimulating its production. This protein is thought to play a key role in bone formation, and plasma concentration correlates with bone formation and mineralization. Other noncollagenous proteins present in bone, including albumin and α-2-HS glycoprotein, are synthesized by the liver and are incorporated into newly synthesized bone matrix. Osteonectin, a noncollagenous glycoprotein identified in bone, is also thought to play a role in the mineralization of bone, though less is known regarding this protein. Fibronectin and thrombospondin are thought to be important for cell attachment, and appear to play a role in the action of osteoclasts as they attach to the cell surface of the bone matrix.

Bone tissue consists of several cell types. Osteoblasts synthesize the extracellular matrix of bone and initiate mineralization. Osteoblasts become encased within the bone matrix and gradually lose their active properties; in this form they are referred to as osteocytes. Osteoclasts, thought to be derived from a different population of precursor cells, are multinucleated and function to resorb bone. Binding with bone in the Howship lacuna, the plasma membrane invaginates to form an irregular border, whereas resorption occurs through a process whereby cysteine-proteinases are secreted into the subosteoclastic portion of bone. This results in a lowering of pH, thus removing mineral from adjacent bone. Lysomal proteinases degrade the matrix. Osteoclasts also require the action of carbonic anhydrase 11 to provide protons for secretion as well as an activation of latent cytokines. Complicating things even further, various hormones and peptides assist in the regulation of bone remodeling. For example, calcitonin inhibits osteoclastic bone resorption by acting directly on G-protein-coupled receptors on the multinucleated osteoclasts.

Structurally, bone is classified into two types of tissue according to the way collagen fibers are formed: woven bone and lamellar bone. Woven bone is found under normal circumstances in the embryo and forms in the adult in response to bone injury. Although it is deposited quickly, it has a rather weak structure and is replaced by lamellar bone over time. Lamellar bone consists of collagen fibers that are arranged in an orderly, parallel manner. There are few osteocytes per unit area of matrix; a uniform distribution of osteocytes is found along lacunae and parallel to the collagen fiber long axis. Lamellar bone is further subdivided into a core of cortex, consisting of circumferential lamellar bone containing vascular canals and cancellous bone in the medulla, referred to as trabecula bone. Cortical bone is deposited in highly ordered arrangements around the longitudinal course of blood vessels. Growth along the length of bones depends on the proliferation of cartilage cells in the growth plate followed by maturation of those cells and endochondral ossification. Growth in the width and thickness of bone is accomplished by forming bone at the periosteal surface and by resorption of bone at the endosteal surface. After the epiphyseal plates close, growth in length ceases; endochondral bone formation can, however, be reactivated under certain conditions. This is referred to as modeling and will lead to the eventual architecture of the skeleton. Modeling ceases at around age 18 with a small increase in total bone mass continuing until age 30–35 when peak bone mass is achieved. Remodeling of bone, however, occurs throughout life and involves all of the bone surfaces, including the periosteal, haversian, and cortical-endosteal portions of bone. This process is credited with the preservation of the mechanical strength of bone. It should be noted that the appendicular skeleton has a slower turnover rate than the axial skeleton, and remodeling of bone is more active adjacent to hematopoietic marrow.

MEASURES OF BONE RESORPTION AND TURNOVER

As mentioned previously, bone is in a dynamic metabolic state throughout life, and continuously is resorbed and formed in a regulated fashion referred to as remodeling. Biochemical markers are available that can be used clinically to assess both bone resorption and bone formation. Bone resorption markers are released into the circulation as byproducts of osteoclastic action on bone. These include urinary hydroxyproline, urinary pyridinoline crosslinks, and plasma tartrate-resistant acid phosphatase (TRAP). Bone formation markers are released during osteoblast synthesis of new bone protein matrix, and include serum alkaline phosphastase, osteocalcin, and procollagen I extension peptides. Although these remain a constant source of study, many have become standard measures for assessing the results of a specific treatment. Pyridinoline crosslinks excreted into the urine have been demonstrated to correlate with bone resorption rates in persons with osteopososis, estrogen replacement therapy, Paget's disease, and hyperparathyroidism (1–3) Newly developed assays using polyclonal antibodies and monoclonal antibodies (MAb) allow direct measurement of these markers in urine by enzyme-linked immunoassays (ELISA) (4). The FDA has approved these immunoassays for biochemical markers of bone resorption. Performed as a simple urine test using a first or second morning sample, values above a "normal" range indicate a rapid rate of bone loss. The Pyrilinks and Pyrilink-D assays measure the excretion of pyridinoline (Pyd) and deoxy-pyridinoline (Dpd), respectively. Dpd is present only in type I collagen of bone and is a very specific measure of bone resorption. Pyd is found in both type I and II collagen found in cartilage. Since bone collagen is the major source of this compound and the turnover of collagen found in cartilage is slower, most Pyd excreted in the urine is derived from bone. The Osteomark assay measures the excretion of crosslinked N-telopeptides (Ntx), one type of peptide-bound pyridinoline. Ntx is highly specific to type I collagen.

Bone alkaline phosphatase is released into the circulation from osteoblasts during bone formation and is a good marker of bone turnover. Since serum alkaline phosphatase assays measure substances derived from both bone and liver, its utility is limited. Specific determinations of bone alkaline phosphatase can be made, however, and can be a specific and reliable marker of bone formation (5). Another marker for bone formation is osteocalcin or bone GLA protein. This noncollagenous protein is found only in bone and dentin, and enters the general circulation where it can be used as a marker and measured using a radioimmunoassay or ELISA. Serum osteocalcin is a sensitive and specific marker for osteoblastic activity, and accurately reflects both gradual age-related and accelerated postmenopausal increases in bone turnover (6). It also decreases rapidly after initiation of glucocorticoid use indicating decreased bone formation. Osteocalcin remains a research tool at this time, though clearly would provide useful information to help monitor the success of specific treatments. Procollagen I extension peptides are formed during the extracellular processing of type I collagen before it is incorporated into bone matrix. These circulate within the blood, and can be determined using radioimmunoassays or ELISA techniques. These remain under study.

Measurements of bone turnover can aid in monitoring response to therapy and in assessing risk of recurrence after discontinuation of therapy. Biochemical markers of bone turnover are preferred over bone density measurements, because they can demonstrate the effects of interventions far in advance of ultimate effects on bone density. Therapy should be aimed at slowing or preventing bone loss as indicated by a return of elevated bone turnover markers to normal, or a 30–60% decrease from pretreatment levels.

MEDICATION-INDUCED METABOLIC BONE DISEASE

Although critical illness of any cause must take priority in determining treatment options, it is important to remember that medications may have side effects capable of affecting bone metabolism with the end result being a loss of bone mass. In the short term, these changes will have minimal consequences; over time, however, bone loss may predispose to fractures, immobility, and increased pain and loss of functional capacity. Although the list of medications capable of affecting the bone is too exhaustive for this chapter, major classes of medications frequently used in the treatment of critical illness will be discussed. As stated previously, the regulatory process of bone remodeling can be disrupted by several mechanisms. There can be an increased frequency of activation or duration of activity of osteoclasts, a decrease in activity or duration of activity of osteoblasts, or some combination of the two. All three mechanism have been observed, and osteopenia may be associated with either a low, normal, or high rate of bone turnover *(7–9)*. Osteomalacia resulting from a loss of mineralized bone owing to a reduction of calcium phosphate levels below those required for normal mineralization of bone matrix must also be considered. A multiplicity of compounds have been associated with bone loss and mineralization defects. Those most related to the treatment of critical illness include glucocorticoids, L-thyroxine, heparin, neuroleptic agents, anticonvulsants, and aluminum binding antacids.

GLUCOCORTICOIDS

Glucocorticoid-induced osteopenia was first reported in 1932 by Cushing in his classic description of hypercortisolism *(10)*. Since glucocorticoids are so widely used, this is a major problem that must be considered in anyone being maintained on this treatment over time. Whether used as an anti-inflammatory or immunosuppressive agent, glucocorticoids exert their effect mostly on trabecular bone; periosteal diameter and intracortical porosity reportedly remain normal *(11)*. Osteopenia is most severe in the vertebrae and ribs with less of an effect on the long bones *(12–14)*. This most often results in fractures of the ribs, pubic rami, and vertebral bodies. Radiographically, this bone loss has been described as "hollow vertebrae" in which vertical and horizontal trabeculae are lost, and in which uniform trabecular thinning produces a thread-like appearance *(15)*. Although the incidence of osteopenia in Cushing's syndrome is 50% *(14)*, the true incidence in iatrogenically induced bone disease is not known. Risk factors include the total cumulative dose, daily dose, gender, age, menopausal status, and duration of therapy. Retrospective analyses of trabecular bone density in the axial skeleton based on dual-photon bone densitometry have demonstrated a 20–50% reduction in bone mineral content of the lumbar spine in women receiving a high daily dose, over 30 mg/d of prednisone equivalent, and large cumulative doses of prednisone of over 22 g over 7 yr *(16)*. Prevalence data suggest that patients receiving doses of <10 mg/d have a 10–12% reduction in bone mineral content of the lumbar spine compared with age-matched controls *(17)*. Annualized loss rates range from 0.3–3.0% *(18)*. Patients receiving a cumulative dose of <10 g were reported to have a 23% incidence of osteopenia and a 22% incidence of fracture. Taking doses between 10 and 30 gs of prednisone was associated with a 40% incidence of osteopenia and a 33% incidence of fracture. Of those taking >30 g of glucocorticoids in prednisone equivalent, 78% had osteopenia and 53% demonstrated radiologic evidence of a previous fracture. Using a fracture threshold of 11% loss of trabecular bone volume, 63% of patients who received glucocorticoid treatment in varying doses for a mean of 5 yr were considered to be at risk of future fracture *(9)*. Prospective data suggest that patients receiving 10–20 mg of prednisone a day had a dose-dependent annual loss of trabecular bone density in the distal tibia and radius of 3.5% *(20)*. Doses <8 mg a day were associated with a loss of 3% in vertebral mineral density compared to those taking 20 mg/d who experienced a 30% loss during the same time interval. Although studies have attempted to correlate short-term bone mineral loss in those treated with steroids for several days with annualized levels of loss, clearly this is not a simplistic calculation owing to coexisting variables. Repeated use of steroids, however, even of short duration, will have an additive effect and must not be forgotten. One study suggested that the rate of bone mineral content declined most during the first 12 wk of high-dose treatment, e.g., 2.5% of distal forearm bone mineral content compared to a rate of loss of 0.6% during the second 12 wk of therapy *(21)*. Another study reported a 20% decrease in trabecular bone after 5–7 mo of glucocorticoid therapy with minimal loss thereafter up to 12 mo *(19)*.

The predisposition to glucocorticoid-induced bone loss is considered to be independent of age, sex, race, and menopausal status *(22)*. That said, in young individuals, the relatively high bone turnover appears to predispose to a more rapid rate of bone loss. Patients who are immobilized and/or postmenopausal with reduced reserve of bone mass will have more fractures as demineralization continues to reduce critical mass and structure. The incidence of fracture in steroid-treated patients ranges form 8–18% *(23)*, two to three times the rate of similarly aged persons not on glucocorticoids. One study reported that whereas premenopausal women treated with low-dose prednisone did not lose cortical or trabecular bone, the same dose resulted in a 2.6% greater bone loss in postmenopausal women. Men on both low- and high-dose glucocorticoid regimens lost bone at an accelated rate with men under 50 yr of age losing more bone than postmenopausal women *(24)*. Owing to great variability among subjects, no one conclusion can be made other than to monitor bone status and attempt to eliminate or at least reduce the dose of steroid treatment as soon as possible.

Studies regarding corticosteroid use have demonstrated many findings, including an increased trabecular resorption surface; increased osteoclast number, activity, and active resorption surfaces; a relative increase in osteoid volume; normal or increased percentage of osteoid surface; and normal or decreased osteoid seam thickness. Dynamic parameters reveal a decreased or normal osteoblast rate, a decreased mineral calcification rate, and a decreased adjusted osteoblast activity rate *(25–27)*.

Major mechanisms proposed in the pathogenesis of glucocorticoid-induced osteoporosis include:

1. Decreased gastrointestinal calcium absorption and increased renal excretion leading to secondary hyperparathyroidism. This mechanism is thought to inhibit osteoblast function directly.
2. Decreased gonadal hormone secretion resulting from an inhibition of pituitary gonodotropin secretion *(28,29)* and direct inhibition of estrogen and testosterone production *(30)*. This will decrease production of prostaglandin E2 and insulin-like growth factor-1 (IGF-1). Prostaglandin E2 has anabolic and antiresorptive effects on bone *(31)*, and can reverse glucocorticoid-induced inhibition of osteoblast synthetic function.
3. Inhibition of IGF-1 production and action. This will increase the sensitivity to parathyroid hormone and 1,25-(OH)2 vitamin D *(32,33)*.
4. Loss of muscle leading to reduced physical stress necessary to maintain bone integrity and a greater osteoclastic activity.

MANAGING GLUCOCORTICOID BONE LOSS

As stated previously, all attempts should be made to reduce or even eliminate glucocorticoid therapy. Supplementation with calcium, vitamin D, and thiazides if possible has been demonstrated to reduce any potential calcium deficit *(34)*. A calcium dose of

1500 mg/d is suggested with some additionally recommending that sodium intake be restricted to 2–3 g/d. Vitamin D supplementation may increase the intestinal calcium absorption, normalize parathyroid levels, and thus reverse resorption and increase mineralization and bone density *(35)*. Caution is advised to avoid toxic doses of vitamin D with its own set of complications, including hypercalcemia, hypercalciuria, and a direct inhibition of bone remodeling. Vitamin D has been shown to be most effective when 24-h urine calcium excretion suggests significant calcium malabsorption. Vitamin D analog can be given to achieve a 24-h urine calcium level of approx 250 mg in women and 300 mg in men. Sodium restriction and thiazide diuretics have been shown to improve gastrointestinal absorption, reduce urine calcium excretion, and decrease cyclic AMP and parathyroid hormone levels in steroid-treated patients *(36)*. Thiazide diuretics in combination with vitamin D can cause hypercalcemia, and thiazides may aggravate corticosteroid-induced hypokalemia. Agents may be used to help increase bone mass. Salmon calcitonin, 100–200 IU subcutaneously or intranasally on a daily or an alternate-day schedule, has been shown to help preserve vertebral bone mineral content while preventing further bone mineral density loss in the lumbar spine *(37–39)* in persons treated with glucocorticoids. This has been shown to be effective for as long as 2 yr *(38)*. Two bisphosphonates have been studied in the setting of glucocorticoid use, pamidronate and etidronate. When given with supplemental calcium, pamidronate was associated with a 19% increase in lumbar bone mineral density over a 12-mo period of time in patients receiving long-term steroid therapy *(40)*. There was a reduction noted in bone formation as well as bone resorption, however. This "low-turnover" state raises concerns over the potential of impaired capacity for microfracture repair. In a study of postmenopausal women receiving high-dose steroid treatment for 1 yr, vertebral bone mineral density was significantly increased after 3, 6, and 12 mo of therapy with pamidronate *(41)*.

In general, anyone on long-term steroid treatment should be carefully monitored with bone density measurement of the lumbar spine at 6-mo intervals for at least the first 2 yr of steroid use. This hopefully will result in early treatment to prevent clinically symptomatic bone disease. Persons who already have osteopenia or precipitating factors other than the steroid use should be approached with more caution and treatment initiated in an attempt to prevent further bone loss. Although short-term studies have demonstrated a beneficial effect from anabolic steroids in postmenopausal women taking glucocorticoids *(42)*, these are not without risk and treatment should be individualized. Dehydeoepiandrosterone (DHEA), a weak androgen when used in combination with calcium and vitamin D, may reduce bone turnover *(43)*. Estrogen use where appropriate may be a useful adjunct to help maintain bone mass in postmenopausal women. Progesterone competes for glucocorticoid receptors in osteoblasts and theoretically may act as a glucocorticoid antagonist *(44)*, thus increasing bone mass. A study of long-acting progestin compounds in steroid-dependent asthmatics demonstrated a 17% increase in vertebral bone mineral density compared to control subjects *(45)*. Although still under study, the synthetic glucocorticoid deflazacort has been shown to have less of a negative effect on the skeleton. There is less suppression of intestinal calcium absorption, less depression of osteoblast function as assessed by osteocalcin levels, and less associated secondary hyperparathyroidism and hypercalciuria *(46–48)*. New compounds continue to show promise, though there is currently no "safe" glucocorticoid available, and prevention is advised above all with early treatment as described above reserved for progressive bone loss.

HEPARIN

Numerous studies have demonstrated a relationship between long-term treatment with high doses of heparin and osteoporosis *(49–51)*. Documented cases of lower dorsal, lumbar, and rib fractures exist, and the development of osteopenia appears to be related to the daily dose and duration of treatment. Spontaneous fractures have been reported only in patients receiving >15,000 IU/d for a period of >4 mo *(52,53)*. This is thought to be owing to an uncoupling of the remodeling mechanism with an increased bone resorption and decreased bone formation *(54)*. The mechanism remains unclear, though heparin has been shown to be capable of changing osteoclast resorption, osteoblast function, bone matrix synthesis, and the level of activity of associated growth factors thought to be influential in bone maintainance *(55,56)*.

CAFFEINE/THEOPHYLLINE

Caffeine and the related compound theophylline are often used in conjunction with medications used in the critical care setting. Chronic ingestion of caffeine equivalent to 16 cups of coffee per day is reported to increase serum bone Gla protein in animal models, suggesting increased bone turnover *(57)*. Epidemiologic data suggest a relationship between bone mineral density and lifetime intake of caffeinated coffee with a decreased bone mineral density noted at both hips and spine in those using more than 2 cups daily. This was an independent variable and appears to be less problematic as long as an adequate amount of calcium is taken as part of the diet *(58)*. Theophylline administration has been associated with a large and sustained increase in urine calcium excretion, a small increase in urine phosphate excretion, and a significant decrease in plasma phosphate *(59)*. These factors may result in an effect on bone remodeling.

CATECHOLAMINES

Epinephrine has been shown to be capable of increasing parathyroid hormone secretion, an effect likely mediated through the β-adrenergic receptor. This effect appears to be transient and is influenced by the level of calcium in surrounding tissue with minimal effects observed under hypercalcemic conditions and exaggerated effects noted in the setting of hypocalcemia *(60)*. Propranolol administration is capable of lowering parathyroid hormone levels acutely in normal subjects *(61)*. Catecholamines with α-adrenergic agonist activity can inhibit parathyroid hormone secretion in vitro, but have little effect in vivo *(62)*. Dopamine has been shown to stimulate the secretion of parathyroid hormone in bovine glands; no action has been observed in human tissue *(63)*. Although the physiological and clinical significance of this remains unclear, theoretically, catecholamines may exert an additive effect to that noted with other medications, as well as synergize the action of other agents, such as thyroid hormone.

ANTICONVULSANTS

Chronic administration of anticonvulsant medication can affect vitamin, mineral, and bone metabolism. Hypocalcemia, decreased intestinal calcium absorption, elevated alkaline phosphatase, decreased serum levels of vitamin D metabolites, increased urine hydroxyproline, increased serum parathyroid hormone levels, decreased bone mass, radiologic changes of osteopenia, and histomorphometric evidence of a spectrum of disorders ranging from mild hyperparathyroidism to a primary mineralization disorder to ostomalacia have all been reported in anywhere from 10–60% of those receiving medications from this class of agents *(64–66)*. Dilantin, phenobarbital, methadione, and paramethadione reportedly produce a dose-related induction of the hepatic microsomal P450 enzyme. This results in an accelerated catabolism of vitamin D and 25-(OH) vitamin D to form metabolically nonactive metabolites, and leads to decreased circulating and tissue levels of biologically active vitamin D metabolites as well as hypocalcemia, decreased intestinal absorption of calcium, hypophosphatemia, increased parathyroid hormone, and alterations in bone remodeling *(67)*. Since the metabolism of vitamin D from its early form of D3 to hydroxylation at the 25 position in the liver increases potency by 100 times, and is further increased 100 times after an additional hydroxy group is added at the 1 position in the kidney, any change in this metabolic pathway will affect bone and mineral metabolism. Although serum drug levels do not appear to correlate directly with either calcium or 25-(OH) vitamin D levels, the incidence of abnormalities increases with the duration of therapy beginning as soon as 6 mo after initiation of treatment *(67,68)*. Evidence suggests that anticonvulsants, especially Dilantin, have a direct effect on bone and mineral metablism at the cellular level. Dilantin has a well-known effect on transcellular ion transport and may decrease calcium absorption *(69)*. It also has been shown to have direct effects on osteoblast and osteoclast activity, as well as inhibit parathyroid hormone-induced bone resorption and calcium mobilization in a dose-dependent manner *(70)*. It has also been shown to have an inhibitory effect on collagen synthesis in vitro possibly capable of influencing bone matrix formation *(71)*. Correction of the vitamin D deficit is necessary, and all attempts should be made to reduce or eliminate the offending medication. Although some argue in favor of vitamin supplements preventively for persons on anticonvulsant treatment, no consensus exists, and most wait until after 6 mo or for proven changes in calcium metabolism, including measures of 25-(OH) vitamin D, the storage form of vitamin D, or some marker of bone turnover.

EFFECT OF DISEASE ON THE SKELETON

Many diseases are capable of influencing the skeleton and may result in situations that may be life-threatening. More commonly, however, these disorders are chronic in nature and become problematic over time. Although the list is too exhaustive to review in this context, examples will be used to illustrate major aspects of the relationship between disease and bone metabolism.

THYROID DISEASE

It is well known that hyperthyroidism is a risk factor for the development of osteopenia, and clinical osteoporosis is a long-term complication of excess thyroid hormone. Increased levels of thyroid hormone for whatever reason, iatrogenic or natural, will result in an increase in bone turnover, increased cortical porosity, and a decrease in cortical and trabecular bone volume *(72–74)*. Studies have demonstrated that hyperthyroidism is associated with an accelerated frequency of activation of bone remodeling units *(75)* and an increased ratio of resorptive to formation surfaces. Osteoblastic activity is enhanced and there is an increase in the rate of calcification and bone formation *(76)*. The negative net balance per remodeling cycle coupled with the increased activation frequency results in a reduction in trabecular thickness and the risk of perforation within the trabecular portion of bone *(77)*.

This perforation leads to a disintegration of the trabecular lattice, and results in a loss of bone and structural integrity. Clinically, symptoms will occur most frequently in those individuals who already have a reduced bone mass or suffer from prolonged hyperthyroidism.

It has been noted that the serum calcium in hyperthyroid patients averaged 0.5 mg/100 mL higher than in a group of age-matched normal control subjects. Serum inorganic phosphorus levels were also high and urinary clearance decreased, suggesting that parathyroid hormone secretion was suppressed *(78)*. The suppression of parathyroid hormone secretion decreases the tubular reabsorption of calcium leading to hypercalciuria. It has also been noted that patients with hyperthyroidism are more sensitive than euthyroid individuals to the hypercalcemic effects of parathyroid hormone *(79)*. Some have suggested that individuals with extremely high levels of calcium are likely to have an underlying parathyroid adenoma and deserve close observation. On return to the euthyroid state, the calcium should also return to normal. Failure to do so should warrant a thorough investigation concerning other possible etiologies for the calcium disturbance.

Data suggest that there may be an age-related difference in the cellular response to thyroid hormone with a more negative bone balance occurring in younger persons *(80)*. Markers of bone turnover, including serum alkaline phosphatase, serum osteocalcin, urine hydroxyproline, and urine pyridinium crosslinks, are elevated in this setting. It is important to note that although hyperthyroidism results in decreased bone density, bone mass will increase after the return to a euthyroid state, though once again to varying degrees depending on other underlying pathology. The finding of patients with subclinical hyperthyroidism either owing to excess endogenous hormone replacement or early stages of hyperthyroidism has allowed additional information to accumulate concerning the effect that excess thyroid hormone has on bone turnover. Even in these cases, a significant change in bone mass has been reported. In premenopausal clinically euthyroid women, L-thyroxine taken as replacement or suppressive therapy for at least 5–10 yr was associated with a 12.8% lower bone mineral density at the femoral neck *(81)*, 10% lower bone density at the femoral trochanter *(81)*, and a 9% reduction in the bone mineral density of the forearm *(82)* compared with age- and weight-matched controls. Lumbar spine density was similar in all groups. Some of those receiving L-thyroxine had increased serum thyroxine concentrations and increased free thyroxine indices, and >50% had suppressed levels of serum thyroid-stimulating hormone (TSH). Those with suppressed TSH levels had significantly lower levels of bone mineral density than those with normal values. Those women treated with L-thyroxine who were older than 35 yr of age with suppressed TSH levels had the greatest loss of bone density. Postmenopausal women treated with thyroid hormone replacement for more than 5 yr were found to have pronounced reduction in bone mineral content primarily within trabecular bone *(83)*. Clearly, TSH should be monitored, and all attempts made to normalize this value even in the setting of clinical euthyroidism or levels of thyroid hormone within the range of normal. Patients placed on suppressive doses of thyroid hormone will be at increased risk for bone loss, and all attempts should be made to minimize the dose of thyroid used as well as monitor bone mass with the goal of introducing methods to help preserve bone.

Although diagnosing hyperthyroidism is simple in many cases, it is especially problematic in elderly persons who are at most risk for bone-related pathology and who have the least reserve of bone mass. An atypical presentation is often the rule with many elderly presenting in a manner referred to as apathetic thyrotoxicosis. In these cases, few classic signs and symptoms are apparent, and only on careful questioning and clinical suspicion does laboratory testing confirm the diagnosis. At this time, the affected person may have had the disease for years with long-term sequelae affecting the bones, muscles, and cardiovascular system. These individuals may be quite ill-appearing, and often are considered terminal or suffering from a severe depression and/or malignancy. As with the case of an iatrogenic thyrotoxicosis, the excess thyroid hormone exerts its effect at the cellular level, causing an imbalance in bone remodeling. A return to euthyroidism is the only way to rectify the situation and bring the skeleton into balance; forming new bone that has been lost remains a more difficult problem.

OSTEOMALACIA AND RICKETS

Osteomalacia and rickets are disorders of mineralization. In osteomalacia, there is a failure to mineralize newly formed organic matric, or osteoid; rickets, a disease of children, results from defective calcification of cartilage involving the growth plate, a disorganization of the cartilage cells, and a thickened growth plate. Clinical manifestations vary with the cause of the pathology; in general, symptoms relate to skeletal pain and deformity, fracture, slippage of epiphyses, and growth disturbances. Hypocalcemia may become symptomatic, though this is usually insignificant. Although causes are numerous, the most common is a vitamin D deficiency. The principal biological action of vitamin D is to enhance intestinal calcium and phosphorus absorption, and increase bone calcium mobilization. Through a series of metabolic conversions, vitamin D is acted on in the skin, liver, and kidney to form the most metabolically active metabolite, 1,25-(OH) vitamin D. Most of the calcium transport is localized in the proximal small intestine, whereas most of vitamin D-mediated phosphorus absorption occurs in the jejunum and ileum. This vitamin metabolite also helps mobilize calcium stores from bone by inducing the dissolution of bone mineral and matrix, and works in concert with parathyroid hormone to remodel bone and maintain serum calcium levels. It induces stem cells to differentiate into osteoclasts. Osteoblasts respond to 1,25-(OH)D by increasing alkaline phosphatase, osteopontin, and osteocalcin as well as a variety of cytokines. It is believed that through this mechanism, bone resorption is mediated *(84–86)*.

Vitamin D deficiency may result from a simple nutritional deficiency state as may occur in individuals who avoid total fat in their diet. Vitamin D is a fat-soluble vitamin. More commonly, vitamin D is deficient secondary to a problem with the absorption of vitamin D, as may occur in persons with celiac disease, or following a partial or total gastrectomy or intestinal bypass procedure for obesity or cancer. Other causes include chronic pancreatic insufficiency, hepatobiliary disease, including cirrhosis, biliary fistula, or biliary atresia, or anything that will affect the metabolism of vitamin D either in the skin, liver, or kidney. Miscellaneous causes include acidosis, phosphate depletion, and hereditary illness. Although any one cause may result in clinical disease if severe enough or present for long periods of time, patients with critical illness frequently have multiple causes for a problem. Lack of sunlight exposure when coupled with long-term anticonvulsant therapy is of concern. Administration of vitamin D to patients with vitamin D-deficient rickets or osteomalacia will result in a healing of the bone. Serum phosphorus levels will climb initially with calcium often lagging behind. There is the potential for hypocalcemia owing to a process called "hungry bone syndrome" or deposition of calcium into bones that have been deficient for long periods of time. Even with treatment, there is a delay in the fall of alkaline phosphatase that accompanies osteomalacia and immunoreactive parathyroid hormone levels may also return only after a period of time. It is common for radiological improvement to take months to show a change.

As with most illness, a high index of suspicion and preventive treatment is suggested as the best way to avoid clinical manifestations of this common problem. Eliminating underlying causes whenever possible may help prevent further pathology; in most cases vitamin D will be required with the dose and form based on the cause of the problem. For example, if there is a problem with hydroxylating vitamin D at the 25 position in the liver, giving this form of vitamin D will bypass the abnormality and treat the problem.

Acidosis has been linked to osteomalacia. The probable mechanism relates to a slow dissolution of the mineral phase of bone in an attempt to buffer retained hydrogen ions. Hypercalciuria is apparent. Maintenance of pH within a critical range is essential for normal mineralization to occur. A decrease in systemic pH can therefore inhibit mineralization by lowering pH at calcification sites. Acidosis also affects phosphate metabolism by altering renal tubular handling of the anion and changing the species of phosphate in solution. Secondary hyperparathyroidism has been postulated as an important factor in the altered phosphate metabolism noted in systemic acidosis. Acidosis may also alter the response to exogenous vitamin D. This form of bone disturbance most commonly is noted in the setting of distal renal tubular acidosis. On correction of the acidosis with sodium bicarbonate alone in doses of 5–10 g/d, bone abnormalities begin to correct. Vitamin D or 1,25-(OH)2 vitamin D can accelerate healing.

PAGET'S DISEASE OF BONE

Paget's disease of the bone was first reported by Sir James Paget in 1876 when he described a single patient in the paper entitled "On a form of chronic inflammation of bones (osteitis deforman)." This disorder is characterized by a localized increase in bone turnover and remodeling. The balance between bone formation and resorption is disordered, resulting in excessive and irregular bone formation. One bone may be affected (monostotic), or several bones (polyostotic) may be involved at the same time. Classically, individuals remain asymptomatic for most if not all of their lives with disease becoming apparent only on coincidental radiologic assessment or some routine blood test. Others have a more dramatic course. Critical, life-threatening illness may be a major component of this disorder, which may go through phases of activity and quiescence. The pelvis, axial skeleton, skull, and weight-bearing bones are affected most commonly. When the disease does become problematic, its two major manifestations are pain and deformities. Other manifestations include increased vascularity, metabolic rate, bone turnover, ischemic ulcers, central nervous system involvement, malignant transformation, and high output cardiac failure.

Pain is the presenting problem in approx 5% of patients. It is usually described as constant, deep, and unrelenting. Worse at night, it often keeps the patient awake. Some report that the pain may be relieved by exercise. There is little correlation between the appearance on X-ray and the severity of the pain. Osteolytic lesions do tend to be associated with more pain. Pain is also more common when the lesion is active with theories regarding why including a possible stretching of the periosteum by the enlarging bone, increased intramedullary pressure from increased bone vascularity, stimulation of nerve endings, and microfractures. Pain may be owing to the disease itself and/or an associated osteoarthritic process. Although rapid response to nonsteroidal therapy has been suggested as more frequently indicating an arthritis accompanying the Paget's disease, the disease itself may also be affected by nonsteroidal agents. Intra-articular injection of lidocaine may be helpful in separating the symptoms of osteoarthritis from Paget's disease with local vs systemic treatment aimed at the underlying pathology. Pain may result from pagetic bone-compressing neighboring nerves. Pain associated with the rare, though always serious complication of osteosarcomatous change is usually quite severe and debilitating, and is often resistant to simple analgesic therapy. Paget's disease of the skull may present with headaches and compression of basilar nerve structures as well as the brain itself, and may be a life-threatening problem.

Paget's disease may result in bone deformities resulting from enlarging and weakened bone. This is particularly noticeable in the long bones and skull. The long bones become larger and bow, the tibia in the anterior position and the femur in the anterolateral direction. The skull may increase in size and become irregular. Cutaneous manifestations are commonly noted over affected bones. Skin overlying pagetic bones may be warmer, especially during periods of active disease. This increased warmth is associated with increased vascularity resulting from increased skeletal blood flow, and to compensatory vasodilatation from an increased metabolic rate and bone turnover. Ischemic ulcers may occur as the blood supply to the skin becomes affected; difficulty in healing may present a problem especially in the setting of skin grafts. Problems with central nervous system involvement may result in lethargy, delirium, or specific cranial nerve involvement. Nerves passing through foramen are subject to compression. The eighth, second, fifth, and seventh nerves are most commonly affected. Hearing loss, monocular visual disturbances, and even blindness may occur. Trigeminal neuralgias may be noted as may a facial palsy or paresis. Although nerve compression is a frequent cause of hearing loss, involvement of the inner ear may occur as the bone changes in density. Patients may also complain of a "roaring" noise, probably owing to the increased blood flow through pagetic bone.

Platybasia, a condition when the base of the skull is affected, may lead to vertebral involvement affecting the long tracts in the spinal cord and lower cranial nerves. Persons affected with platybasia tend to have a short neck with the chin lying on the chest. Radiological examination correlates with the finding of spinal stenosis and arthropathy of the facets. Paget's disease has also been reported to be associated with a cauda equina syndrome, paraparesis, and even paraplegia.

A shunting of blood from the internal to the external carotids may lead to a relative brain anoxia. Hydrocephalus may also be present with altered mental function, gait, and urinary incontinence noted in late stages. Patients with generalized active disease may complain of easy fatigability or have symptoms of congestive heart failure owing to the high output state.

Fractures are the most common complication of Paget's disease. Usually occurring at right angles to the long axis of the bone, they are most common in the femur, tibia, and forearm. Trauma may precipitate the fracture, though even the weight of one's own body may become problematic in this weakened bone. Most fractures present with localized pain, tenderness, and signs of local inflammation at the site. Fracture rates vary from 1.5–6.6 fractures/100 patient yr *(87)*. Fractures occur most commonly during the osteolytic phase of the disease and are associated with a high mortality risk, e.g., 18% at 3 mo *(88)*.

Malignant transformation is rare, but when it occurs, is life-threatening. Affecting approx 0.15% of patients, the pelvis and femoral bones are most commonly involved. Men are affected most with lesions appearing most commonly in those with polyostotic disease. Approximately 50% of patients with osteosarcoma die within 6 mo of diagnosis; approx 10% survive >5 yr. Usually heralded by severe pain and swelling, diagnosis is confirmed by biopsy.

Although cardiovascular complications may occur as a result of Paget's diease, diffuse disease is necessary. Since this is a disease occurring most commonly during later life, coexisting illness will have a significant effect on the degree of difficulty one has with the increased vascularity, and whether one can support the often increased blood volume and blood flow.

Most individuals with Paget's disease will require no treatment for most of their lives. The main reason to treat is to relieve symptoms attributable to the disease, such as pain, discomfort, or complications of the disease. Therapy has also been suggested prior to orthopedic surgery on an affected bone to reduce vascularity. Treatment should never be initiated solely based on radiologic or biochemical measures, though some advocate treatment when measures of bone turnover reflect severe and active disease. Analgesic therapy is the mainstay of treatment in most cases. Depending on the site of the lesion, response to analgesic medications, neurological abnormality, or progression of deformity treatment should also be considered in an attempt to arrest disease progresion. The bisphosphonates are currently the preferred medication. Bisphosphonates are pyrophosphate analogs that bind to the bone mineral surface and act as inhibitors of osteoclast-mediated bone resorption. Etidronate, the first bisphosphonate used in clinical practice in Paget's disease, is an effective agent that has been shown to reduce pagetic activity *(89)*. It has been shown to inhibit the mineralization process completely, resulting in osteomalacia. They affect bone resorption in a dose-dependent fashion and begin to exert an effect within days of administration. Alkaline phosphatase and urinary hydroxyproline are reduced in relation to the disease activity, and bone is histologically returned to normal. There is a decrease in bone resorption and bone formation associated with a decrease in bone blood flow and a decrease in marrow fibrosis. Because of its effectiveness, oral route of administration, safety profile, and relatively low cost, etidronate has received a great deal of support as initial therapy. The recommended dose is 5–10 mg/kg/d for 3–6 mo with higher doses used to suppress the activity of the disease in a more rapid time frame. Repeat courses are usually as effective as the initial dose. Its use, however, has been limited by its relatively narrow therapeutic range with 5 mg/kg/d being associated with focal defects in bone mineralization. Doses in excess of 10 mg/kg/d have been shown to inhibit completely the mineralization process, resulting in osteomalacia. Approximately one-third of persons with Paget's disease fail to respond to bisphosphonate therapy, and approx 15% of persons treated with these agents complain of gastrointestinal symptoms, including diarrhea. This also is usually dose-dependent and can be reduced by dividing the dose into two equal doses given at different times of the day. Etidronate may induce a rise in serum phosphate levels that is dose-dependent owing to an increased renal tubular reabsorption of phosphate. In certain cases, the dose may need to be reduced owing to this effect. For this reason primarily, doses are limited in magnitude and for no more than 6 mo at a time. Because of this interference with bone mineralization, etidronate is not recommended in the presence of extensive osteolytic disease of long bones, particularly those that are weight-bearing. Since this agent is excreted essentially unchanged in the urine, a reduced dose is recommended in the setting of renal insufficiency. Alendronate sodium is another bisphosphonate that is a highly potent and specific inhibitor of osteoclastic bone resorption.

Both oral and iv preparations have been demonstrated to reduce serum alkaline phosphatase and pagetic activity. Since it is at least 1000 times more potent an inhibitor of bone resorption than etidronate, it does not interfere with bone mineralization in doses that are effective against Paget's disease, 40 mg/d *(90)*.

Calcitonin has been used extensively in treating Paget's disease *(91–93)*. Unlike the bisphosphonates whose effects are long-lasting even beyond therapy, calcitonin's effects are short-lived. Calcitonin is a 32 amino acid hormone that has as its main action a goal of preventing hypercalcemia. Calcitonin reduces the rate of bone resorption and therefore the activity of Paget's disease. It specifically inhibits the activity of the osteoclasts as well as reduces their number. Regular administration of calcitonin reduces levels of urinary hydroxyproline, followed by a decrease in serum alkaline phosphatase. The newly formed bone under the effects of calcitonin is more lamellar in form. Several types of calcitonin are available, including human, salmon, and porcine. Salmon calcitonin may have a greater analgesic effect, though both human and salmon have wide acceptance. Antibodies may form and use may become limited. This resistance cannot be predicted and may occur after months or years of continuous therapy. High titers, over 1:1500, of neutralizing antibodies against calcitonin in the presence of a biochemical response to another type of calcitonin implies resistance. Recent development of a nasal spray delivery system has revitalized interest in this agent, long limited by its parenteral requirements. Human calcitonin has been associated with more side effects than salmon, with flushing, vomiting, diarrhea, local pain if injected, nausea, and frequency of urination being the major ones.

Patients in need of rapid treatment, as is the case with a progressive paraplegia or deteriorating neurological status, may benefit from plicamycin *(94)*. Plicamycin is a cytotoxic antibiotic that inhibits RNA synthesis and had been around even before the bisphosphonates became available. It requires iv administration, and a single course can induce remissions lasting up to several years, though most will relapse shortly after treatment is discontinued. Adverse effects are many, and include hepatotoxicity, renal impairment, thrombocytopenia, nausea, diarrhea, and vomiting. Hypocalcemia may occur immediately following treatment and may last as long as 36 h. Administration of calcium and vitamin D is advised for at least 1 d after the infusion.

HYPERCALCEMIA

There are numerous causes of hypercalcemia, an often life-threatening illness. The most common cause is a metastatic malignancy, though primary hyperparathyroidism, milk-alkali syndrome, hyperthyroidism, and hypervitaminosis D are other frequent causes. Although clinical presentations vary greatly, lethargy, volume depletion, renal calculi, bone pain, cardiac arrhythmias, hypertension, peptic ulcer disease, and pancreatitis may be noted. Hypercalcemia may be a metabolic emergency, especially when serum calcium levels exceed 14 mg/dL and clinical instability exists. Primary hyperparathyroidism is believed to be more common than previously thought, largely because of the large number of individuals receiving automated measurements of blood chemistries that uncover asymptomatic cases. Fortunately, most persons affected will have only slight elevations of calcium owing to "equilibrium hypercalcemia" *(95)*, an adjustment of the set point regulating the parathyroid gland. This is not the case when the cause of the hypercalcemia is outside of the parathyroid gland. Therefore, hypercalcemia resulting from a malignancy is referred to as "dysequilibrium hypercalcemia" *(96)*. In this case, hypercalcemia may be associated with a decreased production of parathormone with a net increase in urinary calcium, an osmotic diuresis, and volume contraction. Nausea and vomiting may occur in this setting with their own side effects, including fluid and electrolyte disturbances. Evaluation rests on establishing whether or not the cause of hypercalcemia is related to an overproduction of parathyroid hormone with radioimmunoassays available to assist in this categorization.

Therapy depends on rapid volume replacement with particular attention to avoid volume overload, especially since many of these patients are elderly with coexisting medical problems. Sodium facilitates calcium diuresis whether it is given intravenously or orally. The use of loop diuretics will also assist in calcium elimination by maintaining the coupling mechanism between sodium and calcium. Thiazide diuretics are contraindicated, since they uncouple the sodium to calcium link, thus potentially increasing calcium levels. In most cases, his treatment will bring a prompt reduction in calcium, though careful monitoring is essential. Patients in renal failure may require dialysis with a zero calcium dialysate preparation *(97)*. There are many pharmacological agents capable of reducing serum calcium levels if the above is not satisfactory. Bisphosphonates, calcitonin, plicamycin, glucocorticoids, and gallium nitrate may be used. Bisphosphonates as a class inhibit osteoclast function. Although pamidronate is the most potent and rapid, and is available in both oral and iv forms, etidronate has also been used extensively. Depending on the level of calcium, iv use is preferred to ensure proper absorption from the gastrointestinal tract. Most cases will respond within 24 h, though calcium may continue to drop for several additional days. Calcitonin is available as both a synthetic human or salmon preparation. It also works by inhibiting osteoclastic bone resorption, produces a mild calciuric effect, and has a rapid action. Although its effect is good, it is rather short-lived and probably best used as adjunctive therapy *(98,99)*.

Plicamycin inhibits cellular RNA synthesis and has a rapid onset of action. Calcium usually normalizes within 1–3 d *(100)*. Gallium nitrate also inhibits bone resorption, though its mechanism remains unknown. Owing to its high degree of nephrotoxicity, it is best reserved for persons who fail on the above *(101)*. Glucocorticoids remain the drug of choice for persons with hypervitaminosis D, hematologic malignancies, such as multiple myeloma and lymphoma, and the hypercalcemia of granulomatous disease *(100)*. High doses are used for several days. The onset of action tends to be slow, and the side effects are many, including psychoses, gastrointestinal disturbances, and immunological effects.

PRIMARY HYPERPARATHYROIDISM

Primary hyperparathyroidism results from an overproduction of parathyroid hormone from the parathyroid glands either from four-gland hyperplasia or a single or multiple benign adenomas. The overall incidence of hyperparathyroidism has been reported to be 27/100,000 persons/y. Prevalence rates are approx 1% higher based on the assumption that the majority of patients with hypercalcemia have hyperparathyroidism. In the majority of patients, the disease presents in a mild manner or is asymptomatic altogether. Less frequently, calcium may reach critical levels, mandating prompt action. Fortunately, the death rate attributable to hyperparathyroidism is extremely low, though clearly depends on treatment and degree of illness. It is diagnosed most commonly between the fifth and seventh decades of life, though it can occur at any age. Parathyroid hormone mobilizes calcium from bone, enhances renal tubular absorption of calcium, promotes 1,25 dihydroxycholecalciferol production in the kidney, and increases phosphate excretion. The end result is an increased level of serum calcium and a reduced level of serum phosphorus. Clinically, patients may present with a wide range of signs and symptoms, including generalized weakness, lethargy, headaches, peptic ulcer disease, pancreatitis, chrondrocalcinosis with or without acute attacks of pseudogout, juxta-articular erosions, subchondral fractures, calcific periarthritis, nephrolithiasis, hypertension, and osteitis fibrosa cystica *(102,103)*. About one-fifth of patients with primary hyperparathyroidism have radiologically demonstrable bone involvement, most commonly manifested as diffuse demineralization. When severe disease is present, osteitis fibrosa cystica may be noted. This is characterized by bone demineralization, bone cysts, fractures and deformities, and bone pain. Histologically, there are reduced bone trabeculae, increased giant multinuclear osteoclasts in scalloped areas on the bone surface, and fibrous tissue replacing cellular and marrow elements. Diffuse demineralization may be radiologically indistinguishable from other forms of osteoporosis, but specific signs of osteitis fibrosa may be recognized, particularly in the hands, skull, and jaw. The most important X-ray to obtain is the postero-anterior view of the hands. This may reveal demonstrable bone lesions, and/or subperiosteal resorption of the radial aspects of the middle phalanges. There is usually evidence of erosion of the outer cortical surfaces of bone, generalized de-mineralization of bones, and localized destructive lesions, often of cystic character. The skull is often described as having a "ground-glass" appearance. Although the initial treatment is medical with the goal of stabilizing serum calcium levels, definitive treatment is surgical.

SECONDARY HYPERPARATHYROIDISM AND RENAL FAILURE

Patients with renal failure have difficulty excreting phosphorus as well as producing 1,25 dihydroxycholecalciferol. This may result in a secondary hyperparathyroidism associated with four-gland hyperplasia and hypercalcemia. The skeletal change is referred to as "renal osteodystrophy," and is characterized by a combination of osteomalacia, osteitis fibrosa cystica, osteosclerosis, and osteoporosis. Although all of these conditions predispose to the development of bone fractures, most commonly the renal failure is of clinical concern with uremia, hypocalcemia, hyperkalemia, and acid-base disturbances mandating continual follow-up and clinical management.

IMMOBILIZATION

Prolonged immobilization as may occur in anyone assigned to complete bed rest, who has a body cast, is in traction, or suffers a spinal cord injury will lead to accelerated resorption of bone with the potential for hypercalcemia *(104)*. Changes may be noted within days to weeks with hypercalcemia more problematic in persons with underlying conditions predisposing to calcium abnormalities, such as primary hyperparathyroidism, underlying metastatic malignancy, renal failure, or Paget's disease. Immobilization increases osteoclast activity and bone turnover. Mobilization promptly reverses the condition as does weight-bearing and shifting gravitational force on the skeleton, such as may result from rotating beds. If this is not possible, medical management with bisphosphanates may be beneficial.

METASTATIC BONE DISEASE

Metastasis to bone may result in changes that are either osteolytic, osteoblastic, or some combination of both. Osteolytic lesions can cause extensive destruction to bone, lead to hypercalcemia, and result in pathological fractures. Cancers of the breast, prostate, thyroid, kidney, and lung most commonly metastasize to bone, though other tumors may also involve the skeleton. In general, tumor cells metastasize to vascularized sites of the skeleton *(105)*, most commonly the axial skeleton, ribs, vertebral bodies, and the proximal ends of the long bones. Clinically, bone pain, pathological fractures, nerve compression, or hypercalcemia may be the first presenting sign that the bone is involved. It is important to remember that hypercalcemia may also result from humoral factors produced by tumors even in the absence of bone involvement. Cancers that tend to produce these humoral factors include lung, head and neck, cervix, and kidney with this mechanism accounting for 75% of hypercalcemia associated with malignancy *(106)*.

MULTIPLE MYELOMA

Multiple myeloma classically causes osteolytic lesions. Hypercalcemia is also common during the later stages of the disease and is thought to be secondary to the production of the cytokine lymphotoxin *(107)*. Other cytokines capable of enhancing bone resorption that have also been associated with the hypercalcemia of multiple myeloma are interleukin-1 and interleukin-6 *(108,109)*. Therapy is once again aimed at controlling symptoms, such as bone pain, fractures, and hypercalcemia, and include conventional treatments as described earlier. Treatment aimed at the underlying malignancy may also prevent further skeletal involvement, with particular attention to avoid nephrotoxic agents in light of the known renal complication of this disease.

SUMMARY

The skeleton is frequently involved in disease states that may present as critical illness. Involvement may result from the underlying pathophysiological mechanism itself or from the initiation of life-sustaining treatment. In most cases, the skeleton becomes clinically affected only after a prolonged period of time, though in the case of malignancy or Paget's disease, may become clinically apparent at the same time the critical problem is detected. Although prompt medical attention will most certainly be directed to the critical and life-threatening condition, failure to recognize the impact that the disease or its treatment may have on the skeleton will only further diminish the potential for meaningful recovery and maintenance of as high a quality of life as possible.

REFERENCES

1. Delmas PD. Clinical use of biochemical markers of bone remodeling in osteoporosis. Bone 1992;13:517–521.
2. Uebelhart D, Gineyts E, Chapuy M-C. Urinary excretion of pyridinium crosslinks: a new marker of bone resorption in metabolic bone disease. Bone Miner 1990;8:87–96.
3. Seibel MJ, Cosman F, Shen U. Urinary hydroxypyridinium crosslinks of collagen as markers of bone resorption and estrogen efficacy in postmenopausal osteoporosis. J Bone Miner Res 1993; 8:881–889.
4. Robin S, Woitge H, Hesley R. A direct enzyme linked immunoassay for urinary deoxypyridinoline as a specific marker for measuring bone resorption. J Bone Miner Res 1994;9:1643–1649.

5. Gomez B, Ardakani S, Ju J. Monoclonal antibody assay for measuring bone-specific alkaline phosphatase actuity in serum. Clin Chem 1995;41:1560–1566.
6. Gomez B, Bally CA, Jenkins DK. An enzyme immunoassay for intact newly synthesized osteocalcin: a marker of bone formation (abs). International Conference on Progress in Bone and Mineral Research, Vienna, Austria, 1994.
7. Meunier PJ, Sellami S, Briancon D. Histological heterogeneity of apparently idiopathic osteoporosis. In: DeLuca HF, Frost HM, Jee WS, eds. Osteoporosis: Recent Advances in Pathogenesis and Treatment. University Park Press, Baltimore, 1980, p. 293.
8. Parfitt AM, Matthews C, Rao D. Impaired osteoblast function in metabolic bone disease. In: DeLuca HF, Frost HM, Jee WS, eds. Osteoporosis: Recent Advances in Pathogenesis and Treatment. University Park Press, Baltimore, 1980, p. 321.
9. Weinstein R, Bryce G, Sappington L. Decreased serum ionized calcium and normal vitamin D metabolite levels with anticonvulsant drug treatment. J Clin Endocrinol Metab 1984;58:1003–1009.
10. Cushing H 1982 Basophile adenomas. J Nerv Ment Dis 76:50.
11. Bressot C, Meunier PJ. Histomorphometric profile, pathophysiology and reversibility of corticosteroid induced osteoporosis. Metab Bone Dis Rel Res 1979;1:303–311.
12. Curtiss PH, Clark WS, Herndon CH. Vertebral fractures resulting from prolonged cortisone and corticotropin therapy. JAMA 1954;156:467–469.
13. Howland WJ, Pugh DG, Sprague RG. Roentgenologic changes of the skeletal system in Cushing's syndrome. Radiology 1958;71:69–78.
14. Sussman ML, Copelman B. The roentgenologic appearance of the bones in Cushing's syndrome. Radiology 1942;39:288–292.
15. Maldague B, Malghem J, Nagant de Deuxchaisnes C. Radiologic aspects of glucocortinephrologist. Kidney Int 1984;38:193–211.
16. Schaadt O, Bohr H. Loss of bone mineral in axial and peripheral skeleton in aging, prednisone treatment and osteoporosis. In: Dequeker JV, Johnston CC Jr, eds. Noninvasive Bone Measurements: Methodological Problems. Oxford, IRL Press, 1982, pp. 207–214.
17. Sambrook PN, Eisman JA, Yates MG. Osteoporosis in rheumatoid arthritis: safety of low dose corticosteroids. Ann Rheum Dis 1986;45:950–953.
18. Mitchell D, Lyles K. Glucocorticoid induced osteoporosis mechanisms for bone loss: evaluation of strategy for prevention. J Gerontol 1990;45:M153–158.
19. LoCascio V, Bonucci E, Imbimbo B. Bone loss in response to long-term glucocorticoid therapy. Bone Miner 1990;8:39–51.
20. Reugsegger P, Medici TC, Anliker M. Corticosteroid induced bone loss: a longitudinal study of alternate day therapy in patients with bronchial asthma using quantitative computed tomography. Eur J Clin Pharmacol 1983;25:615–620.
21. Rickers H, Deding A, Christiansen C. Corticosteroid induced osteopenia and vitamin D metabolism: effect of vitamin D_2, calcium phosphate and sodium fluoride administration. Clin Endocrinol 1982;16:409–415.
22. Dykman T, Gluck O, Murphy W. Evaluation of factors associated with glucocorticoid induced osteopenia in patients with rheumatic diseases. Arthritis Rheum 1985;23:361–365.
23. Curtiss PH, Clark WS, Herndon CH. Vertebral fractures resulting from prolonged cortisone and corticotropin therapy. JAMA 1954;156:467–469.
24. Nagant de Deuxchaisnes C, Devogelaer JP, Esselinckx W. The effect of low dose glucocorticoids on bone mass in rheumatoid arthritis: a cross-sectional and a longitudinal study using single photon absorptiometry. Adv Exp Med Biol 1984;171:210–239.
25. Dempster D. Perspectives: bone histomorphometry in glucocorticoid induced osteoporosis. J Bone Miner Res 1989;4:137–150.
26. Dempster DW, Arlot MA, Meunier PJ. Mean wall thickness and formation periods of trabecular bone packets in corticosteroid induced osteoporosis. Calcif Tissue Int 1983;35:410–417.
27. Meunier PJ, Dempster DW, Edouard C. Bone histomorphometry in corticosteroid induced osteoporosis and Cushing's syndrome. Adv Exp Med Biol 1984;171:191–200.
28. Hseuh AJ, Erickson GF. Glucocorticoid inhibition of FSH induced estrogen production in cultured rat granulosa cells. Steroids 1978;32:639–648.
29. Sakakura M, Takebe K, Nakagawa S. Inhibition of leutinizing hormone secretion induced by synthetic LRH by long-term treatment with glucocorticoids in human subjects. J Clin Endocrinol Metab 1975;40:774–779.

30. Macadams MR, White RH, Chipps RE. Reduction of serum testosterone levels during chronic glucocorticoid therapy. Ann Intern Med 1986;104:648–651.
31. Raisz LG, Kream BE. Regulation of bone formation. N Engl J Med 1983;30:83–89.
32. Gourmelen M, Girard F, Biuoux M. Serum somatomedin/insulin like growth factor (IGF) and IGF carrier levels in patients with Cushing's syndrome or receiving glucocorticoid therapy. J Clin Endocrinol Metab 1982;54:885–892.
33. Reid I. Pathogenesis and treatment of steroid osteoporosis. Clin Endocrinol 1989;30:83–103.
34. Hahn T, Henden B, Scharp C. Effect of chronic anticonvulsant therapy on serum 25-hydroxycalciferol levels in adults. N Engl J Med 1972;287:900–904.
35. Bijlsma JW, Raymakers JA, Mosch C. Effect of oral calcium and vitamin D on glucocorticoid induced osteopenia. Clin Exp Rheumatol 1988;6:113–119.
36. Suzuki Y, Ichikawa Y, Saito E. Importance of increased urinary calcium excretion in the development of secondary hyperparathyroidism of patients under glucocorticoid therapy. Metabolism 1983;32:151–156.
37. Emkey R, Reading W, Procaccini P. The effect of calcitonin on bone mass in steroid induced osteoporosis. In: Abstracts of the Annual Scientific Meeting of the American College of Rheumatology, Minneapolis, 1994, p. S183.
38. Montemurro L, Schiraldi G, Zanni D. Two years' treatment with calcitonin nasal spray: effective protection against corticosteroid induced osteoporosis. In: Kovergaard, Christiansen C, eds. Proceedings Third International Symposium in Osteoporosis. Denmark, Glastrup Hospital, 1990.
39. Ringe J, Welzel D. Salmon calcitonin in the therapy of corticoid induced osteoporosis. Eur J Clin Pharmacol 1987;33:35–39.
40. Reid IR, Alexander CJ, King AR. Prevention of steroid induced osteoporosis with (3-amino-1-hydroxylpropylidene) -1, 1-bisphosphonate (APD). Lancet 1988;1:143–146.
41. Mulder H, struys A. Intermittent cyclic etidronate in the prevention of corticosteroid induced bone loss. Br J Rheumatol 1994;33:348–350.
42. Need AG. Corticosteroids and osteoporosis. Aust NZJ Med 1987;17:267–272.
43. Lee YSL, Kohlmeier L, Van Vollenhoven RF. The effects of dehydroepiandrosterone (DHEA) on bone metabolism in healthy postmenopausal women. In: Abstracts of the Annual Scientific Meeting of the American College of Rheumatology, Minneapolis, 1994, p. S182.
44. Reid I. Pathogenesis and treatment of steroid osteoporosis. Clin Endocrinol 1989;30:83–103.
45. Grecu E, Weinshelbaum A, Simmons R. Effective therapy of glucocorticoid induced osteoporosis with medroxyprogesterone acetate. Calcif Tissue Int 1990;46:294–299.
46. Fucik RJ, Kukreja SG, Hargis GK. Effects of glucocorticoids on function of the parathyroid glands in man. J Clin Endocrinol Metab 1975;40:152–155.
47. Imbimbo B, Tuzi R, Porzino F. Clinical equivalence of a new glucocorticoid deflazacort and prednisone in rheumatoid arthritis and SLE patients. In: Avioli L, Gennari C, Imbimbo B, eds. Glucocorticoid Effects and Their Biological Consequences. Plenum, New York 1983, p. 234.
48. Gennari C, Imbimbo B. Effects of prednisone and deflazacort on vertebral bone mass. Calcif Tissue Int 1985;37:592–593.
49. Avioli L. Heparin-induced osteoporosis: an appraisal. Adv Exp Med Biol 1975;52:375–387.
50. Rupp WM, McCarthy HB. Risk of osteoporosis in patients treated with long-term intravenous heparin therapy. Curr Probl Surg 1982;39:419–422.
51. Griffith GC, Nichols G, Asher JD. Heparin osteoporosis JAMA 1965;193:85–88.
52. Squires JW, Pinch LW. Heparin induced spinal fractures. JAMA 1979;241:2417–2418.
53. Wise PH, Hall AS. Heparin induced osteopenia in pregnancy BMJ 1980;281:110–111.
54. Megard M, Cuche M, Grapeloux. Osteoporose de l'heparinotherapie: Analyse histomorphometrique de la biopse ossuse une observation. Nouv Presse Med 1982;11:261–264.
55. Canalis E, McCarthy T, Centrella M. The role of skeletal growth factors in skeletal remodeling. Clin Endocrinol Metab 1989;18:903–919.
56. Schreiber AB, Kenny J, Kowalski WJ. Interaction of endothelial cell growth factor with heparin: Characterization by receptor and antibody recognition. Proc Natl Acad Sci USA 1985.
57. Glajchen N, Ismail F, Epstein S. The effect of chronic caffeine administration on serum markers of bone mineral metabolism and bone histomorphometry in the rat. Calcif Tissue Int 1988;43:277–280.
58. Barrett-Connor E, Chang JC, Edelstein SL. Coffee associated osteoporosis offset by daily milk consumption: The Rancho Bernardo Study. JAMA 1994;271:280–283.
59. Prince R, Monk K, Kent G. Effects of theophylline and salbutamol on phosphate and calcium metabolism in normal subjects. Miner Electrolyte Metab 1988;14:262–265.

60. Blum JW, Fischer JA, Hunziker WH. Parathyroid hormone responses to catecholamines and to changes of extracellular calcium in cows. J Clin Invest 1978;61:1113–1122.
61. Kukreja SC, Hargis GK, Bowser EN. Role of adrenergic stimuli in parathyroid hormone secretion in man. J Clin Endocrinol Metab 1975;40:478–481.
62. Metz SA, Deftos LJ, Baylink DG, Robertson RP. Neuroendocrine modulation of calcitonin and parathyroid hormone in man. J Clin Endocrinol Metab 1978;47:151–159.
63. Brown EM, Gardner DG, Windeck RA. B-Adrenergically stimulated adenosine 3′, 5′-monophosphate accumulation in and parathyroid hormone release from dispersed human parathyroid cells. J Clin Endocrinol Metab 1979;48:618–626.
64. Mulder H, Struys A. Intermittent cyclic etidronate in the prevention of corticosteroid induced bone loss. Br J Rheumatol 1994;33:348–350.
65. Rodbro P, Christiansen C, Lund M. Development of anticonvulsant osteomalacia in epileptic patients on phenytoin treatment. Acta Neurol Scand 1974;50:527–532.
66. Tolman KG, Jubiz W, Sannella J. Osteomalacia associated with anticonvulsant drug therapy in mentally retarded children. Pediatrics 1975;56:45–51.
67. Jubiz W, Meikle AW, Levinson RA. Effect of diphenylhydantoin on the metabolism of dexamethasone: mechanisms of the abnormal dexamethasone suppression in humans. N Engl J Med 1970;283:11–14.
68. Hahn T, Birge S, Scharp C. Phenobarbital induced alterations in vitamin D metabolism J Clin Invest 1972;51:741–748.
69. Koch HV, Kraft D, Von Herrath D. Influence of diphenylhydantoin and phenobarbital on intestinal calcium transport in the rat. Epilepsia 1972;13:829–841.
70. Hahn T, scharp C, Richardson C. Interaction of diphenylhydantoin (phenytoin) and phenobarbital with hormonal mediation of fetal rat bone resorption in vitro. J Clin Invest 1978;62:496–414.
71. Dietrich J, Duffield R. Effects of diphenylhydantoin on synthesis of collagen and noncollagen protein in tissue culture. Endocrinology 1980;106:606–610.
72. Krolner B, Jorgensen JV, Nielsen SP. Spinal bone mineral content in myxedema and thyrotoxicosis: effects of thyroid hormones and antithyroid treatments. Clin Endocrinol 1983;18:439–446.
73. Meunier P, Bianchi G, Edouard C. Bony manifestation of thyrotoxicosis. Orthop Clin North Am 1972;3:745–774.
74. Toft A. Thyroxine therapy. N Engl J Med 1994;331:174–181.
75. Mosekilde L, Eriksen EF, Charles P. Effects of thyroid hormones on bone and mineral metabolism. Endocrinol Metab Clin North Am 1990;19:35–63.
76. Mosekilde L, Melsen F, Bagger JP. Bone changes in hyperthyroidism: interrelationships between bone morphometry, thyroid function and calcium phosphorus metabolism. Acta Endocrinol 1977;85:515–525.
77. Eriksen EF, Mosekilde L, Melsen F. Trabecular bone remodeling and bone balance in hyperthyroidism. Bone 1985;6:421–428.
78. Burman KD, Monchik JM, Earll JM. Ionized and total serum calcium and parathyroid hormone in hyperthyroidism. Ann Intern Med 1976;84:668–671.
79. Manicourt D, Demeester-Mirkine N, Brauman H. Disturbed mineral metabolism in hyperthyroidism: good correlation with triiodothyronine. Clin Endocrinol 1979;101:407–412.
80. Stall G, Harris S, Sokoll L. Accelerated bone loss in hypothyroid patients overtreated with L-thyroxine. Ann Intern Med 1990;113:265–269.
81. Paul T, Kerrigan J, Kelly AM. Long-term L-thyroxine therapy is associated with decreased hip bone density in premenopausal women. JAMA 1988;259:3137–3141.
82. Ross D, Neer R, Ridgway EC. Subclinical hyperthyroidism and reduced bone density as a possible result of prolonged suppression of the pituitary thyroid axis with L-thyroxine. Am J Med 1987;82:1167–1170.
83. Adlin EM, Maurer AM, Marks AD. Bone mineral density in postmenopausal women treated with thyroxine. Am J Med 1991;90:360–366.
84. Baylink D, Stauffer M, Wergedal J, Rich C. Formation mineralization and resorption of bone in vitamin-D deficient rats. J Clin Invest 1970;49:1122–1134.
85. Barnes MJ, Constable BJ, Morton LF, Kodicek E. Bone collagen metabolism in vitamin-D deficiency. Biochem J 1973;132:113–115.
86. Frame B, Parfitt AM. Osteomalacia: current concepts. Ann Intern Med 1978;89:966–982.
87. Kanis JA. Pathophysiology and Treatment of Paget's Disease of Bone. Carolina Academic Press, London.

88. Dove J. Complete fractures of the femur in Paget's disease of bone. J Bone Joint Surg 1980;62B:12–17.
89. Boonekamp PM, van der Wee Pals LJA, van Wij-van Lennep MLL. Two modes of action of biophosphonates on osteoclastic resorption of mineralized matrix. Bone Miner 1986;1:27–39.
90. Siris E, Weinstein RS, Altman R, Conte JM, Favus M, Lombardi A, Lyles K, et al. Comparative study of alendronate versus etidronate for the treatment of Paget's disease of bone. J Clin Endocrinol Metab 1996;81:961–967.
91. Chesnut CH III. Review of calcitonin-present: current status of calcitonin as a therapeutic agent. Bone Miner 1992;16:211–212.
92. Devogelaer JP. Comparison of the acute biological action of injectable salmon calcitonin and an injectable and oral calcitonin analogue. Calcif Tissue Int 1994;55:71–73.
93. Luboshitzky R, Bar-Shalom R. Calcitonin nasal spray for Paget's disease of the bone. Harefuah 1995;128:358–362.
94. Wimalawansa SJ. Dramatic response to plicamycin in a patient with severe Paget's disease refractory to calcitonin and pamidronate. Semin Arthritis Rheum 1994;23:267.
95. Consensus Development Conference Panel. Diagnosis and management of asymptomatic primary hyperparathyroidism: consensus development conference statement. Ann Intern Med 1991;114:593–597.
96. Parfitt AM. Equilibrium and disequilibrium hypercalcemia: new light on an old concept. Metab Bone Dis Relat Res 1979;1:279–293.
97. Kaiser W, Biesenbach G, Kramar R. Calcium free hemodialysis: an effective therapy in hypercalcemic crisis—report of 4 cases. Intens Care Med 1989;15:471–474.
98. Binshock ML, Mundy GR. Effect of calcitonin and glucocorticoids in combination on the hypercalcemia of malignancy. Ann Intern Med 1980;93:269–272.
99. Ljunghall S, Rastad J, Akerstrom G. Comparative effects of calcitonin and clodronate in hypercalcemia. Bone 1987;8:S79–S83.
100. Mundy GR, Wilkinson R, Health DA. Comparative study of available medical therapy for hypercalcemia of malignancy. Am J Med 1983;74:421–432.
101. Warrell RP, Israel R, Frisone M. Gallium nitrate for acute treatment of cancer-related hypercalcemia: a randomized, double-blind comparison to calcitonin. Ann Intern Med 1988;108:669–674.
102. Mallette LE, Bilezikian JP, Heath DA. Primary hyperparathyroidism: Clinical and biochemical features. Medicine 1974;53:127–146.
103. NIH. NIH Consensus Development Conference Statement: Diagnosis and management of asymptomatic primary hyperparathyroidism. Ann Int Med 1991;114:593–597.
104. Stewart AF, Adler M, Byers CM, Segre GV, Broadus AE. Calcium homeostasis in immobilization: an example of resorptive hypercalciuria. N Engl J Med 1982;306:1136–1140.
105. Galasko CSB. Skeletal metastases. Clin Orthop 1990, (September):18–30.
106. Poste G. Pathogenesis of metastatic disease: Implications for current therapy and for the development of new therapeutic strategies. Cancer Treat Rev 1986;70:183–199.
107. Garrett RI, Durie BGM, Nedwin GE. Production of the bone resorbing cytokine lymphotoxin by cultured human myeloma cells. N Engl J Med 1987;317:526–532.
108. Cozzolino F, Torcia M, Aldinucci D. Production of interleukin-1 by bone marrow myeloma cells. Blood 1989;74:387–390.
109. Bataille R, Jourdan M, Zhang Xue-Guang. Serum levels of interleukin-6, a potent myeloma cell growth factor as a reflection of disease severity in plasma cell dyscrasias. J Clin Invest 1989;84:2008–2011.

14 Testicular Function in Critical Illness

Stephen R. Plymate, MD, *and Robert E. Jones,* MD

CONTENTS

> INTRODUCTION
> PHYSIOLOGY OF THE HPT AXIS
> EVALUATION OF THE SUSPECTED HYPOGONADAL PATIENT
>   WITH CRITICAL ILLNESS
> EFFECTS OF MEDICATIONS ON THE HPT AXIS
> ACKNOWLEDGMENT
> REFERENCES

INTRODUCTION

Like other regulated endocrine axes, the hypothalamo–pituitary–testicular (HPT) axis in men is subject to modification from external influences. Both acute and chronic illnesses as well as numerous medications can profoundly affect levels of circulating testosterone and can inhibit spermatogenesis *(1)*. In certain instances, such as hemochromatosis, the alteration in gonadal function is a well-recognized concomitant of the disease process, whereas in other circumstances, the apparent modification of gonadal function may simply represent a nonspecific effect of illness on the HPT axis *(2)*. It is generally accepted that virtually any illness, whether acute, self-limited, or chronic, may have an impact on testicular function. The purpose of this chapter is to explore, specifically, the effects of critical illness and medications on the HPT axis. As well as discussing the possible pathologic consequences owing to these modifications of testicular function *(3)*.

PHYSIOLOGY OF THE HPT AXIS

The production of testosterone by Leydig cells and the generation of spermatozoa by the seminiferous tubules are regulated by an elaborate mechanism of feedback between the testes and the hypothalamic–pituitary unit. Luteinizing hormone (LH) and follicle-stimulating hormone (FSH) are dimeric glycoproteins synthesized and secreted from the anterior pituitary under the influence of a hypothalamic decapeptide, gonadotropin-releasing hormone (GnRH). Although cells containing GnRH are found throughout the central nervous system and other tissues including the gonads, the principal sites of GnRH synthesis destined to regulate pituitary gonadotropin production are the paraventricular and supraoptic hypothalamic nuclei.

From *Contemporary Endocrinology: Endocrinology of Critical Disease*
Edited by K. P. Ober   Humana Press Inc., Totowa, NJ

GnRH is secreted in discrete pulses into the hypophyseal portal system. Both peptidergic and adrenergic neurons modify the secretion of GnRH. β-endorphin and γ-aminobutyric acid (GABA) inhibit GnRH secretion, whereas norepinephrine enhances GnRH secretion. The roles of dopamine and serotonin in modulating GnRH pulse generation are less well defined *(4)*.

The gonadotropins, FSH and LH, are secreted in direct response to the GnRH pulses. As a result, approx 8–14 gonadotropin secretory pulses can occur in normal males over a 24-h period. A variety of factors influence both the height and frequency of these secretory bursts. In addition, the frequency of GnRH bursts has a differential effect on LH and FSH secretion. More frequent GnRH pulses increase LH secretion, whereas slower pulses favor FSH secretion. Consistent with a classic feedback loop, both androgens and estrogens, through distinct mechanisms, appear to decrease LH pulse frequency in men. Similarly, opiates and glucocorticoids also reduce the frequency of pituitary LH secretory pulses *(5)*. FSH secretion is governed by a protein heterodimer, inhibin, secreted from the Sertoli cells and by sex steroids. The relative contributions of either inhibin or sex steroids on FSH production are controversial; however, both seem to work in conjunction as part of the native feedback mechanism *(3)*.

LH stimulates the production of testosterone by the Leydig cells, whereas FSH regulates Sertoli cell function and, consequently, spermatogenesis. Following synthesis, testosterone is rapidly bound to sex hormone binding globulin (SHBG) or to other binding proteins like albumin. The binding of testosterone to carrier proteins is essential because of the relative insolubility of testosterone in an aqueous environment. SHBG is a high-affinity, low-capacity binding protein produced in the liver and, to a lesser extent, in other androgen-sensitive tissues. Approximately 2% of testosterone circulates free in the serum, whereas 40% is bound to SHBG. The remaining portion of testosterone is associated with albumin or other circulating proteins. The nonprotein-bound testosterone is referred to as free testosterone, and the albumin-associated hormone is designated as weakly bound. Together they comprise a circulating pool of hormone called bioavailable testosterone. SHBG is the specific transport protein, and its production ultimately governs the amount of circulating testosterone. Hepatic SHBG synthesis is stimulated by thyroid hormone *(14)* and sex steroids, and is inhibited by insulin or insulin-like growth factor-1. Thus, total testosterone levels may be reduced in hyperinsulinemic states like obesity or noninsulin-dependent diabetes mellitus, or may be elevated in hyperthyroidism. Similarly, nutritional protein deficiency or protein-wasting syndromes may reduce the amount of SHBG and, therefore, circulating total testosterone *(6)*. In normal young men, there is a concordant pronounced diurnal variation of testosterone and SHBG. Highest levels are seen in the morning, whereas the nadir is observed in the early evening. In healthy aging men, the diurnal pattern is markedly dampened, and peak levels of testosterone are significantly lower *(7)*. Although testosterone is the major circulating androgen in men, it may also serve as a prohormone and be either converted through the action of 5-α reductase to a 5-α-reduced androgen, dihydrotestosterone, or aromatized via aromatase to an estrogen, estradiol. Both of these enzymatic steps are irreversible. 5-α-reductase activity is concentrated in skin, liver, and in the accessory sex organs, and the activity of this enzyme is regulated by the amount of available substrate (testosterone) or by thyroid hormone. Aromatase is found in the testes and in adipose tissue. Testicular aromatase activity appears to be regulated by FSH.

The biological effects of sex steroids are mediated through the interaction of the hormone with its high-affinity nuclear receptor. There is a single androgen receptor that has a higher affinity for dihydrotestosterone than testosterone. Similarly, the ability of the dihydrotestosterone–androgen receptor complex to bind to DNA is greater than the testosterone-occupied androgen receptor. In addition to its role in testosterone transport, SHBG may play an additional role (or roles) in modulating reproductive function. Cell-surface receptors for SHBG have been identified and, in the case of the prostate, may play an autocrine role in cell growth.

EVALUATION OF THE SUSPECTED HYPOGONADAL PATIENT WITH CRITICAL ILLNESS

Evaluation of the critically ill man for hypogonadism should be considered if there is reason to believe that treatment of the hypogonadism with testosterone replacement will alter the course of the disease. Especially if the patient has a pre-existing hypogonadal state, treatment with testosterone will provide the benefit of an anabolic agent that would be available to the normally eugonadal man to survive the illness. Pre-existing hypogonadism may be suspected if the patient's history and physical exam are suggestive of a decreased androgen state. The physical and history findings that are suggestive of hypogonadism that has occurred either before or after the onset of puberty are presented in Table 1.

Especially if findings of hypogonalism are present, then the physician may decide to proceed with a laboratory evaluation to confirm the hypogonadal state. The minimal evaluation of a male suspected as being hypogonadal should include a serum testosterone and a simultaneous LH determination. Because of the dramatic circadian variation in testosterone, levels should be obtained in the morning. The theoretical concern of spontaneous LH pulsatility and the concurrent risk of misclassifying a patient by sampling during an LH peak or nadir have little clinical relevance. Therefore, a single LH should yield adequate diagnostic information. Owing to the high probability of concurrent alterations in testosterone transport proteins from common intercurrent medical problems like malnutrition, liver disease, or insulin-resistant states, measurement of SHBG or bioavailable testosterone is frequently helpful. Measuring prolactin is critical in determining the coexistence of significant pituitary pathology if low testosterone levels are observed in conjunction with low or "inappropriately" normal levels of LH. In the setting of considerable physiologic stress or the stress of illness, this type of hypogonadism, hypogonadotropic hypogonadism, is the nearly universal form of hypotestosteronemia noted. When the illness is self-limited, testosterone levels will return to normal in 4–6 wk following recovery; therefore, in most cases, it is prudent to delay therapy or further evaluation until the patient has convalesced. In the case of a chronic or debilitating illness, at least two separate laboratory evaluations of gonadal function should be performed. If both assessments are concordant and document hypogonadism, a critical history and physical examination to complement the laboratory findings should be coupled with sound clinical reasoning to determine whether further testing should be performed or whether therapy with androgens might be beneficial given the clinical setting. However, the issue during the acute illness is not necessarily whether the hypogonadism is primary or secondary, but that it existed prior to the acute disease and should possibly be treated to provide the hypogonadal man with similar anabolic residual to withstand the acute insult to his eugonadal counterpart.

Table 1
Clinical Findings in Men Suggesting Hypogonadism that Occurred Either Before or After the Onset of Puberty

Testicular failure occurring prior to onset of puberty: Clinical characteristics
- Testes <2.5 cm long, volume <5 mL
- Penis <3–5 cm long
- Lack of scrotal pigmentation and rugae
- Peripheral subcutaneous fat distribution over hips, face, and chest
- Eunuchoidal skeletal proportions: crown to pubis/pubis to floor ratio <1
- Arm span >6-cm height (normally black men have a decreased crown to pubis/pubis to floor ratio and a longer arm span than whites)
- Female escutcheon
- No terminal facial hair, decreased body hair
- No temporal hair recession
- High-pitched voice
- Decreased muscle mass
- Delayed bone age
- Small prostate
- Crosshatching over skin lateral to the orbits
- Decreased libido
- Osteoporosis later in life

Postpubertal testicular failure: clinical characteristics
- Normal skeletal proportions and penile length
- Loss of libido
- Decrease in strength and muscle mass
- Normal distribution of pubic hair
- Testes are soft; volume <15 mL
- Prostate is usually adult size, and BPH or prostate cancer are unusual
- No change in voice
- History of diminished aggressiveness
- Decreased amount of axillary and pubic hair
- Osteoporosis later in life

EFFECTS OF MEDICATIONS ON THE HPT AXIS

In addition to the disease or injury, medications that are used in treatment may cause a decrease in testosterone. A variety of medications from virtually all classes of drugs may have diverse effects on the HPT axis. Drugs may influence this system by altering gonadotropin release, by a direct action on testosterone synthesis, changing testosterone transport by influencing SHBG production, by modifying the metabolic clearance rate of testosterone, by affecting mechanisms of feedback at the hypothalamus or pituitary, or by interacting with the androgen receptor. In Table 2 are a few of the drugs from several classes that could either inhibit testosterone at the receptor level, inhibit testosterone synthesis, or suppress gonadotropin release.

Table 2 is not an extensive list of drugs that may affect testosterone metabolism, since that sort of list would encompass more than the space allotted for this entire chapter. However, it will provide an indication that when a low serum testosterone level is measured during an acute illness, the medications given to the patient need to be assessed regarding possible contributors to the process.

Table 2
Drugs That May Alter or Depress the HPT Axis

Drugs that affect the HPT unit

Drugs that inhibit steroid synthesis
- Spironolactone
- Ketoconazole *(8)*
- Aminoglutethimide
- Antineoplastic drugs *(9)*
  - Cyclophosphamide
  - Melphalan
  - Chlorambucil
  - Busulfan
  - Procarbazine
- Ethanol

Drugs that inhibit release on LH or FSH
- calcium channel blockers
- Reserpine
- Amiodarone
- ACE inhibitors
- Tricyclic antidepressants
- Dopamine (↑ and ↓ depending on concentration)
- Neuroleptics
- Major tranquilizers
- Morphine and other narcotics
- Ethanol
- Isoniazide
- Penicillamine
- Corticosteroids

Drugs that block the androgen receptor
- Spironolactone
- Cimetidine
- Digoxin

Drugs that may either increase the metabolism of testosterone or alter the levels of SHBG
- Diphenylhydantoin (phenytoin)-↑ SHBG and ↑ metabolism
- Phenobarbital-↑ SHBG and ↑ metabolism
- Insulin-↓ SHBG
- Thyroid hormone-↑ SHBG

Systemic Diseases Associated with Hypogonadism

This chapter is intended to be directed toward gonadal function in acute critical illness; however, a few more acute and chronic systemic disease states that are associated with hypogonadism will be presented to give a broader sense of the effects of illness on gonadal function. As has been mentioned, any disease state or physical stress that can become severe enough to lead to an acute hospital or ICU admission may result in hypogonadism *(10)*. In fact, the incidence of hypogonadism in a hospitalized population is greater than the so-called euthyroid sick syndrome *(11,12)*.

Pulmonary

Pulmonary diseases, especially chronic obstructive pulmonary disease (COPD), are commonly associated with low serum testosterone levels *(13)*. Although the disease itself causes a decrease in testosterone secretion, there is an even greater degree of secondary hypogonadism that occurs when these men are treated with corticosteroids, which cause further hypothalamic–pituitary–gonadal suppression *(14)*. Additionally, low testosterone levels in men with COPD present a treatment dilemma. These patients often become weak and cachectic, which further impairs their respiratory functioning. On the other hand, as will be discussed later, testosterone impairs the respiratory drive to hypoxia *(15–17)*. Unfortunately, no controlled studies with testosterone have been done on patients with COPD to determine if this potentially beneficial therapy would be either effective or safe.

Renal Disease

Acute renal failure is associated with a decrease in gonadotropin secretion and sunsequent decrease in serum testosterone levels. Several etiologies for the defect in the HPT axis have been identified in renal disease *(18,19)*. One possibility is an increase in prolactin, which affects LH secretion. A second that is seen in the absence of hyperprolactinemia is a change in the LH pulsatility, which suggests an alteration in the hypothalamic pulse generator.

Chronic renal disease is associated with similar defects to those seen with acute renal disease. Interestingly, the defects are not corrected with dialysis, but do correct following renal transplantation if corticosteroid administration is not needed.

Leprosy

The *Mycobacterium leprae* organism has been demonstrated to invade the testes in 75% of cases of leprosy, resulting in hypogonadism *(20)*. Leprosy differs from other forms of testicular infection causing hypogonadism, because leprosy has been shown to affect selectively either the seminiferous tubules or the Leydig cells; by contrast, most other infections are targeted to the seminiferous tubule compartment alone. As a result, these men may appear with monotropic increases in either LH or FSH. Because adequate intratesticular levels of testosterone are necessary for normal spermatogenesis, sperm production will be decreased in all cases. Lepromatous and borderline leprosy are associated with the greatest degree of testicular involvement, whereas tuberculoid disease has lesser involvement.

Testicular Trauma

Obviously the traumatic loss of both testes results in hypogonadism, which necessitates testosterone replacement. In addition, a common reason for loss of a single testis is testicular torsion. It should also be noted that the torsion of a testis may have an effect (possibly immune) on the opposite testis, resulting in infertility.

Malignancy

In addition to the issues that arise with either chemotherapy or irradiation and testicular function, malignancies themselves have a significant effect on gonadal function *(21)*. Men with lung cancer have serum testosterone levels that are significantly lower than their age-matched controls, even at early stages of the tumor when there are no apparent systemic effects from the tumor *(22)*. This may be the result of tumor cytokines, such as tumor necrosis factor-alpha (TNF-α). A similar situation has been shown to exist in men with Hodgkin's disease, when sperm counts and testosterone are decreased before chemotherapy or irradiation has been used *(9,21)*.

Cranial Trauma

Head injury with transection of the pituitary stalk will often result in secondary gonadal failure. This outcome may be suspected clinically following head injury. When the patient has had an episode of either diabetes insipidus or SIADH, even transiently, it suggests that the pituitary stalk has suffered significant disruption *(12)*.

Cranial Irradiation

In addition to testicular irradiation, radiation to the head for brain tumors often results in significant radiation to the hypothalamic–pituitary area. In a recent study, 61% of patients who were postpubertal demonstrated secondary hypogonadism *(23)*.

Hepatic Cirrhosis

Both cirrhosis and ethanol intoxication affect testicular function *(24)*. One pathway for ethanol's acute affect on testicular function stems from its higher affinity for alcohol dehydrogenase than retinol, which prevents formation of retinoic acid. This may occur at a serum ethanol level >0.10 mg/dL causing testosterone production to decrease and serum LH to increase. These findings revert to normal soon after serum ethanol levels return to normal.

Cirrhosis of the liver secondary to the long-term ingestion of ethanol increases both serum estradiol and SHBG. The increased estradiol levels result in decreased gonadotropin levels and lower serum testosterone. In addition, the elevated SHBG levels further decrease the levels of free testosterone.

Neurological and Muscular Diseases

The classic neurologic disease that is associated with hypogonadism is temporal lobe epilepsy. Although the epilepsy may be controlled with appropriate anticonvulsant therapy, correction of the hypogonadism requires testosterone replacement. As was noted in the list of drugs that affect androgen metabolism, two common drugs used to treat epilepsy, diphenylhydantoin and phenobarbital, can affect testosterone metabolism, although it is unusual for them to cause hypogonadism without other suppression of the HPT axis.

Among the neuromuscular diseases, myotonic dystrophy, a sex-linked form of muscular dystrophy, results in decreased Leydig cell function in men, with the disorder beginning in the third and fourth decades of life. Recently, Griggs et al. have demonstrated the need for carefully controlled studies when testosterone replacement is considered *(25)*. In studies of myotonic dystrophy, Griggs et al demonstrated that testosterone replacement significantly increased muscle mass but had no effect on muscle strength, regardless of mass. These studies point out the pitfalls of anabolic replacement during illness, and that catabolism may not be reversed unless the underlying disease process is reversed.

Gastrointestinal Disease

When associated with malnutrition, decreased serum testosterone levels have been found in gastrointestinal diseases, such as celiac sprue *(26–28)*. Otherwise, unless associated with a complication causing an acute systemic crisis, gastrointestinal disease is not commonly associated with decreased serum testosterone levels. However, drugs used to treat gastrointestinal disease have been clearly demonstrated to result consistently in hypogonadism (e.g. cimetidine, azulfidine, and glucocorticoids) *(29–32)*.

Sickle Cell Disease

Men with sickle cell disease often appear to have characteristics of prepubertal hypogonadism *(33)*. They display eunuchoidal skeletal proportions, have decreased muscle mass, and small testes. However, if they are black men, their skeletal proportions may be normal for their race. Some men with this disease do have low serum testosterone levels and inappropriately normal serum gonadotropin levels, suggesting a secondary form of hypogonadism; however, since they also display an abnormal response to hCG, some form of primary testicular dysfunction also occurs.

Hemochromatosis

In this disease, manifest by iron overload, there may be both secondary and primary elements of gonadal failure which is owing to specific organ iron overload, and which may be corrected by iron removal *(2)*.

Human Immunodeficiency Virus-1 (HIV-1)

As in other acute and chronic diseases, hypogonadism has been seen in HIV disease *(34,35)*. However, in HIV without AIDS, hypogonadism is not a universal finding, and increased testosterone levels have been reported by some, but not all investigators. The levels of both total and free testosterone in men with HIV disease have been inversely correlated with markers of the severity of disease *(36)*. CD4 count, fever, and weight loss have been demonstrated to correlate with the decrease in testosterone levels in HIV disease *(8,37)*. These correlations suggest that the decreased serum testosterone in HIV is not unique to the disease, but as with any other illness, is related to the severity of the disease.

A block in 17-ketosteroid reductase has been demonstrated in men with HIV and low serum testosterone levels. As will be discussed later, this block in testosterone biosynthesis may also be associated with increased production of cortisol as a survival pathway.

Recently, several testosterone treatment studies have been reported in men who are HIV-positive with low serum testosterone levels. These studies have shown that replacement improves libido and mood, but no increase in body weight, lean body mass, CD4 counts or other clinical manifestations of the disease were seen to improve significantly *(38)*. Unfortunately, no placebo treatment arm was included in these studies. Therefore, at the present time, there is no unequivocal evidence to indicate that correcting the low serum testosterone levels in men with HIV will result in a significant degree of clinical improvement.

Etiology of Decreased Testosterone Levels in Acute Illness

The etiology of the decrease in testosterone during acute illness remains obscure. There are multiple factors that have been identified in acute illness that could lead to a decrease in serum testosterone level *(39)*. Multiple studies have suggested that the primary defect begins with suppression of the hypothalamic–pituitary unit with a secondary diminution in testosterone secretion. However, a recent study by Spratt et al. *(40)* disputes this notion. In the study, men without prior gonadal disease who were admitted to an ICU were sequentially followed. In the first few days following admission, testosterone levels declined, and both LH and FSH levels increased, suggesting primary gonadal failure. However, 3–4 d following admission, gonadotropins began to fall below the normal range, whereas the serum testosterone levels remained low. During the next 10–14 d during the course of recovery or progression to death, the gonadotropin levels returned to the normal range, but testosterone levels remained suppressed. This latter phenomenon has also been observed to occur in severely burned men *(41)* at approximately the same time-point following thermal injury. Thus, during the course of acute illness, both hypergonadotropic hypogonadism and hypogonadotropic hypogonadism may occur in the same individual.

Studies have evaluated the steroid secretory patterns in acutely ill men. The biosynthesis of steroids appears to shift away from the production of androgens and mineralocorticoid, and favor the synthesis of glucocorticoids *(5)*. This phenomenon has been observed clinically in studies that have shown that the severity of illness correlates with an increase in glucocorticoid secretion and a decrease in serum testosterone. Although the precise mechanism underlying these alterations in steroid biosynthesis has not been fully determined, recent studies have shown that cytokines can regulate steroidogenic enzymes. For instance, TNF-α can downregulate the messenger RNA for cytochromes P450 2CII and 3A2 in the male rat liver, and TNF-α, interleukin-2 (IL-2), and interferon-γ (INF-γ) inhibit several steroidogenic enzymes involved in testosterone production, including 17-ketosteroid *(42)*. Hales has further demonstrated in a mouse Leydig call preparation that IL-1 inhibits testosterone production primarily by inhibiting 17-α a hydroxylase/C17–20 lyase cytochrome P450 expression *(43)*. In contrast, Warren et al. *(44)* noted that both IL-1 and TNF-α stimulated testosterone secretion in Leydig cell preparations. In clinical studies in men admitted to an ICU, IL-6 has been found to be inversely correlated with serum testosterone. Furthermore, IL-6 was elevated above normal, and testosterone was decreased in men admitted with cranial trauma. This relationship was more pronounced following brain death *(45)*. In men receiving IL-2 infusions for the treatment of renal cell carcinoma or melanoma cortisol levels rose and testosterone levels fell, whereas both LH and FSH levels were not significantly altered *(46)*. These studies clearly demonstrate a correlation between changes in levels of various cytokines and serum testosterone levels in acutely ill men. However, the effects of the individual cytokines on isolated Lydig cell preparations are not obvious, which has led some investigators to the conclusion that the effects of compounds, such as IL-2, may be indirect, acting through additional cytokine mediators. As an example, macrophage-conditioned media (MCM) has been shown to decrease testosterone production by Leydig cells; however, none of the individual components of the media, including TNF-α, IL-α, IL-β, IL-2, IL-6, INF-α, or INF-β, had a similar effect *(47,48)*. Whether any or all of the cytokines described above are the cause of the primary defect in acute illness remains to be determined, but it is evident that there is an abundance of candidate effectors in acutely ill men that may cause a direct decrease in testosterone secretion.

Data from our laboratory as well as others have shown that secondary hypogonadism (i.e., a decrease in gonadotrophin or GnRH secretion) also occurs in acutely ill men *(41)*. Again, multiple candidates for these changes have been identified. The principal candidate is the increase in cortisol, which suppresses both gonadotropin and GnRH secretion. Corticotropin-releasing hormone (CRH) as well as proopiomelanocortin (POMC) products have been shown to inhibit both GnRH and gonadotropin secretion. The increase in serum estrogen levels that occurs in acutely ill men may also result in a diminution in serum testosterone levels owing to the suppressive effect of estrogen on the hypothalamic–pituitary axis. In addition, the cytokines IL-1 and IL-2, TNF-α, and IL-6 also may suppress LH and FSH secretion. It is likely that a combination of these factors could result in the defect in the HPT axis in acutely ill men. Further investigation into the time-course and the activities of these factors, as well as their relative contributions to hypogonadism, are areas for future investigation.

Age may be another contributing cause to the hypogonadism of severe illness in men. Because age is associated with a decline in serum testosterone and because the possibility that an acute illness increases with age, it is likely that the effects of both age and illness are additive in affecting the diminution in serum testosterone levels *(49)*. It has been shown that at any given age, serum testosterone was decreased at least 10% with the association of illness *(49)*.

Treatment

Other than the previously cited study on the effects of supplemental testosterone in HIV disease, there has been no investigation that has evaluated the use of testosterone in acutely ill men. This is even more surprising given that other more recently developed anabolic agents, such as insulin-like growth factor, have been evaluated in this clinical setting. The two questions that need to be answered in order to determine if supplemental testosterone could be efficacious in acutely ill men are: (1) would the anabolic effects of androgen replacement improve the catabolic state of these individuals, and (2) would androgen replacement be deleterious to these men? It is clear that treatment of hypogonadal men with testosterone causes a significant increase in lean body mass and a decrease in fat mass. This anabolic action also occurs in older men with myotonic dystrophy *(25)*. Therefore, if the catabolic state of the acute illness is complicating recovery, and if treatment of the associated hypogonadism reverses this phenomenon, further studies of the use of testosterone in acutely ill men may be justified *(39)*. In certain types of acute illness, men may not require replacement. For instance, a period of decreased serum testosterone levels may occur following myocardial infarction or elective surgery, but chances of recovery from the insult are high, and consequently there would appear to be little need for therapeutic intervention with testosterone *(12,50,51)*.

On the other hand, appropriate measures need to be in place to ensure that replacement causes no harm to men. An example of a problem that has been well described with testosterone treatment is an aggravation of sleep apnea *(16,17)*. Although clinically significant sleep apnea is uncommon when testosterone is administered to normal men, severe hypoxia can occur as testosterone is given to men with either a predisposition or the full syndrome of sleep apnea. Studies have shown that respiratory drive to hypoxia is measurably diminished *(15,17)*. Thus, in this group of men, testosterone replacement could have significant deleterious effects. In some situations with a high mortality, such as burns, a major component of recovery relates to the degree of cachexia and catabolism. Perhaps by reversing the cachexia and catabolic state with testosterone replacement, survival could be improved *(39,41)*. However, diseases associated with severe cachexia and catabolism may not respond to the anabolic actions of testosterone, because the cachexia may be a direct consequence of the increased circulating cytokines.

In summary, acute illness in men is frequency accompanied by low serum testosterone levels. The cause of the hypotestosteronemia is multifactorial and is related to the number of cytokines that are increased in response to illness. Patient survival is inversely correlated with the decrease in testosterone. It is unknown whether or not testosterone replacement in acutely ill men will enhance or complicate the recovery from illness. Because of this uncertainty, testosterone replacement is not recommended in acutely ill men unless a previously documented hypogonadal state is present or until a controlled study documents efficacy.

ACKNOWLEDGMENT

This work was supported by a Veteran Affairs Merit Review Grant to S. R. P.

REFERENCES

1. Dong Q, Hawker F, McWilliam D, Bangah M, Burger H, Handelsman DJ. Circulating immunoreactive inhibin and testosterone levels in men with critical illness. Clin Endocrinol 1992;36:399–404.
2. Cundy T, Butler J, Bomford A, Williams R. Reversibility of hypogonadotropic hypogonadism associated with genetic hemochromatosis. Clin Endocrinol 1993;38:617–620.
3. Plymate S, Paulsen C, McLachlan R. Relationship of serum inhibin levels to FSH and sperm production in normal men and men with a varicocele. J Clin Endocrinol Metab 1992;74:859–864.
4. Van den Berghe G, de Zegher F, Lauwers P, Veldhuis J. Luteinizing hormone secretion and hypoandrogenaemia in critically ill men: effect of dopamine. Clin Endocrinol 1994;41:563–569.
5. Reincke M, Lehmann R, Karl M, Magiaou A, Chrousos GP, Allolio B. Severe illness:neuroendocrinology. Ann NY Acad Sci 1995;771:556–569.
6. Goussis O, Pardridge W, Judd H. Critical illness and low testosterone: effects of human serum on testosterone transport into rat brain and liver. J Clin Endocrinol Metab 1983;56:710–714.
7. Plymate S, Tenover J, Bremner W. Circadian variation in testosterone, sex hormone binding globulin, and calculated non-sex hormone binding globulin bound testosterone in healthy young and elderly men. J Androl 1989;10:366–371.
8. Raffi F, Brisseau J, Planchon B, R'emi J, Barrier J, Grolleau J. Endocrine function in 98 HIV-infected patients: a prospective study. AIDS 1991;5:729–733.
9. daCunha M, Meistrich M, Fuller L, al. e. Recovery of spermatogenesis after treatment for Hodgkin's disease: limiting dose of MOPP chemotherapy. J Clin Oncol 1984;2:571–577.
10. Semple C, Gray C, Beastall G. Male hypogonadism—a non-specific consequence of illness. Q J Med 1987;64:601–607.
11. Jarek MJ, Legare EJ, McDermott MT. Endocrine profiles for outcome prediction from the intensive care unit. Crit Care Med 1996;21:543–550.
12. Woolf P, Hamill R, McDonald J, Lee L, Kelly M. Transient hypogonadotropic hypogonadism caused by critical illness. J Clin Endocrinol Metab 1985;60:444–450.
13. Blackman M, Weintraub B, Rosen S, Harman S. Comparison of the effects of lung cancer, benign lung disease, and normal aging on pituitary-gonadal function in men. J Clin Endocrinol Metab 1988;66:88–95.
14. MacAdams M, White R, Chipps B. Reduction in serum testosterone levels during chronic glucocorticoid therapy. Ann Int Med 1986;104:648–651.
15. Schneider B, Pickett C, Zwillich C, Weil J, McDermott M, Santen R, Varano L, White, D. Influence of testosterone on breathing during sleep. J Appl Physiol 1986;61:618–623.
16. Sandblom R, Matsumoto A, Schoene R, Lee K, Giblin E, Bremner W, Pierson D. Obstructive sleep apnea induced by testosterone administration. N Engl J Med 1983;308:508–510.
17. Matsumoto A, Sandblom R, Schoene R, Lee K, Giblin E, Pierson D, Bremner W. Testosterone replacement in hypogonadal men:effects on obstructive sleep apnea, respiratory drives, and sleep. Clin Endocrinol 1985;22:713–721.

18. Handelsman D. Hypothalamic-pituitary-gonadal dysfunction in chronic renal failure, dialysis, and renal transplantation. Endoc Rev 1985;6:151–182.
19. Levitan D, Moser S, Goldstein D, Kletzky O, Lobo R, Massry S. Disturbances in the hypothalamic-pituitary-gonadal axis in male patients with acute renal failure. Am J Nephrol 1984;4:99–106.
20. Shilo S, Livshin Y, Sheshkin J, Spitz I. Gonadal function in Lepromatous Leprosy. Lepr Rev 1981;52:127–136.
21. Chlebowski R, Heber D. Hypogonadism in male patients with metastatic cancer prior to chemotherapy. Cancer Res 1981;42:2495–2498.
22. Aasebo U, Bremnes R, deJong F, Aakvag A, Slordal L. Pituitary-gonadal dysfunction in male patients with lung cancer. Association with serum inhibin levels. Acta Oncol 1994;33:177–180.
23. Constine L, Woolf P, Cann D, et al. Hypothalamic–pituitary function after irradiation for brain tumors. N Eng J Med 1983;328:87–92.
24. Baker H, Burger H, deKretser D, et al. A study of the endocrine manifestations of hepatic cirrhosis. Q J Med 1976;45:145–178.
25. Griggs R, Pandya S, Florence J, et al. Randomized controlled trial of testosterone in men with myotonic dystrophy. Neurology 1989;39:219–222.
26. Farthing M, Edwards C, Rees L, Dawson A. Male gonadal dysfunction in coeliac disease: 1. Sexual dysfunction, infertility, and semen quality. Gut 1982;23:608–618.
27. Farthing M, Edwards C, Rees L, Dawson A. Male gonadal dysfunction in coeliac disease: 3. Pituitary regulation. Clin Endocrinol 1983;19:661–671.
28. Green J, Goble H, Edwards C, Dawson A. Reversible insensitivity to androgens in men with untreated gluren enteropathy. Lancet 1977;1:280–282.
29. Birnie C, McCleod T, Watkinson G. Incidence of sulfasalazine-induced male infertility. Gut 1981;22:452–455.
30. Consentino M, Chey W, Takihara H, Cockett A. The effects of sulphasalazine on human male fertility and seminal prostaglandins. J Urol 1984;57:682–686.
31. Knigge U, Dejgaard A, Wollesen F, et al. The acute and long term effect of the H2-receptor antagonists cimetidine and ranitidine on the pituitary–gonadal axis in men. Clin Endocrinol 1983;118:307–318.
32. van Thiel D, Gavaler J, Smith W, Paul G. Hypothalamic–pituitary–gonadal dysfunction in men using cimetidine. N Eng J Med 1979;300:1012–1015.
33. el-Hazami M, Bahakim H, al-Fawaz I. Endocrine functions in sickle-cell anemia patients. J Trop Pediatr 1991;38:307–313.
34. Croxon T, Chapman W, Miller L, et al. Changes in the hypothalamic-pituitary-gonadal axis in human immunodeficiency virus-infected homosexual men. J Clin Endocrinol Metab 1989;68:317–321.
35. de Paepe M, Waxman M. Testicular atrophy in AIDS:a study of 57 autopsy cases. Hum Pathol 1989;20:210–214.
36. Poretsky L, Can S, Zumoff B. Testicular dysfunction in human immunodeficiency virus-infected men. Metabolism 1995;44:946–953.
37. Wagner G, Rabkin J, Rabkin R. Illness stage, concurrent medications, and other correlates of low testosterone in men with HIV illness. J Acquired Immune Defic Syndrome Hum Retrovirol 1995;8:204–207.
38. Rabkin JG, Rabkin R, Wagner G. Testosterone replacement therapy in HIV illness. Gen Hosp Psychiatry 1995;17:37–42.
39. Luppa P, Munker R, Nagel D, Weber M, Engelhardt D. Serum androgens in intensive-care patients: correlations with clinical findings. Clin Endocrinol 1991;34:305–310.
40. Spratt DI, Bigos ST, Beitins I, Cox P, Longcope C, Orav J. Both hyper- and hypogonadotroic occur transiently in acute illness: bio- and immunoactive gonado tropins. J Clin Endocrinol Metab 1992.
41. Plymate S, Vaughn G, Mason A, Pruitt B. Central hypogonadism in burned men. Horm Res 1987;27:152–158.
42. Nadin L, Butler A, Farrell G, Murray M. Pretranslational downregulation of cytochromes P 450 2c11 and 3A2 in male rat livers by tumor necrosis factor alpha.Gastroenterology 1995;198–205.
43. Hales D. Interleukin-1 inhibits Leydig cell steroidogenesis primarily by decreasing 17 alph-hydroxylase/C17-20 lyase cytochrome P450 expression. Endocrinology 1992;131:2165–2172.
44. Warren D, Pasupuleti V, Lu Y, Platler B, Horton R. Tumor necrosis factor and interleukin-1 stimulate testosterone secretion in adulte male rat Leydig cells in vitro. J Andol 1990;11:353–360.

45. Amado J, L'opez-Espadas F, Vazquez-Barquero A, Salas J, Lopez-Cordovilla J, Garcia-Unzueta M. Blood levels of cytokines in brain-dead patients: relationship with circulating hormones and acute-phase reactants. Metabolism 1995;44:812–816.
46. Meikle A, Cardoso de Sousa J, Dacosta N, Bishop D, Samlowski W. Direct and indirect effects of murine interleukin-2, gamma interferon, and tumor necrosis factor on testosterone synthesis on mose Leydig cells. J Androl 1992;13:437–443.
47. Barak V, Mordel N, Holzer H, Zajicek G, Treves A, Laufer N. The correlation of interleukin-1 and tumor necrosis factor to oestradiol, progesterone, and testosterone levels in periovulatory follicular fluid of in-vitro fertilization. Hum Reprod 1992;7:462–464.
48. Watson M, Newman R, Payne A, Abdelrahim M, Francis G. The effect of macrophage conditioned media on Leydig cell function. Ann Clin Lab Sci 1994;24:84–95.
49. Gray A, Feldman HA, McKinley JB, Longcope C. Age, disease, and changing sex hormone levels in middle-aged men: Results of the Massachusetts male aging study. J Clin Endocrinol Metab 1991;73:1016–1025.
50. Wang C, Chan V, Yeung R. Effect of surgical stress on pituitary-testicular function. Clin Endocrinol 1978;9:255–266.
51. Wang C, Chan V, Yeung R. Effect of acute myocardial infarction on pituitary-testicular function. Clin Endocrinol 1978;9:249–253.

15 The Female Gonadal Response to Critical Disease

Mark D. Nixon, MD, PhD, and Robert W. Rebar, MD

CONTENTS

INTRODUCTION
CHRONIC LIVER DISEASE
CHRONIC RENAL DISEASE
ACQUIRED IMMUNE DEFICIENCY SYNDROME (AIDS)
MALIGNANCIES
RADIATION AND CHEMOTHERAPY
MISCELLANEOUS DISORDERS
SUMMARY
REFERENCES

INTRODUCTION

Although reproductive changes that occur in women in response to critical disease are poorly detailed in the medical literature, it is possible to consider the spectrum of responses that may result. That these changes do in fact occur is based on anecdotal reports and the experience of clinicians.

In general, reproductive function in women remains normal only as long as the individual is healthy, but individual variation is marked. Thus, some women who are critically ill may continue to ovulate and menstruate normally. It is important to recognize that pregnancies can and do occur in women who are critically ill.

Most women will become anovulatory in the face of critical disease. In most cases, central mechanisms will result in anovulation, with the women developing so-called hypothalamic amenorrhea. In this disorder, pulsatile secretion of gonadotropin-releasing hormone (GnRH) from neurons within the hypothalamus is reduced, presumably as a result of inhibition by neurotransmitters. In some serious diseases, anovulation may result from disrupted steroid feedback, producing a clinical picture more similar to that found in polycystic ovarian syndrome (PCO). Such individuals may present with oligomenorrhea or amenorrhea, but may also present with profound bleeding owing to endometrial thickening from unopposed estrogen. This PCO-like picture may be seen in hepatic or renal dysfunction in which there is altered gonadotropin and steroid metabolism, and in disorders, such as Cushing's syndrome, in which adrenal steroids are secreted in excess.

A few studies have attempted to document the alterations in the reproductive axis that occur in response to critical illness. In patients suffering from various acute insults (head injury, stroke, myocardial infarction, and surgery), there is a rapid (within 24 h) fall in gonadotropins and in sex steroids regardless of the type of insult *(1)*. In fact, Gebhart and colleagues *(2)* noted that luteinizing hormone (LH) and follicle-stimulating hormone (FSH) were appropriately elevated in only 31% of critically ill postmenopausal women and were in the hypogonadotropic range (<5 mIU/mL) in 25% *(2)*. In addition, these women had blunted responses to GnRH stimulation. It has also been noted that estradiol levels decrease acutely in response to the stress of insulin-induced hypoglycemia in normal menstruating women *(3)*. It appears that the amount of suppression of these reproductive hormones correlates roughly with the severity of the critical illness *(4)*. Together these findings provide evidence for hypothalamic–pituitary dysfunction in critical disease.

This chapter represents an effort to consider some of the more common serious illnesses present in young women and their effect on gonadal function. In addition, the effects of each illness on any resulting pregnancy will be considered as well.

CHRONIC LIVER DISEASE

Chronic liver disease apparently may result in either amenorrhea or menorrhagia *(5,6)*. At this point, it is not clear if the bleeding pattern that results is related to the severity of the disease or to the specific liver pathology involved. It appears that end-stage liver disease is most frequently associated with amenorrhea, perhaps because of the general debilitated state of the individual patient, and may well be owing to hypothalamic–pituitary dysfunction *(6)*. At least early in the course of primary biliary cirrhosis, however, menorrhagia is the predominant initial menstrual abnormality *(5)*. The menorrhagia does not appear to be owing to any specific coagulation defects, but rather to prolonged unopposed estrogen action in anovulatory women. In one series of women undergoing hysterectomy for the menorrhagia, 5 of 21 (24%) had endometrial hyperplasia. Moreover, 24 of 87 women with primary biliary cirrhosis presented with menorrhagia, compared to 3 of 45 patients with chronic active hepatitis and 2 of 35 patients with alcoholic liver disease *(5)*. Retrospective analysis of individuals with severe liver disease undergoing orthotopic liver transplant suggests that amenorrhea occurs in 30–60% of women in the year prior to transplantation *(6)*. Pregnancy only rarely occurs in chronic, untreated, progressive liver disease *(7)*.

Menstrual disorders and infertility improve with adequate treatment of chronic liver disease. Following liver transplantation, regular menses may resume in over 90% of previously amenorrheic women *(6)*. On the other hand, in another survey, there was no evidence of any dramatic increase in percentage of women having regular menses following transplantation, and liver function did not correlate with menstrual pattern *(8)*. Given the crude survey nature of these studies, such discrepancies may be expected. Together the data suggest that liver transplantation has the potential for improving reproductive function in women with chronic liver disease.

Because conception has occurred prior to the resumption of menstruation in previously amenorrheic women *(9)*, contraception should be provided to sexually active women. Although there is no evidence that engrafted livers have any increased risk of estrogen-induced cholestasis, the possibility of estrogens causing abnormal liver enzymes has led to a recommendation that combination oral contraceptive pills not be used for 6 mo following transplantation *(10)*.

There is no evidence that immunosuppressed patients posttransplant are more likely to contract sexually transmitted diseases, but the consequences of herpes viral infections may be greater in patients receiving antirejection medications. Unlike for patients with chronic liver disease secondary to hepatitis B, women undergoing transplantation who are infected with hepatitis C rarely transmit the virus either to their sexual partner *(11)* or their offspring *(12)*.

Pregnancy following liver transplantation is often successful *(10,13–15)*. However, higher rates of premature rupture of membranes, preterm labor and delivery, preeclampsia, and cesarean section have been reported among transplant patients *(10,14)*. Graft rejection does not appear to be increased by pregnancy, and most pregnancies are managed without changing the immunosuppressive medications. No data suggest any increased risk of teratogenicity with use of the well-established immunosuppressive drugs, but data are scanty when newer agents, such as FK 506, are used *(9)*.

Immunosuppressed women in general are recognized as being at increased risk of developing cytological abnormalities of the cervix, perhaps because of the frequency of human papillomavirus (HPV) infection in the general population. In any case, in one series, only 60% of women acknowledged having a Pap smear after liver transplantation, and over 7% were found to have cervical abnormalities *(8)*. These findings emphasize the importance of regular gynecological examinations in such individuals.

CHRONIC RENAL DISEASE

Women with chronic renal failure often have abnormalities of the hypothalamic–pituitary–ovarian axis and chronic anovulation *(16)*. The anovulation is manifested by menstrual disturbances ranging from amenorrhea to menorrhagia *(17)*, but the majority of patients are amenorrheic. Although some women may resume cyclic menses after beginning dialysis *(17,18)*, approx 35–60% of women remain amenorrheic *(19)*. Abnormal bleeding is also common in patients undergoing dialysis from unopposed estrogenic stimulation of the endometrium.

The endocrine abnormalities found in patients with chronic renal failure undergoing dialysis have been studied in some detail. Hyperprolactinemia is present in 50–90% of such individuals *(19,20)*. Basal concentrations of LH but not FSH are elevated as well *(20,21)*. Pulsatile gonadotropin secretion is often absent *(22)*, and administration of exogenous GnRH results in prolonged and exaggerated gonadotropin secretion *(21–23)*, probably because of decreased metabolic clearance of GnRH *(23)* and perhaps of gonadotropins as well. Serum levels of estradiol are generally low or similar to levels found in normal women in the early follicular phase of the menstrual cycle *(19,22)*. It has been reported that patients with hyperprolactinemia have the lowest estradiol levels and commonly present with amenorrhea *(19)*. The ramifications of estrogen deficiency, including development of osteoporosis and atherogenic lipid changes, have not been investigated in patients with chronic renal failure.

In patients with chronic renal failure who suffer from anovulatory uterine bleeding, the disorder is poorly tolerated. The blood loss contributes to the chronic anemia present in these patients; in addition, such women may have uremia-associated qualitative platelet abnormalities with prolonged bleeding times. Anovulatory bleeding in normal women is frequently treated with combination oral contraceptives, but there is little information about their use in women in chronic renal failure. In one study of the pharmacokinetics of low-dose oral contraceptives in women with chronic renal failure undergoing peritoneal dialysis *(24)*, there was decreased apparent clearance of oral ethinyl estradiol, leading to slightly higher serum concentrations compared with women with normal renal function. The clearance of norethindrone was the same in the patients undergoing peritoneal dialysis and in normal women. These findings led to the conclusion that low-dose combination oral contraceptive preparations may be used in women with chronic renal failure undergoing peritoneal dialysis to manage anovulatory bleeding or to prevent hypoestrogenism. Although additional studies are clearly needed, lowering the dose of ethinyl estradiol may prove beneficial in approximating serum levels found in normal subjects.

At the present time, it is commonly believed that with the exception of certain specific diseases, including systemic lupus erythematosus, renal polyarteritis nodosa, and scleroderma, obstetric outcomes are usually successful, especially if renal function is only moderately compromised and hypertension is absent or minimal *(25)*. Pregnancy in women with chronic renal disease is accompanied by an increase in such complications as hypertension and proteinuria, and by increases in prematurity and fetal loss *(26)*. Although fertility is clearly decreased in women with advanced renal disease, pregnancy sometimes occurs. As already noted, transplantation restores fertility to many women with end-stage renal disease, so contraception should be provided when appropriate.

ACQUIRED IMMUNE DEFICIENCY SYNDROME (AIDS)

Individuals with advanced AIDS would be expected to be amenorrheic because of hypothalamic–pituitary dysfunction. Although few studies have been conducted in women, studies in men suggest that both primary hypogonadism and hypogonadotropic hypogonadism can occur relatively early in the disease process in men *(27,28)*. It is generally believed that the reproductive dysfunction present in HIV-infected patients is related more to cachexia and advanced disease than to HIV or opportunistic infections *(28)*. In any case, it is clear that HIV-infected women can and do conceive, and the need for contraception among those who are sexually active is well recognized. The effectiveness of zidovudine (AZT) in reducing transmission of the virus to the fetus is well documented *(29)*.

MALIGNANCIES

The debilitation that accompanies advanced malignancies is typically associated with anovulation and amenorrhea, most probably because of hypothalamic–pituitary dysfunction. However, many women with less advanced malignancies do in fact conceive. Clearly both surgical removal of any neoplasm and irradiation are possible during pregnancy, but because of transplacental transport, administration of any chemotherapeutic agents can have profound effects on and result in the death of the fetus. Once the diagnosis is made, the dilemma is whether to terminate the pregnancy and treat the patient with such agents, or limit treatment until delivery has been effected. Such decisions must be made with the input of the patient.

There is no evidence that growth of most malignancies is accelerated by pregnancy. This is even true of breast cancer, a malignancy considered to be hormonally responsive.

There is no difference in survival when pregnant women with breast cancer are matched to nonpregnant women by age and stage of disease; moreover, termination of pregnancy is not associated with improved survival *(30)*. Although it is recognized that pregnant women have a 2.5-fold greater risk of metastases, the reason is later diagnosis at a later stage because of the breast changes associated with pregnancy *(31)*. Moreover, a pregnancy, after diagnosis and appropriate therapy for breast cancer, has no negative impact on prognosis *(32)*.

RADIATION AND CHEMOTHERAPY

Radiation therapy and chemotherapy for the treatment of both malignant and benign disease have been important in inducing remissions and cures. A variety of disorders are amenable to treatment with these modalities separately or in combination, as well as in an adjuvant role. Cancers that primarily affect children and young adults have been successfully treated in many cases, resulting in long-term remissions and cures. Thus, a relatively large number of young women of reproductive age have a history of chemotherapy and/or radiation therapy. There were an estimated 125,000 adult survivors of childhood cancers in 1987 *(33)*.

The toxicities of therapy are both acute and delayed. Acute toxicities are primarily related to damage to rapidly dividing cells present in the gastrointestinal tract, skin, and bone marrow. These result in effects such as nausea, vomiting, diarrhea, stomatitis, alopecia, and pancytopenia. For the most part, these are temporary changes that totally resolve within a short period of time. Some effects of therapy are delayed, such as cardiomyopathy from doxorubicin or pulmonary fibrosis from bleomycin. The delayed impact on reproductive function has received attention as experience has accumulated in both the male and female *(34–39)*.

Radiation effects on the human ovary have been recognized for over 50 years. Jacox demonstrated that 500 rads (cGy) of radiation to the ovaries produced 6–18 mo of amenorrhea and rendered women over 40 sterile *(40)*. Acute and chronic damage resulting from radiation, including infertility, in survivors of the atomic bomb explosions in Hiroshima and Nagasaki increased concern over the effects of therapeutic radiation *(41)*. Radiotherapy has been used successfully in the treatment of multiple types of cancers, including but not limited to Hodgkin's disease, leukemia, sarcomas, neuroblastoma, nephroblastoma, and cervical cancer. In addition, it is frequently used for palliation in many other tumors *(38,39)*. Older uses of radiation in women for nonmalignant disease included treatment for infertility *(42)*, uterine bleeding *(43)*, and induction of menopause for menorrhagia *(44)*.

The gonadal toxicity of radiation depends on multiple factors. There are differences in sensitivity between the testes and ovaries, as well as between individuals *(45)*. The state of development of the germ cell at the time of exposure is important *(46)*. In addition, the total dose of radiation and fractionation of the dose impact the susceptibility of germ cells to damage. Direct irradiation of the gonad has more effect than scattered radiation *(37,47)*.

The age of the woman is an important determinant of ovarian sensitivity. *In utero*, germ cells migrate to the gonadal ridge and differentiate into oogonia, then enlarge, and proliferate to become primary oocytes. Primordial follicles are primary oocytes surrounded by stromal cells (granulosa cells). At birth, there are approx 150,000–500,000 primordial follicles and 2 million oocytes, which are arrested in the diplotene stage of prophase. Follicular growth is then continuous, and ovulation is cyclic from puberty to menopause. The most radiosensitive phases are when oogonia undergo mitosis and during preovulatory maturation. In general, small primordial oocytes are more sensitive than oocytes in Graafian follicles *(46)*. The number of germ cells drops from 2 million at birth to essentially none in menopause. Thus, as a woman ages, she is more likely to be rendered amenorrheic or sterile by a given dose of ovarian radiation *(38,45)*. At 60 cGy or less, no deleterious effects are noted. From 60–150 cGy, there is some risk of sterilization, especially for women over 40 yr of age. From 250–500 cGy, effects are variable with 100% of women over 40 sterilized by over 400 cGy, and 60% of women 15–40 yr of age sterilized by 250–500 cGy, with some temporary amenorrhea in others. From 500–800 cGy, 100% of women over 40 yr old are sterilized, and 70% of women 15–40 yr old are sterilized, with high rates of temporary amenorrhea in the rest. Over 800 cGy results in 100% sterilization. There is also evidence to suggest that ovarian injury owing to irradiation can result in delayed puberty *(48,49)*, whereas cranial irradiation may lead to earlier menarche *(50)*.

The ovaries undergo morphological changes with therapy *(51)*. Irradiation leads to a decrease in the number of developing follicles and to a reduction in the number of small, nongrowing follicles. On examination by electron microscopy, the oocyte becomes pyknotic, followed by condensation of chromatin, and finally disruption of the nuclear envelope *(52)*. Eventually, scar tissue replaces the damaged oocytes. With destruction of all oocytes, LH and FSH levels increase to the range found in postmenopausal women, and estradiol falls to very low levels *(53)*.

The effect of scattered radiation was examined by Madsen et al. *(47)*. Thirty-six women with normal menstrual function at the time of diagnosis with Hodgkin's disease were followed. They underwent subtotal lymphoid irradiation to the mantle and para-aortic fields of 4000–4400 cGy. The calculated scatter radiation dose to the ovaries was 320 cGy. One of 36 subjects (2.7%) had premature menopause at age 33, a rate similar to nonirradiated women *(54)*. Eighteen women had a total of 38 pregnancies, all with normal offspring.

A large study by Byrne et al. *(55)* estimated the effects of treatment on fertility in long-term survivors of childhood or adolescent cancer in a retrospective cohort study from five cancer registries. Patients were treated with radiation therapy or chemotherapy with alkylating agents or both. There were 637 women analyzed who met inclusion criteria. A sibling control group was used to compare relative fertility rates. Subjects known to be sterile were excluded, including seven women with primary amenorrhea, 21 with secondary amenorrhea, and 32 with sterilizing operations (only two controls were sterile). Excluding these sterile women somewhat alters their data. Radiation therapy was described as above or below the diaphragm, without specific information on dosing, fields, shielding, or other factors. The overall data showed a decrease in relative fertility rates in survivors vs controls. For radiation below the diaphragm, this rate was 0.78. Adding an alkylating agent to this did not change the relative fertility rate (0.81). The no-radiation and no-chemotherapy (i.e., surgery only) group did not differ from controls, and alkylating agents alone had similar rates to controls. These data generally support the concept that radiation therapy below the diaphragm decreases female fertility and that alkylating agents have a lesser effect. Men were more affected than women for all forms of therapy combined, but especially for the combination of alkylating agents and radiation below the diaphragm (relative fertility 0.38 vs controls for men, 0.81 for women). There were differences among the sites of cancer as well. Surprisingly, the 26 female genital cancer patients had a relative fertility rate of 1.04 vs controls. The 253 Hodgkin's disease survivors had a rate of 0.77 vs controls (men and women), whereas most of the other cancers were between this and 1.0. However, this large study had a heterogeneous population that makes it more difficult to draw definitive conclusions.

Cervical cancer is frequently treated with radiation therapy, using intracavitary or intracavitary/external beam therapy followed by surgery. The ovarian endocrine function was studied in a group of women 24–38 yr old who received at least 8500 cGy of radiation for cervical cancer *(56)*. Based on circulating levels of LH, FSH, and estradiol, ovarian function diminished shortly after treatment was begun, and hormone levels approximated those of postmenopausal women. All patients subsequently had a radical hysterectomy and bilateral lymphadenectomy.

Attempts have been made to reduce the ovarian damage when radiation therapy is needed. Lateral ovarian transposition to the paracolic gutter peritoneum in patients with early stage cervical cancer (I-IIA) has been used *(57)*. Despite ovarian transposition, it appears that about 20–80% of women develop menopausal symptoms of hot flushes and/or vaginal dryness within the first 2 yr after beginning irradiation, with ovarian failure being documented by elevated FSH levels *(58–61)*.

The use of GnRH agonists to protect the ovary from radiation toxicity also has been suggested *(62)*. However, in contrast to findings in the rat *(63)*, Ataya and colleagues were unable to show that a GnRH agonist offered any protective effect in the rhesus monkey. Controlled trials in humans have not been reported.

It has also become apparent that various chemotherapeutic agents alone may produce either temporary or permanent ovarian failure *(34,48,64–67)*. The alkylating agents have been studied most extensively and appear particularly prone to affect reproductive function. Chemotherapeutic agents definitely affecting gonadal function include cyclophosphamide, chlorambucil, L-phenylalanine mustard, nitrogen mustard, busulfan, and procarbazine *(38)*. Those probably related to infertility include doxorubicin, vinblastine, cytosine arabinoside, cisplatin, nitrosoureas, m-AMSA, and etoposide. Agents unlikely to be related include methotrexate, fluorouracil, mercaptopurine, and vincristine. The effects of bleomycin are unknown.

In general, because the human ovary is not easily accessible to biopsy, the ability to assess the effects of cytotoxic agents directly on ovarian histology have been limited. Functional status has been evaluated primarily by obtaining menstrual and reproductive histories, and measuring LH, FSH, and estradiol concentrations in the circulation. As is true for radiation therapy, the younger the individual patient at the time of therapy, the more likely it is that ovarian function will not be compromised by the chemotherapeutic agents. As noted in considering the effects of radiation therapy, it may be that the number of oocytes in the ovaries at the time of therapy is important in determining if ovarian function will persist after therapy. It appears as if most chemotherapeutic agents administered prior to age 20 have no effect on any subsequent pregnancies *(68)*. In this one series, Green and associates *(68)* found no increased risk of congenital anomalies in resulting offspring, except that one particular agent, dactinomycin, may be associated with an increased risk of congenital structural cardiac anomalies. Future studies to address this question are clearly needed.

There have been efforts to evaluate the effects of bone marrow transplantation on subsequent fertility as well. However, because most individuals are treated with high-dose chemotherapy and sometimes radiation before transplant, it is difficult to sort out the effects of the transplant itself. In any case, perhaps one in seven women of reproductive age resume normal menses after therapy, including bone marrow transplantation *(69)*. In resulting pregnancies, the incidences of preterm delivery and low birthweight infants appear increased.

MISCELLANEOUS DISORDERS

Cystic Fibrosis

An increasing number of women with cystic fibrosis are surviving well into the reproductive years. It has been estimated that cystic fibrosis occurs in 1 in 1000–2000 live births in the US and is the most frequent lethal hereditary disorder in white populations, with 1 in 20 being carriers *(70)*. Although perhaps 95% of men with cystic fibrosis are sterile, many women with cystic fibrosis apparently do not have problems with fertility *(71)*. Among those who suffer from infertility, the cause is believed to be related to the altered cervical mucus with decreased water content caused by the disease *(72)*. One case of a young woman with cystic fibrosis and infertility in which the infertility was successfully treated with intrauterine insemination has been reported *(72)*. These observations emphasize the importance of providing contraception to women who are sexually active. The only study of combination oral contraceptive use in women with cystic fibrosis found no detrimental effects in 10 women aged 15–24 yr over a period of 6 mo *(73)*, but in the absence of additional studies, hormonal contraception should be used with caution.

Inflammatory Bowel Disease (IBD)

Except for women with inanition secondary to severe IBD, there is no evidence that fertility is decreased in IBD. In one study comparing 177 women with Crohn's disease and 84 with ulcerative colitis to healthy control women, decreased birthrate was found to be secondary to the woman's choice rather than effect of the disease process *(74)*. Thus, fear of getting pregnant from warnings by physicians or others may be a factor. A small percentage of women with Crohn's disease will be infertile secondary to fistulization to fallopian tubes with resultant tuboovarian abscesses *(75)*. In addition, perineal or labial abscesses and fistulas, as well as pain, may discourage intercourse. Individuals undergoing intra-abdominal surgery also have reduced fertility for any of several reasons *(76)*. In general, pregnancy has not been shown to alter significantly the course of IBD, but exacerbations can and do occur; these exacerbations occur more commonly in the first and second trimesters in women with ulcerative colitis and in the third trimester in Crohn's disease *(70)*. Problems during pregnancy tend to be related to the activity of the disease process during the pregnancy. The risk of preterm birth appears increased about threefold in IBD *(74)*, and there is increased fetal wastage in those with active disease at conception *(70)*. Sulfasalazine does cross the placenta and inhibit the metabolism of folic acid, but there is no evidence of fetal harm *(70)*. Thus, sulfasalazine may be used when needed during pregnancy, but its continued use is not recommended for pregnant women in remission. Perhaps of even greater concern are the possible consequences of azathioprine and mercaptopurine during pregnancy. These agents are teratogenic in animals, but data in humans are scant and conflicting *(70)*. Azathioprine has been associated with lymphopenia, leukopenia, thrombocytopenia, hypogammaglobulinemia, and thymic aplasia *(77)*, and should be avoided during pregnancy.

With regard to contraception, there does not seem to be any strong evidence that hormonal contraceptives will cause a flare in women with IBD. There is evidence of reduced bioavailability of the synthetic progestins contained in oral contraceptives in individuals with reduced small-bowel-absorbing surface because of surgical removal or diarrhea *(70)*. In such individuals, parenteral administration of depomedroxyprogesterone acetate or the use of implantable levonorgestrel pellets would be preferred.

Diabetes Mellitus

There is no question that uncontrolled diabetes mellitus can affect fertility in both men and women. Studies in women have shown that diabetes can delay the onset of menarche, and increase the prevalence of primary amenorrhea, secondary amenorrhea, and oligomenorrhea *(78)*. The effects of pregnancy on the progression of the diabetes remain uncertain and controversial, and should be discussed with patients, especially those with long-standing disease and with evidence of vascular and renal disease *(70)*. It is known that women developing gestational diabetes have a markedly increased risk of becoming overtly diabetic later in life *(79)*. That women with diabetes mellitus are at a greater risk of maternal morbidity and fetal mortality as well as morbidity including congenital malformations, with the caudal regression syndrome being characteristic of infants of diabetic mothers, is now commonly known *(79)*. Pre-eclampsia, preterm delivery, and cesarean sections are increased in diabetic women *(79)*. Because preconception counseling and good glycemic control can reduce the incidence of spontaneous abortions *(80)* and major congenital malformations *(81,82)*, pregnancy planning is essential. Contraceptive counseling is essential as well. The use of hormonal forms of contraception in diabetic women is controversial. The risk of contraception must be balanced against the risks of pregnancy, which are significant in diabetic women. In general, it is believed that combination oral contraceptives can be used by diabetic women <35 yr old who do not smoke and are otherwise healthy, especially in the absence of diabetic vascular complications *(83)*. A case-control study of young women with insulin-dependent diabetes mellitus was unable to detect any differences between oral contraceptive users (of 1–7 yr in duration) and nonusers with respect to longitudinal hemoglobin A1c levels, cholesterol levels, and evidence of retinopathy or nephropathy *(84)*.

Thyroid Disease

Thyroid dysfunction can affect menses and fertility. Both hypothyroidism and hyperthyroidism can be associated with anovulatory bleeding, amenorrhea, and anovulation *(85)*. Because treatment of thyroid disease can lead to resumption of ovulation, effective contraception should be provided.

Untreated hyperthyroidism in pregnancy is associated with very high rates of fetal wastage, and women with untreated hypothyroidism who do conceive have a 30–50% incidence of spontaneous abortion *(86)*. Either methimazole or propylthiouracil can be used to treat hyperthyroidism in pregnancy, but obviously radioactive ^{131}I should be avoided because it can cross the placenta and ablate the fetal thyroid. Although hormonal contraceptives can impact on laboratory tests of thyroid function, there is little evidence that they affect thyroid disease *(70)*.

Rheumatological Diseases

Overall, reproductive function does not appear to be impaired by systemic lupus erythematosus (SLE), but as is true for other disorders, it is likely that women who are seriously ill have an increased incidence of anovulation. There is no universal agreement about the effects of pregnancy on the course of SLE *(70)*. It appears likely that women with more inactive disease do better than those with active SLE. Most studies have documented increased fetal morbidity and mortality among pregnancies of women with SLE, especially among those with lupus nephritis *(70)*. The use of combination oral contraceptives is generally discouraged because of potential vascular side effects of estrogens; progestin-only hormonal contraception may be considered.

Similarly, reproductive dysfunction does not appear to be decreased among women with rheumatoid arthritis. Sexuality and libido may be affected by pain or a significant limitation in joint motion. Rheumatoid arthritis most commonly remits during pregnancy, but there is frequently a postpartum flare *(70)*. There is no real evidence for any increase in risk to a pregnancy or to the fetus as a consequence of rheumatoid arthritis. Many of the medications used to treat rheumatoid arthritis may have detrimental effects on pregnancy and the fetus, and preconception counseling is important. There is no evidence that any form of contraception is contraindicated in women with rheumatoid arthritis.

Cardiac Disease

There is little information regarding the effects of cardiac disease on reproductive function in women. In general, the more severe the cardiac disease, the greater should be the likelihood of impaired reproductive function. This premise is supported by one study examining menstrual patterns in women with congenital heart disease *(87)*. In aggregate, the women with congenital heart disease, virtually all of whom underwent attempts at surgical correction early in life, had menstrual patterns similar to those of the general population. However, for patients remaining cyanotic, menarche is delayed, and there is an increased incidence of menstrual irregularity compared to those women with acyanotic congenital heart disease and the normal population.

Similarly, there is little information regarding reproductive and sexual function in women following cardiac transplantation. One would anticipate that both would improve after successful transplantation. In men, it is clear that sexual dysfunction is common among heart transplant recipients despite improvement in cardiovascular function *(88)*. Whether this is true in women as well remains to be determined.

As a general rule, use of combination oral contraceptives is discouraged in women, such as those with mitral stenosis, who have an increased risk of thromboembolic phenomena. On the other hand, there should be no increased risk of oral contraceptives for women who are anticoagulated.

Severe heart disease may be a contraindication to pregnancy because of the increased cardiac demands. Providing effective contraception must be balanced against the risks of any unplanned pregnancy.

SUMMARY

Although there is not much information regarding the effects of critical disease on gonadal function in women, it is clear from the data that exist that variability clearly is most apparent. Some women continue to have regular menses, whereas others become anovulatory. In general, the more severe the disorder and the poorer the health of the individual patient, the more likely she is to be anovulatory. In most cases, the anovulation that results is central in origin. However, some disorders appear to be associated primarily with chronic anovulation owing to inappropriate feedback, i.e., polycystic ovarian syndrome-like presentation. In addition, some disorders and some medications may be associated with early ovarian failure. It is important to individualize therapy and care for all individuals who are critically ill. It is also important to warn them about the possibility of ovulation and pregnancy and to provide effective contraception when warranted.

REFERENCES

1. Woolf PD, Hamill RW, McDonald JV, Lee LA, Kelly M. Transient hypogonadotropic hypogonadism caused by critical illness. J Clin Endocrin Metab 1985;60:444–450.
2. Gebhart SS, Watts NB, Clark RV, et al. Reversible impairment of gonadotropin secretion in critical illness. Observations in postmenopausal women. Arch Intern Med 1989;149:1637–1641.
3. Bing-You RG, Spratt DI. Serum estradiol but not gonadotropin levels decrease acutely after insulin-induced hypoglycemia in cycling women. J Clin Endocrinol Metab 1992;75:1054–1059.
4. Spratt DI, Cox P, Orav J, et al. Reproductive axis suppression in acute illness is related to disease severity. J Clin Endocrinol Metab 1993;76:1548–1554.
5. Stellon AJ, Williams R. Increased incidence of menstrual abnormalities and hysterectomy preceding primary biliary cirrhosis. Br Med J 1986;293:297–298.
6. Cundy TF, O'Grady JG, Williams R. Recovery of menstruation and pregnancy after liver transplantation. Gut 1990;31:337–338.
7. Varma RR. Course and prognosis of pregnancy in women with liver disease. Semin Liver Dis 1987;7(1):59–66.
8. Mass K, Quint EH, Punch MR, Merion RM. Gynecological and reproductive function after liver transplantation. Transplantation. 1996;62:476–479.
9. O'Grady JG, Williams R. Postoperative care: long-term. In: Maddey WC, Sorrell M, eds. Transplantation of the Liver, 2nd ed. Appleton and Lange, Norwalk, 1995, pp. 207–224.
10. Ghent CN. Survival following liver transplantation. In: Maddey WC, Sorrell MF, eds. Transplantation of the Liver, 2nd ed. Appleton and Lange, Norwalk, 1995, pp. 541–555.
11. Everhart JE, DiBisceglie AM, Murray LM. Risk for non-A, non-B (type C) hepatitis through sexual or household contact with chronic carriers. Ann Int Med 1990;112:544–545.
12. Reinus JF, Leikin EL, Alter HJ. Failure to detect vertical transmission of hepatitis C virus. Ann Intern Med 1992;117:881–885.
13. Scantlebury V, Gordon R, Tzakis A. Childbearing after liver transplantation. Transplantation 1990;49:317–321.
14. Laifer SA, Darby MJ, Scantlebury VP. Pregnancy and liver transplantation. Obstet Gynecol 1990;76:1083–1088.
15. Ville Y, Fernandez H, Samuel D, Bismuth H, Frydman R. Pregnancy after hepatic transplantation. J Gynecol Obstet Biol Reprod 1992;21:691–696.
16. Handelsman DJ. Hypothalamic–pituitary–gonadal dysfunction in renal failure, dialysis and renal transplantation. Endocr Rev 1985;6:151–182.
17. Rice GG. Hypermenorrhea in the young hemodialysis patient. Am J Obstet Gynecol 1973;166:539–542.
18. Ferraris JR, Domene HM, Escobar ME, Caletti MG, Ramirez JA, Rivarola MA. Hormone profile in pubertal females with chronic renal failure: before and under haemodialysis and after renal transplantation. Acta Endocrinol 1987;115:289–296.
19. Lim VS, Henriquez C, Sievertsen, Frohman LA. Ovarian function in chronic renal failure: evidence suggesting hypothalamic anovulation. Ann Intern Med 1980;93:21–27.
20. Lim VS, Kathpalia SC, Frohman LA. Hyperprolactinemia and impaired pituitary response to suppression and stimulation in chronic renal failure: reversal after transplantation. J Clin Endocrinol Metab 1979;48:101–107.
21. Hasegawa K, Matsushita Y, Hirai K, et al. Abnormal response of luteinizing hormone, follicle stimulating hormone, and testosterone to luteinizing hormone-releasing hormone in chronic renal failure. Acta Endocrinol 1978;87:467–475.

22. Swamy AP, Woolf PD, Cestero RVM. Hypothalamic-pituitary-ovarian axis in uremic women. J Lab Clin Med 1979;93:1066–1072.
23. Pimstone B, Epstein S, Hamilton SM, LeRoith D, Hendricks S. Metabolic clearance and plasma half disappearance time of exogenous gonadotropin releasing hormone in normal subjects and in patients with liver disease and chronic renal failure. J Clin Endocrinol Metab 1977;44:356–360.
24. Price TM, Dupuis RE, Carr BR, Stanczyk FZ, Lobo RA, Droegemueller W. Single- and multiple-dose pharmacokinetics of a low-dose oral contraceptive in women with chronic renal failure undergoing peritoneal dialysis. Am J Obstet Gynecol 1993;168:1400–1406.
25. Davison JM, Lindheimer MD. Renal disorders. In: Creasy RK, Resnik R, eds. Maternal-Fetal Medicine: Principles and Practice, 3rd ed. Saunders, Philadelphia, 1994, pp. 844–864.
26. Hou S. Pregnancy in women with chronic renal disease. N Engl J Med 1985;312:836–839.
27. Croxson TS, Chapman WE, Miller LK, Levit CD, Senie R, Zumoff B. Changes in the hypothalamic-pituitary-gonadal axis in human immunodeficiency virus-infected homosexual men. J Clin Endocrinol Metab 1989;68:317–321.
28. Raffi F, Brisseau FM, Planchon B, Remi JP, Barrier JH, Grolleau JY. Endocrine function in 98 HIV-infected patients: a prospective study. AIDS. 1991;5:729–733.
29. Conner EM, Sperling RS, Gelber R, et al. Reduction of maternal-infant transmission of human immunodeficiency virus type 1 with zidovudine treatment. Pediatric AIDS Clinical Trials Group Protocol 076 Study Group. N Engl J Med 1994;331:1173–1180.
30. Zemlickis D, Lishner M, Degendorfer P, et al. Maternal and fetal outcome after breast cancer in pregnancy. Am J Obstet Gynecol 1992;166:781–787.
31. Nugent P, O'Connell TX. Breast cancer and pregnancy. Arch Surg 1985;120:1221–1224.
32. Ribeiro G, Jones DA, Jones M. Carcinoma of the breast associated with pregnancy. Br J Surg 1986;73:607–609.
33. Byrne J, Kessler LG, Devesa SS. The prevalence of cancer among adults in the United States, 1987. Cancer 1992;69:2154–2159.
34. Damewood MD, Grochow LB. Prospects for fertility after chemotherapy or radiation for neoplastic disease. Fertil Steril 1986;45:443–459.
35. Gradishar WJ, Schilsky RL. Effect of cancer treatment on the reproductive system. Crit Rev Oncol Hematol 1988;8:153–171.
36. Chapman RM, Sutcliffe SB, Malpas JS. Male gonadal dysfunction in Hodgkin's disease. JAMA 1982;245:1323–1328.
37. Shapiro E, Kinsella TJ, Makuch RW, et al. Effects of fractionated irradiation on endocrine aspects of testicular function. J Clin Oncol 1985;3:1232–1239.
38. Gradishar WJ, Schilsky RL. Ovarian function following radiation and chemotherapy for cancer. Semin Oncol 1989;16:425–436.
39. Nicholson HS, Byrne J. Fertility and pregnancy after treatment for cancer during childhood or adolescence. Cancer 1993;71(10):3392–3399.
40. Jacox HW. Recovery following human ovum irradiation. Radiology 1939;32:538–545.
41. Miller RW. Delayed effect occurring within the first decade after exposure of young individuals to the Hiroshima atomic bomb. Pediatrics 1956;8:1–17.
42. Kaplan II. The treatment of female sterility with X-ray therapy directed to the pituitary and ovaries. Am J Obstet Gynecol 1958;76:447–453.
43. Dickson RJ. The late results of radium treatment for benign uterine haemorrhage. Br J Radiol 1969;42:582–594.
44. Smith PG, Doll R. Late effects of X-irradiation in patients for metropathia haemorrhagica. Br J Radiol 1976;49:224–232.
45. Ash P. The influence of radiation on fertility in man. Br J Radiol 1980;53:271–278.
46. Baker TG. Radiosensitivity of mammalian oocytes with particular reference to the human female. Am J Obstet Gynecol 1971;110:746–761.
47. Madsen BL, Guidice L, Donaldson SS. Radiation-induced premature menopause: a misconception. Int J Radiat Oncol Biol Phys 1995;32:1461–1464.
48. Siris EJ, Leventhal BG, Vaitukaitis JL. Effects of childhood leukemia and chemotherapy on puberty and reproductive function in girls. N Engl J Med 1976;249:1143–1146.
49. Hamre MR, Robinson LL, Nesbit ME, Sather HN, Meadows AT, Ortega TA. Effects of radiation on ovarian function in long-term survivors of childhood acute lymphoblastic leukemia: a report from the Children's Cancer Study Group. J Clin Oncol 1987;5:1759–1765.

50. Quigley C, Cowell C, Jimenez M, et al. Normal or early development of puberty despite gonadal damage in children treated for acute lymphoblastic leukemia. N Engl J Med 1989;321:143–151.
51. Himmelstein-Braw R, Peters H, Faber M. Influence of irradiation and chemotherapy on the ovaries of children with abdominal tumors. Br J Cancer 1977;36:269–275.
52. Parsons DF. An electron microscopy study of radiation damage in the mouse oocyte. J Cell Biol 1962;14:31–48.
53. Ogilvy-Stuart AL, Clark DJ, Wallace WHB, et al. Endocrine deficit after fractionated total body irradiation. Arch Dis Child 1992;67:1107–1110.
54. Cohen I, Speroff L. Premature ovarian failure update. Obstet Gynecol Survey 1991;46:156–162.
55. Byrne J, Mulvihill JS, Myers MH, et al. Effects of treatments on fertility in long-term survivors of childhood or adolescent cancer. N Engl J Med 1987;317:1315–1321.
56. Janson PO, Jansson I, Skryten A, et al. Ovarian endocrine function in young women underlying radiotherapy for carcinoma of the cervix. Gynecol Oncol 1981;11:218–223.
57. Feeney DD, Moore DH, Look KY, Stehman FB, Sutton GP. The fate of the ovaries after radical hysterectomy and ovarian transposition. Gynecol Oncol 1995;56:3–7.
58. Hodel K, Rich WM, Austin P, DiSaia PJ. The role of ovarian transposition in conservation of ovarian function in radical hysterectomy followed by pelvic radiation. Gynecol Oncol 1982;13:195–202.
59. Anderson B, Buller R, Turner D, Chapman G. Ovarian transposition in cervical cancer. Gynecol Oncol 1992;45:81.
60. Ray GR, Trueblood HW, Enright LD, Kaplan HS, Nelsen TS. Oophoropexy: a means of preserving ovarian function following pelvic megavoltage radiotherapy for Hodgkin's disease. Radiology 1970;96:175–180.
61. Thibaud E, Ramirez M, Brauner R, et al. Preservation of ovarian function by ovarian transposition performed before pelvic irradiation during childhood. J Pediatr 1992;121:880–884.
62. Ataya K, Pydyn E, Ramahi-Ataya A, Orton CG. Is radiation-induced ovarian failure in rhesus monkeys preventable by luteinizing hormone-releasing hormone agonists?: preliminary observations. J Clin Endocrinol Metab 1995;80:790–795.
63. Jarrell J, YoungLai EV, McMahon A, Barr R, O'Connell G, Belbeck. Effect of ionizing radiation and pretreatment with [D-leu 6, des Gly 10] luteinizing hormone-releasing hormone ethylamide on developing rat ovarian follicles. Cancer Res 1987;47:5005–5008.
64. Horning SJ, Hoppe RT, Kaplan HS, et al. Female reproductive potential after treatment for Hodgkin's disease. N Engl J Med 1981;304:1377–1382.
65. Koyama H, Wada T, Nishizawa Y, et al. Cyclophosphamide-induced ovarian failure and its therapeutic significance in patients with breast cancer. Cancer 1977;39:1403–1409.
66. Stillman RJ, Schinfeld JS, Schiff I, et al. Ovarian failure in long-term survivors of childhood malignancy. Am J Obstet Gynecol 1981;139:62–66.
67. Whitehead E, Shalet SM, Blackledge D, et al. The effect of combination chemotherapy on ovarian failure in women treated for Hodgkin's disease. Cancer 1983;52:988–993.
68. Green DM, Zevon MA, Lowrie G, Seigelstein N, Hall B. Congenital anomalies in children of patients who received chemotherapy for cancer in childhood and adolescence. N Engl J Med 1991;325:141–146.
69. Sanders JE, Hawley J, Levy W, et al. Pregnancies following high-dose cyclophosphamide with or without high-dose busulfan or total-body irradiation and bone marrow transplantation. Blood 1996;87:3045–3052.
70. Neinstein LS. Issues in Reproductive Management. Thieme Medical, New York, 1994.
71. Seale TW, Flux M, Rennert OM. Reproductive defects in patients of both sexes with cystic fibrosis: A review. Ann Clin Lab Sci 1985;5:152–158.
72. Kredentser JV, Pokrant C, McCoshen JA. Intrauterine insemination for infertility due to cystic fibrosis. Fertil Steril 1986;45:425–426.
73. Fitzpatrick SB, Stokes DC, Rosenstein BJ, Terry P, Hubbard VS. Use of oral contraceptives in women with cystic fibrosis. Chest 1984;86:863–867.
74. Baird DD, Narendranathan M, Sandler RS. Increased risk of preterm birth for women with inflammatory bowel disease. Gastroenterology 1990;99:987–994.
75. Zeldis JB. Pregnancy and inflammatory bowel disease. West J Med 1989;151:168–171.
76. Wikland M, Jansson I, Asztely M, et al. Gynaecological problems related to anatomical changes after convention proctocolectomy and ileostomy. Int J Colorectal Dis 1990;5:49–52.
77. Lawson DH, Lovatt GE, Gurton CS, Hennings RC. Adverse effects of azathioprine. Adverse Drug React Acute Poisoning Rev 1984;3:161–174.

78. Burkart W, Fischer-Guntenhoener E, Standl E, Schneider HP. Menarche, menstrual cycle and fertility in diabetic patients. Geburtshilfe Frauenheilkd 1989;49:149–154.
79. Moore TR. Diabetes in pregnancy. In: Creasy RK, Resnik R, eds. Maternal-Fetal Medicine: Principles and Practice. Saunders, Philadelphia, 1994, pp. 934–975.
80. Rosenn B, Miodovnik M, Combs CA, Khoury J, Siddiqi TA. Pre-conception management of insulin-dependent diabetes: Improvement of pregnancy outcome. Obstet Gynecol 1991;77:846–849.
81. Steel JM, Johnstone FD, Hepburn DA, Smith AF. Can prepregnancy care of diabetic women reduce the risk of abnormal babies? Br Med J 1990;301:1070–1074.
82. Kitzmiller JL, Gavin LA, Gin GD, Jovanovic-Peterson L, Main EK, Zigrang WD. Preconception care of diabetes: Glycemic control prevents congenital anomalies. JAMA 1991;265:731–736.
83. Speroff L, Darney PD. A Clinical Guide for Contraception, 2nd ed. Williams and Wilkins, Baltimore, 1996, pp. 25–117.
84. Garg SK, Chase HP, Marshall G, Hoops SL, Holmes DL, Jackson WE. Oral contraceptives and renal and retinal complications in young women with insulin-dependent diabetes mellitus. JAMA 1994;271:1099–1102.
85. Becks GP, Burrow GN. Thyroid disease and pregnancy. Med Clin North Am 1991;75:121–150.
86. Seely BL, Burrow GN. Thyroid disease and pregnancy. In: Creasy RK, Resnik R, eds. Maternal-Fetal Medicine: Principles and Practice. Saunders, Philadelphia, 1994, pp. 979–1003.
87. Canobbio MM, Rapkin AJ, Perloff JK, Lin A, Child JS. Menstrual patterns in women with congenital heart disease. Pediatr Cardiol 1995;16:12–15.
88. Mulligan T, Sheehan H, Hanrahan J. Sexual function after heart transplantation. J Heart Lung Transplant 1991;10:125–128.

16 Effects of Aging on the Hormonal Response to Stress

*Gary A. Wittert, MD
and John E. Morley, MB, BCh*

CONTENTS
> THE AGING PROCESS
> THE EFFECTS OF AGING
>   ON THE HYPOTHALAMIC–PITUITARY ADRENAL (HPA) AXIS
> HYPOTHALAMIC–PITUITARY–GONADAL AXIS
> HYPOTHALAMIC–PITUITARY–HYROID AXIS
> PROLACTIN
> GROWTH HORMONE (GH)
> CONCLUSION
> REFERENCES

THE AGING PROCESS

During aging, a progressive decline in the ability of an organism to maintain homeostasis occurs. The mechanism by which senescence of the endocrine system occurs is not known, but presumably involves both genetic and environmental components. In the hypothalamus, morphological changes occur in association with the aging process. In the rat, neurons are lost from areas that regulate temperature and gonadotropin secretion *(1)*. In humans, there is marked enlargement of neurons in the supraoptic and paraventricular nuclei, but no loss of neurons from these areas *(2)*. Parvicellular corticotropin-releasing hormone- (CRH), containing neurons in the paraventricular nucleus have been observed to be activated during the course of aging *(3)*. However, with aging the number of neurons in the suprachiasmatic nucleus decreases *(3)*.

THE EFFECTS OF AGING ON THE HYPOTHALAMIC–PITUITARY–ADRENAL (HPA) AXIS

Studies on the effects of aging on the HPA axis in humans have produced variable results. Methodological issues may account for these inconsistencies, since many studies include only small numbers of subjects who were of variable health status and age range. In addition, variable end points have been studied (e.g., different times of day and different sampling protocols). On balance, however, based on the current literature,

From *Contemporary Endocrinology: Endocrinology of Critical Disease*
Edited by K. P. Ober   Humana Press Inc., Totowa, NJ

there is evidence to suggest that HPA axis changes in aging humans are similar to those occurring in rodents and primates. However, these changes may not be an inevitable consequence of the aging process, senescence of the HPA axis may either be delayed or occur minimally in those individuals who age more "successfully."

The most consistent and earliest feature of HPA axis senescence may be the delay of recovery of the HPA axis after activation, which may be the earliest manifestation of loss of glucocorticoid feedback owing to decreased numbers of hippocampal type 1 glucocorticoid receptors. Increased secretion of cortisol during the nadir of the circadian rhythm and basal hypercortisolemia may occur in the elderly. By contrast, direct activators of pituitary or adrenal function have similar effects in young and old subjects, consistent with the hypothesis of a central defect at the hypothalamic level. There is evidence, however, for delayed recovery of the axis after activation, an observation which would be consistent with the decrease in hippocampal corticosteroid receptors.

A number of studies in humans have failed to demonstrate any change in basal cortisol levels with aging *(4–16)*. Methodological variables in these studies have included time of day, health status, and community vs hospital-based populations. Nevertheless, the consistent lack of age-related difference in plasma cortisol levels between young and elderly in these studies suggest that age, in general, does not have a major impact overall on basal cortisol levels. However, in a recent longitudinal study performed over a 4-yr period in a large number of healthy elderly subjects, a variable pattern of HPA axis activity was observed. Although overall there were no major changes in basal cortisol levels, distinct subgroups could be identified. Furthermore, those subjects who showed high basal cortisol levels and a significant increase in cortisol over the years also showed impairment on tasks measuring explicit memory and selective attention (functions reliant on an intact hippocampus), whereas those who showed a decline in cortisol levels over the years performed as well as young subjects *(17)*. These findings are consistent with animal data on the role of the hippocampus in HPA dysfunction and cognitive impairment. A direct relationship between the degree of dementia and activity of the HPA axis has been found in a number of studies, where increased activity of the HPA axis is associated with both the severity of cognitive impairment and the degree of hippocampal atrophy *(18,19)*.

Although a number of studies have failed to show a change in circadian rhythm with aging for either adrenocorticotropic hormone (ACTH) *(6,20)* or cortisol *(6,9,20,21)*, these studies had either very small sample sizes, insufficiently frequent sampling protocols, or both. More recently, evidence is accumulating that significant changes in circadian variations in ACTH and cortisol secretion do occur with aging.

Cortisol secretion is closely linked to sleep processes. During rapid eye movement (REM) sleep the secretory activity of the HPA axis is inhibited *(22)*. In elderly people a decline in time spent in slow-wave sleep (SWS) and a decrease in REM sleep have been reported, associated with diminished nocturnal growth hormone surges and a phase advance in the nocturnal maximum of cortisol secretion when compared to younger subjects *(23)*. The cortisol nadir occurring within the first two nor-REM/REM sleep cycles of undisturbed sleep and mean cortisol concentrations during the night have been found to increase linearly with increasing age *(24)*. However, the age-related increase in cortisol nadir concentrations were found to be independent of the decrease of SWS and REM sleep; this suggest that separate mechanisms are responsible for these changes, and that they do not simply reflect a generalized defect of the circadian pacemaker *(24)*. Ferrari et al. *(25)* also demonstrated that elderly subjects exhibit higher plasma cortisol values during the evening and night hours when compared to young subjects, and these values are significantly age-related. In both studies, a coexistence of relatively high levels of both ACTH and cortisol suggested reduced sensitivity to steroid feedback. Animal data suggests that this change in activity of the HPA axis with aging is the consequence of loss of hippocampal type 1 corticosteroid receptors *(26)*. The observation that blocking type 1 corticosteroid receptors in young subjects with canrenoate will increase basal cortisol secretion during the first half of nocturnal sleep *(27)* is supportive of such a mechanism in humans.

In healthy elderly subjects, reduced sensitivity to glucocorticoid feedback, using dexamethasone suppression testing, has been found in some *(25,28–30)*, but not all studies *(31,32)*. An association among advancing age, impaired glucocorticoid feedback, and cognitive dysfunction has been demonstrated *(33)*. Dexamethasone has much greater affinity for type 2 corticosteroid receptors, and results may have been different if the response to hydrocortisone was determined instead.

A number of studies have examined the response of the HPA axis to CRH in young and elderly subjects with variable results. Two studies, both carried out in the morning, have shown no difference in the peak response of ACTH and cortisol between elderly and younger subjects *(16,34)*. Two studies have been done in the late afternoon. In one *(13)* the peak ACTH response was greater in older compared to the younger subjects, but in the other *(35)* the peak cortisol response was greater in the young. However, in the latter study, basal cortisol levels were greater in the younger subjects, and analysis of the data by area under the curve shows no significant difference between young and elderly subjects. Three significant additional observations were made in this study. First, elderly subjects with diseases such as diabetes or hypertension had greater responses of cortisol to CRH than healthy elderly subjects. Second, elderly women had greater responses than elderly men, an observation that is consistent with rodent data on sexual dimorphism of HPA axis responsiveness with aging *(36)*. Finally, when the pattern of recovery of the HPA axis after stimulation was analyzed, a longer period was required for cortisol levels to return to baseline in the elderly compared to the young. A similar observation can be made on the analysis of the data by Waltman et al. *(16)*. Furthermore, the elderly show more prolonged activation of the HPA axis in response to challenge by surgery *(37)* or metyrapone challenge *(38)*. A more prolonged pattern of HPA activation would be consistent with decreased corticosteroid feedback. Changes in cortisol binding globulin or clearance of cortisol has not been demonstrated in relation to aging.

The response of the HPA axis to acute stress in elderly subjects does not differ from that of young controls. Malarkey et al. *(39)* found that in a group of 19 men ages 53–74 yr that ultraendurance stress produced an increase in plasma ACTH and cortisol that was similar to that observed in the young controls. The recovery levels of ACTH and cortisol were also similar in the two groups. The response of the HPA axis to surgery and anesthesia has also been observed to be similar in young and elderly subjects *(37,40,41)*. Furthermore, the response of the HPA axis to insulin hypoglycemia *(42)* or the cold pressor test *(43)* does not differ significantly between young and elderly subjects. The response of the HPA axis to metyrapone has also been shown to be similar in young and elderly subjects *(38)*. By contrast, the pharmacological stimuli physostigmine *(44)* and naloxone *(45)* (which activate the HPA axis by increasing central cholinergic activity and inhibiting central mu opioid receptors respectively) result in greater cortisol responses in elderly subjects. However, these findings may reflect altered function of the central chatecholaminergic and opioid neuroendocrine systems per se rather than any primary change in activity of the HPA axis. Similarly, the 5-HT_{1a} agonist ipsapirone produces different effects on the HPA axis in elderly subjects than in young subjects; the response was reduced in elderly men, but increased in elderly women (46).

HYPOTHALAMIC–PITUITARY–THYROID AXIS

With aging there is a decrease in thyroxine (T_4) production rate and a decrease in plasma clearance rate (47). As a result, thyroxine levels do not decrease with age. Triiodothyronine (T_3) levels decline with aging as production rate decreases by 25% without any change in plasma clearance rate. There is a decrease in the thyroid-stimulating hormone (TSH) response to thyrotropin-releasing hormone in men, but not women, with advancing age. Even the stress of extreme old age has minimal effects on the thyroid axis, with healthy centenarians showing no change in free thyroxine levels, a small decrease in free T_3 and suppression of TSH levels (48).

There are very few studies specifically examining the effects of various stressors on the hypothalamic–pituitary–thyroid axis in older persons. Acute near-maximal exercise in persons with coronary artery disease failed to alter T_4, T_3, reverse T_3, or TSH (49). A heat stressor (8 MH_2 local radiofrequency hyperthermia) in patients with bladder cancer resulted in a decrease in thyroxine binding globulin, but no changes were observed in free thyroxine, free triiodothyronine, or reverse T_3. Patients receiving fetanyl-oxygen anesthesia for cardiac surgery had marked declines in free T_3 and total T_3 and lesser declines in free T_4 and total T_4 (50). In another study T_3 also declined after abdominal surgery, but T_4 and reverse T_3 increased when enflurane and halothane were used (but not with other anesthetics) (51); this suggests that changes in thyroxine after surgery may be more dependent on the anesthetic used than on the surgical stress.

Acute and chronic illness as a stressor is well recognized to alter thyroid hormone level (as described in Chapter 8). Mild illness decreases T_3 and increases rT_3 levels by decreasing the activity of the 5′ mono-iodinase that converts T_4 to T_3 (52). Early in an illness there may be a small increase in total T_4 levels, and free thyroxine levels may increase (53,54). In severe illness serum inhibitors reduce the binding of T_4 to thyroxine-binding globulin. Very low thyroxine levels have been found in severely ill patients in the intensive care unit and appear to predict subsequent mortality (55,56). In severe illness there is a decrease in serum TSH levels (57). Because many older persons have a variety of chronic stressors associated with the production of cytokines, the supersensitive TSH assays are poor markers of hyperthyroidism or secondary hypothyroidism (see ref. 58, 110 for a review of this literature). In healthy humans recombinant human interferon alpha therapy decreased TSH and T_3 while increasing reverse T_3 (59). Other cytokines, such as interleukin-6, also decrease TSH levels (60).

Gregerman and Solomon (61) compared the half-life of thyroxine in 12 young and 7 old (60–83 yr of age) patients with pneumococcal pneumonia. During the acute illness there was a marked reduction in thyroxine half-life to 2.4 ± 1.2 d in the older group and a similar decrease was observed in the younger group. On recovery, the mean T_4 half-life in the older group rose to 11.9 d and a similar decrease in T_3 turnover rate was seen in the two older subjects studied. Clearly, severe stress produces major changes in thyroid hormone turnover, which can be offset by increased thyroid hormone production in response to the stress, even in the elderly.

Acute psychiatric illness is also associated with alterations in thyroid function. Acute psychotic episodes are associated with increases in serum T_4 and free T_4 and/or free T_3

(62,63). This condition has been called "stress hyperthyroxinemia" and may be related to increased central phenylethylamine secretion *(62,62,64)*. Psychiatric illness is also associated with a low T_3 syndrome similar to that seen in persons with the euthyroid sick syndrome *(62)*.

Overall, the available studies suggest that acute physiological stressors in older persons have little effect on circulating thyroid hormone levels, because the thyroid gland appears to be capable of compensating by increased production of thyroid hormone. On the other hand, acute and chronic physical illnesses can produce major changes in thyroid hormone economy. However, there is little evidence that older persons respond to these severe stressors differently from younger persons.

PROLACTIN

In men there is a small increase in prolactin with aging *(65,66)*. In women, prolactin levels fall until 80 yr of age, after which there is a small increase. Prolactin levels increase in response to surgery *(67,68)*. Older persons (56–75 yr) have a lesser prolactin response to inguinal herniorrhaphy than do younger persons. Spinal blockade with epidural anesthesia significantly attenuates the differences between younger and older persons in the prolactin response, and Segawa et al. *(69)* demonstrated that epidural analgesia at the level of C8 to T_2 blocks the increase in prolactin seen at the time of skin incision.

In persons who develop syncope during tilt-table testing, there is an increase in prolactin that is not observed in persons who do not develop severe hypotension *(70)*. Electroconvulsive therapy (ECT) increases prolactin levels within 2–4 min after the seizure onset *(71)*. Clark et al. *(72)* examined the affect of ECT on prolactin in 15 depressed geriatric inpatients. Bilateral ECT produced higher prolactin levels than unilateral ECT. Patients who had a greater prolactin response to ECT tended to have a better therapeutic response. Not surprisingly, grand-mal seizures are also associated with increased prolactin levels *(73,74)*. Zautra et al. *(75)* measured prolactin levels in 33 women from ages 37–78 yr who had rheumatoid arthritis or osteoarthritis, depression and interpersonal conflicts were positively related to prolactin levels in the patients with rheumatoid arthritis.

In younger persons prolactin levels increase after treadmill exercise *(76)* and after running a marathon *(77)*, but studies of the effect of exercise on prolactin response in older persons are not available. In older persons there is some evidence that there may be an attenuated response of prolactin to stress, but there are insufficient studies to make any absolute conclusions at present.

HYPOTHALAMIC–PITUITARY–GONADAL AXIS

Women

In women, the menopause is marked by the cessation of menses, a decrease in estrogen and inhibin levels, and an increase in luteinizing hormone (LH) and follicle-stimulating hormone (FSH) levels. Peak LH and FSH levels are seen after 2–3 yr, with a decline over the next three decades to approximately half the level seen at their peak *(78,79)*. A number of stress-related factors can produce an earlier menopause, including undernutrition, hard physical work, poverty, smoking, and alcohol consumption *(80–83)*. Age of menopause is positively associated with age of death *(84)*.

Endogenous opioids inhibit LH secretion *(85)*, but the administration of an opioid antagonist fails to increase LH in postmenopausal women *(86)*. When postmenopausal women are replaced with conjugated estrogens, the ability of naloxone to increase LH is restored *(87)*. This suggests that stress (using opioid response as a marker) does not play a role in the gonadotropin changes associated with menopause.

In young women, exercise decreases LH levels while having a minimal effect on FSH levels *(88)*; excessive exercise is associated with amenorrhea. The effects of stress on gonadotropin responses in the postmenopausal women have been poorly studied.

Men

In contrast to women, men have a slower decline in hormonal levels with aging. Testosterone levels decline linearly from 40 yr of age *(89)*. There are greater decreases in free testosterone and bioavailable testosterone *(90,91)*. There is a small increase in sex hormone binding globulin with aging *(92)*.

LH levels rise minimally early in the aging process *(92)*. This is the result of a decrease in LH secretory bursts *(93)*. There is some evidence that the failure to see an increase in LH in middle age is caused by increased opioid tone *(94)*; a longitudinal study suggests that LH levels eventually increase in the old-old *(58)*, which is in keeping with naloxone's failure to increase LH in older individuals *(95)*. FSH levels increase and inhibin levels decrease with aging *(96)*. FSH levels increase independently of LH levels, showing that FSH is under different regulation from LH in the aging man.

Physical exercise decreases LH levels in young men *(97)*. In middle-aged males (ages 55–70 yr of age) resistive exercises had no effect on testosterone *(98)*. Master's athletes have extremely low testosterone levels (Kaiser, Morley, and Korenman, unpublished studies). Psychological stressors, such as depression, decrease testosterone levels *(99)*. This is thought to be the result of an increase in CRH that inhibits LH release *(100)*. The role of stressors in the production of the secondary hypogonadism in middle-aged men is not established. However, there is sufficient tantalizing evidence to suggest that this is a possible contributor to the pathophysiology of the "low testosterone syndrome".

GROWTH HORMONE (GH)

GH is secreted in bursts predominantly at night. In older persons, there is a decrease in the bursts of GH that occur during sleep *(101)*. There is a decrease in GH response to GH-releasing hormone (RH) with aging. In addition to alterations in the release of GH at the pituitary level, there is evidence of decreased release of GH-RH and an increase in the inhibitory hormone, somatostatin, from the hypothalamus with aging. In women, the decrease in GH with aging is owing, at least in part, to estrogen lack. Many of the effects of GH are produced secondary to the release of insulin growth factor-I (IGF-I). IGF-I levels are reduced in older men and women.

Insulin hypoglycemia is a classical stress test. Insulin hypoglycemia increases GH by inhibiting somatostatin release from the hypothalamus. The studies to date on the effects of insulin hypoglycemia on GH have produced an unclear picture to date. Some suggested a blunted response, but others have found no difference *(42,102,103)*. There is a blunted response of GH to stressful stimuli that act by increasing GH-RH, such as heat *(104)* and apomorphine *(105)*.

Physical exercise of the endurance type (70% of maximal O_2 consumption) increases GH in young adults. In older persons the GH response to this form of exercise has been demonstrated to be attenuated *(106)*. A similar decrease in GH response with aging has also been demonstrated to maximal exercise *(108)*. Similarly, the GH response to resistance exercise seen in younger persons is markedly diminished in older persons *(108)*.

Overall, GH decreases with age, and it would appear that most stressors fail to produce the same maximum response in older persons compared to those seen in younger persons. Ongoing studies of GH replacement in older persons have failed to demonstrate that the attenuation of GH with aging has a major physiological impact *(109)*.

CONCLUSION

Overall, there tends to be a blunted GH and prolactin response to stress with aging. Little difference in response of the other hormones reviewed in this chapter to stress have been reported. There is unfortunately minuscule data examining the impact of these hormonal alterations on the ability of the older person to respond to stressful situations.

REFERENCES

1. Hsu HK, Peng MT. Hypothalamic neuron number of old female rats. Gerontology 1978;24:434–440.
2. Buttlar-Bretano K. Zur Lebensgeschichte des Nuclear basilis, tubermauanalasis, suproopticus und paravenricular unter normalen und pathogenen Bedingungen. J Hirnforsch 1954;1:337–419.
3. Swaab DF, Hofman MA, Lucassen PJ, Purba JS, Raadsheer FC, Van de Nes JA. Functional neuroanatomy and neuropathology of the human hypothalamus (Review). Anat Embryol Berl 1993;187:317–330.
4. West CD, Brown H, Simon EL, Carter DB, Kumagai LF, Englert E. Adrenocortical function and cortisol metabolism in old age. J Clin Endo Metab 1961; 21:1197–1207.
5. Friedman M, Green MF, Sharland DE. Assessment of hypothalamic-pituitary adrenal function in the geriatric age group. J Gerontol 1969;24:292–297.
6. Jensen HK, Blichert-Toft M. Serum corticotrophin, Plasma cortisol and urinary excretion of 17-ketogenic steroids in the elderly (age group:66–94 years). Acta Endocrinol 1971;66:25–34.
7. Weitzman ED, Fukushima D, Nogeire C, Roffwarg H, Gallagher TF, Hellman L. Twenty-four hour pattern of the episodic secretion of cortisol in normal subjects. J Clin Endocrinol 1971;33:14–22.
8. Zumpff B, Fukushima DK, Weitzman ED, Kream J, Hellman L. The sex difference in plasma cortisol concentration in man. J Clin Endo Metab 1974; 39:805–808.
9. Colucci CF, Dalessandro B, Bellastella A, Montalbeti N. Circadian rhythm of plasma cortisol in the aged (Cosinor method). Geront Clin 1975;17:89–95.
10. Lakatua DJ, Nicolau Gy, Bogdan C, Petrescu E, Sackett-Lundeen LL, Irvine PW, Haus E. Circadian endocrine time structure in humans above 80 years of age. J Gerontol 1984;39:648–654.
11. Linkowski P, Mendlewicz J, Leclerq R, Brasseur M, Hubain P, Golstein J, Copinschi G, Van Cauter E. The 24-hour profile of adrenocorticotropin and cortisol in major depressive illness. J Clin Endocrinol Metab 1985;61:429–438.
12. Sherman B, Wysham C, Pfohl B. Age-related changes in the circadian rhythms of plasma cortisol in man. J Clin Endocrinol Metab 1985; 61:439–443.
13. Pavlov EP, Harman SM, Chrousos GP, Loriaux DL, Blackman MR. Responses of plasma adrenocorticotropin, cortisol, and dehydroepiandrosterone to ovine corticotropin-releasing hormone in healthy aging men. J Clin Endocrinol Metab 1986;62:767–772.
14. Jensen BA, Sanders S, Frolund B, Hjortup A. Adrenocortical function in old age as reflected by plasma cortisol and ACTH test during the course of acute myocardial infarction. Arch Gerontol Geriat 1988;7:289–296.
15. Sharma M, Palacios J, Schwartz G, Iskandar H, Thakur M, Quirion M, Nair NPV. Circadian rhythms of cortisol and melatonin in aging. Biol Psychiatry 1989;25:305–319.
16. Waltman C, Blackman MR, Chrousos GP, Riemann C, Harman SM. Spontaneous and glucocorticoid-inhibited adrenocorticotropic hormone and cortisol secretion are similar in healthy young and old men. J Clin Endocrinol Metab 1991;73:495–502.
17. Lupien S, Roch Lecours A, Lussier I, Schwartz G, Nair NPV, Meaney MJ. Basal cortisol levels and cognitive deficits in human aging. J Neurosci 1994;14:2893–2903.

18. Gurevich D, Siegel B, Dumlao M, Perl E, Chaitin P, Bagne C, Oxenkrug G. HPA-axis responsivity to dexamethasone and the cognitive impairment in dementia. Prog Neuropsychopharmacol Biol Psychiatry 1990;14:297–308.
19. De Leon MJ, McRae T, Tsai JR, George AE, Marcus DL, Freedman M, Wolf AP, McEwen B. Abnormal cortisol response in Alzheimer's disease linked to hippocampal atrophy. Lancet 1988;13:391–392.
20. Rolandi E, Franceschini R, Marabini A, Messina V, Cataldi A, Salvemini M, Barreca T. Twenty-four hour beta endorphin secretory pattern in the elderly. Acta Endocrinol (Copenh) 1987;115:441–446.
21. Dean S, Felton SP. Circadian rhythm in the elderly: a study using cortisol specific radioimmunoassay. Age Aging 1979;8:243–245.
22. Born J, Kern W, Bieber K, Kehm-Woldfsdorf G, Schiebe M, Fehm HL. Night plasma cortisol secretion is associated with specific sleep stages. Biol Psych 1986;21:1415–1424.
23. Van Coeverden A, Mockel J, Laurent E, Kerkhofs M, L'Hermite-Baleriaux M, Decoster C, Neve P, Van Cauter E. Neuroendocrine rhythms and sleep in aging men. Am J Physiol 1991; 260:E651–E661.
24. Kern W, Dodt C, Born J, Fehm HL. Changes in cortisol and growth hormone secretion during nocturnal sleep in the course of aging. J Gerontol A Biol Sci Med Sci 1996;51A:M3–M9.
25. Ferrari E, Magri F, Dori D, Migliorati G, Tiziana N, Molla G, Fioravanti M, Solerte SB. Neuroendocrine correlates of the aging brain in humans. Neuroendocrinology 1995;61:464–470.
26. Jacobsen L, Sapolsky R. The role of the hippocampus in feedback regulation of the hypothalamo–pituitary–adrenocortical axis. Endocr Rev 1991;12:118–134.
27. Dodt C, Kern W, Fehm HL, Born J. Antimineralcorticoid canrenoate enhances secretory activity of the hypothalamo-pituitary adrenocortical (HPA) axis in humans. Neuroendocrinology 1993; 58:570–574.
28. Oxenkrug GF, Pomara N, McIntyre IM, Braconnier RJ, Stanley M, Gershon S. Aging and cortisol resistance to suppression by dexamethasone: a positive correlation. Psychiatry Res 1983;10:125–130.
29. Sharma RP, Pandey GN, Janicak PG, Peterson J, Comaty JE, Davis JM. The effect of diagnosis and age on the DST: a meta-analytic approach. Biol Psychiatry 1988; 24:555–568.
30. Weiner MF. Age and cortisol suppression by dexamethasone in normal subjects. J Psychiatr Res 1989; 23:163–168.
31. Tiller JWG, Maguire KP, Schweitzer I, et al. The dexamethasone suppression test: a study in a normal population. Psychoneuroendocrinology 1988;13:377–384.
32. Hunt GE, Johnson GFS, Caterson ID. The effect of age on cortisol and plasma dexamethasone levels in depressed patients and controls. J Affect Disord 1989;17:21–32.
33. O'Brien JT, Schweitzer I, Ames D, Tuckwell V, Mastwyk M. Cortisol suppression by dexamethasone in the healthy elderly: effects of age, dexamethasone levels, a cognitive function. Biol Psych 1994;36;389–394.
34. Ohashi M, Fujio N, Kato K, Nawata H, Ibayashi H. Aging is without effect on the pituitary adrenal axis in men. Gerontology 1986;32:335–339.
35. Greenspan SL, Rowe JW, Maitland LA, McAloon-Dyke M, Elahi D. The pituitary–adrenal glucocorticoid response is altered by gender and disease. J Gerontol 1993;48:M72–M77.
36. Brett LP, Levine R, Levine S. Bidirectional responsiveness of the pituitary-adrenal system in old and young male and female rats. Neurobiol Aging 1986;7:331–335.
37. Blichert-Toft M, Hippe E, Jensen HK. Adrenal cortical function as reflected by plasma hydrocortisone and urinary 17 ketogenic steroids in relation to surgery in elderly patients. Acta Chir Scand 1967;133:591–599.
38. Blichert-Toft M, Hummer L. Serum immunoreactive corticotrophin and response to metyrapone in old aged man. Gerontology 1977;23:236–243.
39. Malarkey BW, Hall JC, Rice RR, O'Toole ML, Douglas PS, Demers LM, Glaser R. The influence of age on endocrine responses to ultraendurance stress. J Gerontol 1993;48:M134–M139.
40. Bowen DJ, Richardson DJ. Adrenocortical response to major surgery and anaesthesia in elderly patients. Br J Anaesth 1974;46:873–876.
41. Furuya K, Shimizu R, Hirabayashi Y, Ishii R, Fukuda H. Stress hormone responses to major intra-abdominal surgery during and immediately after sevoflurane-niruous oxide anaesthesia in elderly patients. Can J Anaesth 1993;40:435–439.

42. Muggeo M, Fedele D, Tiengo A, et al. Human growth hormone and cortisol response to insulin stimulation in aging. J Gerontol 1975;39:546–551.
43. Casale G. Pecorini M, Cuzzoni G, de Nicola P. Beat -endorphin and cold pressor test in the aged. Gerontology 1985;31:101-105.
44. Raskind MA, Peskind EA, Veith RC, Wilkinson CW, Federighi D, Dorsa DM. Differential effects of aging on neuroendocrine responses to physostigmine in normal men. J Clin Endocrinol Metab 1990;70:1420–1425.
45. Coiro V, Passeri M, Volpi R, Marchesi M, Bertoni P, Fagnoni F, Schianchi L, Bianconi L, Marcato A, Chiodera P. Different effects of aging on the opioid mechanisms controlling gonadotrophin and cortisol secretion in man. Horm Res 1989;32:119–123.
46. Gelfin Y, Lerer B, Lesch K.-P, Gorline M, Allolio B. Complex effects of age and gender on hypothermic, adrenocorticotrophic hormone and cortisol responses to isapirone challenge in normal subjects. Psychopharmacology 1995;120:356–364.
47. Mooradian AD, Morley JE, Korenman SG. Endocrinology in aging. Disease-A-Month 1988; 34:393–461.
48. Mariotti S, Barbesino G, Caturegli P, Bartalena L, Sansoni P, Fagnoni F, Monti D, Fagiolo U, Franceschi C, Pinchera A. Complex alteration of thyroid function in healthy centenarians. J Clin Endocrinol Metab 1993;77:1130–1134.
49. Siddiqui AR, Hinnefeld RB, Dillon T, Judson WE. Immediate effects of heavy exercise on the circulating thyroid hormones. Br J Sports Med 1983;17:180–183.
50. Imberti R, Maira G, Confortini MC, Preseglio I, Domenegati E. Effect of fentanyl-oxygen anesthesia during cardiac surgery on serum thyroid hormones. Acta Anaesthesiologica Belgica 1988;39:217–222.
51. Chikenji T, Mizutani M, Kitsukawa Y. Anaesthesia, not surgical stress, induces increases in serum concentrations of reverse triiodothyronine and thyroxine during surgery. Exp Clin Endocrinol 1990;95:217–223.
52. Chopra IJ, Hershman JM, Pardridge WM, Nicoloff JT. Thyroid function in nonthyroidal illnesses [Review]. Ann Intern Med 1983;98:946–957.
53. Britton KE, Quinn V, Ellis SM, Cayley AC, Miralles JM, Brown BL, Ekins RP. Is "T4 toxicosis" a normal biochemical finding in elderly women? Lancet 1975:2:141, 142.
54. Burrows AW, Shakespear RA, Hesch RD, Cooper E, Aickin CM, Burke CW. Thyroid hormones in the elderly sick. "T4 euthyroidism," Br Med J 1975;4:437–439.
55. Slag MF, Morley JE, Elson MK, Crowson TW, Nuttall FQ, Shafer RB. Hypothyroxinemia in critically ill patients as a predictor of high mortality. JAMA 1981;245:434–435.
56. Kaptein EM, Weiner JM, Robinson WJ, Wheeler WS, Nicoloff JT. Relationship of altered thyroid hormone indices to survival in nonthyroidal illnesses. Clin Endocrinol 1982;16:565–574.
57. Bhakri HL, Fisher R, Khadri A, MacMahon DG. Longitudinal study of thyroid function in acutely ill elderly patients using a sensitive TSH assay-defer testing until recovery. Gerontology 1990;36:140–144.
58. Morley JE, Kaiser FE, Perry HM, Baumgartner R, Vellas B, Garry P. Longitudinal changes in testosterone luteinizing hormone and follicle stimulating hormone in healthy older males. Metabolism, in press.
59. Corssmit EP, Heyligenberg R, Endert E, Sauerwein HP, Romijn JA. Acute effects of interferon-alpha administration on thyroid hormone metabolism in healthy men. J Clin Endocrinol Metab 1995;80:3140–3144.
60. Jones TH, Kenneth RL. Cytokines and hypothalamic–pituitary function. Cytokine 1993;5:531–538.
61. Gregerman RI, Solomon N. Acceleration of thyroxine and triiodothyronine turnover during bacterial pulmonary infections and fever: implications for the functional state of the thyroid during stress and in senescence. J Clin Endocrinol Metab 1967;27:93–105.
62. Morley JE, Shafer RB. Thyroid function screening in new psychiatric admissions. Arch Intern Med 1982;142:591–593.
63. Roca RP, Blackman MR, Ackerley MB, Harman SM, Gregerman RI. Thyroid hormone elevations during acute psychiatric illness: relationship to severity and distinction from hyperthyroidism. Endocrine Res 1990;16:415–447.
64. Morley JE, Shafer RB, Elson MK, Slag MF, Raleigh MJ, Brammer GL, Yuwiler A, Hershman JM. Amphetamine-induced hyperthyroxinemia. Ann Intern Med 1980;93:707–709.
65. Sawin CT, Carlson HE, Geller A, Castelli WP, Bacharach P. Serum prolactin and aging: basal values and changes with estrogen use and hypothyroidism. J Gerontol 1989;44:M131–M135.

66. Tennekoon KH, Karunanayake EH. Effect of age on serum prolactin concentration in presumably fertile men in Sri Lanka. Ceylon Med J 1994;39:11–13.
67. Arnetz BB. Endocrine reactions during standardized surgical stress: the effects of age and methods of anaesthesia. Age Ageing 1985;14:96–101.
68. Arnetz BB, Lahnborg G, Eneroth P, Thunell S. Age-related differences in the serum prolactin response during standardized surgery. Life Sci 1984;35:2675–2680.
69. Segawa H, Mori K, Kasai K, Fukata J, Nakao K. The role of the phrenic nerves in stress response in upper abdominal surgery. Anesth Analg 1996;82:1215–1224.
70. Oribe E, Amini R, Nissenbaum E, Boal B. Serum prolactin concentrations are elevated after syncope. Neurology 1996;47:60–62.
71. Whalley LJ, Rosie R, Dick H, Levy G, Watts AG, Sheward WJ, Christie JE, Fink G. Immediate increases in plasma prolactin and neurophysin but not other hormones after electroconvulsive therapy. Lancet 1982;2:1064–1068.
72. Clark CP, Alexopoulos GS, Kaplan J. Prolactin release and clinical response to electroconvulsive therapy in depressed geriatric inpatients: a preliminary report. Convulsive Ther 1995;11:24–31.
73. Culebras A, Miller M, Bertram L, Koch J. Differential response of growth hormone, cortisol, and prolactin to seizures and to stress. Epilepsia 1987;28:564–570.
74. Abbott RJ, Browning MC, Davidson DL. Serum prolactin and cortisol concentrations after grand mal seizures. J Neurol Neurosurg Psychiatry 1980;43:163–1967.
75. Zautra AJ, Burleson MH, Matt KS, Roth S, Burrows L. Interpersonal stress, depression, and disease activity in rheumatoid arthritis and osteoarthritis patients. Health Psychol 1994;13:139–148.
76. Sowers JR, Raj RP, Hershman JM, Carlson HE, McCallum RW. The effect of stressful diagnostic studies and surgery on anterior pituitary hormone release in man. Acta Endocrinologica 1977;86:25–32.
77. Tanaka H, Cleroux J, de Champlain J, Ducharme JR, Collu R. Persistent effects of a marathon run on the pituitary–testicular axis. J Endocrinol Invest 1986;9:97–101.
78. Chakravarti S, Collins WP, Forecast JD, Newton JR, Oram DH, Studd JW. Hormonal profiles after the menopause. Br Med J 1976;2:784–7.
79. Rossmanith WG, Scherbaum WA, Lauritzen C. Gonadotropin secretion during aging in postmenopausal women. Neuroendocrinology 1991;54:211–218.
80. Frisch RE. Body fat, menarche, fitness and fertility. Hum Reprod 1987;2:521–533.
81. Garrido-Latorre F., Lazcano-Ponce EC, Lopez-Carrillo L, Hernandez-Avila M. Age of natural menopause among women in Mexico City. Int J Gynaecol Obstet 1996;53:159–166.
82. Torgerson DJ, Avenell A, Russell IT, Reid DM. Factors associated with onset of menopause in women aged 45–49. Maturitas 1994;19:83–92.
83. Kato I, Tominaga S, Suzuki T. Factors related to late menopause and early menarche as risk factors for breast cancer. Jpn J Cancer Res 1988;79:165–172.
84. Snowdon DA. Early natural menopause and the duration of postmenopausal life. Findings from a mathematical model of life expectancy. J Am Geriatr Soc 1990;38:402–408.
85. Morley JE. The endocrinology of the opiates and opioid peptides. Metabol: Clin Exp 1981;30:195–209.
86. Petraglia F, Porro C, Facchinetti F, Cicoli C, Bertellini E, Volpe A, Barbieri GC, Genazzani AR. Opioid control of LH secretion in humans: menstrual cycle, menopause and aging reduce effect of naloxone but not of morphine. Life Sci 1986;38:2103–2110.
87. Melis GB, Paoletti AM, Gambacciani M, Mais V, Fioretti P. Evidence that estrogens inhibit LH secretion through opioids in postmenopausal women using naloxone. Neuroendocrinology 1984;39:60–63.
88. Elias AN, Wilson AF. Exercise and gonadal function (Review). Hum Reprod 1993;8:1747–1761.
89. Gray A, Feldman HA, McKinlay JB, Longcope C. Age, disease, and changing sex hormone levels in middle-aged men: results of the Massachusetts Male Aging Study. J Clin Endocrinol Metab 1991;73:1016–25.
90. Nankin HR, Calkins JH. Decreased bioavailable testosterone in aging normal and impotent men. J Clin Endocrinol Metab 1986;63:1418–1420.
91. Korenman SG, Morley JE, Mooradian AD, Davis SS, Kaiser FE, Silver AJ, Viosca SP, Garza D. Secondary hypogonadism in older men: its relation to impotence. J Clin Endocrinol Metab 1990;71:963–969.
92. Baker HW, Burger HG, de Kretser DM, Hudson B, O'Connor S, Wang C, Mirovics A, Court J, Dunlop M, Rennie GC. Changes in the pituitary-testicular system with age. Clin Endocrinol 1976;5:349–372.

93. Veldhuis JD, Iranmanesh A, Lizarralde G, Urban RJ. Combined deficits in the somatotropic and gonadotropic axes in healthy aging men: an appraisal of neuroendocrine mechanisms by deconvolution analysis. Neurobiol Aging 1994;15:509–517.
94. Billington CJ, Shafer RB, Morley JE. Effects of opioid blockade with nalmefene in older impotent men. Life Sci 1990;47:799–805.
95. Mikuma N, Kumamoto Y, Maruta H, Nitta T. Role of the hypothalamic opioidergic system in the control of gonadotropin secretion in elderly men. Andrologia 1994;26:39–45.
96. Haji M, Tanaka S, Nishi Y, Yanase T, Takayanagi R, Hasegawa Y, Sasamoto S, Nawata H. Sertoli cell function declines earlier than Leydig cell function in aging Japanese men. Maturitas 1994;8(2):143–153.
97. Remes K, Kuoppasalmi K, Adlercreutz H. Effect of physical exercise and sleep deprivation on plasma androgen levels: modifying effect of physical fitness, Int J Sports Med 1985;6:131–135.
98. Nicklas BJ, Ryan AJ, Treuth MM, Harman SM, Blackman MR, Hurley BF, Rogers MA. Testosterone, growth hormone and IGF-I responses to acute and chronic resistive exercise in men aged 55–70 years. Int J Sports Med 1995; 16:445–450.
99. Yesavage JA, Davidson J, Widrow L, Berger PA. Plasma testosterone levels, depression, sexuality, and age. Biol Psychiatry 1985; 20:222–225.
100. Barbarino A, De Marinis L, Folli G, Tofani A, Della Casa S, D'Amico C, Mancini A, Corsello SM, Sambo P, Barini A. Corticotropin-releasing hormone inhibition of gonadotropin secretion during the menstrual cycle. Metabol: Clin Exp 1989;38(6):504–506.
101. Kelijman M. Age-related alterations of the growth hormoneinsulin-like-growth-factor I axis. JAGS 1991;39:295–307.
102. Kalk WJ, Vinik AI, Pimstone BL, et al. Growth hormone response to insulin hypoglycemia in the elderly. J Gerontol 1973;28:431–433.
103. Wakabayashi I, Shibasaki T, Ling N. A divergence of plasma growth hormone response between growth hormone-releasing factor and insulin-induced hypoglycaemia among middle-aged healthy male subjects. Clin Endocrinol 1986;24:279–283.
104. Leppaluoto J, Tapanainen P, Knip M. Heat exposure elevates plasma immunoreactive growth hormone-releasing hormone levels in man. J Clin Endocrinol Metab 1987;65:1035–1038.
105. Lal S, Nair NPV, Thavundayil JX, et al. Growth hormone response to apomorphine, a dopamine receptor agonist, in normal aging and in dementia of the Alzheimer type. Neurobiol Aging 1989;10:227–231.
106. Hagberg JM, Seals DR, Yerg JE, Gavin J, Gingerich R, Premachandra B, Holloszy JO. Metabolic responses to exercise in young and older athletes and sedentary men. J Appl Physiol 1988;65:900–908.
107. Silverman HG, Mazzeo RS. Hormonal responses to maximal and submaximal exercise in trained and untrained men of various ages. J Gerontol A Biol Sci Med Sci 1996;51:B30–B37.
108. Pyka G, Wiswell RA, Marcus R. Age-dependent effect of resistance exercise on growth hormone secretion in people. J Clin Endocrinol Metab 1992;75:404–407.
109. Yarasheski KE, Zachwieja JJ, Campbell JA, Bier DM. Effect of growth hormone and resistance exercise on muscle growth and strength in older men. Am J Physiol 1995;268:E268–276.
110. Morley JE. Aging. In: Bagdade JD, ed. Yearbook of Endocrinology 1992. Mosby, St. Louis, MO, 1992, pp. 61–94.

INDEX

A

Acetylcholine, 9, 37, 69
Acidemia/Acidosis, 29, 48, 49
    osteomalacia, 259
Acquired immune deficiency syndrome
    (AIDS), 16, 54, 148, 180–183, 288
Acromegaly, 75, 77
Adenosine monophosphate, cyclic (cAMP), 91
Adenosine triphosphate (ATP)
Adrenal cortex,
    embryology, 30–34
Adrenal hemorrhage, 128, 129, 148
Adrenal medulla,
    embryonic development, 35–37
α-Adrenergic,
    blocking drugs, 114
    receptors, 71, 90, 147
β-Adrenergic,
    blocking agents, 114, 223
    receptors, 90
    symptoms, 221
Adrenergic receptors, 91, 98
Adrenergic symptoms, 219
Adrenocortical insufficiency, 16, 91,
    128–132, 181, 182, 237
    hypercalcemia, 242
    hyponatremia, 185, 186
    therapy, 132
Adrenocorticotropin (ACTH), 1–17, 27–29,
    32, 123, 140
    aging, 300
    CRH-ACTH-cortisol axis, 123–132
    secretion in fetus/newborn, 28–30
    stimulation test, 130
Adrenomedullin, 97
Aging, 178
    effects on hormonal response to stress,
        299–305
    process, 299
Akee fruit, 227
Alcohol, 5, 6
Alcoholism, 6, 237

Aldosterone, 16, 30, 32, 137–154
    escape, 141
Alendronate, 262, 263
Alkaline phosphatase, 252
Alzheimer's disease, 8
Amenorrhea,
    hypothalamic, 285
    in critical illness, 285–295
Amygdala, 5,6
Androgen, 13,16
    excess, 58
    receptor, 273
Anencephaly, 28–30, 32, 36
Anesthesia, 73, 111, 127, 302
Angiotensin-converting enzyme
    inhibitors, 144, 146
Angiotensinogen, 139
Anorexia, 235
Anorexia nervosa, 9, 159
Anticonvulsants, 256, 257
Antidiuretic hormone (ADH),
    syndrome of inappropriate, 177, 180, 190,
        191
Apache II scoring system, 160
Apgar score, 235
Arcuate nucleus, 6, 25
Arginine vasopressin (AVP), 2, 8, 10, 13,
    27, 123, 176–192
    inappropriate secretion, 29
    secretion in fetus/newborn, 28–32
    V1 receptors, 176
    V2 receptors, 176, 177
Aromatase, 272
Arrhythmia, 236
Asphyxia,
    neonatal 29
Asthma, 13, 51, 108
Atrial fibrillation, 163
Atrial natriuretic factor (ANF), 96, 144
Autoimmune disease, 6, 10, 12, 13, 75, 239
Autonomic,
    nervous system, 1, 35
    symptoms, 219

B

Bartter's syndrome, 143
Beclomethasone, 51
Biofeedback, 113
Birth, 98
Bisphosphonates, 245, 262, 264
Blindness, 4
Blood–brain barrier, 10
Bone,
    cortical, 251
    disease,
        metabolic, medication-induced, 252, 253
    lamellar, 251
    modeling, 251
    physiology, 250, 251
    remodeling, 251, 252
    resorption, 245, 251, 252
    turnover, 251, 252
    woven, 251
Brainstem, 1, 5, 6
Breast cancer, 241
Bromocriptine, 74, 75
Bronchopulmonary dysplasia, 34
Burns, 142, 161
Butyrophenones, 67

C

C-peptide, 222
Caffeine, 256
Calcitonin, 52, 245, 255, 263, 264
Calcium, 233–246
    bound, 235
    complexed, 235
    free, 235
    homeostasis, 14, 234, 235
    intake, 54
    ionized, 235
    metabolism, 233–246
    supplementation, 52
    therapy, 242
Cancer, 73, 266
    hypocalcemia, 236, 237
    diseases, 105–108
Cardiac arrest, 127
Cardiac disease, 53, 54, 294
Cardiac function,
    calcium, 242
Cardiopulmonary resuscitation (CPR), 112
Carpopedal spasm, 235
Catabolic states-catabolism, 76
Catecholamine(s), 1, 10, 37, 87–115, 256

    conjugation, 101
    degradation, 93
    measurement, 100–102
    metabolites, 101, 102
    mobilization, survival value of, 103–105
    responses to stress, 95, 96
    synthesis, 91, 92
Catechol-*O*-methyltransferase (COMT), 93
Celiac disease, 54, 259, 278
Central nervous system, 1
    hypercalcemia, 237
    hypocalcemia, 236
    hypoglycemia, 212–214
Chemotaxis, 75
Chemotherapy, 49, 51, 289–292
Chlorpheniramine, 71
Chlorpropamide, 176, 225
Cholecystokinin, 69
Cholesterol, 124
    synthesis, 32
Chromogranin A, 36, 96
Chronic fatigue, 6
Chronic obstructive pulmonary disease, 190, 276
Chvostek's sign, 236
Circadian rhythm, 4, 5
Cirrhosis, 144, 145, 187, 188, 204, 277
    primary biliary, 286
Clonidine, 9, 114
Cold, 97
    adaptation, 99
    exposure, 110, 111
Collagen, 250
Congenital adrenal hyperplasia, 148
Congestive heart failure, 145, 163, 186, 187, 224
    catecholamine response, 105
Constitutional delay of growth and adolescence (CDGA), 46, 52
Cooling,
    activation of neonatal thyroid hormone production, 39
Corticostatins, 11, 130
Corticosteroid therapy, for adrenal insufficiency, 132
Corticotropin release inhibiting factor (CRIF), 15
Corticotropin releasing factor receptor, 7
Corticotropin releasing hormone (CRH), 1–17, 26–28, 123, 280
    CRH-ACTH adrenal axis, 123–132, 161
    immune, 7, 13
    receptors, 8
    reproductive, 7

response in elderly, 301
testing, 131
Cortisol, 2, 3, 16, 30, 32, 161, 166, 280
    binding globulin, 3, 125
    circadian variation, 4
    counterregulation, 219
    CRH-ACTH cortisol axis, 123–132
    deficiency and hypoglycemia, 224
    immune system, 124, 125, 127
    production, 123, 124
    secretion, 300
Counterregulation of hypoglycemia, 217–220
Counterregulatory hormones, 199, 203
Craniopharyngioma, 50
Crohn's disease, 54
Cushing's disease/syndrome 4, 5, 10, 11, 56, 58, 124, 253
Cyclosporin, 75
Cyproheptadine, 71
Cystic fibrosis, 52, 292
Cytokines, 4, 10, 11, 13, 16, 75, 124, 160, 162, 277, 279, 280

D

Dawn phenomenon, 75
Death of spouse, 110
Deflazacort, 255
Dehydration, 236
Dehydroepiandrosterone (DHEA), 32
Dehydroepiandrosterone sulfate (DS), 30, 31, 110
    sulfotransferase (DST), 32
Dementia and HPA axis, 300
Dental surgery, 113
Deoxycorticosterone, 35
17-Deoxysteroids, 181
Depression, 2, 5, 9, 13, 110, 304
Dexamethasone, 5, 51
    supression testing, 301
Diabetes insipidus, 179, 180, 182
Diabetes mellitus, 13, 227
    effects of pregnancy, 293
    hepatogenous, 204
    type I (insulin-dependent), 54, 108, 212
    type II
Dialysis, 49
Diarrhea,
    infectious, 225
Diazepam, 113
Diencephalon, 25
DiGeorge's syndrome, 240

Dihydrotestosterone, 272
Dihydroxyphenylalanine (DOPA), 91
Dihydroxyphyenylglycol (DHPG),
Dilantin, 257
Diuresis,
    osmotic, 143
Diuretics, 143
    calcium, 244, 245
Diurnal rhythm, 15
Dopamine, 67, 71, 91, 92, 165
    receptors, 71
    D_2, 67
Dorsal spinal column stimulation, 97
Dorsomedial nucleus, 25
Down syndrome, 47
Dwarfism,
    psychosocial, 47

E

Earthquake, 111
"Ebb phase" of traumatic injury, 197, 199
Edema-forming states, 186–189
Electroconvulsive therapy (ECT),
    prolactin, 303
Encephalopathy,
    hyponatremic, 191
β-Endorphin 13, 28, 29, 96
Endorphins, 96
Epinephrine, 4, 36, 88–115, 219
Estradiol, 13
Estrogen, 13, 255
Ethanol, 226, 277
Etidronate, 245, 262
Euthyroid sick syndrome, 155, 275
Exercise, 74, 101, 108, 113, 217, 303
    catecholamine levels, 97
    growth hormone, 304, 305
    menstual disturbance, 72, 304
    testosterone, 304

F

Famotidine, 52
Fasting, 161, 217
Fetal,
    endocrine system 25–44
    growth retardation, 32
    stress
    zone of adrenal cortex, 30, 32
Fibromyalgia, 6
Fibronectin, 251
"Fight or flight" response, 87, 90, 93, 101

"Flow phase" of traumatic injury, 198, 199
Fludrocortisone, 149
Follicle stimulating hormone (FSH), 13, 28, 271, 272, 276, 279, 280, 286, 303, 304
Fractures, 261
Furosemide, 245

G

GABA, 9, 68
Galanin, 69
Gallium nitrate, 245, 264
Gastrointestinal hemorrhage, 235
Gastrointestinal disease, 54, 278
General adaptation syndrome, 1–17, 88
Gitelman's syndrome, 143
Gla protein, 250
Glucagon, 200, 219, 228
Glucocorticoid(s),
   deficiency, 4, 185, 186
   excess, 127
   -induced bone loss, 253, 254
   inhaled,
      effect on growth, 52
   management, 254, 255
   molecular actions, 2–4
   receptors, 3, 16, 125
   physiologic actions, 126, 127
   response element (GRE), 3, 15, 125
   side effects, 58
   skeletal effects, 253–255
   stress in, 2–4, 127, 128
   therapy with, 48, 50, 51, 52, 54, 129, 131, 132, 165
   treatment of hypercalcemia, 245
Gluconeogenesis, 98, 158, 159, 200, 216, 223, 224, 225
   disorders of, 224
Glucose, 211–228
   maintenance, 215–217
   measurement, 227
   normal, 216
   production, 200, 201
   transporters, 201, 202, 212, 213, 225
   uptake and utilization, 201–203
      insulin-mediated glucose uptake (IMGU), 201
      noninsulin-mediated glucose uptake (NIMGU), 201, 203
Glycogenolysis, 98, 200, 216, 223
Glycolysis, 200
   aerobic, 202

Gonadotropin associated peptide (GAP), 67, 68
Gonadotropin-releasing hormone (GnRH), 13, 69, 271, 272, 285
   deficiency, 50
Granulocyte macrophage colony-stimulating factor, 200
Granulomatous disease, 242
Growth and critical disease, 45–59
Growth and development, 45, 46
   regulation of, 47
Growth hormone, 13, 15, 47, 48, 56, 75
   aging, 304, 305
   deficiency, 48, 51, 56, 77
      diagnosis of, 57
      hypoglycemia, 224
   exercise, 304, 305
   hypoglycemia counterregulation, 219
   immune system, 77, 78
   intermediary metabolism, 76, 77
   secretion, 69–71, 73, 74
   therapy, 48, 49, 57, 59
Growth hormone-releasing hormone (GHRH), 13, 69, 73, 77
Guanine nucleotide binding protein, 71, 237

H

Heart, 99
Heart disease,
   congenital, 53, 294
Heat, 111
Hemochromatosis, 278
Hemorrhage and renin-angiotensin-aldosterone system, 142
Heparin, 149, 256
Hepatorenal syndrome, 145
Histamine, 9
   receptors, 71
Homeostasis, 1, 87
Human chorionic gonadotropin, 30
Human immune deficiency virus, 128, 278
   thyroid effects, 167
"Hungry bone syndrome," 239, 259
3β-Hydroxysteroid dehydrogenase, 32
11-Hydroxysteroid dehydrogenase, 4, 5
Hyperaldosteronism,
   primary, 141
   secondary, 141–146
      classification, 142
Hypercalcemia, 233–246, 263, 264, 266
   "equilibrium," 263

Hypercapnea, 189, 190
Hyperemesis gravidarum, 168
Hyperglycemia, 197–206
  management, 205, 206
Hyperinsulinemia, 220
Hyperlactatemia, 202
Hyperparathyroidism,
  primary, 236, 241, 264, 265
  secondary, 255, 260, 265
Hyperphosphatemia, 244
Hypertension, 33, 96, 100, 105–108, 145, 237
  accelerated/malignant, 145, 146
  "white coat," 111
Hyperthyroidism,
  in pregnancy, 293
  skeletal effects, 257–259
Hyperthyroxinemia and stress, 302
Hypoalbuminemia, 144, 235
Hypoaldosteronism, 147–149
  hyperreninemic, 148
  hyporeninemic, 147, 148, 182
  treatment, 149
Hypocalcemia, 233–244
  causes, 237–241
  clinical manifestations, 236, 237
  prevalence, 235, 236
  treatment, 242–244
Hypoglycemia, 38, 72, 73, 104, 108, 109, 198, 211–228
  adverse effects/consequences, 214
  awareness/unawareness, 214
  brain, 219, 220
  clinical manifestations, 214–221
  diagnosis, 220, 221
  differential diagnosis, 221–227
  factitious, 222
  growth hormone, 304
  insulin autoimmune, 222
  insulin-induced, 221
  ketotic, 224
  therapy, 227, 228
Hypogonadism,
  effect of age, 280
  evaluation, 273, 274
  hypogonadotropic, 54, 57, 163, 273
  secondary, 279, 280
  treatment, 280
Hypomagnesemia, 144, 235, 240, 242
Hyponatremia, 140, 175–192
  drug-induced, 177
  encephalopathy, 191
  postoperative, 191

Hypoparathyroidism, 237, 239, 240
Hypophosphatemia, 240
Hypopituitarism, 57
Hypotension, 4, 16, 105–108, 236
Hypothalamic-pituitary-adrenal axis, 1–17, 123–136
  effects of aging, 299, 302
  immune system, 9–12
  neural control, 8, 9
  supression, 34
Hypothalamic-pituitary axis,
  development, 25–30
Hypothalamus, 1, 6
  embryological development, 25–30
Hypothermia, 98
  of hypoglycemia, 215
Hypothyroidism, 56, 58, 162
  hypothalamic, 163
  water metabolism, 183–185
Hypoxemia/Hypoxia, 29, 32, 37, 108, 189, 190, 214, 280

I

IgA deficiency, 54
Immobilization, 241, 265
  stress model, 95
Immune,
  diseases, 110, 111
  response following stress, 110
  system, 2, 16, 71
    effect of cortisol, 124, 125
    effect of GH, 77
Immunological disease, 54
Infection/Infectious diseases, 16, 54, 110, 111, 224, 227
  pulmonary or respiratory, 29, 48, 52, 191
Inflammation, 4, 10
Inflammatory bowel disease, 54, 292, 293
Inflammatory diseases, 110, 111
Injury,
  "flow" phase of, 76
  traumatic, 197
Insulin, 216
  excess, 221
  receptors, 203
  resistance, 74–76, 203, 204
Insulin-like growth factor-1 (IGF-1), 47, 48, 54, 56, 57, 69, 75, 77
Insulin-like growth factor-2 (IGF-2), 32, 223
Insulin-like growth factor binding protein-2 (IGF-BP2), 223

Insulin-like growth factor binding protein-3 (IGF-BP3), 48, 54, 56, 57, 223
Insulinoma, 222
Integrated endocrine response, 168, 169
Interferon, 10, 16, 75, 124
Interleukins, 10, 13, 16, 74, 75, 124, 192, 279, 280
Intubation, 111, 190
Iron, 54

J

Jamaican vomiting illness, 227
Jet lag, 4

K

Ketoacidosis, 143
Ketones, 158
17-Ketosteroid reductase, 278

L

Labetalol, 114
Labor and delivery, 37
Laron syndrome, 56
Leprosy, 276
Leptin, 9
Leukemia, 51, 239
  acute lymphoblastic, 49
Leukocytes, 10
Leydig cells, 13, 271, 272
Light, 4
Lipolysis, 76
β-Lipotropin, 29
Liver disease,
  amenorrhea, 286, 287
  hypogonadism, 273
  hypoglycemia, 224, 227
  thyroid effects of, 167
Locus ceruleus (LC), 5, 9
  LC-norepinephrine system, 88, 93, 110
Luteinizing hormone (LH), 13, 28, 30, 271–273, 276, 279, 280, 286, 303–304
Lymphocytes, 74, 77
  B-cell, 77
  T-cell, 10, 13, 74, 75, 77
Lymphoma, 237, 239, 241

M

Macrophage, 77
  activating factor(s), 74
Magnesium replacement therapy, 242, 243
Magnocellular neurons, 27

Malabsorption, 54
Malaria, 224
Malignancy, 49, 235
  amenorrhea, 288, 289
  hypercalcemia, 241, 242
  hypogonadism, 276, 277
  SIADH, 191
Malnutrition, 223, 227, 274
Mauriac syndrome, 54
Median eminence, 25, 67
Meningococcemia, 149
Menopause, 303, 304
6-Mercaptopurine, 54
Metadrenalines, 191
Metastatic bone disease, 266
Metyrapone, 7
Mifepristone, 5
Mineralocorticoid(s),
  deficiency, 186
  receptor, 4, 140
Monoamine oxidase (MAO), 93
Multiple myeloma, 266
Multiple sclerosis, 16
Myotonic dystrophy, 277

N

Naloxone, 72, 131
Nausea, 235
Neocortical zone of adrenal cortex, 30
Nephropathy,
  sodium-losing, 143
Nephrotic syndrome, 144, 188, 189
Neural crest, 35
Neuroblasts, 35, 36
Neuroglycopenic symptoms, 219
Neuropeptide(s), hypothalamic and posterior pituitary,
  biochemical development, 26, 27
Neuropeptide Y, 9, 96
Neurophysin-1, 27
Neuropsychological disorders, 109, 110
Neurosteroids, 97
Neurotensin, 69
Nonislet cell tumors, 222, 223
Nonsteroidal antiinflammatory drugs, 147
Nonthyroidal illness, 155–170
Norepinephrine, 4, 36, 88–115
Nutrition, 47–49, 53, 113, 161, 162

O

Obesity, 9, 109
Obsessive-compulsive disorder, 9
Octopamine, 106
Opioid(s), 69, 96
    receptors, 71, 72, 96
Orthostatism, 108
Osteoarthritis, 13
Osteoblast, 52, 250, 251
Osteocalcin, 252
Osteoclasts, 251
Osteodystrophy,
    renal, 48
Osteomalacia, 253, 259, 260
Osteonectin, 250
Osteopenia,
    glucocorticoid-induced, 253–255
Osteoporosis, 17
Osteosarcoma, 262
Ouabain-like compound (OLC), 97
Ovarian function in critical illness, 285–295
Oxytocin, 27, 69

P

Paget's disease, 260–263
Pain, 35, 73
Pamidronate, 245, 255
Pancreatic insufficiency, 52
Pancreatitis, 204, 235, 237
Panic disorder, 110
Paracrine function, 37
Parathyroid crisis, 241
Parathyroid hormone (PTH), 234, 236–242
    -related protein (PTHrP), 242
Paraventricular nucleus, 5, 71
Parvocellular neurons, 27
Peptide histidine methionine (PHM), 69
Periventricular nucleus, 25, 71
Phagocytosis, 75, 160
Phenolsulfotransferase (PST), 93
Phenobarbital, 257
Phenothiazines, 67
Phenylethanolamine N-methyl transferase (PMNT), 36, 91
Pheochromocyte, 35
Pheochromocytoma, 101
Phosphate, 239
    intravenous, 245
Phosphodiesterase (PDE), 99
Pimozide, 71

Pituitary, 25–30, 67–86
    development of hormones, 27, 28
    insufficiency, 91
    response to stress, 67–86
    stalk, 277
Placenta, 27, 34, 47
Plicamycin, 245, 263, 264
Pneumocystis carinii, 131, 167, 181
Pneumothorax, 29
Polyarteritis nodosa, 145
Polycystic ovarian syndrome, 285
Polydipsia,
    dipsogenic, 179
    primary, 179
    psychogenic, 179
Positive end expiratory ventilation, 190
Post-traumatic stress syndrome, 91
Potassium, 140
Prednisone, 51
Pre-eclampsia, 146
Pregnancy, 6, 27, 33, 139, 146
    liver transplant, 287
    thyroid function, 168
Pregnenolone, 32, 124
Prematurity, 34, 35, 39
Progesterone, 13, 35, 255
Prolactin, 15
    aging, 303
    carbohydrate metabolism, 74
    exercise, 72, 303
    hyperprolactinemia in renal disease, 287
    hypoglycemia, 72
    hypogonadism, 273, 276
    immune system, 74–76
    inhibitory factors, 67, 68
    lymphoblastoid, 76
    releasing factors, 67
    secretion, 67–69, 71, 72
Proopiomelanocortin (POMC), 8, 26–29, 32, 280
Prosencephalon, 25
Prostacyclin, 115
Prostaglandin deficiency, 147
Pseudohypoaldosteronism, 143
Pseudohypoparathyroidism, 237
Psychiatric disease, 5, 9
    thyroid function, 168, 302, 303
Puberty, 46, 47, 50, 58
    growth hormone therapy, 57
    precocious, 50
Public speaking, 97

Pulmonary disease, 51–53, 105–108, 276
Pyridinoline crosslinks, 252

Q

Quinine, 224, 226

R

Radiation, 50, 51, 58, 240
    cranial, 277
    gonadal toxicity, 50, 289–291
Rathke's pouch, 25
Reiter's syndrome, 75
Relaxation therapy, 113
Renal artery stenosis, 145
Renal disease,
    amenorrhea, 287
    growth, 48–49
    hypocalcemia, 239
    hypoglycemia, 223, 227
    hypogonadism, 276
    thyroid function, 167, 168
Renal failure, 227, 265
Renal insufficiency, 48, 235
Renal osteodystrophy, 265
Renal tubular acidosis, 49, 260
Renin, 138, 139
    synthesis, 138, 139
Respiratory distress syndrome, 34, 39, 131
Respiratory failure, 189–191
Reyes syndrome, 224
Rhabdomyolysis, 239
Rheumatoid arthritis, 13, 294
Rheumatological diseases, 294
Rickets,
    vitamin-D deficient, 58, 259, 260
    X-linked hypophosphatemic, 58
Russell-Silver syndrome, 47

S

Salicylate poisoning, 226
Seizures, 242, 303
Sella turcica, 25
Sepsis, 16, 73, 128, 201, 224, 225, 235, 239
Serotonin, 9
    receptors, 71
Sertoli cell, 272
Severe combined immunodeficiency syndrome (SCID), 54
Sex hormone binding globulin (SHBG), 272, 273, 274
Sexual dimorphism,
    in stress response, 13, 14
Sickle cell disease, 278
Skeletal metabolism, 249–266
Sleep, 300
    apnea, 280
    REM, 300
Sodium-potassium ATPase, 99, 141
Somatomedin C, 13, 69
Somatostatin, 13, 15, 54, 69, 73, 77
    receptors, 71
Spermatogenesis, 13, 271, 272
Spironolactone, 146
Starvation, 54
    "intracellular," 56
Steroid(s), adrenal
    fetal production, 31–34
    secretion in newborns, 34, 35
Stress, 2, 6, 8
    adaptive adjustment, 98–100
    definition, 1, 89, 90
    homeostatic response, 90
    mechanisms, 91–93
    operative, 35
    pituitary response, 67–86
    psychological, 90
    sympathoadrenomedullary response, 89–105
Substance P, 9, 12, 69, 97
Sulfonylureas, 222, 225, 226
Surgery, 37, 54, 73, 161, 235
    cortisol response, 127
    stress, 111
Supraoptic nucleus, 27
Sympathetic nervous system, 1, 9, 113
Sympathoadrenal activity in fetus and newborn, 37, 38
Sympathoadrenomedullary response, 87–122
Systemic lupus erythematosis, 75, 294

T

Telencephalon, 25
Temperature, 98
Temporal lobe,
    epilepsy, 277
Testicular function in critical illness, 271–281
Testicular trauma, 276
Testosterone, 13
    bioavailable, 272
    decreased levels in acute illness, 278–280
    effects of medications, 274, 275

levels, 272
   with aging, 304
   production, 271, 272
   replacement, 280, 281
Tetany, 233, 236, 242
Tetrahydrobioptin (BH_4), 95
Tetralogy of Fallot, 53
Theophylline, 256
Thermal stress, 111
Thirst mechanism, 178, 179
Thrombospondin, 250
Thyroid,
   embryology of, 38
   response to critical illness, 155–173
Thyroid hormone, 47, 97, 109
   production in fetus and newborn, 38, 39
Thyroiditis, 13
Thyroid-stimulating hormone (TSH), 13, 28, 163–166
   in aging, 302
   regulation, 162, 163
   secretion in fetus and newborn, 28–30
Thyrotropin releasing hormone (TRH), 13, 14, 15, 25, 68, 162
Thyrotoxicosis, 162
   apathetic, 258
Thyroxine (T_4), 13, 38
   aging effects, 302, 303
   skeletal effects, 257–259
Thyroxine binding globulin (TBG), 38, 159, 160
   "slow," 160
Thyroxine-binding prealbumin (TBPA), 38
Tolbutamide, 52
Toxic shock syndrome, 239
Transfusion, blood, 38, 235, 239
Transplantation, 112
   cardiac, 294
   liver, 286, 287
Transposition of the great arteries, 53
Trauma, 73, 75, 111
   cranial, 277
Tricyclic antidepressants, 5
Triiodothyroacetic acid (T_3AC), 156–158
Triiodothyronine (T_3), 13, 38, 302, 303
   low T_3 state, 156–159, 302, 303
   low T_3-T_4 state, 159–162, 302
   reverse (rT_3), 38, 302
   sulfate (T_3S), 157, 158

Trousseau's sign, 236
Tuberculosis, 10, 190
Tumor necrosis factor (TNF), 10, 13, 77, 124, 279
Turner syndrome, 47, 48
Tyrosine hydroxylase, 36, 91

U

Ulcerative colitis, 54
Urocortin, 7, 13
Urotensin, 7
Uveitis, 74

V

Vacor, 227
Vasoactive intestinal peptide (VIP), 69, 92
Vasopressin, 69
Ventromedial nucleus, 25, 67
Vitamin A, 113, 242
Vitamin B_1, 54
Vitamin B_6, 54
Vitamin C, 54
Vitamin D, 54, 234, 239
   deficiency, 240
   25-OH, 234, 240
   1,25-OH, 234, 239, 240
   resistance, 240
   therapy, 244
   toxicity, 242, 245
Volume,
   effective arterial blood, 187
   effective blood, 187
   loss, 142–144, 146

W

Water metabolism, 175–192
   effects of age, 178, 179
   effects of drugs, 176, 177
   normal physiology, 175, 176
Wernicke-Korsakoff syndrome, 226
Whipple's triad, 221

Y

Yohimbine, 9

Z

Zona fasciculata, 2, 30
Zona glumerulosa, 30, 139, 148
Zona reticularis, 30, 32